Exotic Animal Medicine
for the
Veterinary Technician

Second Edition

Exotic Animal Medicine
for the
Veterinary Technician

Second Edition

Edited by
Bonnie Ballard, DVM
and Ryan Cheek, RVTg VTS (ECC)

WILEY-BLACKWELL

A John Wiley & Sons, Inc., Publication

First edition first published 2003
Second edition first published 2010
© 2010 Blackwell Publishing

Blackwell Publishing was acquired by John Wiley & Sons in February 2007. Blackwell's publishing program has been merged with Wiley's global Scientific, Technical, and Medical business to form Wiley-Blackwell.

Editorial Office
2121 State Avenue, Ames, Iowa 50014-8300, USA

For details of our global editorial offices, for customer services, and for information about how to apply for permission to reuse the copyright material in this book, please see our website at www.wiley.com/wiley-blackwell.

Library of Congress Cataloging-in-Publication Data

Exotic animal medicine for the veterinary technician / edited by Bonnie Ballard and Ryan Cheek. – 2nd ed.
    p. ; cm.
Includes bibliographical references and index.
  ISBN-13: 978-0-8138-2206-8 (alk. paper)

  1. Exotic animals–Diseases.   2. Wildlife diseases.   3. Pet medicine.   4. Veterinary nursing.   I. Ballard, Bonnie M.   II. Cheek, Ryan.
  [DNLM: 1. Animal Diseases.   2. Animals, Wild.   3. Animal Technicians.   4. Veterinary Medicine–methods.   SF 997.5.E95 E96 2010]
  SF997.5.E95C44 2010
  636.089′073–dc22
      2009035848

A catalog record for this book is available from the U.S. Library of Congress.

Set in 10 on 12 pt Sabon by Toppan Best-set Premedia Limited
Printed and bound in Malaysia by Vivar Printing Sdn Bhd

Disclaimer
The contents of this work are intended to further general scientific research, understanding, and discussion only and are not intended and should not be relied upon as recommending or promoting a specific method, diagnosis, or treatment by practitioners for any particular patient. The publisher and the author make no representations or warranties with respect to the accuracy or completeness of the contents of this work and specifically disclaim all warranties, including without limitation any implied warranties of fitness for a particular purpose. In view of ongoing research, equipment modifications, changes in governmental regulations, and the constant flow of information relating to the use of medicines, equipment, and devices, the reader is urged to review and evaluate the information provided in the package insert or instructions for each medicine, equipment, or device for, among other things, any changes in the instructions or indication of usage and for added warnings and precautions. Readers should consult with a specialist where appropriate. The fact that an organization or Website is referred to in this work as a citation and/or a potential source of further information does not mean that the author or the publisher endorses the information the organization or Website may provide or recommendations it may make. Further, readers should be aware that Internet Websites listed in this work may have changed or disappeared between when this work was written and when it is read. No warranty may be created or extended by any promotional statements for this work. Neither the publisher nor the author shall be liable for any damages arising herefrom.

6   2013

Table of Contents

See the supporting companion Web site for this book: www.wiley.com/go/ballard.

See the supporting companion Web site for this book: www.wiley.com/go/ballard.

See the supporting companion Web site for this book: www.wiley.com/go/ballard.

See the supporting companion Web site for this book: www.wiley.com/go/ballard.

See the supporting companion Web site for this book: www.wiley.com/go/ballard.

See the supporting companion Web site for this book: www.wiley.com/go/ballard.

Preface

The second edition was written to provide the veterinary technician with important information about a variety of species commonly seen in exotic practice, reflecting changes in this branch of medicine that have occurred since the first edition. This text is beneficial to the technician who would like to work with these animals but may have graduated years ago, before this area of medicine was popular. This text is also helpful to the technician who works for a veterinarian who would like to add exotic species to his/her practice. While it was not written for veterinarians, they may find it beneficial as well.

With the help of this book, the technician will know what questions to ask to obtain an adequate history, be able to educate the client about husbandry and nutrition, be able to safely handle and restrain common species, and be able to perform necessary procedures when needed. Because the field of exotic animal medicine is a dynamic one, new knowledge is constantly emerging about many of the species kept as pets, and new information can, in some cases, contradict what was thought to be true before. For many species, exotic animal medicine can be said to be in its infancy. We realize that for some of the species featured in this book, the information presented may need to be modified in the future. Further, because what we know about exotic animal medicine is forever changing and much has not been scientifically proven, it is common to find contradicting information from one reputable source to the next. This can create frustration but also provide the challenge of working in a cutting edge area of medicine. This is the major reason why it is paramount to attend continuing education in this area of medicine. Veterinary technicians working in exotic medicine must engage in lifelong learning to be up to date on the latest information.

New contributors as well as new chapters have been added to this edition. Although some of the contributors have provided drug dosages and formularies, we do not take responsibility for what this information. We also realize that while technicians do not make decisions about what drugs to use in any animal, they are required to be familiar with different pharmaceuticals, know where to find a dosage, and know how to calculate it.

This book was written with the assumption that the technician already is educated in topics such as anatomy, physiology, medical terminology, pathology, and pharmacology. We present only what is unique to the species featured here.

We hope this book proves to be beneficial to all technicians interested in exotic animal medicine.

Acknowledgements

I would like to thank all of our new contributors who gave their time to provide additional information to enhance this edition. Appreciation also goes to the original contributors who took time to update their original chapters. I would like to thank my husband Brian Kershaw for continually being supportive and understanding when I had to take my precious little free time to work on the book!

Bonnie Ballard

This second edition has seen many changes. I would like to thank my family and friends for the support they have given me throughout this entire process. I would also like to acknowledge the many technicians working in the field of exotic animal medicine. This is an ever-changing and evolving field that requires dedication and patience. Your commitment to this field is truly inspiring.

Ryan Cheek

Contributors

Bonnie Ballard, DVM, has worked in veterinary medicine since 1974, starting as a veterinary assistant, becoming a technician in 1979, and earning a DVM in 1994. In 1997, she started the veterinary technology program at Gwinnett Technical College. The program has been AVMA accredited since 2000. Dr. Ballard currently is the program's director and one of two full time faculty members. She has won numerous teaching awards and has received many accolades for the program. She also practices small animal and exotic medicine at Winder Animal Hospital in Winder, Georgia.

Denise I. Bounous, DVM, PhD, Diplomate ACVP, was a professor of clinical pathology at the University of Georgia College of Veterinary Medicine before her move into the pharmaceutical industry. Her academic interests included avian and reptilian clinical pathology, and her research was in avian immunomodulation.

Ryan Cheek graduated from Gwinnett Technical College in 1999 with an Associate's Degree in Applied Technology in veterinary technology, where he focused his studies on exotic animal medicine. He worked at Zoo Atlanta and then at a small animal/exotic animal practice for four years. He has worked in emergency and critical care for the past eleven years. He completed his Veterinary Technician Specialist in Emergency and Critical Care in 2005 and his Bachelor's of Applied Science Degree in veterinary technology from St. Petersburg College in 2007. He has taught full time at Gwinnett Technical College since 2007; he teaches many subjects including exotic, wildlife, zoo, and laboratory animal medicine.

Maria M. Crane, DVM, received her MS in exercise science from Georgia State University and her DVM from the University of Georgia in 1994. She worked as a veterinarian at Zoo Atlanta, providing clinical and surgical care, and later as vice president of animal health, managing veterinary and nutritional services. She has also practiced small and exotic animal medicine.

Lillian Gerhardt, LVT, graduated from the State University of New York. She has been a technician at the University of Tennessee College of Veterinary Medicine in the Avian and Zoological Medicine Service for eighteen years. She has presented seminars at the Avian Veterinarian Annual Conferences several times. She has always had a special interest in birds and has shared the last twenty-three years of her life with a sulphur crested cockatoo named Sugar.

Cheryl B. Greenacre, DVM, Diplomate ABVP-Avian, graduated from the University of Georgia College of Veterinary Medicine in 1991 and taught avian and exotic animal medicine at UGA for ten years and at the University of Tennessee College of Veterinary Medicine for nine years. Dr. Greenacre is the immediate past chair for the UT Institutional Animal Care and Use Committee, and is currently a professor at the University of Tennessee. She divides her work time between teaching veterinary students and residents, providing clients and referring veterinarians with service, and studying thyroid testing in birds and pain relief in reptiles.

Tarah Hadley, DVM, Diplomate ABVP-Avian, is a graduate of Dartmouth College and Tufts University, where she received her DVM. She completed an internship in small animal medicine and surgery at Rowley Memorial Animal Hospital in Massachusetts and a residency in avian medicine and surgery at the University of Tennessee. During her residency, Dr. Hadley was also trained in exotic animal and zoological medicine. She currently serves as director of the Atlanta Hospital for Birds and Exotics and is a member of the veterinary staff at Zoo Atlanta.

Melanie Haire, VMT, received an AS degree in veterinary technology from Wilson College in 1987 and worked for six years in an Atlanta small animal clinic following graduation. She has spent the last fifteen years on the veterinary staff at Zoo Atlanta, where she is the senior veterinary technician and hospital manager. She is federally licensed to rehabilitate migratory bird species and raptors and has a state permit to rehabilitate wild mammals, including rabies vector species. She volunteers at the local wildlife rehabilitation center, Atlanta Wild Animal Rescue Effort (AWARE), where she is also a board member.

Anne E. Hudson, LVT, LAT, graduated from Blue Ridge Community College with an AAS in veterinary technology and received AALAS certification. She has worked as a biological laboratory technician for the Department of Defense's Clinical Investigation and Research Department. She teaches veterinary assisting to high school students interested in pursuing careers in the veterinary field.

Michael J. Huerkamp, DVM, Diplomate ACLAM, earned his DVM from The Ohio State University and did postdoctoral training in the specialty area of laboratory animal medicine at the University of Michigan. He is a professor of pathology and laboratory medicine in the Emory University School of Medicine, where he also serves as director of the Division of Animal Resources. Dr. Huerkamp has twenty-two years of experience in the medical care and management of laboratory animals, including rabbits.

Michael Duffy Jones, DVM, received a BS from Notre Dame and DVM from Tufts University. He completed an internship at Georgia Veterinary Specialists. He worked for five years at Bells Ferry Animal Hospital before opening his own practice, Peachtree Hills Animal Hospital, in Atlanta in 2005. He has a particular interest in the use of ultrasound as a diagnostic tool, which he uses regularly in his practice and which he teaches to other veterinarians.

Vanessa Lee, DVM, obtained her veterinary degree from the University of Georgia in 2005. She was an associate veterinarian in a small animal and exotic companion animal private practice for two years and is currently in a laboratory animal medicine residency at Emory University in Atlanta, Georgia.

Trevor Lyon, RVT, graduated from Maple Woods Community College with an AA in veterinary technology. Focusing on internal medicine, he has lectured at several veterinary conferences around the country. He is a technician supervisor and co-owner of Bells Ferry Veterinary Hospital. He has worked with wildlife rehabilitation programs and participated in programs to educate the public about wildlife.

David Martinez-Jimenez, DVM, was born in Spain, where he completed his veterinary degree in 2002. After graduation, he performed several externships in exotic pet, zoo, and wildlife medicine. In 2004, he completed a Master's Degree in Wild Animal Health at the Royal Veterinary College and Institute of Zoology of London. He then moved to the USA, where he completed an internship in exotic, zoo, and wildlife medicine at the University of Georgia College of Veterinary Medicine. Dr. Martinez-Jimenez is currently practicing in zoo, wildlife, and exotic medicine

Julie Mays, LVT, graduated from Snead State Community College with an AA in veterinary technology. She has long had an interest in exotic animal medicine and surgery.

James R. McClearen, DVM, graduated from the University of Georgia with a BS in agriculture. He received his DVM from the University of Georgia College of Veterinary Medicine, where he worked for several years in raptor rehabilitation. He sold Bells Ferry Veterinary Hospital, his small animal and exotic pet practice, in 2007, although he still works there. He is active in the Georgia Veterinary Medical Association and served as its president in 2008.

Deborah Mook, DVM, Diplomate ACLAM, received her DVM from the University of Wisconsin-Madison in 1998 and became board-certified in laboratory animal medicine in 2004. She worked with pet rabbits in the clinical setting and rabbits as research models in the medical school setting. Her primary expertise lies in the field of laboratory animal medicine, with a focus on murine infectious disease.

Shannon Goldsmith, CAT, operates a reptile and amphibian rescue program and is active in the community, providing educational programs related to these wonderful creatures.

Samuel Rivera, DVM, Diplomate ABVP-Avian, graduated from Kansas State University College of Veterinary Medicine. He later received a Masters of Science in veterinary pathobiology. After practicing in an avian and exotic practice for several years, he now serves as an associate veterinarian at Zoo Atlanta.

April Romagnano, PhD, DVM, Diplomate ABVP, obtained her PhD from the Universitæ de Montræal in 1987, and a DVM from the University of Florida in 1992. She completed an internship in wildlife/small animal medicine at the University of Florida in 1993, a residency in non-domestic avian medicine at North Carolina State University in 1995, and a post doctoral appointment in BCL2 transgenic mice at the Howard Hughes Medical Institute Research Lab at Washington University in St. Louis, Missouri, in 1988. In 2001 she opened an animal clinic and serves as the avian specialist there. She also serves as the full-time director of animal resources at Scripps Florida, a consultant veterinarian for Lion Country Safari in Loxahatchee, Florida, and a courtesy clinical assistant professor at the College of Veterinary Medicine at the University of Florida.

Douglas K. Taylor, DVM, MS, Diplomate ACLAM, received his Veterinary Degree from Michigan State University in 1995 and practiced small animal medicine for five years afterward. He received his specialty training in laboratory animal medicine at the University of Michigan, where he also earned his MS. He is currently the director of surgery and anesthesia services and the assistant director of the residency training program at Emory University in Atlanta, Georgia.

Brad Wilson, DVM, is a veterinarian and partner in two private practice veterinary clinics in north Atlanta. He received his BS in zoology and his DVM from the University of Georgia. He is the consulting veterinarian for the largest wholesale importer and distributor of fish, reptiles, amphibians, pocket pets, ferrets, and birds in north Georgia as well as for the Atlanta Botanical Garden, which has an extensive collection of dendrobatid and Central and South American hylid frogs. He has personally maintained and captively bred many species of snakes and frogs.

Disclaimer

Because exotic animal dosages are based largely on empirical data and not researched facts, the editors and contributors make no guarantees regarding the results obtained from dosages used in this textbook.

Exotic Animal Medicine
for the
Veterinary Technician

Second Edition

Section 1
Introduction

CHAPTER ONE

The Role of the Veterinary Technician in Exotic Animal Medicine

Bonnie Ballard

Welcome to the world of exotic animal medicine! For those who practice it, it is the variety that provides the spice to veterinary life. In a practice that sees exotics, it is not uncommon to see a dog for vaccines, a diabetic cat, an iguana with metabolic bone disease, a ferret for a physical examination, a rabbit with hair loss, and a feather-picking cockatoo all in one day. The challenge for those in this field lies in the vast differences in the species seen (Figure 1.1).

In the world of veterinary medicine, an exotic animal is any animal that isn't a dog, cat, horse, or cow. Exotic animals include wildlife species, animals commonly used in research that are kept as pets, and animals native to various regions of the world such as South America, Australia, and Africa. Owners of "pocket pets" such as mice, rats, gerbils, and hamsters commonly seek veterinary care for their pets.

There are several scenarios in which a technician faced with exotics may find this book helpful. For instance, a technician might take a job in a practice that sees exotics but she knows little about them because she graduated before exotics became popular pets. Another technician may work for a veterinarian who wants to add exotics to the practice but doesn't have hands-on experience with them. Alternatively, a technician who finds employment at a zoological park or works with a wildlife rehabilitator may want to brush up on current ideas about exotics. While this book does not cover zoo species specifically, knowledge of exotic animals, their treatment, and their care is desirable in the zoo environment.

It is essential that a technician who works for a veterinarian who would like to add exotics to the practice help the veterinarian understand how the practice will need to change to accommodate these species. One must accept the fact that a fifteen- or twenty-minute appointment will not suffice. In many cases appointments of thirty minutes or longer are required. Because husbandry and nutrition are typically the two most common causes of illness in exotics, a thorough history in these areas is essential. Furthermore, more time may be required to perform a physical examination due to the delicate nature of some of the species. In many cases it is necessary to allow adequate time to educate the owner about how to keep his/her pet healthy.

The front office staff must be knowledgeable and interested in exotic pets because they will be the first people the pet owner sees in the office. The worst thing that can happen for a snake owner, for example, is to step up to the front desk and see the receptionist recoil in horror. Not only is this behavior unprofessional, but it also calls into question the knowledge of the doctors. Likewise, if a receptionist does not know the difference between a macaw and a cockatoo, it may give the impression that the clinic doesn't see many birds.

Housing is another consideration in the decision to treat exotic pets. Because many pocket pets are prey

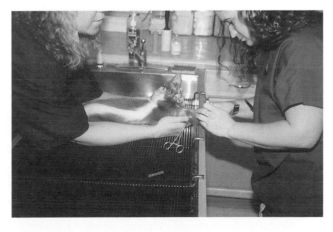

Figure 1.1. A technician drawing blood from a skunk. (Photo courtesy of Ryan Cheek.)

animals, their housing in relation to that of dogs and cats must be considered. For example, a rabbit should not be caged where a cat patient can watch it. This alone can create undue added stress for a rabbit patient, which is already stressed by being in the hospital environment. An exotic pet should not have to add the fear of being eaten to its worries during a hospital stay.

While the average animal hospital has most of the necessary equipment needed to treat exotics, some items will need to be purchased. For example, a gram scale is required to weigh many of the very small patients. Microtainer blood collection tubes are also essential. A list of equipment that is useful in exotic practices appears in Appendix 12.

The technician's role in exotic animal medicine is the same as it is in small or large animal medicine. One of the most important roles is that of a meticulous history taker. As each chapter illustrates, a simple history will not do. Detailed questions must be asked about how and where the pet was acquired. Wild-caught species can have different health problems than those raised in captivity. How the pet is housed is vitally important, and this means not only asking what it is housed in but the cage size, construction, substrate used, and where it is kept in the house. If the animal is not brought in the cage it is housed in, the technician, after gathering the history, should be able to create a mental picture of what the cage at home looks like.

The same is true for gathering adequate information about the pet's diet. It is not good enough to ask what is fed, because that may not be what is consumed. For example, an owner may report that his Amazon parrot's daily diet is made up of fruits, vegetables, and seeds. When asked how much of each is consumed each day, the answer may be mostly seeds, which is an inadequate diet.

In many cases, owners of exotics may have been misinformed about their pets' care by the pet shops where the pets were purchased. Although some pet shop employees are knowledgeable, many simply do not know the correct information about the species they sell. In addition, an owner may have read information from a less than reputable source. The veterinary technician should be able to give owners the correct information about husbandry and nutrition without chastising them for their mistakes. Many owners honestly may not know that what they were doing was wrong. They may have obtained books that are not written by reputable sources or found information on the Internet that is inaccurate. Clients value information about how to keep their pets healthy, and their veterinary clinic should be the source of that information.

The technician can also provide valuable information about what type of exotic pet a client should buy. For example, an iguana is considered to be a difficult reptile to keep because its housing and nutrition requirements are demanding. A bearded dragon may be a better choice. A parakeet may be a better choice than a macaw for a first-time bird owner, because macaws can be noisy and messy. The topic of conservation of species is important here as well. New exotic pet owners should be encouraged to acquire captive-raised species rather than wild-caught if possible. In many exotic species, the numbers in the wild are diminishing. This is especially true of many avian species. Most exotic species that are desirable as pets can be obtained from captive-raised sources.

One should never underestimate the strength of the human-animal bond that exists between owners and their exotic pets. An owner can be as bonded to a mouse or a snake as another owner is to a dog or horse. Just as one should never assume what an owner is willing to spend for medical care on dogs, cats, and horses, one should never assume what exotic pet owners will spend for their pets. It is not uncommon to see a devoted owner spend hundreds of dollars for a surgical procedure for a pet rat.

Some veterinary practices see primates and venomous species. Because of the dangers to humans, these veterinarians typically set "rules of engagement" regarding the care and treatment of these animals. For example, the veterinarian may only see a primate or venomous snake after hours, when all employees and clients are gone. Likewise, a veterinarian may require that an owner of a venomous snake provide in-date antivenin along with the snake.

Some veterinarians will not see large exotic cats due to safety concerns. And yes, there are people who have permits to keep them. Others will see these animals on the owner's premises as long as handling equipment, such as squeeze cages, is provided. It is important that all employees know the clinic's protocol for seeing primates, venomous species, and large cats.

Every state has different laws regarding which species are legal to keep as pets and which are not. It is up to the veterinarian to decide whether she will see animals that may in fact be illegal pets, and to communicate this information to the technicians and other staff.

Continuing education is an important part of a graduate technician's professional enhancement, and its importance in exotic medicine cannot be overemphasized. What is known about the care and treatment of exotic animals is forever changing as more and more is learned. What was described as the proper diet for a particular lizard one year may be something different the next. More and more drugs are being tried in exotics. This type of cutting-edge information is often presented at conferences and in professional publications. This presents an added challenge to practices that see exotic animals because information is forever changing.

In response to this challenge, we have assembled here for the veterinary technician a survey of the most recent practices in the area of exotic animal care. Exotic animal medicine provides a veterinary technician with the opportunity to use all of his skills and knowledge in a way that has a direct benefit to the practice and to the patients. Enjoy!

Section 2
Avian

CHAPTER TWO

Psittacines and Passerines

Cheryl B. Greenacre and Lillian Gerhardt

INTRODUCTION

The Class Aves consists of more than 8,500 species of birds and 29 orders of birds. Two orders commonly kept as pets in the United States are the Psittaciformes (parrots) (Table 2.1) and the Passeriformes (canaries and finches) (Figures 2.1, 2.2). Anatomically and physiologically there is no generic bird, meaning that each species is different in its anatomy, hematology (lymphocytes may predominate in some species), and drug metabolism. Avian medicine has many similarities to canine and feline medicine, as well as some definite differences. The similarities include use of similar, albeit smaller, equipment, similar drugs, and similar techniques. Most differences encountered in caring for birds relate to the drastically different anatomy and physiology, especially respiratory physiology, and this in turn dictates a different approach to restraint, pro-

Table 2.1. Examples of common species of birds encountered in practice.

Common name	Scientific name	Color plate number	Common name	Scientific name	Color plate number
Cockatoo			**Conure**		
Moluccan	*Cacutua moluccensis*		Blue-crowned	*Aratinga acuticaudata*	
Umbrella*	*Cacatua alba*	3.1	Sun	*Aratinga solstitialis*	
Sulfur-crested	*Cacatua sulphurea*		Half-moon	*Aratinga canicularis*	
Macaw			Maroon (Red)-bellied	*Pyrrhura frontalis*	
Blue and gold*	*Ara ararauna*	3.6	Nanday	*Nandayus nenday*	
Scarlet	*Ara macao*		Green-cheeked	*Pyrrhura molinae*	
Hyacinth	*Anodorhynchus hyacinthinus*	3.7	Mitred	*Aratinga mitrata*	
Military	*Ara militaris*	3.8	Lovebird, Peach-faced	*Agapornis rosicollis*	
Green-winged	*Ara chloroptera*		Cockatiel*	*Nymphicus hollandicus*	
Amazon parrot			**Parakeet**		
Yellow-naped*	*Amazona ochrocephala*	3.10	Standard budgie*	*Melopsittacus undulates*	
Red-lored	*Amazona autumnalis*		Grey-cheeked	*Brotogeris pyrrhopterus*	
Orange-winged	*Amazona amazonica*		Quaker (Monk)	*Myiopsitta monachus*	
Double yellow-headed	*Amazona ochrocephala*		**Finch**		
Blue-fronted	*Amazona aestiva*	3.11	Zebra	*Poephila castanotis*	
Mexican red-headed	*Amazona viridigenalis*		Lady Gouldian	*Poephila gouldiae*	
Lory, Rainbow	*Trichoglossus haematodus*		**Parrot**		
			African grey*	*Psittacus erithacus*	3.4
			Eclectus	*Eclectus roratus*	3.2

Source: Forshaw and Cooper (1989).
*Most commonly encountered species.

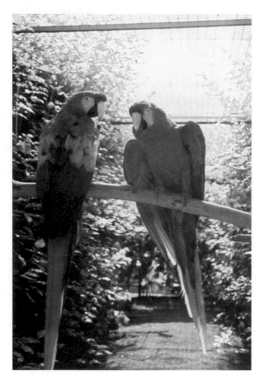

Figure 2.1. *Two scarlet macaws* (Ara macao) *in an outdoor aviary. This is an example of a psittacine bird, or parrot.*

viding air to the lungs, and supportive care. Once these differences are recognized, avian medicine is quite straightforward and rewarding.

ANATOMY AND PHYSIOLOGY

The anatomy and physiology of birds is drastically different from mammalian anatomy and physiology. These differences are usually due to an adaptation that helps enable flight or relates to development within an egg.

Integumentary System
Feathers are made of keratin and are used for flight, insulation, and attracting a mate. There are various types of feathers including primaries, also known as wing remiges and tail rectrices (very large feathers that originate from the carpus and metacarpus, and pygostyle, respectively), secondaries (large feathers that originate from the radius and ulna), contour (over the body), and down feathers (produce powder down). Feathers lay in feathered tracts called pterylae, and the non-feathered tracts are called apterylae. The main shaft of the feather is called the rachis; barbs are attached to the rachis, and barbules are attached to the

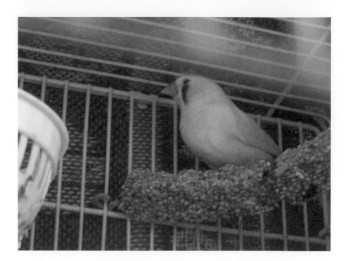

Figure 2.2. *A female fawn-colored zebra finch* (Poephila castanotis). *This is an example of a passerine, or soft billed, bird.*

barbs at a 45-degree angle that hook with nearby barbules at a 90-degree angle (Figure 2.3).

The very thin skin (two to four cell layers thick in feathered areas) is difficult to suture, usually requiring 4-0 or 5-0 suture. There is very little, if any, subcutaneous tissue. The feet are an exception in that they usually have thick, prominent scales in the non-feathered regions to protect them from trauma. The wing web of a bird is called a patagium. There are only two proper glands in birds, the bi-lobed uropygial (preen) gland that helps waterproof the feathers, which are absent in some birds (such as in Amazon parrots), and the ear gland, which is absent in most birds. Birds have no external ear pinna and no sweat glands. Birds bruise green because they lack biliverdin reductase, which converts biliverdin to bilirubin. Do not confuse a bright green bruise on a bird for gangrene.

Musculoskeletal System
Unlike mammals, birds can have a variable number of cervical vertebrae; they have eight to twenty-five instead of seven (King 1984) (Figure 2.4). Birds use their long, flexible necks to gain access to food and to reach the uropygial (preen) gland to preen their feathers. The remainder of the spine is fused in many areas to provide a stable body part for flight. A keel along the sternum provides for attachment of the large pectoral (flight) muscles. The notarium is a fusion of the first thoracic vertebrae. The synsacrum is a fusion of the caudal thoracic, lumbar, sacral, and caudal vertebrae. The pygostyle is a distal fusion of the caudal vertebrae for tail muscle attachment. The sternum has a prominent keel for pectoral muscle attachment. The

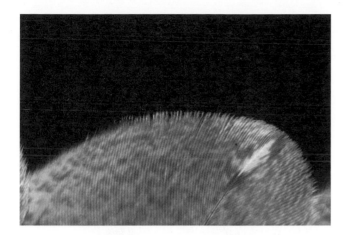

Figure 2.3. *The central main shaft of the feather is called the rachis. Barbs extend from each side of the rachis at a 45-degree angle. Microscopically, barbules extend from each side of the barb a 45 degree angle. Barbules on the leading edge of a barb hook onto the barbules of the trailing edge. When birds preen their feathers, they are realigning these barbules.*

pectoral girdle consists of the unique coracoid bone, that acts as a strut enabling flight, the clavicle, and the scapula. Bones of the wing from proximal to distal include humerus; radius; ulna; ulnar and radial carpal bones; and major and minor metacarpals, phalanges, and alula (remnants of a thumb). Bones of the hind limb from proximal to distal include femur, tibiotarsus, tarsometatarsus, and phalanges.

Most important clinically is that the femur, humerus, and some vertebrae are pneumatic bones—bones filled with air—which connect directly to the respiratory tract to lighten the bones for flight. Intraosseous catheters should not be placed in pneumatic bones because any fluid administered could go directly to the lungs and drown the bird.

Cardiovascular System

Birds, like mammals, possess a four-chambered heart, but unlike mammals, birds lack a diaphragm, therefore the apex of the heart is directly surrounded by liver (Figure 2.5). The avian heart is comparatively one and a half to two times larger than a mammalian heart. Unlike mammals, the mean electrical axis of birds is

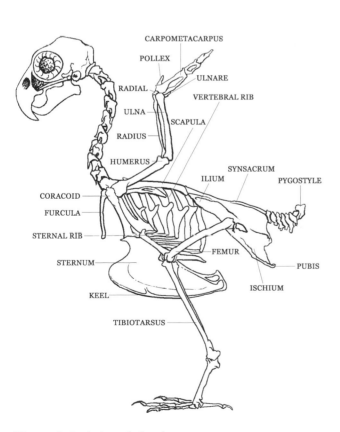

Figure 2.4. *Avian skeletal anatomy.*

CARPOMETACARPUS
POLLEX
RADIAL
ULNARE
VERTEBRAL RIB
ULNA
SCAPULA
RADIUS
HUMERUS
SYNSACRUM
ILIUM
PYGOSTYLE
CORACOID
FURCULA
STERNAL RIB
FEMUR
STERNUM
PUBIS
KEEL
ISCHIUM
TIBIOTARSUS

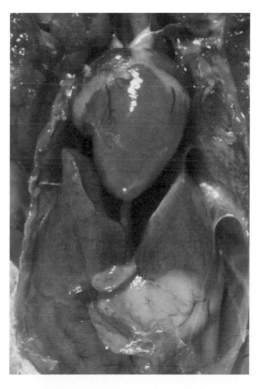

Figure 2.5. *Birds, like mammals, possess a four-chambered heart, but because birds lack a diaphragm, the apex of the heart is directly surrounded by liver.*

Table 2.2. Representative heart and respiratory rates for various species of birds.

Species	Weight (grams)	HR (rest)	HR (restraint)	RR (rest)	RR (restraint)
Cockatiel	100	200	500–600	40–52	60–80
Amazon	400	150	200–350	25–30	40–60
Macaw	1000	125	150–350	15–20	25–40

Source: Ritchie, Harrison, and Harrison (1994).
Note: HR = heart rate, RR = respiratory rate.

negative 90 degrees (in dogs it is positive 90 degrees). Birds do not possess lymph nodes, but they do have lymph vessels. Phlebotomy sites in birds include the right jugular vein (the right one is two-thirds larger than the left), basilic (or cutaneous ulnar) vein, and medial metatarsal vein. The cutaneous ulnar vein, as it crosses the proximal ulna, is an excellent vein for determining vein refill time; if the vein can be seen to refill this is considered slow and suggestive of dehydration or shock. Through a renal-portal system, birds can choose to shunt blood from the caudal half of the body through the kidneys first before going through the heart. Therefore, it is better to give parenteral medications in the front half of the body (i.e. give IM injections in the pectoral muscles rather than the in the leg) (Table 2.2).

Renal System
Birds possess a renal portal system in which blood from the caudal half of the body may pass through the kidneys first before reaching the heart. This means that any drug administered in the caudal half of the body may go undiluted directly to the kidneys before going to the heart. Parrots have three divisions to their kidneys (cranial, middle, and caudal) and the kidneys are located dorsally in a concavity of the sacrum. Avian kidneys produce both urine (from their mammalian-type nephrons) and urates (from their reptilian-type nephrons that lack a loop of Henle). Urates consist of uric acid. Therefore, uric acid concentrations and not BUN are evaluated to determine renal function in birds.

Neurology and Ophthalmology
Birds possess a large optic nerve compared to mammals. In fact, the two optic nerves together are larger than the bird's spinal cord. Olfactory lobes are small in most birds because sense of smell is not an important sense in most birds. The eyes of a bird constitute approximately 15% of their body weight, whereas in humans they constitute 1%. The avian iris consists of voluntary, striated muscle, rather than smooth muscle as in mammals; therefore, atropine is ineffective at dilating the pupils. Birds have a well-developed third eyelid that closes over the eye in a craniodorsal to

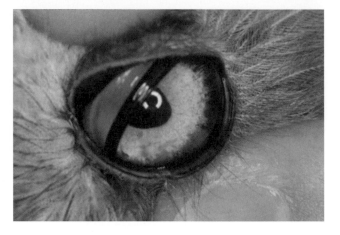

Figure 2.6. Birds have a well developed third eyelid that closes over the eye in a craniodorsal to caudal ventral direction.

caudal ventral direction (Figure 2.6). A unique pigmented structure called the pecten, which is attached to the retina, supplies nutrients to the vitreous. Birds have no tapetum, but they have an avascular retina.

Respiratory System
The cere is an area at the base of the upper beak that surrounds the nostrils (nares) (Figure 2.7). Just inside the nares in parrots is a keratinized flap of tissue called the operculum. Birds possess an extensive infraorbital sinus; in fact, most of their head is sinus. Compared to mammals, birds have a very large trachea, allowing birds to inhale more air than do mammals. The opening to the trachea is called a glottis (Figure 2.8). Birds have complete tracheal rings; therefore uncuffed endotracheal tubes must be used to avoid pressure necrosis inside the trachea. Again, birds lack a diaphragm; therefore, they must be allowed to move their sternum up and down or they will suffocate. Old stories of birds dying right after being restrained were probably due to accidental sternal compression and secondary suffocation.

The syrinx is responsible for sound generation in the bird, not the larynx, as in mammals. Because the syrinx is just past the tracheal bifurcation, birds can still vocalize even when intubated. The path of air

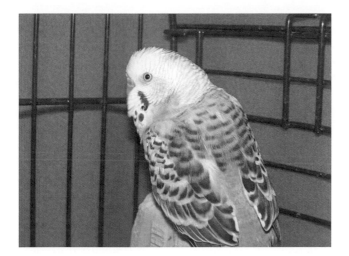

Figure 2.7. *The cere is an area at the base of the upper beak that surrounds the nostrils (nares). In adult male budgerigars, such as this one, the cere is blue. In adult female budgerigars the cere is a brownish pink.*

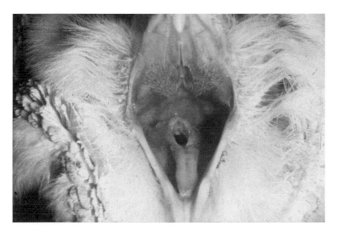

Figure 2.8. *The opening to the trachea in birds is called a glottis. The glottis is usually located directly caudal to the base of the tongue in most birds. This is the glottis of a barn owl. Also note the V-shaped opening on the roof of the mouth called the choana.*

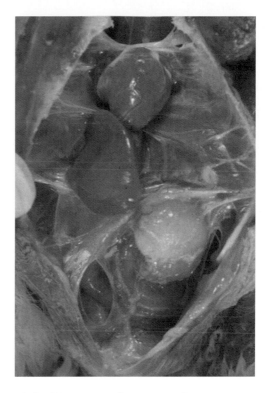

Figure 2.9. *Necropsy of a parrot demonstrating clear, normal air sacs. Air sacs warm and store air. Because air from the caudal air sacs shown here go directly to the lungs, air, oxygen, or anesthesia can be delivered through a tube (air sac tube) placed into one of these air sacs.*

through the lungs goes from the trachea or air sacs to the primary bronchus to the secondary bronchus to the parabronchi to the air capillaries. Birds have air capillaries that are 3 microns in diameter, whereas mammals have alveoli that are approximately 10 microns in diameter. Therefore, birds have a comparatively greater lung surface area than mammals. Birds also have air sacs, usually nine of them, that store and warm air (Figure 2.9). Because air can go from the air sacs to the lungs, as well as from the trachea to the lungs, oxygen exchange occurs on both inspiration and expiration, increasing oxygen use in birds compared to mammals.

Digestive System

Birds lack a diaphragm, so they possess a coelomic cavity, not an abdominal cavity. Birds do not have teeth; instead, they have a beak that is variable between species. Parrots are sometimes called hookbills because of their strong, hooked beak. The tongue is quite variable among bird species; parrots have a muscular tongue. The esophagus in birds is divided into two sections (cervical esophagus and thoracic esophagus) by an out-pouching of the esophagus called the crop (ingluvies). The ingluvies stores food and has waves of peristalsis that occur at a rate of at least one per minute. Birds possess a proventriculus (true glandular stomach) and a ventriculus (the gizzard) (Figure 2.10). Some birds possess a cecum (chickens) while others lack one (parrots). Some birds possess a gall bladder, while others lack one (parrots).

The feces of parrots contains mainly (90% or more) Gram-positive organisms (purple); waterfowl, raptors, and poultry can have mostly Gram-negative organisms

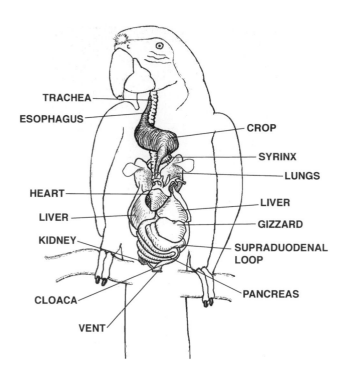

Figure 2.10. Avian viscera.

(pink). Typically, passerine birds have very little bacteria in their feces, and it is Gram-positive. Clostridium spp. should not be seen in parrot feces and is characterized by a septic tank smell to the feces and the characteristic safety-pin or racket shape seen on a Gram stain (Color Plate 2.1). The cloaca is the end point for three systems: gastrointestinal, reproductive, and urinary. The cloaca is divided into three parts: the copradeum receives feces from the rectum, the urodeum receives urine and urates from the ureter and sperm or eggs from the vas deferens and uterus/vagina, respectively, and the proctodeum is the area just before the opening (vent).

Reproductive System

The male bird possesses two intra-abdominal testis and a phallus (a rudimentary fold of tissue that is either intromittant or non-intromittant). The female bird usually possesses only one left ovary (the right ovary usually fails to develop). The female reproductive tract consists of an infundibulum, magnum, isthmus, uterus (shell gland), and a very short vagina. Parrots are not usually sexually dimorphic; therefore, surgical sexing or blood sexing must be performed to determine the gender of a bird. Surgical sexing involves visualizing the gonads and reproductive tract via a rigid endoscope placed in the abdominal air sac. Blood sexing involves evaluating 0.2 ml of blood via an ELISA test for a heterogamete (female is ZW) or homogamete (male is ZZ).

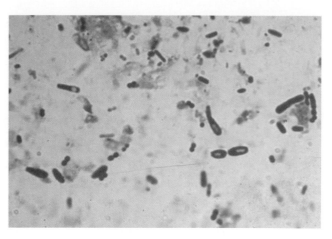

Plate 2.1. Clostridial overgrowth is apparent in this fecal Gram stain from a parrot. Clostridium shown here is a large Gram-positive rod with no spore, a clear central spore (safety pin shape), or clear end spore (racket shape). (See also color plates)

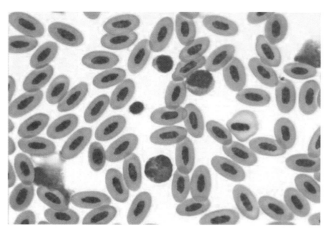

Plate 2.2. A Diff-Quick stained blood smear from a parrot. Note that birds have nucleated red blood cells. The cell at the twelve o'clock position is a lymphocyte, the two o'clock position is a monocyte, the six o'clock position is a heterophil (like a neutrophil), and the nine o'clock position is a normally occurring nucleated thrombocyte. (See also color plates)

COMPARATIVE CLINICAL PATHOLOGY

The blood glucose of birds is twice that of mammals. Birds possess heterophils instead of neutrophils; they are called heterophils due to the different, eosinophilic staining of the rod-shaped cytoplasmic granules. Birds, like reptiles, have nucleated RBCs and thrombocytes (not platelets). Some parrots are lymphocytic species like cows (Amazon parrots, cockatiels, budgies, eclectus, etc.) Birds can show up to 8% polychromasia since their RBC lifespan is so short (thirty-eight days compared to the 120 days of most mammals) (Color Plate 2.2).

NUTRITION

Species of birds kept as pets come from all over the world. Their diets are as varied as they are and the environments they come from. The specific dietary requirements for all these species are not well known.

Historically, psittacines (hookbilled birds or parrots) and passerines (canaries and finches) kept in captivity readily accepted seed diets, which then became the basis of diets available for pet birds. Seed-based diets provide poor nutrition—they are low in calcium, vitamins, and protein, and they are high in fat (Color Plate 2.3). Consequently, rather long-lived birds on all seed diets, such as Amazon parrots (possibly 50+ years) are seen dying from effects associated with chronic malnutrition as young as ten to fifteen years of age. Most nutritional research is still based on the dietary requirements of chickens (Brue 1994).

The introduction of pelleted foods for avian species has made it possible to dramatically improve the overall health of companion and caged birds (Color Plate 2.4). Balanced nutrition can be provided by pellets with the same ease of feeding as a seed diet.

Two methods are used to manufacture pelleted diets. "Bound" pellets are not usually cooked and are finely ground. The ingredients are mixed under pressure with a substance that, when pressed, forms the pellets. Much of the color and smell of the food used is retained in bound pellets. "Extruded" pellets are made of food ingredients that have been cooked and mixed together. The mixture moves through a processing machine that presses the food into various shapes. Color and vitamins are added afterward to the shapes and many have a sweet smell.

The current recommendation is to feed parrots a quality pelleted food that makes up 80% of their total intake. Fresh dark green and dark yellow vegetables (leafy greens, carrots, sweet potatoes) should make up the other 20%. Fruits and seeds are to be offered as treats. Some quality nuts (preferably in their shells) such as almonds, brazil nuts, or pine nuts can also be offered. Avoid peanuts because they may contain aflatoxins, which over time affect the liver. Budgerigars and cockatiels are the exception and require seed as part of their daily diet (up to 50%). Pellets alone may provide protein levels that are too high for these species.

Passerine birds (songbirds, i.e. canary and finches) require seed as part of their basic diet (up to 50%). Canary/ finch diets contain millet, rape, hemp, sesame, and linseed among other types of seed. These seed

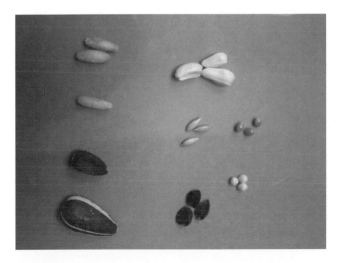

Plate 2.3. Examples of seeds found in seed diets. The left column, from top to bottom, is oat groats, small black sunflower seed, and large white striped sunflower seed. The right column, from top to bottom, is safflower seeds, red millet, white millet, and rape seeds. (See also color plates)

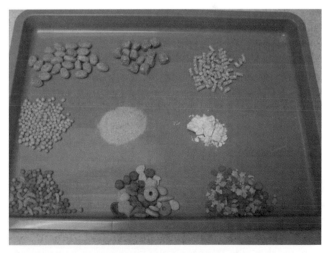

Plate 2.4. The introduction of pelleted foods for avian species has made it possible to dramatically improve the overall health of companion and caged birds. Various brands of natural and artificially colored pelleted food marketed for birds are shown here. Finely ground formulas are available to mix with water for hand or tube feeding. (See also color plates)

mixes, along with pellets and fresh vegetables, form a complete diet. Many of the rarer species of finches not commonly kept as pets also require insects or fruit as part of their regular diet.

Special need diets have been created for some species. Lories and lorikeets from Australia and the South Pacific Islands eat mainly nectar, fruits, and pollen. Fresh fruits and powdered diets commercially available for lories should be the basic diet for these species. Toucans, mynah birds, and some lories are predisposed to iron storage disease of the liver (hemochromatosis). Diets with low iron composition have been specially formulated for these species. Care must be taken with the choice of vegetables and fruit added for these species. For example, grapes are high in iron and should not be fed to mynah birds or toucans and others susceptible to iron storage disease (Tully 2009). Food high in vitamin C also should be avoided because vitamin C enhances absorption of iron.

Some foods can be toxic to birds. Do not feed chocolate (toxic theobromine) or avocados. Foods high in salt, sugar, or caffeine should also be avoided. Peanuts should be avoided for the aflatoxins that are invariably present.

Birds in the wild spend long hours foraging for food. They eat a wide variety of foods that change with each season and have many colors, textures, and tastes, creating a diverse diet that stimulates a bird psychologically and provides a lifetime of health. In the hospital setting a variety of diets should be kept on hand, such as the commonly used pelleted foods, as well as seed diets appropriate for various species. During hospitalization is not the time to change diets. During illness and the stress associated with a hospital stay it is often difficult to keep a bird eating enough to maintain weight. Having familiar diets available can encourage the avian patient to eat. This includes fresh vegetables and fruits.

Should a bird's appetite decrease or stop during hospitalization it is necessary to supplement nutrition via gavage feeding. Gavage tubes come in a number of sizes. There are various critical care diets available to readily pass through a gavage tube (see the techniques section). Hand feeding formulas designed for neonates also work well. Weighing the bird becomes a critical part of care to ensure that enough nutrition and calories are provided to maintain body weight. Ideally the patient should be weighed every morning before food or treatments are given.

Fresh clean water should be provided daily. Birds are able to tolerate municipal tap water. Well water may be clean coming out of the ground, but may be easily contaminated by bacteria colonizing the pipes leading to the faucet. Some owners choose bottled water. Spring or drinking water can be used, but do not use distilled water, because this lacks necessary salts and minerals.

HISTORY, RESTRAINT, AND PHYSICAL EXAMINATION

Often a bird's illness has been developing much longer than the owner realized and by the time signs are noticed the problem may be advanced. As with all species of animals, acquiring a through history is the first step. Obtaining an adequate avian history may involve more time than that of a dog or a cat patient. Birds should always be enclosed in a carrier or travel cage when arriving for their appointments (Figure 2.11). There are too many opportunities for harm to

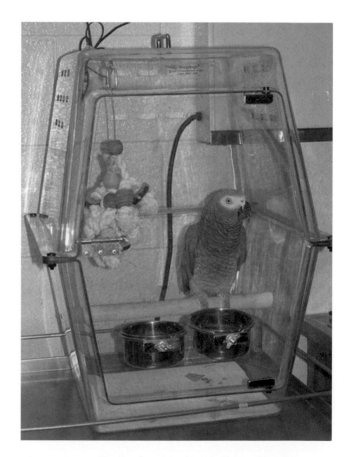

Figure 2.11. Birds should always be enclosed in a carrier or travel cage when arriving for their appointments. A towel can be used to cover a cage, especially a clear one such as this, to provide visual security for the bird.

come to the bird in an unfamiliar environment. Be sure the owner is made aware of this when the appointment is made.

History

The following questions should be asked during the history taking:

How old is the bird?

How long has it been owned and where was it acquired (breeder/pet store/ bird fair)?

Have there been any previous problems?

Has the bird been tested for chlamydiosis or psittacine beak and feather disease?

Has it been vaccinated against polyomavirus?

Have there been any changes in the bird such as voice change, attitude or weight change, or a change in the droppings (increase or decrease, color changes, more or less urine or urates) (Color Plates 2.5, 2.6, 2.7, 2.8, 2.9).

When was the last molt and has the bird been given any medications or herbal supplements?

What is the problem today?

How long has the illness been occurring?

When, if at all, has the bird been to a veterinarian?

Next, move to questions about the animal's environment:

What is the bird fed and what does it actually eat out of what is offered?

What is the cage like: size, perching?

What materials are used to make the cage (lead/zinc)?

What type of substrate is used, how often is it cleaned, and with what?

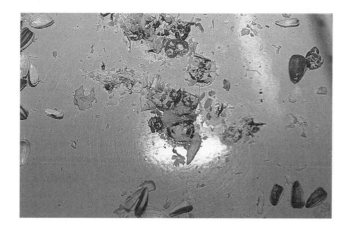

Plate 2.6. Normal feces. (See also color plates)

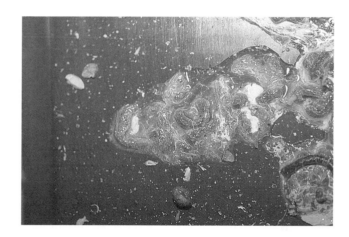

Plate 2.7. Normal feces. (See also color plates)

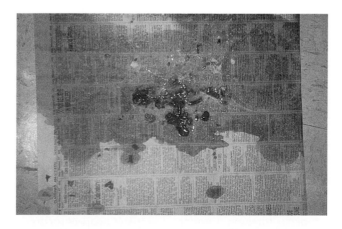

Plate 2.5. Polyuria (See also color plates)

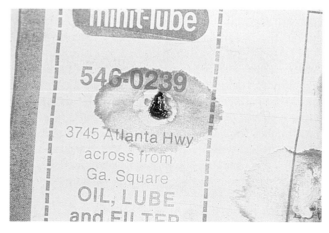

Plate 2.8. Hematuria and melena (See also color plates)

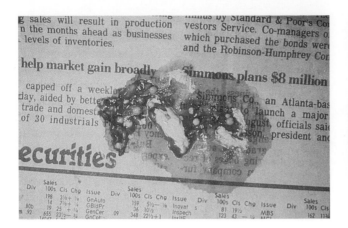

Plate 2.9. Undigested seeds. (See also color plates)

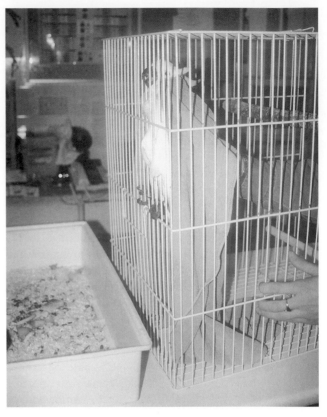

Figure 2.12. Capturing a bird while in its cage.

Does the bird spend time outdoors?

What is the temperature where the cage is kept and are there any drafts?

Is the bird let out of the cage and is it supervised during that time?

What type of enrichment is used (toys)?

How much sleep does the bird get? Sleep is very important to a bird and approximately twelve hours of sleep each night is required for good health. This should not be in a covered cage in a room where the television is on or family members are still talking, but somewhere quiet.

With these questions you can also develop an idea of the general knowledge that the owner has regarding bird care.

When a complete history has been attained move to the physical exam. Begin by observing the bird from afar. Birds are prey animals and they work at looking normal, especially in an unfamiliar environment. A bird in the hospital should never be sitting fluffed or with closed eyes. This indicates a very sick animal. Observe the bird's behavior, attitude, posture, breathing, skin and feather quality, and neurological status. Look for symmetry. Look at the droppings in the cage bottom or for regurgitated food. Dyspnea in a bird usually manifests as a "tail bob" movement of the tail up and down with each breath. After observing the bird from a distance, a physical exam can be performed with the bird restrained in a towel.

Restraint

After the bird has been observed and deemed able to withstand a hands-on examination it can be restrained in a towel. Restraint is needed to perform a thorough examination. Capture and restraint are perhaps the most traumatic events for the avian patient. If the bird will step up on to a perch it can be removed from the cage or carrier, set on the floor in a corner, and then caught using a towel. Setting the bird on the floor should only be done if the bird has clipped wing feathers and cannot become airborne. If the bird will not come out of its enclosure, the towel can be used to reach in and secure the animal. The towel is used to help protect the hands and to have the bird associate being restrained with the towel, not the hands. Never attempt to capture a bird when it is being held by the owner. The owner could be bitten and it is possible that this could affect the bond between the owner and bird.

Approach the parrot with a towel-covered hand and attempt to quickly wrap the fingers around the bird's neck. An ideal opportunity to grasp the neck is when the bird is attempting to move away from the towel, using its beak to hold onto the cage or carrier (Figure 2.12). Coming from behind, wrap the fingers around the neck, forming a collar. When the head is secured, bring the towel around the body with the other hand meeting the two ends of the towel across the front of the bird (Figure 2.13 A and B). This controls flapping of the wings. Remember, birds use the muscle around the sternum to move air through the respiratory system (they lack a diaphragm), and therefore care must be taken not to put pressure on the sternum because suffocation can occur (Figure 2.14). Proper hand placement is shown in Figure 2.15. The towel can be moved to expose sections of the bird as the examination progresses. When dealing with small cage birds (canaries, budgerigars), it is helpful to have one person at the light switch while another puts his hand into the cage. Make note of where the bird is just before the lights are turned off and then grab the bird quickly before it has time to adjust to the darkness.

Restraint time should be kept to a minimum (preferably less than two to four minutes). Before the bird is caught up, all of the material needed for diagnostic sample collection, examination, and grooming should

be anticipated and in place. During restraint it is commonly the responsibility of the holder to monitor the well being of the bird. When signs of excessive stress including panting, eye closing, weakness, and generally any change from when the bird was initially restrained appear, the bird should be released and given the opportunity to recover. Speaking to the bird in a soothing voice can help reduce the stress during handling.

Physical Examination

Once the bird has been restrained the physical examination of the avian patient is no different from that of another animal. The examination begins at the head and ends at the vent. Look straight on at the head and beak. Examine for symmetry and normal alignment of the beak and check for swelling or bruising, pitting on surface of beak, or fractures (Harrison 1994). Look at the nares (nostrils) to check for symmetry and any

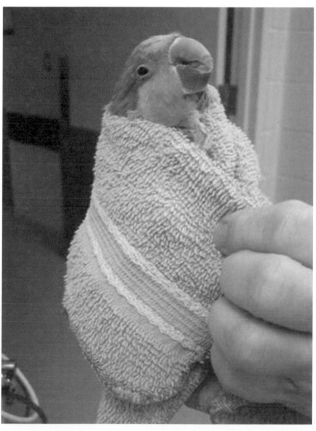

A

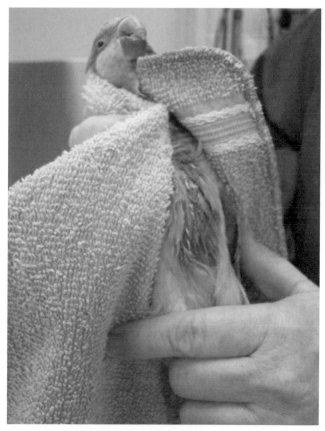

B

Figure 2.13. (A) A bird that is properly restrained within a towel. The neck and wings are under control. (B) The towel can be manipulated to gain access to various areas while still restraining the bird.

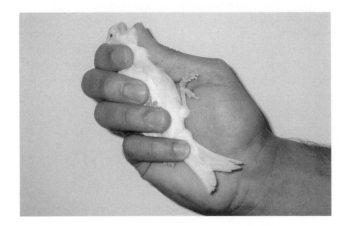

Figure 2.14. *Restraint of a small bird.*

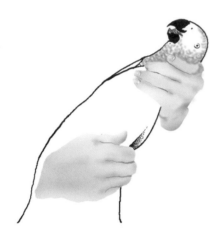

Figure 2.15. *Restraint of a bird.*

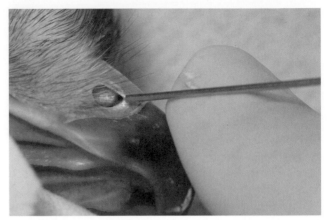

Figure 2.16. *Just inside the nares (nostril) is a fleshy part called the operculum that warms and regulates air. Most birds, including this red-tailed hawk, have an operculum and it should not be mistaken for something that needs to be removed because disturbing this structure causes bleeding.*

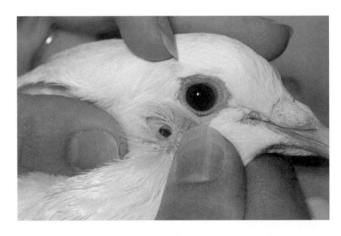

Figure 2.17. *Birds do not have an external ear pinna. The ears are located caudal and ventral to the lateral canthus of the eye. The ears may be observed by moving the feathers cranially, as is shown on this white Carneaux pigeon.*

discharge, debris, or blood. Because most birds have feathers near the nares, matting of the feathers above the nares will occur with a discharge.

Note: It is normal for a structure to be present just inside the nares; this is called the operculum (Figure 2.16). Disturbing this structure can cause bleeding. The eyes are also checked for discharge (again the matting of feathers will be present), lens opacity, blood, or disruption of normal anatomy. Hydration can be assessed using ocular parameters, such as moisture of the cornea (dull appearance when dehydrated) and the position of the globe (recessed when dehydrated).

While there is seldom disease in the ears of birds, the ears should still be examined. There is no external pinna and the ears are located caudal and ventral to the lateral canthus of the eye. The ears may be observed by moving the feathers (Figure 2.17).

The oral cavity and choanal slit can be viewed with the help of an avian speculum. The cloacal slit is the V-shaped opening on the roof of the mouth. Care must be taken when using a speculum to prevent iatrogenic trauma to the beak (Figures 2.18 A and B). A normal choanal slit is lined with papillae (pointed projections). Lack of vitamin A can cause the papillae to become blunted or disappear completely in severe cases. The tongue is a prominent feature in the oral cavity. The glottis is at the base of the tongue. The tissue in the oral cavity should be dry and smooth. Abnormal findings can include abscesses, fungal plaques, and excessive moisture.

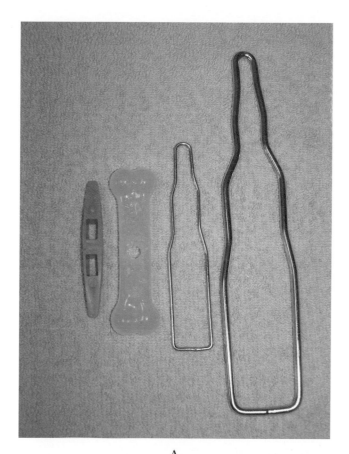

A

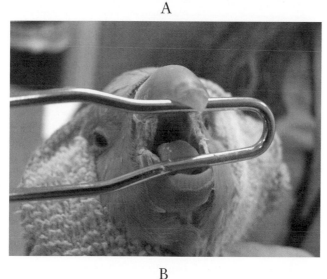

B

Figure 2.18. (A) A variety of speculums are available. (B) Care must be taken when using any speculum in a bird because beak damage can occur.

Next, palpate the thoracic inlet. Check the crop for foreign objects, crop burns (in young birds being handfed), distention, or crop stasis. Crop stasis can be noted by parting feathers and watching for movement

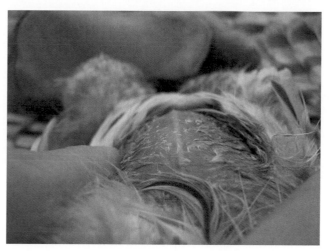

Figure 2.19. A Cooper's hawk restrained with gloves in dorsal recumbancy showing normal pectoral muscle mass on either side of the bony keel, forming a slight V-shape. This view is from the head of the bird looking caudally. Less pectoral muscle mass and a more prominent keel would have suggested a thin bird.

(regular contractions occur in the crop). There should be at least one wave of movement across the crop per minute.

Palpating the pectoral muscles can determine the body condition of the avian patient (Figure 2.19). A score of one to five is used; one signifies a very emaciated animal and five is considered to be overweight. Normally, the edge of the keel can be palpated between the rounded pectoral muscles that slope slightly on either side. The feathers should be examined over the body. Feathers should have a bright iridescent appearance. Wings and legs should be gently flexed, and extended to evaluate joint function. Check the plantar surface of the feet. Erosion of the bottom of the feet may be associated with a diet deficient in vitamin A and/or improper perches. Erosions can lead to ulcerative dermatitis, commonly known as bumblefoot (Figure 2.20). Also look for necrotic areas, swelling, abscesses, or gout (an accumulation of white uric acid under the skin). Examine the cloaca (vent), looking for masses, irritation (hyperemic), prolapse of the tissue, and the presence of matted fecal material (the feathers around the vent should be clean).

The caudal coelomic cavity can be palpated. Organs cannot be easily palpated due to the sternum extending over most of the coelomic cavity, although a large liver or the presence of an egg can be palpated and should be considered as abnormal findings. Normally the liver

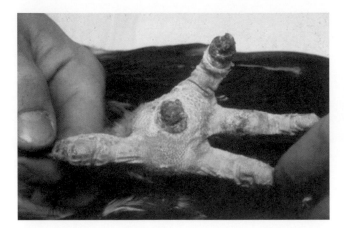

Figure 2.20. *Plantar surface of a raptor foot demonstrating ulcerative pododermatitis, as known as bumblefoot. This lesion can start as a smooth, pink, erosive, or flattened area on the plantar surface of the foot. In psittacine birds this can be due to poor quality perches or vitamin A deficiency.*

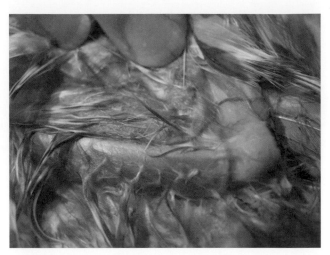

Figure 2.21. *Elbow area of a bird showing the cutaneous ulnar (basilic) vein crossing superficial to the proximal ulna. This vein is used to determine hydration status in a bird, for phlebotomy, and IV injections.*

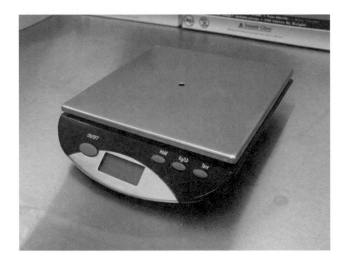

Figure 2.22. *A digital gram scale should be used to accurately determine the weight of birds. The scale should be able to weigh in 1-gram increments.*

does not extend past the level of the sternum. The uropygial gland (preen gland) can be found at the extreme caudal dorsal surface and should be examined for symmetry and overall appearance. Remember, not all birds kept as pets have a uropygial gland.

The bird should be ausculated to access heart health and respiratory condition. Placing a pediatric stethoscope over the lateral body wall allows auscultation of the heart. Listening over the craniodorsal body wall is best to assess the respiratory condition. Hydration can be assessed with a "vein refill time" using the basilic (cutaneous ulnar) vein. In a normally hydrated bird this vein should instantaneously refill; by the time a finger is off the vein to see it, it should have refilled. If the basilic vein can be seen refilling, it is estimated that the bird is about 5% dehydrated. If the vein requires one second to refill, the bird is severely dehydrated (10%) or is in shock (low blood pressure) (Figure 2.21).

Obtain the bird's weight at the end of the exam, before it is placed back into the carrier. Use a digital gram scale that has a maximum weight of 4 to 5 kilograms and weigh in 1-gram increments (Figure 2.22).

COMMON DISEASES

Infectious Diseases

Avian Chlamydiosis

Avian chlamydiosis is one name given the disease in birds caused by the organism *Chlamydophila psittaci*; other names include ornithosis, chlamydiosis, and chlamydophilosis. The term "psittacosis" refers to the disease in people originating from a parrot (a psittacine bird), whereas the term ornithosis refers to the disease in people originating from any species of bird. Note that *Chlamydophila psittaci* should not be confused with a related organism in people, *Chlamydia trachomatis*, which causes a sexually transmitted disease, or another related organism, *Chlamydophila pneumoniae*, a common mild respiratory pathogen of people. Changes in nomenclature in 1999 reflected recent advances in DNA testing that revealed differences between organisms that were previously thought to be the same. What used to be just one genus, *Chlamydia*, is now described as two, *Chlamydia* and *Chlamydophila*. A word of caution, therefore, when reading any literature on chlamydial organisms prior to 1999—the reader may not be 100% certain as to which of the newly categorized organisms was being referred to in the document. The term *Chlamydophila psittaci* is used throughout this document to refer to the organism formerly known as *Chlamydia psittaci*.

The organism has been found in more than 130 species of birds worldwide and a variety of mammals, including humans, and is therefore a zoonotic disease. Numerous potential avian species may act as a source of infection for people. The most common source of infection (70% of all cases in the 1980s) is exposure to a recently acquired psittacine bird. Other birds can be a potential source of infection, such as domestic or wild pigeons, passerines (soft-billed birds), or poultry. People at occupational risk include pet store employees, veterinarians, veterinary technicians, laboratory workers, workers in avian quarantine stations, farmers, wildlife rehabilitators, zoo workers, and employees of poultry (usually turkey) slaughtering and processing plants. Occasionally exposure to wild pigeon roosts is a source of infection to the general public.

The *Chlamydophila psittaci* organism is transmitted by inhalation or ingestion of the spore-like elementary body phase of the organism. Shedding in birds can be activated by stress, such as shipping, crowding, chilling, and breeding. Person-to-person transmission has been suggested, but never proven. Those individuals that are immunosuppressed are more susceptible to the disease and its effects. The organism *Chlamydophila psittaci* is relatively resistant, surviving in the soil for three months or within a bird dropping for up to one month.

Clinical signs can differ based on species of bird. Some birds present quite ill, whereas others exhibit very subtle signs of disease. Generally, a parrot with psittacosis presents with depression, lethargy, anorexia, dyspnea, nasal or ocular discharge, conjunctivitis, and biliverdinuria (green urates). Rarely, birds present comatose, which has been observed in sensitive species such as macaws. Commonly both the spleen and liver are enlarged. Pigeons and passerines seem to exhibit little if any clinical signs of disease while infected with the *Chlamydophila psittaci* organism and therefore are sometimes referred to as asymptomatic carriers of the disease.

A suggestive diagnosis can be made by radiographs showing splenomegaly, ± hepatomegaly. A CBC showing a heterophilic, monocytic leukocytosis and a mild non-regenerative anemia are also suggestive. A plasma electrophoresis may be suggestive of either acute or chronic disease.

Diagnostic testing is varied. There are tests to detect antibodies in the serum (elementary body assay [EBA] and immunofluorescent antibody [IFA]) and tests to detect antigen in the feces or blood (enzyme linked immunofluorescent antibody assay [ELISA] and polymerase chain reaction [PCR]). It is best to perform a panel of three tests including PCR of blood, PCR of feces, and IFA of serum. In addition, a fluorescent antibody (FA) test can be performed on tissue such as liver tissue from a biopsy or necropsy. For legal purposes, cell culture from the feces is the best test, but the organism does not consistently grow, and shedding of the organism in the feces is intermittent. There is also risk to laboratory personnel when the organism is grown in the laboratory.

The Texas Medical Diagnostic Laboratory is currently the only laboratory commercially offering culture. Addresses and phone numbers of laboratories that test for *Chlamydophila* and definitions that have been accepted by the American Veterinary Medical Association (AVMA) and the Association of Avian Veterinarians can be found in the Compendium of Measures to Control *Chlamydophila psittaci* (formerly *Chlamydia psittaci*) Infection Among Humans (Psittacosis) and Pet Birds (Avian Chlamydiosis), 2004, by the National Association of State Public Health Veterinarians (NASPHV) http://www.avma.org/pubhlth/psittacosis.asp.

Treatment of birds, which should be supervised by a licensed veterinarian, consists of doxycycline for forty-five days. A lower dose is used in macaws to prevent regurgitation. Avian chlamydiosis is usually a reportable disease, but it depends on the state. Most states require that veterinarians report any diagnoses of psittacosis in a bird to the state veterinarian or public health department.

Other Bacterial Infections

Bacterial infections in birds can be localized or systemic and can involve any system, but commonly involve the liver or GI or respiratory systems. Usually Gram-negative organisms, such as *E. coli*, *Klebsiella*, *Enterobacter*, or *Pseudomonas*, are involved, but infections involving Gram-positive organisms or anaerobes can occur as well. Treatment is based on culture and sensitivity and cytological findings (such as an in-house Gram stain), but usually involves the use of broad-spectrum, bacteriocidal antibiotics such as enrofloxacin, trimethoprim-sulfa, and cephaolsporins. Macaws commonly regurgitate after trimethoprim-sulfa or doxycycline administration.

Canary Pox

Poxviruses are the largest of viruses and the genus Avipoxviruses are found worldwide in more than twenty families of birds. There are many species of Avipoxvirus, such as psittacine pox, canary pox, pigeon pox, falcon pox, and fowl pox. Each species of pox has varied host specificity, but typically the most severe clinical signs are seen in its natural host. Pox used to be common in recently imported Amazon parrots, especially blue-fronted Amazon parrots, macaws and pionus, but is rarely seen today. Occasionally an older imported bird presents with old pox scars on the eyelids, nostrils, and face.

Today canary pox is the most commonly seen pox. The virus is transmitted via mosquito or mechanical means through broken skin. Birds can show blepharitis, ocular discharge, rhinitis, and conjunctivitis associated with raised papules ten to fourteen days post infection. Clinical signs can be divided into "dry" pox, which consists of cutaneous papular lesions, and "wet" pox, which consists of mucosal papular lesions of the oropharynx. Occasionally birds may display neurological signs.

Diagnosis is based on typical clinical signs and histological finding of Bollinger bodies, which are intracytoplasmic inclusion bodies, of skin or mucosal cells, and is considered pathognomonic. Treatment consists of providing supportive care. Leave scabs to heal naturally to lessen scarring. Vaccines have been created for chickens, pigeons, turkeys, canaries (Poximmune, Biomune, Lenexa, KS), quail, waterfowl, falcons, and Amazon parrots. It is recommended to vaccinate before the breeding and/or mosquito season. Maximum protection occurs three to four months after vaccination. Some canary breeders vaccinate every six months.

Polyomavirus

Polyomaviruses are rather host specific and cause subclinical disease in mammals, but in psittacine birds they cause severe clinical disease in a wide variety of psittacine and other species of birds. Immature psittacine birds commonly present with acute disease with an approximate mortality rate of 27% to 41%. The disease is characterized by twelve to forty-eight hours of depression, anorexia, delayed crop emptying, regurgitation, diarrhea, dehydration, SQ hemorrhage, dyspnea, and polyuria. The SQ hemorrhages are most easily seen over the crop, carpi, or cranium.

Transmission of polyomavirus is through exposure to excretions and secretions, especially urine.

Polyomavirus is a non-enveloped virus and therefore very stable in the environment and difficult to destroy. A DNA probe (PCR) test is available to detect viral DNA in tissue or feces. Antibody tests are available and a positive result denotes exposure has occurred and that the bird probably sheds virus intermittently. Many birds in aviaries are subclinically affected and are a constant source of infection for all birds in the aviary and are a particular danger for young birds. Therefore, all birds should be vaccinated. Psittamune (Biomune, Lenexa, KS) is a commercially available, licensed vaccine for use in psittacine birds. The vaccine is administered SQ and has been proven to be safe and effective. It is an inactivated vaccine; therefore, optimum protection occurs two weeks after the second vaccine. There is no treatment for the disease. The prognosis is grave if clinical signs are present in a young bird.

Proventricular Dilation Disease

The causative organism of this disease has been identified as an 89 nm virus, but of unknown type. The route of transmission is via fecal-oral and appears to affect birds of many orders, including psittacine birds. Clinical signs include severe, chronic weight loss, regurgitation, delayed crop emptying, ravenous appetite, undigested food in stool, and neurological signs (i.e. falling off perch) in an adult bird. The virus paralyzes the nerves in the proventriculus and the bird essentially starves to death, despite a good appetite, due to the inability to process its food. Suggestive diagnostic testing includes radiographs demonstrating proventricular dilation and whole undigested food particles or seeds in the feces.

Note that many diseases can cause proventricular dilation, including disease from parasites, yeast, megabacterium, mycobacterium, foreign bodies, neoplasia, and lead and zinc toxicosis. Definitive diagnostic testing includes a crop biopsy demonstrating lymphoplasmocytic ganglioneuritis. Birds usually die within two years of developing clinical signs, but recently treatment with the NSAID celecoxib (Celebrex®, a COX-2 inhibitor) or any other COX-2 inhibitor has been described; however, the mechanism against the virus is unknown. Prevention currently consists of avoiding exposure to known infected birds.

Psittacine Beak and Feather Disease (PBFD)

This disease of parrots is caused by a circovirus. These non-enveloped viruses are among of the smallest yet described, at 14 to 16 nm. PBFD virus is shed in feces, feather dander, and various excretions and secretions. Asymptomatic birds can shed the virus for years before exhibiting any clinical signs. Because the virus is non-enveloped, it is very stable and can survive years in the environment and is resistant to destruction by common disinfectants.

Generally the progression of the disease is dictated by the age of the bird when clinical signs first appear. Younger birds have a faster progression of the disease. Most birds present with chronic PBFD, which is characterized by symmetrical, slowly progressive dystrophy of developing feathers that worsens with each successive molt. The feather dystrophy includes retained feather sheaths, hemorrhage within the pulp, curled feathers, and circumferential constrictions of the feather shaft. Usually the down and contour feathers are affected first, and then the primaries. Birds can go on to develop complete alopecia and sometimes beak abnormalities consisting of progressive elongation of the beak and necrosis of the palate rostrally, near the upper beak. These birds are often immunocompromised and die of secondary bacterial or fungal infections.

The PBFD DNA probe tests are performed on whole blood and detect viral DNA; therefore, a positive result means there was PBFD viral DNA in the blood. In a bird with no clinical signs, it is recommended to retest the bird in ninety days to see if the viral DNA is still present. If so, then the bird is infected, but if not, then the bird was transiently infected and overcame the infection. Any bird displaying feather abnormalities should have a feather follicle biopsy and DNA in situ hybridization performed in addition to the DNA probe blood test, since some clinical birds are so viremic that they will have a negative blood test.

This can also occur if a bird is extremely leukopenic. A DNA probe test can be used to detect viral DNA on a swab of the environment to assist in determining the effectiveness of disinfection efforts. Treatment consists of supportive care and antimicrobials for secondary infections. Once clinical signs develop the disease is always fatal (Color Plate 2.10).

Papillomatosis Caused by Herpesvirus

Papillomatosis, or wart-like GI lesions caused by a herpesvirus, should not be confused with facial warts caused by papillomavirus. Species most commonly affected include the Amazon parrots and macaws. Amazon parrots are prone to developing concomitant bile duct or GI tract carcinoma that has recently been associated with PHV-1, genotype 3.

Clinical signs of papillomatosis include wart-like masses observed anywhere along the GI tract, but most commonly in the cloaca and oropharynx (Figure 2.23).

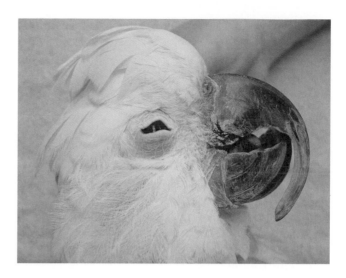

Plate 2.10. Bird with PBFD. (See also color plates)

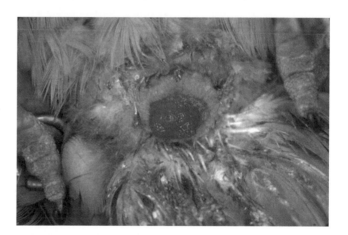

Figure 2.23. Clinical signs of papillomatosis (caused by a herpesvirus) include wart-like masses observed anywhere along the GI tract, but most commonly in the cloaca, as seen in this Amazon parrot, and oropharynx.

Birds may exhibit weight loss, signs of straining to defecate, soiled vent, or blood in the stool. Some cases have GI obstruction with associated clinical signs. Because the virus is latent, birds that have been previously treated may have a recurrence of lesions and signs with stress. Amazon parrots with bile duct carcinoma may exhibit biliverdinuria and lethargy, and bile acid levels may be high. Diagnosis is suggestive based on gross appearance and location. Definitive diagnosis is based on histology. Treatment involves removing the wart-like growth. In the author's experience it is best to apply silver nitrate to the lesion, or half of the lesion if it is circumferentially involving the cloaca, every week under anesthesia until gone.

Butorphanol is also administered at 1 to 2 mg/kg IM once before the procedure.

West Nile Virus

West Nile virus is caused by a flavivirus. West Nile virus is endemic in other countries, but in the late 1990s it was found within the eastern U.S. and has since spread across the country. Crows, jays, and raptors, as well as horses, are susceptible species, whereas poultry are considered resistant. The WNV virus is spread by mosquitoes. If people or dogs are affected they are usually older or immunosuppressed. Clinical signs range from none in resistant species such as poultry to neurologic signs (ataxia, circling, head tilt, and seizuring) and death in susceptible species. A CBC is usually normal or a lymphocytosis is present. A serum antibody test is available. Treatment consists of supportive care. Recently the use of alpha interferon has seemed to result in better success in people. This disease has already spread throughout the U.S. so it is too late to prevent the disease in this country. A conditionally licensed vaccine is available for use in horses that is currently being used intramuscularly in birds at the same or a reduced dose.

Aspergillosis

The two most common etiological agents associated with aspergillosis in birds are *Aspergillus flavus or fumigatus*. Predisposing factors associated with the disease are immunosuppression, including hypovitaminosis A, and being exposed to massive quantities of fungal spores which can easily occur when corn cob or wheat or pine straw is used as bedding. Aspergillosis is more common in African Grey parrots, macaws, and raptors. The location of the infection is most commonly in the bifurcation of the trachea near the syrinx or in the caudal thoracic air sac, and occasionally in the sinuses. A suggestive diagnosis is based on a very elevated CBC (usually above 40,000), with a heterophilic leukocytosis and monocytosis. Serum antigen and antibody tests are available, but are just suggestive of the disease. A definitive diagnosis is usually obtained by direct visualization and sampling via endoscopy of either the trachea or the air sac, and cytology or culture of those samples. Treatment consists of antifungals such as the conazoles, including ketaconazole, itraconazole, and fluconazole. Itraconazole is the best, but should not be used in African Grey parrots (or used at very low doses). Also amphotericin-B is good, but can only be given IV or through nebulization and it is quickly renal-toxic. Months of treatment are necessary, so early and proper diagnosis is imperative. Any underlying cause of immunosupression or overexposure should also be corrected.

Candidiasis

Candidiasis is caused by the yeast organism *Candida albicans*. Clinical signs include regurgitation, delayed crop emptying, and white plaques in oral cavity. The crop is the most common organ affected and the crop contents have a yeasty, sweet smell. Young birds/neonates are the most severely affected. If adults have clinical signs of candidiasis, look for some cause of immunosuppression. Diagnosis is easily done by identifying the organism on a Gram stain of crop or fecal material. Treatment of mild cases consists of antifungal therapy with oral nystatin, which acts topically in the GI tract. If the candidiasis is severe and invading the mucosa, then in addition to nystatain, a systemic antifungal such as one of the conazoles is necessary to attack the infection from the vascular system as well as topically.

Non-infectious Diseases

Heavy Metal Toxicosis

Heavy metal toxicosis is usually caused by ingestion of lead or zinc. Sources of lead include fishing weights, curtain weights, bullets, paint, and costume jewelry. Sources of zinc include pennies minted after 1986, Monopoly® game pieces, powder coating, paint, and costume jewelry. The ventriculus (gizzard) of birds retains heavy particles for grinding food, but in the case of heavy metal particles, they are retained and slowly digested, allowing constant absorption of the toxins. Clinical signs include depression, weakness, regurgitation, and sometimes neurological signs.

Diagnosis is usually made by visualizing the metal-dense particles on radiographs, but a definitive diagnosis can be made on only 0.2 ml of blood for lead or 0.2 ml of serum for zinc at the Louisiana Veterinary Medical Diagnostic Laboratory (Figures 2.24 A and B). Toxic levels of lead in the blood are greater than 0.2 ppm, and greater than 2 ppm for serum zinc. Treatment consists of a chelating agent such as CaEDTA or dimercaptosuccinic acid or d-penicillamine to bind with the heavy metal, rendering it harmless; it then can be urinated out of the body. Stressful procedures such as surgery or endoscopy to remove a large particle should be done after some chelation therapy, because stress can cause lead to move suddenly from the bone where it is stored to the blood and worsen clinical signs. Other products such as lactulose to assist the liver with toxicosis, lubricants such

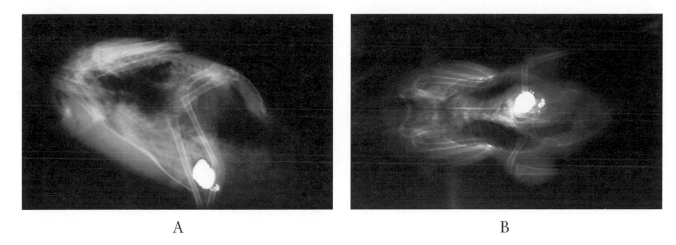

Figure 2.24. (A) *Lateral standing radiograph in a duck showing heavy metal in the ventriculus. Later, 97 cents worth of various coins were removed endoscopically. (B) Ventrodorsal view of the same duck.*

as corn oil or peanut butter, or bulking agents such as psyillium can also be given.

Hypovitaminosis A

A diet deficient in vitamin A, such as an all seed diet, can lead to hypovitaminosis A. Clinical signs include choanal papillae in the oral cavity that are blunted, plantar erosions on the feet, and poor quality skin and feathers (darkened areas on the feathers of the wings). A diagnosis is made based on history and clinical signs. Secondary bacterial or fungal infections involving the respiratory tract are common. Sometimes a Gram stain of a choanal swab shows increased epithelial cells and basophilic staining. Treatment includes an increase in dietary vitamin A by providing the bird with dark yellow vegetables (sweet potato, carrot, commercial bird pellets). One could also give one injection of vitamin A. Avoid giving too much vitamin A because it is a fat-soluble vitamin that can result in hypervitaminosis A.

Hypocalcemia of African Grey Parrots

Adult African grey parrots, especially those on a low calcium seed diet rather than a healthy pelleted diet, can present with seizures due to hypocalcemia. A total calcium level, and even better, an ionized calcium as well, diagnoses the disease. Treatment consists of calcium gluconate IM. Oral calcium can be administered later in the form of calcium glubionate. Of course treatment also includes improving the diet by supplementing with calcium and slowly changing to a pelleted diet.

Non-stick Cookware Toxicosis

Non-stick cookware, such as Teflon®, is made of polytetrafluoroethylene (PTFE). If burned and heated to above 540°F, the PTFE fumes are released, causing immediate pulmonary hemorrhage and death in birds anywhere in the household. Rarely, immediately supplied fresh air and steroids prevent death.

Egg Binding

Some birds, such as cockatiels, chronically lay eggs, and especially those on an all seed diet that is low calcium can present with egg binding. The egg is stuck in the uterus because the uterine muscles lack enough calcium to contract and push the egg out. The egg puts pressure on the kidneys, causing the bird to go into shock, and it can die within hours to days without removal of the egg. Other birds may have egg binding due to an abnormally large egg. If the egg is normal size and there are no obstructions such as scarring of the uterus, then hormones, such as oxytocin or prostaglandin F2 alpha, can be given to stimulate contractions, but only after calcium has been absorbed IM so the uterine muscles have enough calcium to contract. In the case of an egg that should not be forced out, it can be imploded by creating negative pressure within the egg by suctioning out the contents with a needle and syringe placed through the egg exposed at the cloaca or through the celomic wall and uterus on the ventral abdomen. This is an emergency procedure performed under anesthesia and is not without risk of hemorrhage or infection. If these procedures are unsuccessful, surgery to perform a salpingohysterectomy (removal of uterus) can be performed. Supportive care with fluids, antibiotics, etc. are also necessary.

Crop Burns

Juvenile birds that are hand fed by humans may sometimes be offered gruel that is too hot (above 105°F), usually heated in a microwave, that causes a burn of the thin crop and overlying skin. It is usually not until ten days later that the effects of the burn are noticed by visualizing the sudden appearance of gruel pouring out of a hole in the crop and running down the breast of the bird. It is only at this ten-day point, after a scab has formed and the body has determined dead from healthy tissue, that surgery should be performed to close the hole. Supportive care, including antibiotics or the mild antifungal nystatin and fluids, etc., are usually needed.

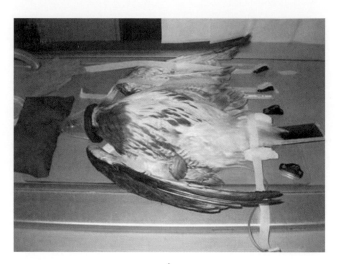

A

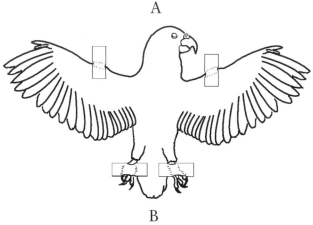

B

RADIOLOGY

Radiographs can be taken awake or under anesthesia depending on the goals. Usually the bird is under anesthesia so that it is absolutely still and in the proper position for accurate evaluation. This also produces the least amount of stress. A bird can be placed in a cardboard box awake to determine if an egg or metal is present, or in the case of a barium series, see the location and speed of barium travel. Most radiogaphs are taken at 500 mAs and 50 Kvp for 1/120 of a second, but each machine is different. Two views are taken: the ventrodorsal, with the keel of the sternum perfectly aligned with the spine, and the lateral, with the coxo-femoral joints and shoulder joints superimposed (McMillan 1994). This positioning allows evaluation of the radiographs (Figures 2.25 A, B, and C and 2.26 A and B).

ANESTHESIA AND ANALGESIA

Isoflurane is the safest gas anesthetic choice in birds (Curro 1994). Sevoflurane has been shown to be just as effective and recovery is slightly faster (Quandt 1999). Birds are usually restrained in a towel and mask induced, usually starting at 2% in healthy birds at 2 l/minute oxygen flow rate. For short procedures, such as immobilization for radiographs that require less than fifteen minutes, most birds are not intubated. For longer procedures, birds can be intubated with an uncuffed endotracheal tube. Once intubated, the oxygen flow rate must be reduced to 1 l/minute so as not to damage the delicate air sacs.

The best method to secure an endotracheal tube in a bird is to tape it to the bottom beak so the mouth can be opened to wipe out excess moisture if necessary.

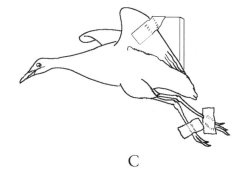

C

Figure 2.25. (A) A red tailed hawk properly positioned for a ventrodorsal radiograph. (B and C) Positioning of an avian patient for radiographs.

Always keep the head and glottis above the level of the crop, because liquid from the crop can trickle into the trachea and drown the bird in an instant. Birds have complete tracheal rings, so an inflated cuffed tube can

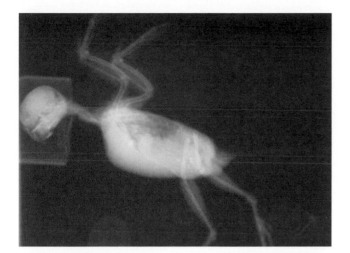

A

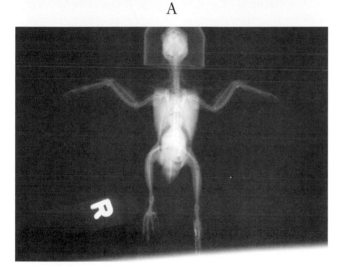

B

Figure 2.26. *(A) An example of a parrot well positioned for a lateral radiograph. Note how the shoulder and hip joints are aligned. (B) An example of a parrot well positioned for a ventrodorsal radiograph. Note how the keel and spine are aligned (superimposed).*

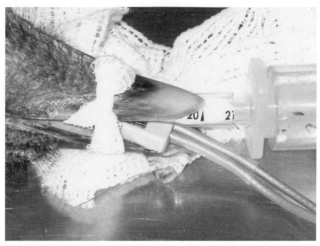

Figure 2.27. *A wild turkey intubated and under anesthesia, showing the placement of a Doppler probe on the roof of the mouth over the palatine artery to monitor heart rate. This can be performed in any species of bird.*

exert too much pressure on the lumen of the trachea that cannot expand and thus cause pressure necrosis and a subsequent diphtheritic membrane. It is important to realize that birds, especially cockatoos, have tracheas that narrow a few centimeters past the glottis, causing an endotracheal tube to initially seem the appropriate size but then after passing it a quarter of the way down the trachea it becomes lodged, causing pressure necrosis. Therefore, pick an appropriate size tube and re-intubate if it feels as if it is lodged. It is

very easy to intubate a parrot because the glottis is very forward at the base of the tongue.

Birds tend to not do well after one hour under anesthesia due to hypothermia, hypoventilation, and respiratory acidosis. The use of forced heated air blankets has greatly improved the attempted maintenance of normal body temperature in birds under anesthesia (Rembert 2001). It is imperative that adequate lubrication is applied to the eyes to prevent dry eye with forced heated air blankets. In addition, the laterally placed eyes of birds should not be allowed to rest on any surface or they can collapse. Although this is usually temporary, it may be a permanent condition. Common monitoring equipment includes a pulse oximeter on the leg, Doppler probe over the radial artery or palatine artery, and ECG (Figure 2.27). Simply listening with a stethoscope and CONSTANT watch of the respiratory rate and depth are absolute minimums in monitoring birds under anesthesia.

When assessing an avian patient for signs of pain, selecting a pain reliever, or determining a dose and the frequency of administration, it must be remembered that there is NO GENERIC PARROT. One must be familiar with the very limited scientific research that has been conducted regarding pain management in psittacine birds. Furthermore, each patient must be evaluated and re-evaluated individually and constantly. Unlike mammals, birds have more kappa than mu opiate receptors; therefore, a partial agonist/antagonist such as butorphanol has been shown to provide pain relief, but at much higher than mammalian doses at 1 to 2 mg/Kg IM (Paul-Murphy 1999). Buprenorphine has not been shown to work as well (Paul-Murphy 2004).

Pollack (2005) recommends the following analgesic doses:

Lidocaine: 1 mg/kg at site, dilute 1:10; 4 mg/kg or higher is toxic

Butorphanol: 0.5–2 mg/kg IM (1 to 2 mg/kg IM every 2 to 4 hours as needed)

Carprofen: 1 to 10 mg/kg IM/PO (most use 2 mg/kg)

Celecoxib: 10 mg/kg PO (used for proventricular dilatation disease)

Meloxicam: 0.1 to 1 mg/kg IM/PO (0.5 mg/kg) (Wilson 2004)

It is very difficult to assess pain in birds and there are no standard methods or assessments available. Therefore, one must rely on past experience, observation, and anthropomorphism (If I had a fractured bone I would want an opiate). Birds are very stoic and do not cry out in pain despite the fact that they can be very loud when they want to be. Birds have a flock mentality, meaning they are a prey species and if they make their illness conspicuous to the rest of the flock they risk being ostracized (so as not to attract the attention of a predator). It is best to observe your patient before it is aware that you are observing it. When it realizes you are there, you will probably observe it straightening up, opening its eyelids more, and it may even turn to partially face you in an attempt to look alert.

Birds do not seem to become profoundly depressed on analgesics, therefore I tend to give analgesics at any hint of pain in a bird. In most cases I tend to give an opiate at surgery, then both an opiate (butorphanol) and an anti-inflammatory (meloxicam) for the first six to forty-eight hours, followed by only the anti-inflammatory for about three to five days.

SURGERY

It is best to remember to use analgesics before pain occurs to prevent "wind up." Butorphanol is best in birds.

Preparation of the skin is similar as for mammals, with three applications in succession of chlorhexidine scrub, but there are some differences, including the use of sterile saline or very sparing amounts of alcohol, patting the skin rather than rubbing so as not to cause subcutaneous petechial hemorrhaging, and plucking of feathers under anesthesia before preparing the skin. Plucking feathers is very painful and usually requires a surgical plane of anesthesia and should be done one feather at a time, pulling in the direction in which it grows. Clear, see-through drapes are a necessity for the anesthetist to be able to assess breathing in the patient. Sticky surgi-drapes or sterile clear plastic wrap can be used.

A radiosurgical unit is preferable to an electrosurgical unit in birds. It can be used in monopolar or bipolar modes. A special "Harrison tip" is a bipolar tip used in birds (Figure 2.28). Birds should be under anesthesia for less than one hour, so having everything possible prepared and ready for use to shorten surgery time is essential in avian surgery. If the celomic cavity is to be breeched, remember that birds do not have a diaphragm and that anesthetic gases will escape the surgery site, causing the bird's anesthetic depth to lighten.

Also be aware that it is easier to "bag" or IPPV (intermittent partial pressure ventilation) a bird once the air sac is incised. If at any time the bird's breathing cannot be assessed it is the anesthetist's responsibility to stop the surgeon to assess breathing. Fluids, such as LRS or Normosol-R, are usually administered at

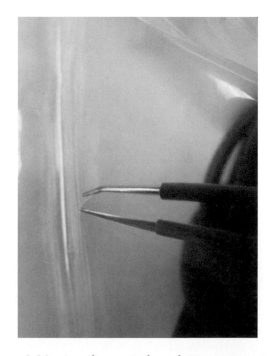

Figure 2.28. A radiosurgical or electrocautery tip used in birds, called a "Harrison tip," is specifically designed for birds with one bent tip for better access. Do not straighten.

10 ml/Kg/hour for the first hour and then at 5 ml/Kg/hour thereafter. A bolus of fluids may need to be given if blood loss is greater than 10% of the blood volume. The suture used is typically 4-0 to 5-0 PDS.

Common surgeries include accessing the crop for a biopsy to definitively diagnose proventricular dilation disease (PDD), repairing a crop burn in a neonate, or removing a foreign body or accessing the proventriculus with an endoscope through the crop. Common surgeries requiring celomic cavity access include salpingohysterectomy (removing the uterus, not the ovary, in a bird), liver biopsy (either directly or endoscopically), proventriculotomy to remove a foreign body, or exploratory laparatomy.

Strictly follow manufacturer's directions on cleaning, maintaining, and handling endoscopes to ensure the long life of this expensive equipment.

PARASITOLOGY

Although ascaridosis is now uncommon, the clinical signs are none or diarrhea; rarely a GI impaction can occur. A diagnosis is easily made on fecal flotation. The treatment can be with ivermectin, fenbendazole, or piperazine. Giardiaisis is caused by the protozoal organism in the *Giardia spp.* Clinical signs can be none or diarrhea and weight loss. A diagnosis can be made on a fecal Gram stain in severe cases, but the motile protozoa are easier to visualize on a direct saline smear, especially with the addition of iodine. An ELISA for giardia Ag is the best current test. Treatment is with metronidazole.

Trichomoniasis is caused by the *Trichomonas* spp. of protozoa and is called "canker" in pigeons and "frounce" in raptors eating pigeons. It is associated with white plaques in the oral cavity. Diagnosis is based on demonstration of the protozoal organisms on direct saline smear of the oral cavity. Treatment is metronidazole. Syngamus is also known as "gape worm" because affected birds gape their mouths open trying to breathe around the physical presence of the large worm in their trachea. The worms are thick bodied and dark red, and the male and female join to form a permanent "Y" shape. It is common in waterfowl and robins, and it is treatable with antiparasiticides. Some have even used endoscopy to retrieve the worms.

Knemidokoptes pilae, or the scaly leg and face mite, causes pitting and scaling of the keratin of the skin and beak of parakeets and other birds, but causes scaling on the legs and feet of canaries and finches (Figure 2.29 A and B). Although the diagnosis can be made by the

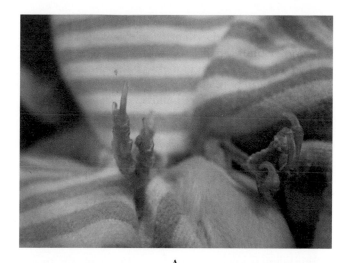

A

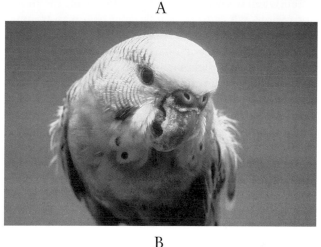

B

Figure 2.29. (A) Knemidokoptes infestation in a canary, manifesting as flaking of skin on feet. (B) Deformed beak from Knemidokoptes. (Courtesy of Cheryl Greenacre.)

typical appearance of the skin and beak, a scraping of the affected area onto a slide with mineral oil reveals the round-shaped mites. The treatment is topical Ivermectin, or similar product, given twice ten to fourteen days apart. Do NOT give ivermectin IM in birds, especially small birds, because they commonly die from an anaphylactic reaction, presumably from the propylene glycol in the product.

GENDER DETERMINATION

Most parrots do not exhibit obvious signs of sexual dimorphism. The gonads in both males and females are internal. If a client wishes to know the gender of her pet bird, a blood test should be recommended. This involves taking a small amount (0.2 ml) of blood or pulling a feather, which are DNA checked for chromosomes. Several companies offer this test. Surgical sexing should only be offered to owners who plan on breeding their birds. The gonads are visualized with a sterile rigid endoscope. Any abnormalities of the gonads or other structures can then be identified. This, of course, carries the low risk of anesthetic complications, hemorrhage, and infection.

GROOMING

Nails

Often when a bird presents for a nail trim, the nail is not overgrown but the points have begun to traumatize the skin of the owner's arm. A stone tip on a roto-tool or an emory board can be used to quickly round and dull the points. If nails are overgrown, human nail clippers or guillotine-type nail trimmers can be used to take the length back. This should then be followed with the roto-tool or emory board to round off any sharp edges created during clipping. If the nail extends in an arc that is more than half a circle it is probably too long (Figure 2.30). The quick differs in length between individuals. Always have silver nitrate sticks or ferric subsulfate powder available to stop hemorrhage if it occurs.

Beak

Knowing the normal beak shape and length for various species is a must before any trimming takes place. Some species of parrots possess a longer beak than others (i.e. compare a macaw to an Amazon parrot). Beak trims can be performed when the bird is awake. A roto-tool (larger parrot) or nail file (birds smaller than a cockatiel) can be used. The tip can be blunted. If the bill tip organ becomes visible (as a row of white dots on the occlusal surface of the beak) do not trim further or hemorrhage and pain will occur. The flaking on the external surface of the beak can be removed with the roto-tool/nail file. When using the power tool be sure to never stop moving, using long, gentle strokes to avoid going too deep and cutting into bone. The beak is a bony structure covered with keratin. Some individual parrots maintain their beak length and never need a trim. A bird with a maloccluded beak needs corrective trimming on a regular schedule. A bird with a fast growing beak that is constantly in need of trimming may have underlying liver disease that needs to be addressed (Figure 2.31).

Wing

Wing trims are performed to prevent the bird from flying freely. Indoors, free flying birds have encounters with ceiling fans, windows, being squeezed into doors, and flying out through an open door or window. An ideal wing trim is symmetrical and allows the bird to gently glide to the floor. Too severe a wing trim can

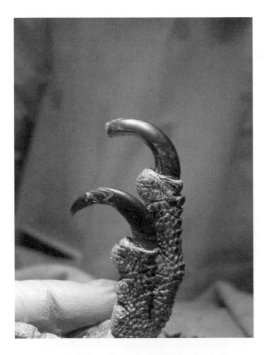

Figure 2.30. A clipped and unclipped nail.

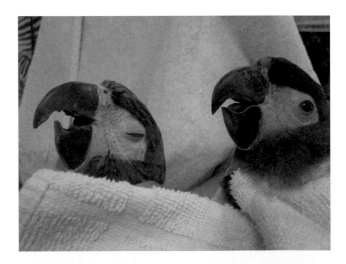

Figure 2.31. Most birds do not need to have their beaks trimmed. The severe macaw on the right has a normal beak, while its clutch mate on the left has an abnormal, thickened beak.

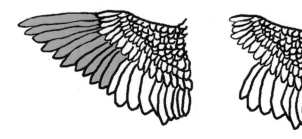

Figure 2.32. Wing trim.

cause trauma, most commonly resulting in damage to the keel.

A correct wing trim depends on the weight (i.e. obese compared to a normal weight bird), body type (i.e. heavy bodied bird compared to an elongated, long tailed bird), and the number of pin (blood) feathers that are growing in at the time of the trim. Only primary feathers (consisting of the first ten wing feathers counting from the tip) should be trimmed. Therefore, depending on the body shape of the bird, a wing trim consists of cutting four to ten primary feathers on each side (Figure 2.32). If, for example, one were trimming an Amazon parrot, which is a heavy bodied, short tailed bird, approximately four or five feathers would be trimmed on both wings. A cockatiel, built very differently than an Amazon, most likely would need all ten primary feathers removed.

To clip the feathers, the wing must be gently extended, and a firm grip should be used, incorporating the carpus and patagial ligament in the hold. This will support the wing if the bird should struggle and help to avoid injury to the wing. Before cutting, check for pin feathers—those that have not finished growing and still have a blood source. If pin feathers are present leave a mature feather on either side of the pin feather to protect the growing feather. If several blood feathers are present it is best to reschedule the trim when they have finished maturing. The feathers are trimmed just behind the tips of the lateral coverts. Care should be taken not to clip the covert feathers because this will leave an unsightly cut line. Always use sharp scissors and be sure not to cut toes straying into the field of the scissors. Birds with properly trimmed wings live safer lives indoors. Owners must be made aware that even a bird with properly trimmed wings can fly away.

EMERGENCY AND CRITICAL CARE

The causes for a bird to have an emergency visit to the veterinarian are similar to those for mammals, but may vary slightly. Examples of emergency cases include trauma (hit by ceiling fan, toe closed in door, big bird/little bird incidents, dog/cat attack, burns), toxins (lead, zinc, PTFE fumes from Teflon®), metabolic disorders (chronic hypovitaminosis A, hypocalcemia in African grey parrots), or infection (due to bacteria, virus, fungus, or Chlamydophila usually involving the liver or GI or respiratory tract). Egg binding (dystocia) due to low total body calcium from a long-term calcium-deficient diet (such as a seed diet) is a common avian emergency.

Unlike mammals, birds usually present with a terminal manifestation of chronic disease that has just recently showed overt acute signs. Subtle clues of disease often go unrecognized by the owner because birds hide signs of disease to avoid being ostracized by the flock (i.e. the flock doesn't want to be around a bird that is attracting a predator). The first approach to an emergency should include, if possible, obtaining a history over the phone so as to be as prepared as possible when the bird arrives. Be familiar with common species problems (i.e. hypocalcemia should be at the top of the rule-out list for a seizuring African grey parrot). Evaluate the history, cage and husbandry, and droppings, and observe the bird for clues about the etiology before pursuing stressful restraint.

Perform a rapid but thorough physical exam and diagnostic collection (±CBC, profile, radiographs, fecal Gram stain). Sometimes the bird may be so stressed that the examination may need to be performed in less than one minute or in stages. Obtain an accurate weight with a gram scale so drugs can be dosed and administered accurately. Provide therapy to stabilize the patient: warmth (85° to 90°F), a stress-free environment (no barking dogs), and ±O₂ (Figure 2.33). Offer familiar/favorite foods and water at an elevated level right in front of the bird, provide ten hours of daylight and fourteen hours of dark, and provide a low perch or none at all (birds insist on perching on the highest available perch, even when severely debilitated.

During the examination for an emergent bird, first check to see that the patient has a patent airway. Is the airway patent or is there a mass or foreign body in the trachea? Examples of a mass include an aspergillus granuloma, neoplasia, or diptheritic membrane. A millet seed in a cockatiel trachea (this can be directly visualized in the trachea with a rigid 1-mm endoscope) is an example of a foreign body.

Second, check to see if the animal is breathing; if not, intubate with an uncuffed endotracheal tube and provide intermittent partial pressure ventilation (IPPV) in birds at one breath/five seconds. Due to the unique respiratory system in birds an air sac tube can be

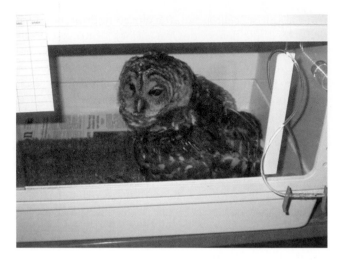

Figure 2.33. *Hospitalized owl in warmed cage. The owl is receiving supplemental oxygen and fluids through an intraosseous catheter.*

placed in the caudal thoracic or abdominal air sac and oxygenated air will flow through the lung. An air sac tube can be connected to O_2 or anesthesia and left in place for five days.

Third, check to see if there is a heartbeat. If a bird experiences cardiac arrest, the prognosis for reversing this situation is poor/grave due to a bird's high metabolic rate and oxygen demands. The following treatments can be attempted to reinitiate heart beat: rapid heart massage and ventilation (100 beats/minute and one breath/five seconds), epinephrine IV or IT (intratracheally), atropine (usually used to prevent bradycardia, though), doxapram IV or IT (stimulates respirations), or bolus IV fluids ±2.5% to 5% dextrose.

Blood Loss

The average blood volume of a bird is approximately 10% of its body weight (BW). For example, a 1-kg blue and gold macaw has an average blood volume of about 100 ml. A healthy bird can lose up to 10% of its blood volume (or 1% of BW) without any adverse side effects. Therefore, a healthy 1-kg blue and gold macaw could lose up to 10 ml without any adverse side effects. Unlike mammals, a healthy bird can usually lose up to 30% of its blood volume without dying due to compensatory mechanisms. Because of these compensatory mechanisms, it is important to realize that the packed cell volume (PCV) in a bird is not accurate (i.e. not equilibrated) for twenty-four hours after a hemorrhagic incident because birds can shunt blood from large skeletal muscle capillary beds and away

from the kidneys via the renal portal system to increase blood flow to central areas. Therefore, an equilibrated PCV < 15% or an immediate PCV < 20% are similar and serious enough to contemplate a blood transfusion. Fluids, hetastarch, oxyglobin, or a blood transfusion (5% of BW) help a bird with severe blood loss. The anemic patient may require vitamin B complex, iron dextran, and vitamin K_1.

Dehydration

Most sick birds are 5% to 10% dehydrated. Severe dehydration is usually > 10%. Clinical signs of dehydration include depression, reduced skin elasticity over digits, sunken eyes, cool digits, and decreased refill time of the basilic (cutaneous ulnar) vein. A general rule of thumb is that a normally hydrated bird has a basilic vein refill time that is instantaneous, such that you cannot see the vein refill after applying digital pressure to it. If you can see the vein refill, the bird is at least 5% dehydrated, and if the vein takes one second or more to refill, the bird is more than 5% dehydrated.

Maintenance fluids are the same for birds as they are for mammals: 50 ml/kg/day. For example, maintenance fluid calculations for a 500-gram Amazon parrot are 0.5 kg × 50 ml/kg/day = 25 ml/day. The dehydration fluid replacement needed for a 500-gram Amazon parrot that is 6% dehydrated is as follows: dehydration replacement in liters is BW (in kg) × % dehydration (expressed as a decimal amount), 0.5 kg × 0.06 = 0.030 liters = 30 ml. The calculated dose for dehydration replacement (30 ml) should be administered over forty-eight hours.

The schedule for administration of maintenance and dehydration fluids given to the above bird in forty-eight hours is as follows: Day 1: 25 ml for maintenance + 15 ml for half the dehydration replacement = 40 ml; Day 2: 25 ml for maintenance + 15 ml for the second half of dehydration replacement = 40 ml.

Fluid therapy is a critical component of emergency therapy. The most commonly used fluids are lactated Ringer's solution or Normosol-R because they most closely resemble the fluid lost. Warm fluids (about 100°F) are imperative. Keep in mind that the body temperature of most birds is 104° to 109°F. Sometimes 2.5% dextrose is added to the SQ or IV fluids.

Mild dehydration may only require conservative management such as oral or SQ fluids. SQ fluids are generally administered into the inguinal area in birds. Severe dehydration or shock requires rapid circulatory expansion with IV or intraosseous (IO) fluids; oral or SQ fluids are inadequate in these cases due to lack of absorption at the administration site. Peripheral indwelling catheters have been avoided in birds because birds have small, fragile veins that easily form hematomas, their dermis is highly mobile (causing difficulties in stabilizing the catheter), and they have refractory temperaments and a powerful beak. Repeated IV bolusing can be attempted, but it is stressful to the birds to be repeatedly restrained and it is damaging to the veins. Switching to oral fluids should be done as soon as possible.

TECHNIQUES

Catheter Placement
Intraosseous Catheters

IO catheters allow continuous access to peripheral circulation, and they provide the ability to administer drugs, fluids, or total parenteral nutrition (TPN). Their use is safe, rapid, and practical. IO catheters are most commonly placed in the distal ulna or proximal tibiotarsus. They should not be placed in a pneumatic bone because pneumatic bones communicate with the respiratory system; therefore, this may drown the bird when fluids are administered. Likewise, intracoelomic fluids should not be administered because this may also drown the bird if fluids get into an air sac. To place the IO catheter, pluck and aseptically prepare the carpus. Position the needle in the center of distal ulna. Support the ulna and rotate the catheter. Once past the cortex, the catheter passes easily. Aspiration should produce a small amount of blood. Anchor the catheter to the soft tissue of the carpus and apply a figure-8 bandage (Figure 2.34 A and B).

Air Sac Tube

To place an air sac tube, make a skin incision over the sternal notch area (borders are the last rib, the femur, and the lateral processes of the vertebrae) and use a pair of hemostats to penetrate body wall, and then insert an ET tube.

Blood Collection

The blood volume of birds is approximately 10% of their body weight. The amount of blood that can be collected safely from a healthy bird is approximately 1% of the body weight (1 ml/100 grams of body weight in a healthy bird). This amount should be reduced with a sick patient. For example, a maximum of 1.2 ml of blood can be removed from a healthy 120-gram (0.12 Kg) sun conure without adverse effects. For a 1,000 gram (1 Kg) healthy macaw a maximum of 10 ml can be removed. For example:

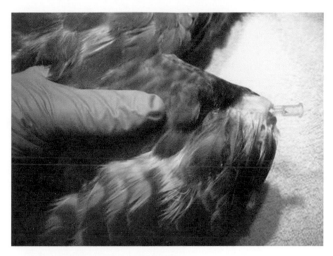

A

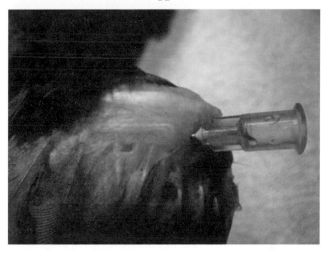

B

Figure 2.34. (A and B) Intraosseous catheter placement into the distal ulna of a Cooper's hawk. A 22-gauge needle or spinal needle can be used. A catheter cap fits on the end. Sterile technique should be used to place a catheter.

cockatiel: 0.120 Kg × 0.01 = 0.001 liters = 1 ml
macaw: 1 Kg × 0.01 = 0.010 liters = 10 ml

There are a variety of sites from which blood can be collected in the avian patient. These include the right jugular vein, basilic vein (also called the cutaneous ulnar vein), and the medial metatarsal vein. The size of the bird influences the site chosen.

Jugular Vein

The right jugular vein is the vein of choice for parrots kept as pets. The right jugular vein is chosen over the left because it is two-thirds larger. To collect from the jugular vein the bird must be restrained in right lateral recumbency with the head and neck gently extended. The vein should be visible when collecting blood. The jugular vein is found in a featherless tract or aptera (featherless area) on the ventrolateral aspect of the cervical area. The vein can be seen by lightly wetting the feathers with alcohol. Bird veins are mobile under the skin and have very elastic vessel walls, which can make needle punctures a challenge. Light digital pressure at the level of the thoracic inlet should be used when holding off the vein. A 1-ml or 3-ml syringe with a 22- to 25-gauge needle is commonly used.

Basilic Vein

The basilic vein (cutaneous ulnar vein) is also a choice for blood collection on medium to large birds and courses over the medial surface of the proximal ulna. This vein is superficial, lacking support tissue to disperse a hematoma, and often small, making it prone to collapse. To collect from this vein the bird should be restrained on its back. The wing should carefully be extended, and it should be supported by grasping the carpus and patagium.

Medial Metatarsal Vein

The medial metatarsal vein is another venipuncture choice. The larger the bird, the more developed the vein is. This vein lies in a groove on the medial side of the tibiotarsus, near the tiobtarsal-tarsaometatarsal joint (hock joint). This vein is a good choice for small amounts of blood, an IV injection, or IV catheter placement. The bird can be restrained in a towel, held upright, and the leg gently extended. Poultry and water fowl have a large metatarsal vein, making it an excellent choice for blood collection in these birds. Small blood tubes, including serum separator tubes, are available for use in small patients (Figures 2.35, 2.36).

ADMINISTRATION OF MEDICATIONS

Most infections in parrots are due to Gram-negative organisms. Most drugs are used empirically, since very few if any pharmacodynamic and pharmacokinetic studies have been performed in any species of bird, or in just a few species of birds. Remember that there is no generic bird; different parrot species react differently to different drugs so, research on each species would take forever.

The goal is to achieve antimicrobial tissue levels at the site of infection that are greater than the MIC, but one must realize that tissue penetrations vary. One must also realize that drug excretion is rapid in birds compared to mammals. Antibiotics can cause immunosuppression and change normal flora, producing a secondary fungal infection. Therefore, antibiotics should only be used when indicated to avoid upsetting the delicate balance of normal flora in birds. Choose bacteriocidal instead of bacteriostatic antibiotics.

Water Additives

The advantages of adding medication to the drinking water are ease of administration, the bird medicates itself, restraint isn't required, and specific water borne diseases may be reduced. The disadvantages, which far out weigh the advantages, include inexact dosing, poor palatability that reduces water and drug intake, instability of some medications in water, the likely possibility of under-dosing, increasing organism resistance, and medication being poorly or slowly absorbed.

Food Additives

The advantages of adding medication to the food include ease of administration, food consumption may be fairly consistent, and ease of treating hand-fed nestlings. The disadvantages again outweigh the advantages and include the same reasons discussed above for adding medication to water. One must also realize that sick birds are often anorectic.

Direct Oral Medication

The advantages of giving medications orally include the fact that a precise dose is given (unless the bird spits the drug out or doesn't swallow), many pediatric suspensions are available, and these medications can be given simultaneously when a bird is gavaged or tube fed. The disadvantages include the stress of capture and restraint, the risk of aspiration of the drug, the drug may be poorly or slowly absorbed through the gastrointestinal tract of very ill birds, or malabsorption (if, for example, the bird is in shock or has a GI disorder) (Figure 2.37).

Intramuscular Injection of Medication

The advantages of giving medication via an intramuscular injection into the pectoral muscle of a bird include the knowledge that the bird will receive an exact dose, it is quick and easy to administer (meaning less stress of handling), and it is quickly absorbed. Among the disadvantages, not all drugs are available for IM use, and pain and necrosis may occur at the injection site. In critically ill birds that cannot initially absorb oral medications, the bird can be started on IM medications and then switched to oral forms later (Figure 2.38).

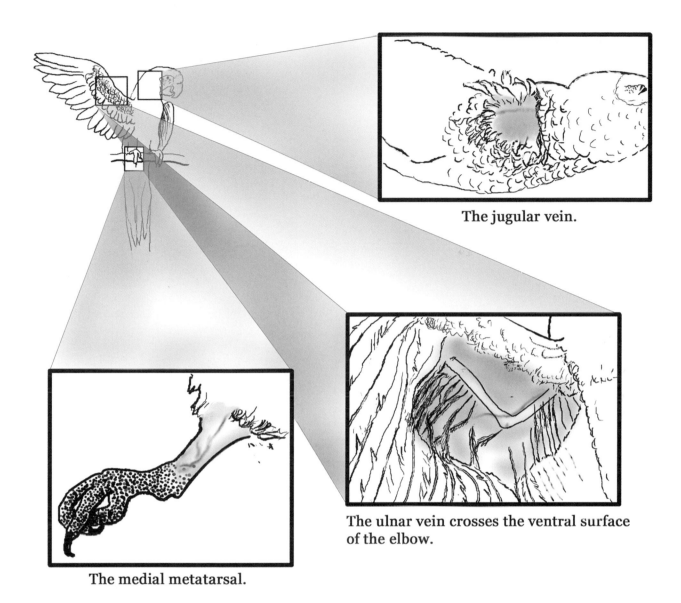

The jugular vein.

The ulnar vein crosses the ventral surface
of the elbow.

The medial metatarsal.

Figure 2.35. Venipuncture sites.

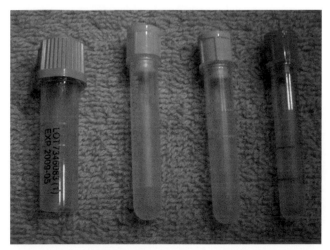

*Figure 2.36. Small blood collection tubes are
available for small patients.*

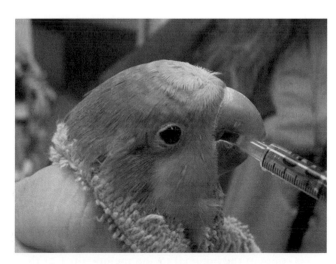

*Figure 2.37. Oral medications being given to a
Quaker parakeet. One drop at a time should be
given under the tongue to avoid aspiration.*

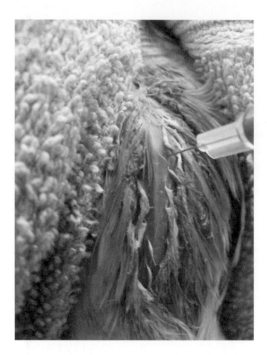

Figure 2.38. Intramuscular injection given into the left pectoral muscle of a bird. The pectoral muscles are found to either side of the bony keel. Use a 25- to 26-gauge needle.

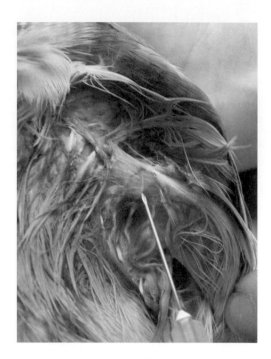

Figure 2.39. Subcutaneous fluids being given to a bird with a 22-gauge needle into the left inguinal area. The left leg is gently pulled caudally. Care should be taken to not abduct (pull laterally on) the leg because bird legs do not abduct much.

Intravenous Medications

The advantages of intravenous medications via the jugular or medial metatarsal or basilic vein are that an exact dose is given, it is rapidly absorbed, and it rapidly reaches therapeutic levels. The disadvantages of IV medications are the stress of prolonged restraint while giving a bolus, the risk of the bird chewing the IV line if it is on an IV drip, and the fragile veins of birds.

Intraosseous Medication

The advantages of giving medications via an intraosseous catheter in the distal ulna or proximal tibiotarsus include the fact that a precise dose is given (and like IV administration it is rapidly absorbed) and the catheter can be left in place up to five days. The disadvantages of IO administration include discomfort or, if not bolus treating, the bird chewing the IV line.

Subcutaneous Medication

The advantages of giving medications via the subcutaneous route in the inguinal region include the fact that a precise dose can be given and it is quick and easy to administer. The disadvantages include the fact that some drugs are irritating when given SQ and some

severely debilitated birds may not absorb SQ fluids or drugs. If fluids pool in the SQ space and are not absorbed within one to two hours then IV or IO fluids are necessary (Figure 2.39).

Topical

In birds, greasy topical compounds should be avoided because this reduces the insulation of the feathers. If ointments must be used, then they should be used sparingly. It is better to use water soluble creams.

Nebulization

Nebulization is used to deliver medications for respiratory infections. Nebulization is a process in which atomization of a liquid into small (<3 microns) droplets occurs so that it can be inhaled. Usually nebulization is performed for ten to thirty minutes by forcing oxygen through a solution containing antibiotics or antifungals, etc.

Sinus/Nasal Flushing

Sinus flushing can be diagnostic (cytology, culture) and/or therapeutic. Warm saline should be used. It is imperative to hold the bird completely vertically upside down to avoid aspiration of fluid into the trachea.

Flushing can be performed in an awake bird or an anesthetized, intubated bird (Figure 2.40).

Tube Feeding

Tube feeding is controversial in critically ill patients (will they process it?). The bird must be hydrated first. Usually one should start with a thin carbohydrate supplement (such as Emeraid) and later use a juvenile parrot hand feeding formula or specially made avian critical care diet (high calorie, easy to digest).

Birds have a high basal metabolic rate with very little in reserve; therefore, if a bird is losing weight, it needs to be tube fed. While hospitalized, a bird is weighed daily in the morning on a gram scale. Tube feeding is necessary if a bird is not maintaining or gaining weight in the hospital. Generally birds are tube fed one to four times/day. The technique consists of restraining the bird in a normal upright position to avoid regurgitation and aspiration. Some prefer a stainless steel feeding needle with ball tip; others use a red-rubber catheter and a speculum to prevent the bird from biting the tube in two (Figure 2.41).

The tube is aimed from the left commissure to the right crop area (Figure 2.42). Care must be taken to avoid the large trachea and excessive force must be avoided to prevent puncturing the esophagus and depositing food into the neck of the bird. Confirm placement of the tube by palpating/visualizing the tube in the crop before administering the formula. If the bird regurgitates at any time, then set it down and let go immediately to allow the bird to concentrate on not aspirating.

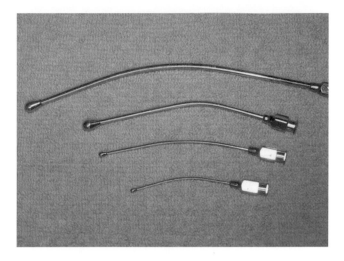

Figure 2.41. *A variety of sizes of stainless steel ball tipped feeding needles used to gavage food directly into a bird's crop.*

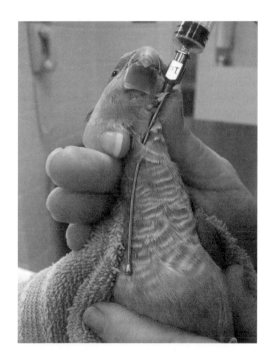

Figure 2.42. *A metal ball tipped feeding or gavage tube is held external to the bird to show the proper placement of the tube internally. The tube should gently enter from the bird's left commissure and aim for the right shoulder area. The crop of a bird is on the right side of the neck and is very thin and subject to puncture.*

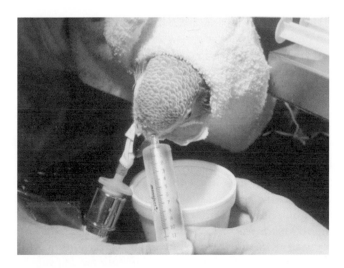

Figure 2.40. *Nasal flush. (Courtesy of Cheryl Greenacre.)*

Approximate Feeding Quantities (Start with Small Amounts, Then Increase to Amount Below)

Budgie: 1 ml
Cockatiel: 3 to 5 ml
Amazon parrot: 15 to 30 ml
Cockatoo: 20 to 40 ml
Macaw: 30 to 60 ml

DIAGNOSTIC SAMPLING

Blood is drawn from the right jugular vein because it is two-thirds larger than the left. No more than 10% of the blood volume, or 1% of the body weight, can be removed from a healthy bird without adverse effects. If a bird is sick or debilitated in any way, less must be taken. Generally, whole blood is placed in a lithium heparin tube for a CBC, but a CaEDTA tube can be used. Plasma from a lithium heparin separator tube is ideal, but other tubes producing plasma or serum can be used. Microtainer tubes that hold less than 1 ml are ideal for small bird patients. Nasal flush and other techniques are covered in the techniques section.

WOUND CARE AND BANDAGING

Wound care is very similar to that of mammals, except that birds are very sensitive to steroids; thus, topical or parenteral steroids should be avoided. Bandaging is also similar except for those below pertaining to the special anatomy of birds. Typical bandage materials simply need to be cut smaller.

Ball or snowshoe bandages are used to protect the plantar surface of the foot and evenly distribute the bird's weight in cases of ulcerative pododermatitis, or bumblefoot. The interdigitating bandage is wrapped around the entire foot between the toes (Figure 2.43). The ball bandage is more ball shaped, and the snowshoe bandage is flatter.

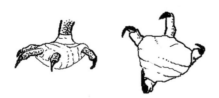

Figure 2.43. Ball foot bandage.

Figure-8 bandages are used to immobilize the wing distal to and including the radius and ulna. They are not used for humeral fractures unless a wrap about the body is included. This bandage is usually for temporary use because the propatagial ligament that extends from the shoulder to the carpus becomes severely contracted after five to seven days (Figure 2.44).

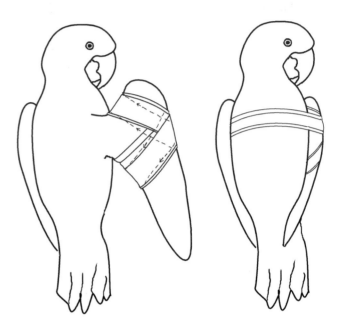

Figure 2.44. Figure-eight bandage.

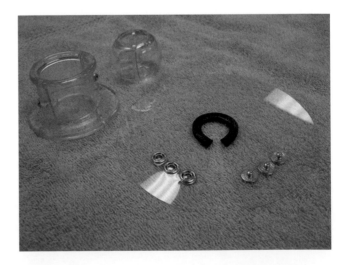

Figure 2.45. Examples of Elizabethan and tube collars used in birds. Generally they are not recommended for use in birds because they are invariably heavy, make eating and preening difficult, and they stress the bird. Exceptions are made for collar use when a bird self traumatizes, i.e. bites its own flesh and bleeds.

Elizabethan or tube collars about the neck are not recommended in birds because they are invariably heavy, make eating and preening difficult, and stress the bird. Exceptions are made for collar use when a bird self traumatizes, i.e. bites its own flesh and bleeds (Figure 2.45).

EUTHANASIA

Any animal should be rendered unconscious prior to euthanasia, regardless of the species. Birds are easily masked under anesthesia with isoflurane and then once unconscious, the euthanasia solution can be given via the intravenous or intracardiac route or in the cisterna magna. AVMA Euthanasia Guidelines 2007 include birds and can be found at http://www.avma.org/issues/animal_welfare/euthanasia.pdf.

REFERENCES

Brue RN. 1994. Nutrition. In: Avian Medicine: Principles and Application, edited by Ritchie BW, Harrison GJ, Harrison LR. Lake Worth: Winger's Publications.

Curro TG, Brunson DB, Paul-Murphy J. 1994. Determination of the ED$_{50}$ of isoflurane and evaluation of the isoflurane-sparing effect of butorphanol in cockatoos (*Cacatua* spp.). *Vet Surg*, 23: 429–433.

Forshaw JM, Cooper WT. 1989. Parrots of the World. 3rd ed. Willoughby, Australia: Landsdown Press.

Harrison GJ, Ritchie BW. 1994. Making distinctions on the physical examination. In: Avian Medicine: Principles and Application, edited by Ritchie BW, Harrison GJ, Harrison LR, Lake Worth: Winger's Publications.

King AS, McLelland J. 1984. Birds, Their Structure and Function. 2nd edition. Eastbourne, England: Bailliere Tindall.

McMillan MC. 1994. Imaging Techniques. In: Avian Medicine: Principles and Application, edited by Ritchie BW, Harrison GJ, Harrison LR, Lake Worth: Winger's Publications.

Paul-Murphy JR, Brunson DB, Miletic V. 1999. Analgesic effects of butorphanol and buprenorphine in conscious African grey parrots (*Psittacus erithacus erithacus* and *P. erithacus timneh*). *Amer J Vet Res*, 60(10): 1218–1221.

Paul-Murphy J, Hess JC, Fialkowski JP. 2004. Pharmacokinetic properties of a single intramuscular dose of buprenorphine in African grey parrots (*Psittacus erithacus erithacus*). *J Avian Med Surg*, 18(4): 224–228.

Pollack C, Carpenter JW, Antinoff N. Birds. 2005. In: Exotic Animal Formulary, 3rd edition, edited by Carpenter JW. St. Louis: Elsevier, pp. 135–346.

Quandt JE, Greenacre CB. 1999. Sevoflurane anesthesia in psittacines. *Journal of Zoo and Wildlife Medicine* 30 (2): 308–309.

Rembert MS, Smith JA, Hosgood G, Marks SL, Tully TN. 2001. Comparison of traditional thermal support with the forced air warmer system in Hispaniolan Amazon parrots (*Amazona ventralis*). Assoc. of Avian Vets Annual Conf, 215–217.

Ritchie B, Harrison GJ, Harrison LR. 1994. Avian Medicine: Principles and Application. Lake Warde: Winger's Publishing.

Tully TN. Birds. In: Mitchell MA, Tully TN. 2009. Manual of Exotic Pet Practice, St. Louis: Elsevier, pp. 250–298.

Wilson GH, Hernandez-Divers S, Budsberg SC. 2004. Pharmacokinetics and use of meloxicam in psittacine birds. Proc Annu Conf Assoc Avian Vet, 7–9.

CHAPTER THREE

Psittacine Behavior, Husbandry, and Enrichment

Tarah Hadley

INTRODUCTION

Psittacine bird species account for approximately 330 of the 9,700 known avian species. These birds, which are primarily found in tropical regions of the world, are classified into three families: the Loriidae (includes lories and lorikeets), the Cacatuidae (cockatoos), and the Psittacidae (includes parakeets and parrots). Birds in each of these families demonstrate distinct physical and behavioral characteristics. Keep in mind that what constitutes normal and abnormal behavior may be heavily influenced by the species, the individual bird, and the environment. In many situations, behavior in captive birds does not always equate with the behavior of those in the wild.

BEHAVIOR OF COMMON PET PSITTACINE SPECIES

Lories and Lorikeets

These birds are extremely energetic and intelligent. They are not good talkers but when excited or stressed they may emit an ear-piercing, high-pitched screech. In the home environment these birds tend to be very curious and may get into trouble going into places they shouldn't. Many of these birds do well in a group of at least two. As individual pets, they can attach themselves to one favorite owner and be very nippy toward anyone else.

In general, due to their wet diet of fruit, nectar, and pollen, these birds are also very messy eaters and it is not unusual to see food splashed around the cage or on floors and walls. Species from this family commonly seen in the pet trade include the black lory, red lory, rainbow lory, and chattering Lory. The brilliance and beauty of their plumage have made these birds attractive as pets. However, they may also be extremely territorial, which may contribute to unwanted biting behavior.

Cockatoos

Like all birds, cockatoos are very intelligent (Color Plate 3.1). Most cockatoos, especially the larger varieties, also tend to be very sweet-natured. This behavioral tendency may encourage some owners to treat them like babies or small children instead of birds. Likewise, many of these same birds become very attached to their owners, contributing to the development of abnormal behavior, such as feather picking.

Smaller cockatoos tend to bite even their owners but some may be sweet-natured. Cockatoos are decent talkers. They are also prone to screaming loudly at certain times of the day, such as dusk or dawn, when they are tired and ready for sleep, or when they become excited. If left unattended or sometimes in plain view, their curiosity may get the best of them and lead to damaged baseboards or other broken items.

Cockatoos cannot distinguish between safe and unsafe items so it is essential to bird-proof the home environment from electrical cords or metallic items such as jewelry. The cockatoo species most commonly kept as pets include the umbrella cockatoo, salmon-crested cockatoo (also known as the moluccan cockatoo), galah (also known as the rose-breasted cockatoo), sulphur-crested cockatoo (including the lesser variety), Goffin's cockatoo, and Ducorp's cockatoo.

In general, the temperament of these pet birds may quickly change from very quiet and observant to very noisy and active. These birds also produce a large amount of dander which coats the beak with a visible layer of fine white powder. In addition, a large amount of feces is produced daily by these birds.

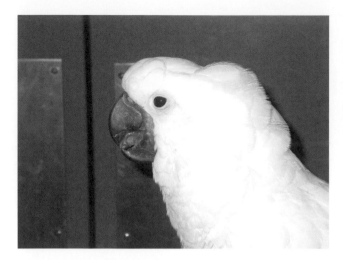

Plate 3.1. Umbrella cockatoo. (Photo courtesy of Dr. Tarah Hadley.) (See also color plates)

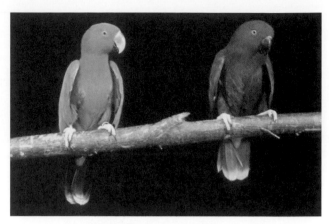

Plate 3.2. Pair of eclectus parrots, one of several sexually dimorphic psittacine species. (Photo courtesy of Dr. April Romagnano.) (See also color plates)

Budgerigar

These small birds are very active and social, especially when grouped with other birds. It is not unusual to see preening or food sharing behavior between birds. As with other birds, they may be trained to step up and obey other commands. If they are not trained they tend to be very flighty when approached and can sometimes be a challenge to capture. These birds may also become nippy during restraint. In most other areas, the behavior of budgerigars is similar to that of other birds. Therefore, it is important to avoid promotion of these birds as "starter birds" for new enthusiasts because their intelligence requires enrichment equal to that of other birds.

Eclectus

These birds are one of the few sexually dimorphic species (males are green and females are red) (Plate 3.2). The male eclectus tends to have a sweeter and calmer disposition compared to the female eclectus, whose behavior seems more cautious and suspicious, especially toward people she does not know. The females also have a reputation for being more aggressive in some situations and more likely to bite than the males.

In general, eclectus birds are quieter and less active than other birds. Like most birds, however, they are very intelligent and curious about their surroundings. As pets, these birds thrive with owners that have a patient hand. With time and practice, they may become adequate talkers. Like the cockatoos, these birds may also develop feather destructive behaviors.

Cockatiel

Cockatiels are sweet, feisty birds with very active social lives (Color Plate 3.3). They may also be very

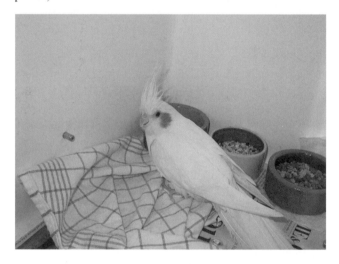

Plate 3.3. Bright orange cheek patches are often more prevalent in male cockatiels, such as the one pictured here. (Photo courtesy of Dr. Tarah Hadley.) (See also color plates)

vocal at times and can be good talkers and singers. They are very trainable to the hand and make good avian pets for first-time bird owners. They enjoy interacting with other cockatiels or people. Female birds kept in a group or alone may be prone to chronic egg-laying, which can be detrimental to their overall health.

African Grey

These birds are extremely intelligent and also very good talkers. (Color Plate 3.4) They tend to be friendly but also may be somewhat cautious depending on the environment. African grey parrots are also one of a few species that commonly present for feather destructive behaviors. Respiratory diseases such as sinusitis and aspergillosis also seem to be prevalent in this

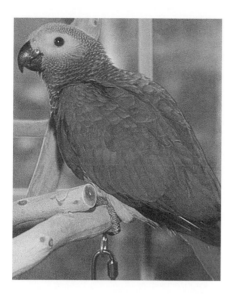

Plate 3.4. *Congo African grey parrot. (Photo courtesy of Cherie Fox.) (See also color plates)*

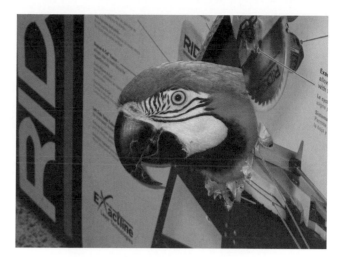

Plate 3.6. *Blue and gold macaw that has chewed its way partly out one side of a cardboard box. (Photo courtesy of Dr. Tarah Hadley.) (See also color plates)*

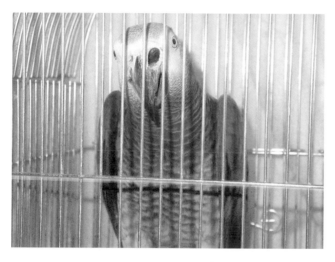

Plate 3.5. *Congo African grey parrot with an enlarged left nare, most likely caused by chronic upper respiratory infections and sinusitis. (Photo courtesy of Dr. Tarah Hadley.) (See also color plates)*

species (Color Plate 3.5). Hence, many of these birds may be more sensitive to aerosolized toxins and other agents. Like other birds, interaction with the owner and environmental enrichment are just some of the ways these birds may be kept stimulated. These birds normally produce a small amount of feather dander that lightly coats their beaks with a fine white powder.

Senegal
These smaller parrots make good pets and seem to thrive in an environment supported by interaction with

the owner. They are fairly good speakers and may also be trained to perform small tricks.

Lovebird
Owners may form close and friendly relationships with these birds on an individual basis. The birds may learn to vocalize some and tend to be fairly active singers. When paired with one or more other lovebirds, these birds may sometimes become less friendly with the owner to the point of biting and may become overly protective of their cage mates.

Macaws
These birds make up some of the largest members of the Psittacidae family. They are very active and vocal and may be adequate to fairly good talkers with encouragement. Sometimes their vocalizations can be ear-piercing. Behavior of these birds may range from friendly to cautious or unfriendly, depending on the background of the bird. (Color Plates 3.6, 3.7, 3.8) On occasion, macaws in stressful environments may exhibit feather destructive behaviors. Due to their large size and particularly long feathers, large cages that permit activity are required to house these birds. Owners should also be aware that they produce large amounts of feces on a daily basis. Their large beaks, another common characteristic of these birds, are used to crack open nuts with the largest and hardest of shells. Many species exist in the pet population, including the hyacinth macaw, blue and gold macaw, scarlet macaw, green-winged macaw, and military macaw.

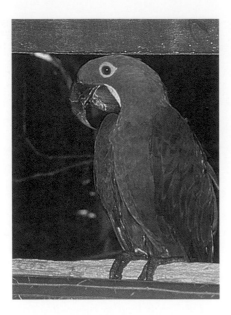

Plate 3.7. Hyacinth macaws. (Photo courtesy of Cherie Fox.) (See also color plates)

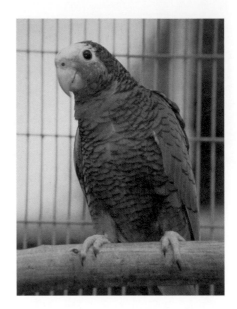

Plate 3.9. Cuban Amazon in outside aviary on a natural wood perch. (Photo courtesy of Dr. April Romagnano.) (See also color plates)

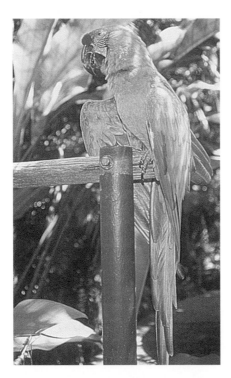

Plate 3.8. Military macaw. (Photo courtesy of Cherie Fox.) (See also color plates)

Conure

These species of birds comprise some of the small to medium-sized parrots. They are extremely active birds and very active singers or talkers. They may sing or screech for several minutes at a time or longer. Hence, the best households are those that can tolerate the loud vocalizations. They may form close relationships with owners and they can also be nippy or bite in certain situations. Common species seen in the pet industry include the mitred conure, sun conure, maroon-bellied conure, and green-cheeked conure.

Parrotlet

Parrotlets include some of the smallest species in the Psittacidae family. They are also extremely intelligent birds with a feisty temperament that belies their body size. They have been known to challenge or defend their territory from birds that are many times larger, which can sometimes get them into trouble. They are not considered very good talkers but will vocalize with encouragement. Parrotlets lead very active lives and tend to be very good fliers. Owners should always be aware of the location of non-caged birds because they can sometimes get underfoot.

Amazon

Amazon bird species are big-bodied birds that are medium in size (Color Plates 3.9, 3.10, 3.11). They may be trained to become very good talkers and may be friendly pets, depending on the individual bird and the environment. They enjoy the interaction with owners as well as playing on their own with toys in their environment.

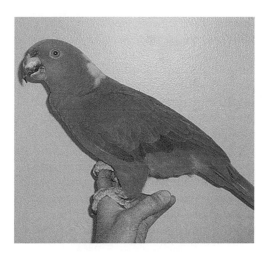

Plate 3.10. *Yellow-naped Amazon. (Photo courtesy of Dr. Sam Rivera.) (See also color plates)*

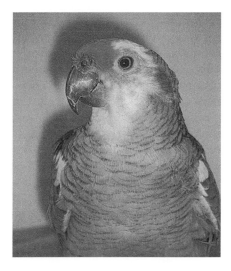

Plate 3.11. *Blue-fronted Amazon. (Photo courtesy of Dr. Sam Rivera.) (See also color plates)*

HUSBANDRY

The Cage Environment

After—and sometimes before—the acquisition of a pet bird, many owners consider the habitat that the bird will live in when it is inside the cage. One of the most important considerations will be the size of the cage. The size should be appropriately matched to the size of the bird. If the cage is for a large parrot species, such as a macaw, the cage should at least be as wide as the wingspan of the bird. An even wider cage provides plenty of room for play and other antics. The height of the cage must also be evaluated such that the long feathers of perched birds have adequate space to prevent damage when the bird moves around. Likewise, smaller birds require cages that are proportional to their wingspans and sizes.

Other considerations include the thickness of the bars and the width between bars. Whereas larger birds may be safely enclosed in cages with wide spaces between bars, owners of small birds need to be careful that the width is not so great that the bird may be able to easily slip through. Precautions should also be taken to ensure that the cages are properly manufactured and do not contain materials such as lead that may harm birds.

Cages should have the ability to separate birds from fecal droppings so that birds that like to go to the bottom of their cages may do so without risk of stepping in their feces. Ideally, the grate above the bottom of the cage is removable for ease of cleaning.

Placement of food bowls within cages should also be considered. Some cages have built-in brackets that hold food and water bowls. Others are flexible and allow the owners to decide where they should be located. Keep in mind that many smaller birds do a better job of leaving the food bowls alone and not trying to remove them from their holders. However, many larger birds continually attempt to dislodge bowls from their holders. For these birds, a system in which the bowl sits in a permanent bracket and cannot be removed when the bowl is inside the cage is a good solution. This also prevents birds from creating more cage mess by wasting food or water on the floor.

There are a tremendous variety of cage styles and designs to choose from. The actual style chosen may depend on multiple factors. Owners should consider the space available for the cage. The shape is also a major consideration because some birds prefer dome-shaped cages over flat-topped cages. The shape of the cage also affects the inside space available to the bird. Owners should wisely choose the preferred height of the cage so that birds on top of cages are not unreachable by the owner. Owners may choose from a variety of cage designs that may include external play and perching areas.

Perches

The appropriate choice of perches is often poorly understood by many owners. There are also many opinions about the best type and size of perch. Many owners forget that birds stand on their feet all day while they are awake and all night while they sleep. Hence, what the bird stands on may have a serious impact on its overall well being in addition to its health. That said, owners may choose from a variety of perch sizes and types. A few considerations for choosing the best perch:

As a general rule, the best perch allows the bird's toes to wrap around about three-fourths of the diameter of the perch. The best perches are also typically made out of natural wood. Owners often ask whether wooden dowels or concrete perches are acceptable types of perches. The answer is likely that most birds will do fine with them as long as they are not the only perches in the cage.

Although they are made out of wood, the downside of wood dowels is that they are flat, sometimes slippery, and lack good texture for gripping. They are a reliable form of transport for birds that travel between water and food bowls at mealtimes. They are not comfortable for long-term perching. Pet stores also sell plastic dowels which fit nicely inside pre-fabricated cages; however, they tend to be more slippery than wood dowels. Smaller and lighter-weight birds do better on plastic dowels but also likely encounter the same problems with discomfort after a period of time.

Concrete perches are often touted as a good alternative to nail trimming in birds of any size. Based upon experience, these perches dull the nails of a select few birds; many more still need to be trimmed regularly. For many birds, particularly those with foot or ankle problems and heavier birds, the concrete may wear away the normal skin layer on some parts of the foot. In its place the skin may become calloused, worn, and unnaturally smooth. This may also lead to extreme discomfort.

Natural wood perches, such as manzanita, may provide the best source of comfort to a bird's feet. These perches come in varying diameters. As long as part of the perch length is an appropriate diameter for the foot size of the bird, changes in the diameter within the same perch provide the best opportunity for a bird to exercise its feet. Foot problems may lead to poor health and increased risk for systemic disease. Healthy feet lead to healthy skin, allow for increased activity and movement, and permit the bird to get better quality rest in the evenings. The number of perches provided is affected by the size of the cage. Avoid having too many perches because that crowds the cage and decreases the available space.

The Cage Bottom

Bird owners far and wide have all received a similar warning: when your bird goes to the bottom of the cage, it is extremely sick. While that is true in some cases, it is not always true. In fact, the cage bottom is just another place where birds may play. Many birds routinely go to the bottom of the cage to play with toys or shred newspaper, and this is completely normal.

Not all birds do this. Some birds are completely terrified of the bottom of the cage. Do not force them to go to the cage bottom.

It is important to provide birds that do play on the cage bottom with appropriate toys or enrichment. If a bird likes to shred newspaper, place a layer of newspaper on top of the grate so the bird has access to it. Do not scold birds that like to play with newspaper for making a mess. That is just part of being an active bird. Some birds may also enjoy paper balls or cardboard boxes. Birds that were previously scolded for shredding newspaper may enjoy accidental access to newspaper. In this scenario, owners may make it a little easier for birds to grab newspaper through the grate while the birds still see it as a challenging and forbidden activity.

Upkeep of the cage bottom is especially important to the overall cleanliness of the cage. Substrate options include newspaper, butcher paper, recycled cardboard, wood shavings, and corn cob bedding. Ideally, the substrate on the cage bottom should be changed daily. This is easier to do when newspaper or butcher paper are used as the substrates. Daily cleaning limits growth of bacteria or fungus and formation of maggots.

Daily cleaning is not so easy or cost efficient when shavings or corn cob bedding are used. Many owners that use these substrates prefer to scoop away fecal piles on a daily basis rather than replace the substrate. The likelihood that bacteria or fungus will grow in these scenarios is higher. Wood shavings with added treatments, such as cedar wood shavings, can be harmful to birds. Young birds that don't know any better or older birds that have a tendency to eat things they shouldn't have been known to ingest the substrate, so it is essential that it be relatively safe.

Toys and Non-toy Enrichment Items

Birds are extremely intelligent animals that need an active, fulfilling environment to match their intensity. Toys tend to be the most common way of providing fulfillment to the inner and outer environment of birds' cages. Toys come in a variety of shapes, sizes, colors, and noise options.

The best toy for a bird depends on its size and personality and available space. Many birds are afraid of new additions to their cages and may need time to get used to new toys. Owners should also avoid the temptation to crowd the cage with several toys. Crowded cages do not allow enough room for birds to stretch or play with toys and may pose an environmental hazard. Toys should be individually assessed for practicality and safeness.

Toys may also be created from safe household items, such as cardboard boxes, cereal boxes, rope, and paper towel rolls. These items are usually cheap to create and are easily replaced. They may also be tailor-made to suit the activity level of the bird. Toys that encourage curiosity on the part of the bird, particularly those that encourage foraging or searching for food, may provide great stimulation to the bird's environment. Other items of enrichment that birds may enjoy include music, television, or videos.

Cage Location

The location of the cage is also important. Owners should choose a location for their bird that will allow daily interaction with owners and provide quiet in the evening for rest. It is not simply enough to cover a bird's cage in the evening and expect that complete rest will occur. As long as activity, noise, and bright light occurs in the environment, birds may also continue to stay awake and not sleep. For this reason many owners have a separate cage in a quiet place to put their bird at night.

As a general rule, birds usually need between ten and twelve hours of sleep each night to be well rested the following day. Birds that don't get enough sleep may become anxious or nippy or may resort to feather destructive behaviors. Safety should also be a consideration. For instance, a kitchen location for a cage may expose birds to undesirable fumes.

NORMAL BEHAVIOR OF PSITTACINE BIRD SPECIES

What constitutes normal behavior tends to be similar across many psittacine bird species, with some minor differences. Many of these behaviors are particular to birds in captivity, although some may be exhibited by birds in the wild that have not had the influence of a captive experience. Bird owners also come to learn that differences in behavior, activity level, and temperament occur among their individual pet birds. Environment and husbandry likely have strong influences on the development of certain behaviors.

Bathing

Some birds enjoy bathing themselves in their water bowl. Bathing may be triggered by loud noises, such as music or a vacuum, or the appearance of natural sunlight on certain portions of the cage, or it may just occur at some time known only to the bird. When a bird is self-bathing it is not uncommon for it to dunk its head, beak, feet and legs, or parts of its tail in the water bowl. After dunking parts of its body, the bird usually shakes off the water and then the behavior is repeated. A bird that is allowed more free flight in the home may fly to the sound of running water and immerse itself underneath the running spout or sprayer.

Playing on the Cage Bottom

Some birds actually enjoy spending time on the cage bottom as much as they do on perches near the top of the cage. The cage bottom is where "illegal" access to newspaper or other substrate may be obtained, which seems to be thrilling for many birds.

Owners are encouraged to place toys, newspaper, or other items on the bottom grate so birds have activities. The healthy bird that plays on the cage bottom may still vocalize and will continue to be very active—all normal behaviors for birds.

Preening and Molting

Preening is a normal grooming activity that birds perform on a daily basis. Birds use their beaks to smooth down erratic-looking feathers all over their body. Often, owners may see birds reaching to the hidden preen gland at the lower back near the base of the tail. The material taken from this area is used by the birds to get their feathers back in shape. As part of the normal preening behavior, it is not usual to see a few old or loose feathers drop from the body.

Molting is another behavior that occurs in birds. As new feathers come in, old feathers are pushed out. Newer feathers may come in singly, as in the case of large wing and tail feathers, or in groups, such as is the case with head feathers. Newer feathers may be surrounded by an opaque sheath that the bird removes during the preening process. When a large tail or wing feather molts on one side of the body, the same feather on the opposite side of the body usually molts at the same time. In general, it is normal for large feathers to molt twice yearly and small feathers such as those covering the chest and head to molt several times yearly.

Sleeping

Many birds sleep through the evening for about nine to twelve hours, depending on the environment and lighting conditions. Birds also take naps periodically during the day. Most birds that are sleeping for an extended period of time usually sleep on their most comfortable perch with one foot clenched and held up near their abdominal area. Their heads are often turned backward a full 180 degrees and their beaks are tucked into the feathers of their back near their wings. Any loud noise or other disturbance may disrupt a bird from this position. Some birds, such as cockatoos, may get upset about disruptions to their sleep time and may vocalize loudly until their environment quiets down. Many birds respond well to having a cover placed around their cages at sleep time.

Regurgitation

Parents that raise chicks in the nest provide nutrition to them in the form of regurgitated food. However, juvenile and adult birds have been known to regurgitate to their owners. Often no food material is expelled but the birds go through the motion of regurgitating food into their mouths and re-swallowing it. This may simply be a sign of a bird's close attachment with an owner and not necessarily mean that the bird is sick.

Eye Movements

Owners often marvel at how quickly and easily birds are able to change the way their eyes look. In most other animals, the size of the colored iris is affected by the amount of light coming into the eye. Hence, these animals have involuntary control of their iris muscles. Birds are uniquely able to directly control the movement of their irises due to the presence of voluntary muscles. Birds that are excited or angry often make the openings of their irises smaller. This is often referred to as "flashing" their eyes.

Body Shivering

Many birds give the appearance of being cold when their bodies start to quiver or shake. Although this is a possibility for birds exposed to cold weather, birds usually quiver or shake when they are nervous or exposed to new environments or people. Some birds appear to do this for no reason in environments where they have been completely comfortable.

Vocalizations

The time of day or situation during which a bird vocalizes depends upon many factors. The species of bird and the personality of the individual bird usually play a role. Stimuli that cause vocalizations by birds may be natural or artificial in origin. Common stimuli for vocalization by birds include bathing time, loud noises such as music or the vacuum cleaner, feeding time, or during dawn and dusk.

ABNORMAL BEHAVIOR

Veterinary staff may pick up on some very obvious signs to determine whether a bird is not feeling well. More subtle clues are usually detected by the owner. That is why it is so important to get a thorough and complete history, which should include asking the same background questions of every avian owner.

Feather Destructive Behaviors

Feather destructive behaviors include medical and non-medical causes of injury to the feathers and surrounding tissue. Birds may destroy parts or all of a feather. They also may directly cause trauma to the underlying skin and muscle. Some birds just pull out feathers. Behaviors that involve feather and tissue destruction are not normal and potential causes should be investigated as early as possible to try to minimize trauma. Any trauma that causes excessive bleeding and/or tissue damage needs immediate attention (Color Plate 3.12).

Sitting on the Cage Bottom

Birds that are extremely ill are often too tired or weak to perch and go to the bottom of the cage. These birds may be distinguished from their healthy counterparts by their dull attitude and overall depression. Sometimes they lean against the side of the cage and keep their eyes closed for extended periods of time, even when attempts are made to stimulate them. This is considered a medical emergency and requires immediate attention by a veterinarian.

Fluffed Feathers and Shivering

Often one of the first signs of illness that owners notice is when their bird's feathers become fluffed and they

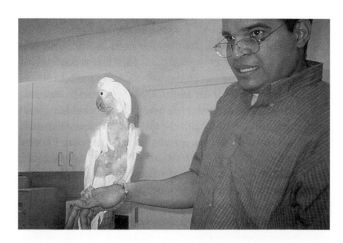

Plate 3.12. *A feather picker. (Photo courtesy of Dr. Sam Rivera.) (See also color plates)*

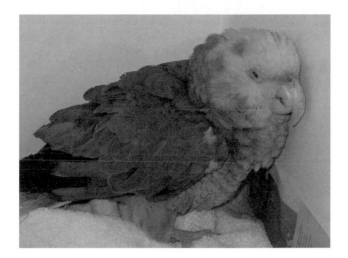

Plate 3.13. Yellow-headed Amazon that presented lethargic with eyes closed and fluffed feathers. (Photo courtesy of Dr. Tarah Hadley.) (See also color plates)

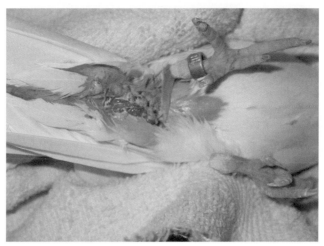

Plate 3.14. Cockatiel with fecal staining of vent area secondary to egg binding. (Photo courtesy of Dr. Tarah Hadley.) (See also color plates)

look puffy (Color Plate 3.13). Many birds often shiver. These are signs that the bird is unable to properly regulate its body temperature and the bird is doing everything it can to trap heat for warmth. Birds in this condition should be evaluated as soon as possible by a veterinarian.

Regurgitation and Vomiting

Regurgitation can be a sign of illness in a bird. Birds often make bobbing motions with their heads as food is moved from the lower gastrointestinal tract to the beak. If the food material is unable to be swallowed, the bird will vomit the contents. A sick bird makes these motions repetitively. Causes of regurgitation and vomiting include an obstruction in the gastrointestinal tract, inflammation, infection, heavy metal toxicosis, and cancer.

Mean Bird Turned Friendly

This is a classic sign observed by owners who notice that their bird is not acting like it usually does. Owners who inquire further will interact with a usually mean bird and are surprised to see that the bird will come out of its cage and onto the owner's hand easily. These birds are likely sick and tend to be more quiet and docile than usual. In addition, some previously unapproachable birds may permit you to touch them.

Decreased or No Fecal Production

Stool production is one of the best indicators of how well or how poorly a bird is eating. That is why it is

a good idea for owners to change the substrate at the bottom of cage frequently so that the amount of fecal production may be regularly evaluated. A bird that is anorexic or has decreased appetite will have scant or no feces in its droppings. Some birds may also have multiple droppings stuck to the underside of their tails, which is usually caused by general weakness and an inability to properly release feces away from the body (Color Plate 3.14).

Open-mouth Breathing and Tail Bobbing

A bird that is breathing abnormally breathes with its mouth open and often its tongue moves in and out of the mouth as it inhales and exhales. Many birds having difficulty breathing also bob their tails up and down as they struggle to bring air into their bodies. These signs should also be treated as medical emergencies and oxygen supplementation may be required as part of the initial treatment.

Falling Off Perch

It is not unusual for most birds to fall of their perches at some point while they are sleeping. However, birds that do this consistently while asleep or awake are not normal. This may actually be a sign of neurologic disease, a nutritional abnormality, or some other illness. Causes of falling off the perch may need further investigation. Until then, it may be safer to lower the perches in these birds' cages or use a smaller cage in which the perches are closer to the bottom.

Inappropriate Molting

Most birds should molt their large wing and tail feathers at least twice yearly while their small covert or covering feathers usually molt more frequently. Birds that fail to molt these feathers on a regular basis may have issues with their nutrition or some other illness affecting their metabolism. Long-standing feathers may become tattered, broken, or dull. Regular baths should be part of the hygiene for all birds to assist them in maintaining their feathers.

ADDITIONAL READING

Bays TB, Lightfoot T, Mayer J. 2006. *Exotic Pet Behavior*. Philadelphia: Saunders.

Forshaw JM. 1977. *Parrots of the World*. Neptune: Doubleday and Company.

Manual of Parrot Behavior, edited by Andrew U. Luescher, 2006. Australia: Wiley-Blackwell.

CHAPTER FOUR

Aviary Design and Management

April Romagnano

INTRODUCTION

The avicultural veterinary team, consisting of the avian technician and avian veterinarian, must know the avian collection, including its size and culture, and be aware of the importance of avicultural management and pediatric care. Good hygiene and impeccable sanitation are important for successful pediatrics and breeding of adult birds, but sound avicultural management must precede it.

This primarily includes good sanitation, effective nutritional protocols for birds of all ages, and preventive avicultural and pediatric medicine. This is a greater challenge in larger aviaries. Second, proper quarantine for new acquisitions is imperative, as are necropsy and histopathology of those lost to the collection. The latter procedures, necropsy and histopathology, are important because a complete preventive medicine program incorporates a thorough pre- and post-mortem evaluation.

AVICULTURE

The avicultural veterinary team must first be aware of the importance of cleanliness, husbandry, avicultural and pediatric medicine, and common sense in aviary management to ensure a successful avicultural collection. The best way to achieve the above is to follow a strict set of rules in the aviary to protect the entire avicultural collection as a whole.

- Consider in advance the number of birds to be acquired.
- Consider in advance the species of birds to be acquired.
- Acquire birds from a reputable source.
- Follow strict quarantine at all times.
- Require extensive testing at pre- and post-purchase examination, as well as yearly for the health of the collection.

- Implement proper management and nutrition (Figures 4.1 and 4.2).
- Routinely practice good hygiene and impeccable sanitation (Figure 4.3).

Infectious disease prevention is best achieved by following the principles mentioned above. Hence, the avicultural veterinary team must first make sure that good medicine, management, husbandry, and hygiene practices are in place. The team must then implement proper quarantine, vaccination, disinfection, necropsy, and histopathology procedures. The latter two procedures are important because a complete preventive medicine program incorporates thorough post-mortem evaluation.

QUARANTINE

Newly introduced birds should undergo strict quarantine in a separate designated quarantine building where

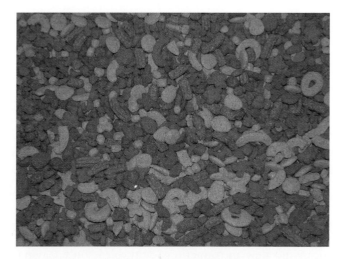

Figure 4.1. High-quality pelleted brands of feed are commonly part of the nutrition for birds in an aviary. (Photo courtesy of Dr. April Romagnano.)

55

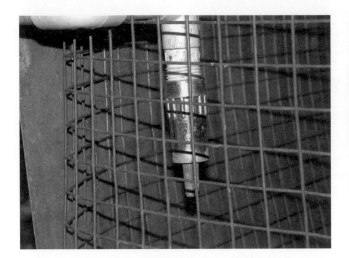

Figure 4.2. Aviary watering system that constantly provides fresh water from a central system into individual cages. Aviary birds learn to operate and drink water from the nozzle, which minimizes bacteria buildup. (Photo courtesy of Dr. April Romagnano.)

extensive testing and a minimum quarantine period of forty-five days are required. Although testing can be cost prohibitive to some, an outbreak would be devastating to all. Management must decide if new acquisitions are worth the risk.

Quarantine is indeed one of the best methods of infectious disease control. When a separate building is unavailable an alternative plan must be instituted. Hence, regardless of the collection size, location, or value, a separate quarantine facility, even if it is a friend's bird-free home, is imperative.

Collections vary and may include large or small psittacines, soft bills, and passerines. All collections warrant constant consistent flock management. A complete health history of all breeding birds in a collection, including baseline blood work and endoscopy, is imperative for ensuring proper reproductive management and optimal reproductive performance. Consideration for maintaining an open or closed aviary is important in the health of the collection. Open aviaries are defined as those in which new birds (thus new potential diseases) can be introduced into the collection.

The "closed aviary concept," in which strict quarantine procedures are practiced, is a must in an effective preventive medicine program. A closed aviary means no new introductions, with birds only leaving the collection. Traffic within the aviary should be managed and controlled, and new introductions must immediately be put into the separate quarantine building. Only dedicated staff that has no contact with

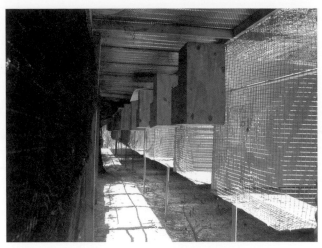

Figure 4.3. Longitudinal aviary cage design permits quick visualization of multiple cages. The cage design provides barriers between individual cages to minimize contact. Mesh cage bottoms permit release of unwanted food, water, and feces away from the cage and onto the ground where appropriate removal may take place. Wooden nest boxes, located for easy access by the veterinary team, may be easily replaced as needed. (Photo courtesy of Dr. April Romagnano.)

other birds or general staff who are at the end of their day and about to leave the property should enter this building.

Further, before entering, employees must gown and put on booties, masks, and gloves. The building should be self-sufficient with its own caging, nets, towels, protective clothing, water source, bowls, and washing facilities. Nothing should ever leave the quarantine building to be re-introduced into the main collection because it may act as a fomite. The only exception should be garbage going directly off the property.

EXAMINATIONS AND DIAGNOSTIC TESTING: NEONATES, JUVENILES, BREEDERS, AND NEW ACQUISITIONS

Neonates and juveniles are examined daily and tested on a case-by-case basis (Figure 4.4). A crop and cloacal culture and fecal Gram stain are considered routine tests in young and very young birds. Yearly examination and testing of breeders and immediate testing of new acquisitions should include a CBC, serum chemistries, fecal float, fecal direct exam, fecal Gram stain and cytology, cloacal culture, polyoma virus swab DNA probe test, PBFD whole blood DNA probe test,

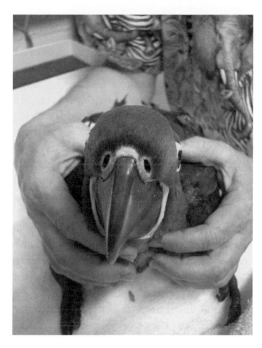

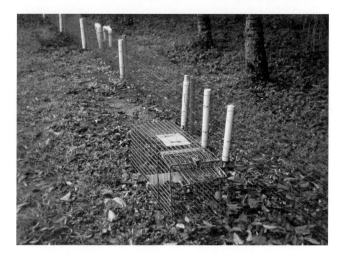

Figure 4.5. Metal traps and hot-wire fencing are just some of the methods used to minimize the introduction of disease into an aviary via indigenous vectors such as opossums and raccoons. (Photo courtesy of Dr. April Romagnano.)

Figure 4.4. Young hyacinth macaw during examination by the veterinary team. (Photo courtesy Dr. April Romagnano.)

chlamydophila serology, and indirect and direct screening for PDD. Additional or alternative testing may be performed and is determined on a case-by-case basis. Again, although testing can be cost prohibitive to some, an outbreak would be devastating to all.

Vaccination protocols are limited in avian medicine, because very few vaccines are available, safe, and effective in psittacine birds. Presently only the polyoma vaccine (Avian Polyoma Virus vaccine, Biomune) is recommended for routine use and is USDA-registered.

DISINFECTION AND DISEASE PREVENTION

Disinfection and infectious disease prevention are very important in an effective preventive medicine protocol because organic matter inactivates most disinfectants. A disinfectant is defined as an agent that destroys many disease-causing microorganisms present on the surface of inanimate objects. Hence, first clean the area by removing all organic debris prior to disinfectant application. The easier an object is to clean the more likely it can be adequately disinfected.

Wood is the perfect example of a difficult-to-clean object; therefore, all wooden perches, nest boxes, and toys should be destroyed and replaced yearly, or imme-

diately if an infectious disease is suspected (Figure 4.3). Enveloped viruses are the most easily inactivated and are susceptible to quaternary ammonia products. Note that chlorhexidine has limited activity against some bacteria, especially *Pseudomonas spp.* and certain Gram negative bacteria, and although it can kill some enveloped viruses, it cannot be considered a reliable viricide. Non-enveloped viruses require phenolic compounds and sodium hypochlorite (bleach) or stabilized chlorine dioxide for inactivation.

Glutaraldehydes inactivate most bacteria, including mycobacteria, many viruses, and chlamydophila, even in the presence of organic debris. As a result, this product is particularly useful for endoscopy disinfection and sterilization. Overall, the most widely recommended and economical disinfectant in avian establishments is bleach (at the dilution of one part bleach to twenty parts of water). Bleach, in any strength, should never be sprayed around birds, because it can be fatal. However, bleach is often used to disinfect floors and bowls in aviculture, once they have been pre-washed with hot water and soap.

The geographic location and whether the birds are housed in or out of doors reflect disease potential and susceptibility. For example, sarcocystosis and eastern equine encephalitis pox are diseases that are introduced by indigenous vectors such as rats, mosquitoes, opossums, raccoons, cockroaches, and snakes in southern states such as Florida. An effective pest-prevention program is required in any aviary (Figure 4.5).

PEDIATRICS FOR THE AVICULTURIST

Pediatric History Evaluation

Note that a chick's health depends on many historical factors, such as its parent's health and breeding history, the condition of its siblings, and any problems the chick may have had during its incubation and hatching. The pediatric diet, its preparation, and the amount and frequency of feedings delivered are also part of the history. Whether the chick's crop is empty for each feeding, especially the first feeding of the day, is also part of the history. It is important to know whether the chick's environment, housing, and substrate were and are clean, safe, and warm choices. A chick's behavior, especially its feeding response, and the colors, consistency, and volume of its feces, urine, and urates are all important historical factors.

Frequent Examination of Young Birds

Physical examination of the chick entails evaluation of available weight charts for daily gain, assessing overall appearance, proportions, and behavior. In neonates, this examination should be performed in a warm room with pre-warmed hands. Knowledge of different species growth rates, development, and behavioral characteristics is helpful.

Psittacine neonates are altricial (hatched with eyes closed, down minimal to absent, and limited mobility), hence nourishment, warmth (93° to 98°F), and a safe place must be provided (Figure 4.6). Neonates normally have a visible liver, duodenal loop, yolk sac, ventriculus, and occasionally lung through their body skin. The lungs and heart should be ausculted. Assess body mass by palpation of elbows, toes, and hips, because keel muscle mass is an unreliable indicator of weight in the very young.

Crops should be examined visually for size and color, and carefully palpated for thickness, tone, burns, punctures, or the presence of foreign bodies. Skin should be evaluated for color, texture, hydration, and the presence of SQ fat. Normally, psittacine chicks should have beige-pink, warm, and supple skin. Dehydration causes a chick's skin to become dry, hyperemic, and tacky. In juveniles, feathers should be examined for stress marks, color bars, hemorrhage, or deformities of shafts and emerging feathers.

The musculoskeletal system should be palpated and assessed for skeletal defects or trauma in chicks of all ages. Until weaning, cockatoo chicks sit back on their hocks and are balanced forward on their large abdomens; macaws prefer to lie down. Chicks normally have prominent abdomens due to a food-filled proventriculus, ventriculus, and small intestine. Beaks should be examined for malformations at rest. Examine the beaks' pump pads for wounds.

Eyes should be examined for swelling, discharge, crusting, or blepharospasm. Normally a clear discharge is noted in the eyes when they are first opening, which typically occurs unilaterally. Nares and ears should be examined for discharge and aperture size. The oral cavity should be examined for plaques, inflammation, or injuries. Generally, a healthy chick or baby bird should elicit a vigorous feeding response when stimulated at the beak's lateral commissures or pump pads.

Pediatric Diagnostics
Clinical pathology:

PCV, TP = lower
WBC = higher
Albumin, uric acids = lower
ALP, CPK = higher

Microbiology
Gram-positive bacteria normal:

Cloacal cultures
Crop cultures
Gram stain

Radiology
Gastrointestinal tract enlarged—endoscopy:

Foreign body retrieval
Syrinx examination
Surgical sexing

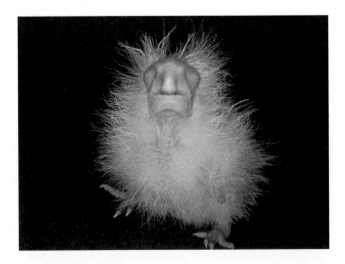

Figure 4.6. Psittacine neonate. (Photo courtesy of Dr. April Romagnano.)

Common Pediatric Problems

Unretracted yolk sac
Stunting
Leg and toe deformities
Constricted toe syndrome
Beak malformations
Regurgitation
Esophageal or pharyngeal punctures
Crop stasis
Crop burns
Foreign body ingestion or impaction

Less Common Pediatric Problems

Intestinal intussusception
Hepatic hematomas
Gout
Wine-colored urine
Hepatic lipidosis

Diseases in the Nursery
Viral diseases:

Polyomavirus
Psittacine beak and feather disease
Proventricular dilatation disease
Pacheco's disease
Poxvirus

Microbial Diseases—Microbial Alimentary and Respiratory Infections

Gram-negative or yeast infections are abnormal

Microbial Diseases—Chlamydophila

Zoonotic disease

CONCLUSION

The aviculture care of breeders and pediatric patients are tightly associated disciplines. A neonate that gets off to a good start has the best chance of becoming a thriving juvenile, and eventually a reproductively successful adult (Figure 4.7). The majority of pediatric problems are associated with avicultural husbandry and hand feeding. Nursery management and veterinary preventive medicine are equally important in the production of healthy baby birds.

Crop stasis is the most common pediatric problem seen, and if managed correctly, it need not be a fatal

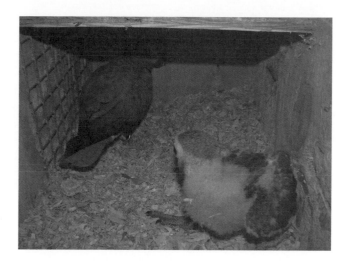

Figure 4.7. Healthy Congo African grey chick (right) and parent in nest box. (Photo courtesy of Dr. April Romagnano.)

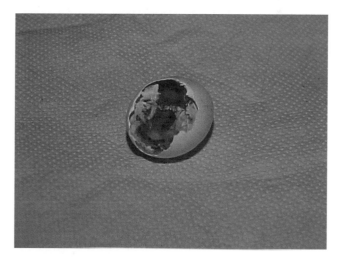

Figure 4.8. Psittacine embryo deceased in egg. Necropsy often includes assessment of the embryo's position in the egg, evaluation of anatomy, and culture when infection is suspected. (Photo courtesy of Dr. April Romagnano.)

condition. Immediate intervention should include a thorough history, physical examination, medical and mechanical therapy, and blood work to help reverse this condition. Fluids (± whole blood) are critical in this reversal process, and lactobacillus and acetic acid may be helpful.

Antibiotic and antifungal medications, although important, should be used cautiously in baby birds. When used correctly, antimicrobials can halt infection and decrease the chance of sepsis. Along with dehydration, sepsis is the most common killer of pediatric patients.

Preventive avicultural medicine and pediatrics are ongoing interactive processes that incorporates thorough routine avicultural team visits as a method of data collection. The aviculturist and the avian veterinarian and technician must know the pet bird and/or the collection (large or small) intricately, and be aware of the importance of psittacine husbandry and management. The team must evaluate, diagnose, and treat the individual pet bird, as well as the entire collection. The necessity of diagnostic testing and therapeutic protocols are established based on the patient's history, the veterinarian's overall observations of the collection, and the physical examination of the individual patient.

Thus, pre-mortem tests are chosen on a case-by-case basis, but post-mortem examination is imperative and should be performed in all cases. Hence, necropsy and histopathology are also necessary for infectious disease prevention, as are quarantine, vaccination, and disinfection (Figure 4.8).

ADDITIONAL READING

Romagnano A. 2006. Mate Trauma. In: Manual of Parrot Behavior, edited by AU. Luescher, Australia: Wiley-Blackwell.

Romagnano A, Wolf S, Garner MM. 2000. Management of diseases and syndromes in a closed psittacine nursery. Proceedings of the 21st Annual Conference of the Association of Avian Veterinarians, Portland, Oregon.

Schubot RM, Clubb KJ, Clubb SL. 1992. Psittacine Aviculture. Loxahatchee: Avicultural Breeding and Research Center.

CHAPTER FIVE

Sex Differentiation and Reproduction

April Romagnano and Tarah Hadley

INTRODUCTION

Veterinary clinics that see birds as patients are likely to have owners who want to know if their pet is male or female, if it isn't visually obvious. Veterinary technicians must be educated in the methods of sexing a bird and able to discuss these options with owners. Veterinary technicians also must be knowledgeable about normal reproductive anatomy and problems that can arise. These topics are addressed in this chapter.

SEX DIFFERENTIATION

Most psittacines are sexually monomorphic—the male and female are visually indistinguishable from each other. Although a few general characteristics may help the aviculturist guess a bird's sex, they are only indicators that are incapable of accurate sexual determination. Such indicators include the size of the head and beak, overall size of the bird, feather color, and aggressive behavior.

Sexual differentiation is paramount for successful psittacine aviculture because the first requirement for successful captive breeding is a heterosexual or true pair. Sexual differentiation is also important for the client who is struggling with his pet bird's identity—should "it" be named Jack or Jill? Whatever the reason, accurate sexual differentiation is important because the clinician is making a diagnosis when providing the veterinary service of sexing. Various options for sexing are now available, so the avian veterinarian can choose the method most suitable to the patient, the client, and her practice.

Visual Sexing
A handful of psittacine species are sexually dimorphic and can be definitively sexed by visual examination. Among these species:

Eclectus parrot: Male is green and female is vibrant red and purple.

White-fronted Amazon parrot: Male has red versus green feathers on the upper wing coverts, the edge of the carpus, and the alula.

Pileated parrot: Males have red feathers on head; females have green.

Red-tailed black cockatoos: Females have spots on head, body, and wing feathers, and tail is barred with yellow-orange feathers. Males lack spots and the tail has red bars.

White-tailed black cockatoos: Females have white ear coverts and light horn-colored beak. Males have gray ear coverts and dark gray beaks.

Gang gang cockatoos: Males have red head and crest feathers; females are totally gray and barred with grayish white (Color Plate 5.1).

White cockatoos: In some of the white cockatoo species iris color is red at maturity in females and dark brown to black in males.

Pesquet's parrot: Males have red feathers behind the eye, which are absent in females.

Australian king parrot: Males have scarlet red feathers on the head, neck, and under parts. Female has green feathers on the head and chest and red feathers on the lower abdomen. The beak is red-orange and black tipped in the male and black in the female.

Vent Sexing
Vent sexing is an accurate sexing method for some avian species, such as the vasa parrot, poultry, waterfowl, ratites, and canaries during the breeding season.

Surgical Sexing
Surgical sexing was first performed in the 1970s. The fasted bird is masked down with isoflurane. The endoscope is inserted through an incision in the left flank between the ribs and the femur. Typically the caudal thoracic air sac is entered first; the lungs are straight

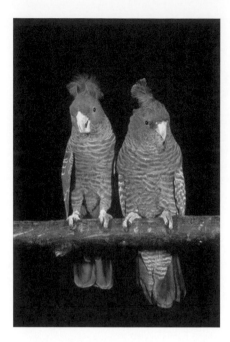

Plate 5.1. Pair of gang gang cockatoos. Note the distinction between the male (left) and the female. (Photo courtesy of Dr. April Romagnano.) (See also color plates)

ahead, the abdominal air sac is to the right, and the cranial thoracic air sac is to the left. The abdominal air sac is entered next, and the gonads are visualized and evaluated, sexing the bird immediately.

The standard protocol is to tattoo the ventral wing web of the sexed bird; males are tattooed on the right, females on the left. In the abdominal air sac, the kidneys, adrenals, spleen, and gastrointestinal (GI) tract should also be examined. Organs visible through the caudal thoracic and cranial thoracic air sacs, including the proventriculus and liver, and the heart and great vessels should be assessed respectively. The main disadvantage of surgical sexing is the inherent, though minimal, surgical risk.

Feather Sexing

Feather sexing was first performed in the 1980s as a non-surgical alternative for sexing birds. Blood feathers are plucked and placed in media for overnight mailing to a cytogenetic laboratory. Chromosomal analysis is performed on cells cultured from the growing blood feathers.

Advantages of cytogenetics include complete karyotype evaluation and identification of chromosomal defects. Cytogenetic defects identified in psittacines include chromosomal inversions, chromosome translocations, triploidy, and ZZ ZW chimerism. These defects significantly reduce fertility. Disadvantages of feather sexing include a two-week turn-around time and the remote possibility of culture failure.

DNA or Blood Sexing

DNA and blood sexing tests, the newest means of non-surgical sex determination in avian medicine, became commercially available in the 1990s. This technique involves acquiring and submitting a very small amount of whole blood preserved in saline and EDTA or blotted on paper to a sexing laboratory. The DNA is run on an electrophoretic gel (southern blot) and the resulting bands are probed and compared with male and female controls. The main disadvantages of blood or DNA sexing are the one-week turn-around time and the requirement of species-specific probes in some cases.

REPRODUCTION

Female

In most species, the female reproductive tract consists of a left ovary and oviduct because the right side regresses before hatch. Exceptions include some raptors and the brown kiwi. In raptors the right ovary and oviduct may be present and even active posthatch. In the kiwi, both ovaries are active, but only the left oviduct receives the ovum by spanning the width of the coelomic cavity with its fimbria.

The avian ovary is located at the cranial pole of the kidney, and is flat and small in young birds and bumpy and large in mature birds. Normally it contains numerous follicles when active and it may be melanistic depending on the species. During lay, the left oviduct enlarges and occupies most of the left abdomen; in the non-breeding season it shrinks considerably in size.

The oviduct consists of five microscopically distinguishable regions: infundibulum, magnum, isthmus, uterus (shell gland), and vagina. Peristaltic activity moves the ovum down and the sperm up. The infundibulum has a funnel shape near the top. Fertilization occurs in the lower tubular part of the infundibulum as does the production of the chalaziferous layer of the albumen and the paired chalazae, which suspends the yolk at both ends of the egg.

In the magnum, the largest part of the oviduct, the egg takes on albumen, sodium, magnesium, and calcium. In the isthmus, it acquires the inner and outer shell membranes. The uterus, or shell gland, produces the egg's shell and its pigment. It also gives the egg salts and water. The vagina is the thickest portion of the oviduct and terminates in the cloaca.

Male

The male reproductive tract consists of paired "tic tac" shaped internal testes located ventral to and near the cranial border of the kidney and the abdominal air sac. Both testes are functional, although one may be larger than the other. Like the ovaries, the testes may be melanistic depending on the species. During the breeding season yellow testes may turn white and black-gray testes turn gray-white. Some species of birds have a phallus or phallus-like protrusion. These include the vasa parrots, various waterfowl, and ratites.

REPRODUCTIVE MEDICINE AND SURGERY

Normal Oviposition

Oviposition includes the processes that occur when the egg is expelled from the body. The muscular uterus pushes the formed egg into the vagina. The bearing down reflex is started when the vagina "senses" the presence of the egg, forcing the egg into the cloaca and then out of the body.

The length of time for oviposition and the time of day when oviposition occurs is different between bird species. However, in most birds the egg laying interval ranges from twenty-four hours to five days. The brown kiwi lies at the opposite end of the spectrum with a laying interval up to forty-four days.

Post Incubation and Hatching

At the end of incubation, the beak of the embryo breaks through the inner shell membrane into the air cell. The lungs start to work at this time. After several hours, the beak "pips" or cracks the outer shell membrane and shell to begin the active part of hatching.

Abnormal Oviposition or Dystocia

Some birds experience difficulty laying eggs. Many of these birds are first-time layers. Others may be chronic egg layers. Avian species overrepresented as problem layers include parakeets, cockatiels, cockatoos, and eclectus. Amazon species may lay their first egg well into their prime and experience multiple problems as a result. Of key importance is that the presence of a male bird is often not required to stimulate egg laying behavior in a female bird.

Improper diets have been partly blamed as a cause for dystocia. Female birds that have been on mostly seed diets may be predisposed to vitamin and mineral deficiencies and have a greater risk of egg-laying difficulties. These diets tend to be low in calcium and other needed nutrients. Inappropriate husbandry may

also play a role, including the lack of a proper nesting area and proper temperature and humidity. The requirements vary between avian species. Some, such as cockatoos, may experience heightened reproductive behavior due to an inappropriate relationship with the human caretaker.

Signs of dystocia in a bird may include decreased or absent fecal production, watery or bloody droppings, anorexia, regurgitation, difficulty breathing, tail bobbing, fluffed feathers, swollen coelomic (abdominal) area, abdominal straining, leg lameness, and sitting on the cage bottom. These signs occur for many reasons. The egg may put pressure on the gastrointestinal tract, preventing the passage of ingesta. This blockage may lead to regurgitation. Other times only liquid products may pass through, resulting in watery droppings.

A large egg may also put pressure on the air sacs, making it difficult for the bird to breathe. Likewise, pressure from the egg on the sciatic nerve unilaterally or bilaterally can cause lameness. Similar pressure on the kidneys may lead to life-threatening renal compromise. Abdominal straining may lead to prolapsed tissues, such as a prolapsed cloaca or prolapsed oviduct (Color Plate 5.2). Other signs seen in these patients may be due to general illness. A basic blood panel can provide the first step in determining the underlying health status of the patient.

Palpation of the abdominal area often reveals skin that is stretched and edematous. A firm egg-shaped swelling can usually be felt beneath. Care must be taken not to stress the patient and to avoid cracking what may be a fragile egg. Radiographs of the bird usually show the outline of an egg in the area of the pelvic canal. The egg may also be just cranial to the pelvis and unable to pass through the canal because it is over large. Sometimes the egg is soft-shelled and difficult to detect radiographically (Figure 5.1).

A bird in dystocia is considered a medical emergency due to the risk that the patient may die while attempting to pass the egg. These patients usually require humidity and a warm incubator heated to 87°F to 90°F. The patient in respiratory distress also requires supplemental oxygen. Other medical treatments include nutritional supplementation, calcium supplementation, antibiotic medication, anti-inflammatory medication, reproductive muscle stimulants, and fluid therapy.

A patient that is early in the dystocia process may successfully pass the egg with this minimal supportive care. An egg that is close to passing may also be lubricated with a water-based lubricant. Sometimes gentle massage of the area may assist with passage of the egg.

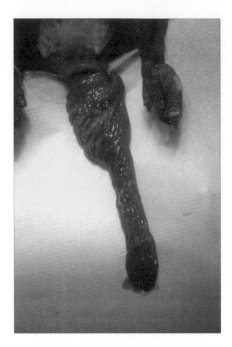

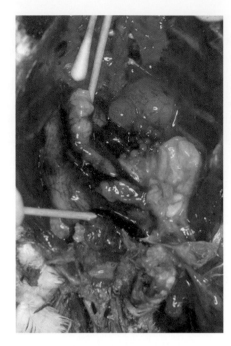

Plate 5.2. Parrot with prolapse of the oviduct. (Photo courtesy of Dr. April Romagnano.) (See also color plates)

Plate 5.3. Egg yolk peritonitis in a parrot. Note the yellow-tinged coelomic cavity contents caused by a ruptured egg. (Photo courtesy of Dr. April Romagnano.) (See also color plates)

More critical patients require faster intervention and possibly more invasive therapy. Over large eggs that will not pass on their own may be collapsed by having their contents expelled with a needle attached to a syringe inserted into the egg. The collapsed egg may be gently removed or allowed to pass on its own.

Other patients, particularly those suspected of having severely infected reproductive tracts, may require surgery to remove egg contents. One of the most challenging circumstances is a patient with soft-shelled eggs. Sometimes the back-up of soft-shelled eggs behind a calcified egg causes parts of the reproductive system to become necrotic. The breakdown of egg components and/or associated soft tissue often leads to peritonitis, a severe inflammation of the coelomic cavity (Color Plate 5.3). The risk of sepsis, or a systemic infection, is increased in these patients.

Many of these procedures require anesthesia, a risk that may need to be taken to save the life of the patient who is already in dire straits. Anesthesia should only be used if there is no other alternative to save the life of the patient and if all possible attempts to stabilize the patient have been taken. The anesthetic risk increases in patients with suspected renal compromise.

Care of the patient after treatment for dystocia is just as important. These birds may need additional

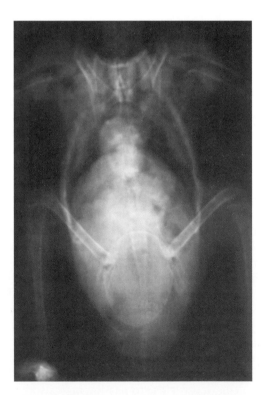

Figure 5.1. Radiograph showing dystocia in a bird. (Photo courtesy of Ryan Cheek.)

supportive care to help them feel better prior to discharge from the hospital. In particular, a plan of action must be formulated for chronic egg layers to break the reproductive cycle. Some birds have experienced successful treatment with human reproductive hormones used to create a negative feedback mechanism. Modifications in diet, light cycle, and relationship with the human caretaker may also go a long way toward improving the bird's reproductive function.

ADDITIONAL READING

Clubb K, Clubb S, Phillips A, Wolf S. 1992. Intraspecific Aggression in Cockatoos. In Psittacine Aviculture: Perspectives, Techniques, and Research, edited by Schubot RM, Clubb KJ, and Clubb SL, Chapter 8. Loxahatchee: Avicultural and Breeding Research Center.

Clubb SL. 1986. Sex Determination Techniques. In Clinical Avian Medicine and Surgery, edited by Harrison GJ and Harrison LR. Philadelphia: WB Saunders.

Harrison GJ. 1986. Reproductive Medicine. In Clinical Avian Medicine and Surgery, edited by Harrison GJ and Harrison LR. Philadelphia: WB Saunders.

Joyner KL. 1994. Theriogenology. In Avian Medicine Principles and Application, edited by Ritchie BW, Harrison GJ, and Harrison LR. Lake Worth: Wingers Publishing.

King AS, McLelland J. 1984. Female Reproductive System. In Birds: Their Structure and Function, Philadelphia: Bailliere Tindall.

Abramson J, Speer BL, Thomsen JB, eds. 1995. The Large Macaws: Their Care, Breeding, and Conservation. Fort Bragg: Raintree Publications. Chapters 3 and 17.

Orosz S, Dorrestein GM, Speer BL. 1997. Urogenital Disorders. In Avian Medicine and Surgery. Philadelphia: WB Saunders.

Section 3
Reptiles

CHAPTER SIX

Lizards

Brad Wilson

INTRODUCTION

From the seemingly impenetrable spines of *Moloch horridus*, the gliding pseudo-wings of *Draco* spp., the color-changing chromatophores of *Chamaeleo* spp., the cryptic cutaneous fimbriations of *Uroplatus* spp., the venomous bite of *Heloderma* spp., to the bipedal water-walking *Basiliscus* spp., the adhesive glass-climbing Gekkonidae, and the legless snake-like Anguinidae, lizards, of the order Squamata in the class Reptilia, exhibit tremendous anatomic, physiologic, nutritional, and behavioral variation that make them the hallmark of diversity among all modern reptiles. When distributed among 3,800 known species (Barten 1996a, de Vosjoli 1992), it becomes obvious that the diagnostic challenge presented to the veterinary clinician and technician can be overwhelming (Color Plates 6.1–6.6).

Though the details may be overwhelming, the basic categories of differentiating lizards based on natural history leads to a basic understanding of husbandry requirements. Technicians familiar with reptile medicine soon learn that many health disorders arise from improper husbandry; therefore, recognizing and correcting improper husbandry techniques may hasten the recovery from disease and prevent unnecessary medicating of debilitated patients.

Representatives of many families of lizards are commonly seen in the pet trade (Table 6.1). The green iguana (*Iguana iguana*) is one of the most popular of all reptile pets and historically has been the first reptile pet of many people new to the hobby of herpetoculture, the care and maintenance of captive reptiles and amphibians. In the past fifteen years the reptile pet industry has exponentially increased in popularity and in recent years the author has observed the popularity of lizards approach, if not exceed, that of snakes as reptile pets. This leads to the question: why keep reptiles as pets? To the dedicated pet owner, the answer is the same as if the question were about keeping a spider, fish, bird, cat, dog, goat, or horse as a pet. For avid reptile pet owners, however, a quote from de Vosjoli (1997) is most appropriate: "the current philosophy in herpetoculture strives towards establishing viable self-sustaining captive-breeding populations through managed field culture and/or through more controlled systems of indoor and outdoor vivaria."

ANATOMY AND PHYSIOLOGY

Integument

Lizard scales commonly overlap and are created by a many-layered epidermis that is shed at regular intervals during the life of the lizard. The shedding of skin, ecdysis, occurs in multiple pieces in lizards, as opposed to snakes, in which the skin is usually shed in one piece. Many lizard species eat the shed skin. Factors that influence ecdysis are age, growth rate, temperature, humidity, and nutrition (Barten 1996a, Goin et al. 1978). Dysecdysis is commonly associated with low humidity and poor nutrition among other health abnormalities.

Reptilian epidermis does not have a respiratory function and contains very few glands (Goin et al. 1978). The skin and scales are relatively impermeable in normal health. The mucous membranes (oral cavity, cloaca, conjunctiva) are quite permeable, however. This consideration is important when considering potential absorption of topical medications applied to these regions (Mader 2000a, Klingenberg 1996). Some reptile vitamin supplements are marketed as sprays to be applied to the skin. These products, though not likely harmful, have little to no systemic physiologic value to reptiles.

Chamaeleo spp. and *Anolis* spp. have chromatophores in the skin that allow change in the reflectivity of visible light, resulting in color change. These changes are influenced by light, heat, and social influences, but not by surrounding environmental color (Barten 1996a, Goin et al. 1978). Many herpetoculturists who raise chameleons can predict color changes of

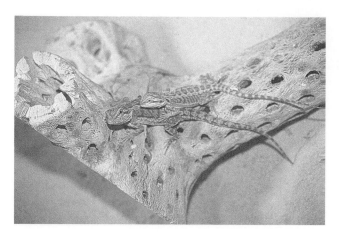

Plate 6.1. Bearded dragon. (Photo courtesy of Ryan Cheek.) (See also color plates)

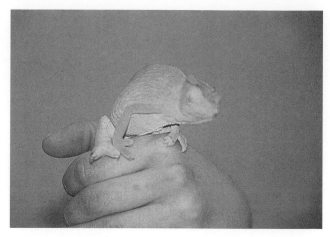

Plate 6.4. Chameleon. (Photo courtesy of Ryan Cheek.) (See also color plates)

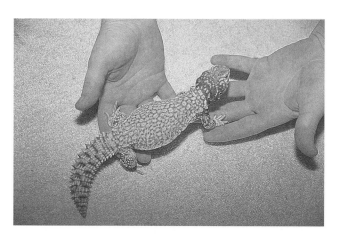

Plate 6.2. Mali uromastyx. (Photo courtesy of Ryan Cheek.) (See also color plates)

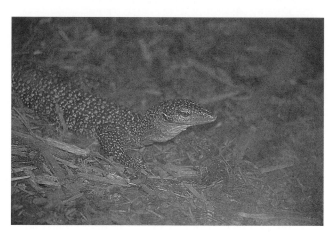

Plate 6.5. Mangrove monitor. (Photo courtesy of Ryan Cheek.) (See also color plates)

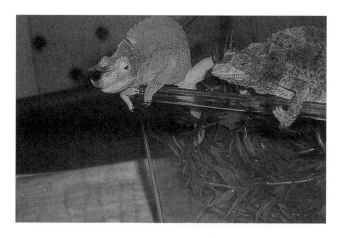

Plate 6.3. Jackson chameleon. (Photo courtesy of Dr. Sam Rivera.) (See also color plates)

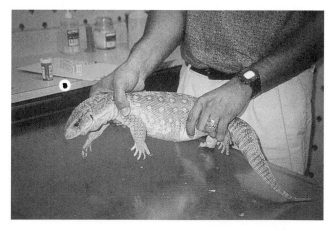

Plate 6.6. Savannah monitor. (Photo courtesy of Dr. Sam Rivera.) (See also color plates)

Table 6.1. Lizards Commonly Seen in Captivity.

Common name/species name	Origin	Habitat	Size (cm)[1]	Temp (d/n)[2]	Repro[3]	Feed[4]	Rest[5]	Handling concerns[6]
Agamidae								
Agamas, *Agama* spp.[10]	Africa	Arid, desert, terrestrial	30–40	30C/20C	oviparous	O/a	yes, no	Occas. aggressive, sturdy
Bearded Dragon, *Pogona* spp.[10,16]	Australia	Arid, terrestrial	to 50	30C/20C	oviparous	O/a	yes	Docile, sturdy
Frilled lizard, *Chlamydosaurus kingi*[10,16]	Australia	Dry, forest, terrestrial	to 100	30C/20C	oviparous	C/a,v	yes	Occas. aggressive, sturdy
Water dragon, *Physignathus coccinus*[10]	SE Asia	Humid, rain forest, arboreal	100	26C/20C	oviparous	O/a,v,n	no	Occas. aggressive, sturdy
Uromastyx, *Uromastyx* spp.[12]	NW Africa, SW Asia	Arid, desert, terrestrial	30–50	37C/22C	oviparous	H,O/a	yes	Docile, sturdy
Anguidae								
Glass lizards, *Ophisaurus* spp.[10]	Worldwide	Dry, rocky forest, terrestrial	to 140	26C/20C	oviparous	C/a,g	yes	Docile, fragile, tail autotomy[+]
Chamaeleontidae								
Veiled chameleon, *Chamaeleo calyptratus*[13]	E Africa	Montane forest, arboreal	50	30C/20C	oviparous	I	no	Docile, fragile to sturdy
Flapneck chameleon, *Chamaeleo dilepis*[10,14]	Africa	Tropical savanna, arboreal	30	30C/20C	oviparous	I	no	Docile, fragile to sturdy
Three-horned chameleon, *Ch. jacksonii*[13]	E Africa	Montane forest, arboreal	30	25C/20C	viviparous	I	no	Docile, fragile to sturdy
Panther chameleon, *Chamaeleo pardalis*[13]	Madagascar	Coastal forest, arboreal	60	30C/20C	oviparous	I	no	Occas. aggressive, sturdy
Gekkonidae								
Day geckos, *Phelsuma* spp.[8]	Indian Ocean Islands	Tropical rain forest, arboreal	to 25	30C/25C	oviparous	O/a,n	no	Docile, tail autotomy, skin slough
Leaf-tailed geckos, *Uroplatus* spp.[6,10,14]	Madagascar	Tropical rain forest, arboreal	to 25	28C/22C	oviparous	I	no	Docile, fragile, tail autotomy[+]
Leopard gecko, *Eublepharis macularius*[9]	Asia	Desert, terrestrial	to 20	30C/25C	oviparous	I	yes	Occas. aggressive, tail autotomy[+]
Tokay gecko, *Gekko gecko*[10]	SE Asia	Tropical rain forest, arboreal	to 30	27C/20C	oviparous	C/a,v	no	Aggressive, sturdy

Table 6.1. Continued

Common name/species name	Origin	Habitat	Size (cm)[1]	Temp (d/n)[2]	Repro[3]	Feed[4]	Rest[5]	Handling concerns[6]
Iguanidae								
Green anole, *Anolis carolinensis*[10]	N America	Temperate forest, arboreal	20	26C/20C	oviparous	I	yes	Docile, tail autotomy
Green iguana, *Iguana iguana*[7]	Central, S America	Tropical rain forest, arboreal	200	31C/22C	oviparous	H	yes	Very aggressive, tail autotomy
Horned lizards, *Phrynosoma* spp.[10]	Central, N America	Arid, desert, savanna, terrestrial	to 20	35C/20C	vivi-,ovi-	I/t	yes	Docile, sturdy
Spiny lizards, *Sceloporus* spp.[10,14]	N, S, Central America	Dry, rocky, forest, arb/terrestrial	to 30	26C/20C	vivi-,ovi-	I	yes	Docile, sturdy
Lacertidae								
Jeweled lizard, *Lacerta* spp.[10]	Europe, Africa	Dry, forest, arboreal/terrestrial	to 40	25C/15C	vivi-,ovi-	O/a,n	yes	Occas. aggressive, sturdy
Scincidae								
Skinks, *Eumeces* spp.[10]	Worldwide	Forest, terrestrial, occas. arboreal	to 30	26C/20C	vivi-,ovi-	I	yes	Docile, tail autotomy
Blue-tongued skinks, *Tiliqua* spp.[10,14]	Australia	Forest, desert, terrestrial	to 50	30C/20C	viviparous	O/a,g	yes	Docile, sturdy
Prehensile-tailed skink, *Corucia zebrata*[15]	Solomon Islands	Tropical forest, arboreal	to 60	30C/24C	viviparous	H	yes	Occas. aggressive, sturdy
Teiidae								
Ameivas, *Ameiva* spp.[10]	Central, S America	Forest, fields, terrestrial	to 50	26C/20C	oviparous	O/a,n	yes	Docile, sturdy
Tegus, *Tupinambis* spp.[10,11]	S America	Forests, terrestrial	to 140	30C/20C	oviparous	C/a,v,e	yes	Occas. aggressive, sturdy

Varanidae								
Nile monitor, *Varanus niloticus*[11]	Africa	Stream, riverbank, terrestrial	to 200	30C/20C	oviparous	C/e,g,v	yes	Very aggressive, sturdy
Savannah monitor, *V. exanthematicus*[11]	Africa	Desert, dry grassland, terrestrial	to 100	30C/20C	oviparous	C/a,g,e,v	yes	Occas. aggressive, sturdy

[1] Average maximum adult size.

[2] Average day and night temperatures for adults of species or typical of genus.

[3] Oviparous (ovi-) = egg laying; viviparous (vivi-) = live birth; parthenogenic (partheno-) = produces offspring without mating.

[4] Diet of the adult lizard *in nature*: O = omnivore, I = exclusive insectivore, C = primary carnivore, H = exclusive herbivore, H,O = some spp. exclusively herbivorous, some spp. omnivorous. Specializations or primary food consumed listed in order of importance for each sp.: a = arthropods, e = eggs, g = gastropods, n = nectar or ripe fruit, t = termites and ants, v = vertebrates.

[5] Does lizard seasonally hibernate or brumate? Yes = successful captive breeding may require cooling/rest period. No = successful breeding does not require cooling/rest period.

[6] Typical response of patient to handling:

Docile: lizards will allow handling with minimal resistance.

Occasionally aggressive: lizards may attempt to bite or claw when handled and can inflict injury upon handler.

Aggressive: lizards will routinely bite, claw, or struggle during or before handling. The Tokay gecko is not particularly dangerous to handle, but is aggressive.

Very aggressive: lizards may bite, scratch, or whip tail *prior* to handling. Large monitors and iguanas should be considered dangerous at all times and handled only by experienced staff.

Sturdy: little to no stress or trauma results from routine handling when healthy.

Fragile: may stress easily when handled for routine examination. Bodily injury to lizard may result from routine restraint or handling.

Tail autotomy: lizards may lose tail when handled (not all spp. capable of autotomy are marked). [+]Tail autotomy in some species may occur even if lizard is not handled, but merely stressed.

Skin slough: lizards with skin that tears easily when minimally restrained or touched.

[7] de Vosjoli, 1992.

[8] McKeown 1993.

[9] de Vosjoli et al. 1997.

[10] Obst et al. 1988.

[11] Balsai 1997.

[12] de Vosjoli 1995.

[13] de Vosjoli & Ferguson 1995.

[14] de Vosjoli 1997.

[15] de Vosjoli 1993.

[16] de Vosjoli 2001.

particular species or individuals based on a variety of environmental or behavioral influences.

Some gecko species can autotomize, tear, or release, the entire skin in response to capture by a predator. These species include the fish-scale geckos (*Geckolepis* spp.) and the day geckos (*Phelsuma* spp.) (Glaw and Vences 1994, McKeown 1993). Skin regeneration occurs in these species but may result in unsightly scars and secondary bacterial or fungal infections.

Foot and toe adaptations are diverse. Integument specialization is quite notable in the fan-like adhesive discs of Gekkonidae. These species are capable of climbing glass and inverted smooth surfaces. Large arboreal and terrestrial lizards usually possess sharp sturdy claws. Lizard claws are similar to those of birds; they have a pulp containing a blood vessel and nerve that is sensitive to short trimming.

Skeletal System

The general lizard skeletal system is quadruped consisting of an ossified skull, vertebral column, ribs, and pelvic and pectoral girdles (Figure 6.1). The ribs of lizards connect ventrally to a cartilaginous sternum that is absent in snakes and turtles (Goin et al. 1978). Lizard teeth are either acrodont or pleurodont. Acrodont teeth attach to the masticating surface of the mandible or maxilla and have no socket. These teeth are not replaced when lost and are characteristic of true chameleons. Pleurodont teeth are attached to the inner or lingual surface of the mandible or maxilla and have no socket. These teeth are replaced through the

life of the lizard and are characteristic of iguanas and monitors.

Locomotion for lizards is apodal, bipedal, or quadrupedal. Most lizards have four legs and five toes, though there are species that are snake-like with no functional legs (*Anguis* spp., *Anniela* spp., *Lialis* spp., *Ophisaurus* spp.) and others with greatly reduced limbs (*Chalcides chalcides*, *Neoseps reynoldsi*, *Chamaesaura* spp.). Bipedal locomotion is observed in basilisks (*Basiliscus* spp.) and frilled dragons (*Chlamydosaurus kingii*) when excited or during escape behavior. This behavior is rarely observed in small enclosures. Old world chameleons (*Chamaeleo* spp.) are zygodactylous, having two toes and three toes fused into a claw-like foot, creating a strong gripping foot for climbing on limbs and branches (Goin et al. 1978).

Tail autotomy, the loss or release of the tail, occurs in many species (Iguanidae, Gekkonidae, some Scincidae). This adaptation (coupled with certain behaviors) creates distraction and allows the tailless lizard to escape as a potential predator investigates the released yet still moving tail. Transverse cleavage plates are present in each caudal vertebrae of these species, allowing release of the tail at multiple locations (Barten 1996a, Goin et al. 1978). Hemorrhage is minimal with tail loss because vertebral vessels are quick to constrict. If the tail stump is undamaged, species capable of autotomy can regenerate tails that are usually smaller with irregular scalation and darker color than the original tail. If species that are not

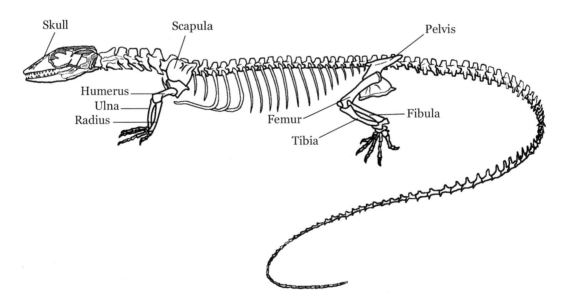

Figure 6.1. Lizard skeletal anatomy.

capable of autotomy (Chamaeleontidae, Varanidae) suffer traumatic tail loss, the tail usually cannot regenerate completely. Some lizards (some Chamaeleontidae and *Corucia zebrata*) use a prehensile tail for stabilization or movement between branches.

It is important to note that touching or manipulating the tail is not necessary to cause its release in some species. The leaf-tailed geckos, *Uroplatus* spp., can only autotomize the entire tail from the first one or two caudal vertebrae so the entire tail is always lost (Glaw and Vences 1994). A common escape behavior in these species is to wave the tail to distract the potential predator and then release it from the body without the lizard being touched or manipulated. Similar behavior can occur in the terrestrial leopard and African fat-tailed geckos (*Eublepharis macularius, Hemitheconyx caudicinctus*) (de Vosjoli 1997).

Cardiovascular System

The heart has three chambers consisting of two atria and one ventricle. Despite the absence of an interventricular septum, the majority of deoxygenated blood is directed to the lungs via the pulmonary aorta and oxygenated blood is directed to the right and left aortic arches to perfuse the body tissues (Goin et al. 1978).

Lizards, like amphibians, possess a large ventral abdominal vein that is intracoelomic along the ventral midline several millimeters dorsal to the body wall. This vein is secured by a thin mesovasorum and travels adjacent to the ventral midline from one-fourth the distance from the cranial aspect of the pubis cranially to the umbilicus and then courses dorsally to join the hepatic vein. Venous collateral circulation parallels the ventral abdominal vein via the caudal vena cava. The ventral abdominal vein is routinely avoided during coelomic surgery, though accidental or intentional transection and ligation of this vessel is compensated by collateral circulation (Mader 2002b).

The caudal tail vein is the optimal site for blood collection from lizards. It is located along the ventral midline of the tail and is accessed approximately one-third (or less) the distance from the cloaca to the tail tip.

Respiratory System

The respiratory system of lizards consists of external nares, internal nares, glottis, trachea, and lungs. The internal nares are located rostrally in the dorsal oral cavity and are contiguous with the external nares. The glottis, located at the base of the tongue, fits into the common opening of the internal nares when the mouth is closed to enable nasal respiration.

The trachea of most lizards bifurcates into the lungs that in some lizards may more resemble air sacs of birds than the familiar mammalian lung. Lizards do not have a diaphragm and therefore have a common coelomic cavity rather than separate thoracic and abdominal cavities. Ventilation in lizards is accomplished with rib expansion by contraction of intercostal muscles.

The lungs of lizards are not as highly derived as those of mammals. The cranial portions of the lungs are more vascular and serve for most respiratory functions and the caudal lungs are more sac-like and may extend to the pelvis (Murray 1996). Unlike birds, lizards do not have pneumatic bones.

Digestive System

The digestive system of most lizards is quite basic and, with the exception of the teeth, follows the design of higher vertebrates. The oral cavity contains several glands that aid in the lubrication of food items for swallowing. The Gila monster and Mexican beaded lizard (*Heloderma suspectum, H. horridum*) have modified bilateral sublingual glands that produce poisonous saliva that is chewed into the prey item rather than hypodermically injected as with venomous snakes (Barten 1996a, Goin et al. 1978).

The tongue of some lizards serves both in scent collection and swallowing. The tongue of anguimorph (legless) lizards serves almost exclusively a sensory function and the tongue of some Chamaeleontidae serves an exclusive food prehension and swallowing function (Goin et al. 1978). Most carnivorous lizards (Varanidae) have snake-like tongues to track prey items and the majority of herbivorous lizards have thick fleshy tongues to aid in swallowing. The sensory tongue retracts into a lingual sheath that lies ventral to the glottis.

The alimentary tract consists of an esophagus, stomach, small and large intestine, and cloaca. The alimentary, respiratory, reproductive, cardiovascular, and reproductive tracts are not separated by a diaphragm and are contained within a pleuroperitoneum or coelomic cavity (coelom). The proximal portion of the esophagus is the only opening to the back of the oral cavity. Thus, by visualizing and avoiding the opening to the glottis on the floor of the mouth, feeding or sampling tubes may be safely passed into the digestive tract with no risk of accidental respiratory intubation. The stomach in most lizards is quite large and does not serve as a gizzard or grinding organ (Barten 1996a, Goin et al. 1978). The small intestine has histologically discrete duodenum, jejunum, and ileum (Frye 1991). A cecum-like sacculation of the colon is present in herbivorous lizards (*Corucia zebrata*, *Iguana* spp., *Uromastyx* spp., and others). The cloaca is the common collecting chamber of the digestive and genitourinary tracts. These openings are the coprodeum and urodeum, respectively. The proctodeum is the common chamber opening to the vent. (Figures 6.2, 6.3).

The liver and gall bladder are present in lizards and located cranial to the stomach in the cranio-ventral abdomen. The gall bladder in anguimorph lizards is observed in a more caudal position, and is usually found in close proximity to the pancreas, as seen in snakes. The pancreas in lizards has both endocrine and exocrine glandular functions.

Large paired fat bodies in the left and right caudal coelomic cavity are not digestive structures, but may be commonly confused with pathologic lesions. These are particularly palpable in bearded dragons and are commonly observed in dorsoventral radiographs.

Excretory System

Paired kidneys are located in the caudo-dorsal coelom and the caudal poles commonly extend into the pelvic canal. Lizards are uricotelic; the majority of nitrogenous waste from purine digestion is excreted from most lizards as insoluble uric acid (Frye 1991). A mesonephric duct collects and transports nitrogenous wastes from each kidney to a urinary bladder. The urinary bladder empties into the cranio-ventral urodeum. In larger lizards the urinary bladder may be catheterized from the cloaca via this opening.

The renal portal system in reptiles is well documented (Barten 1996a, Frye 1991, Innis 2000). The system allows blood to flow from the caudal portion of the body directly to the kidneys prior to returning to the heart. Historically, this physiology has led to the conclusion that the reptile kidney may reduce the concentration of chemotherapeutics injected into the caudal body prior to their entry into the general circulation, thus leading to a decreased concentration in the blood and tissues. Also, suspicion was raised that injections of potentially nephrotoxic drugs should be avoided in the region. Several pharmacologic studies in turtles have revealed that the presence of this system does not necessarily indicate that all blood flow follows this theorized pathway and there may be no impact on drug metabolism when injected into the caudal body of tortoises (Innis 2000).

Reproductive System

Lizards have intracoelomic paired testes or ovaries, and oviducts. Female lizards have no true uterus, but in live-bearing (ovoviviparous or viviparous) lizards,

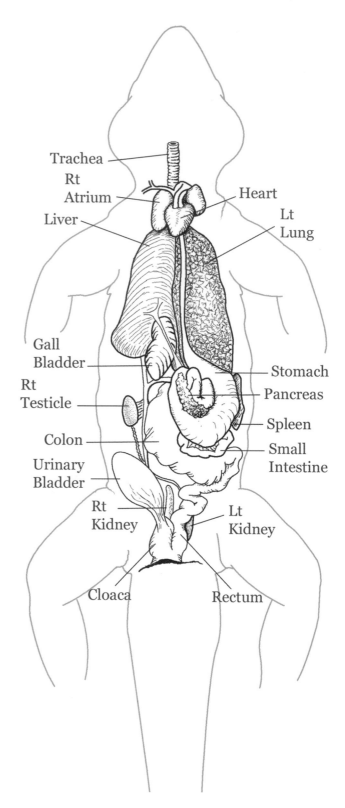

Figure 6.2. *Lizard visceral anatomy.*

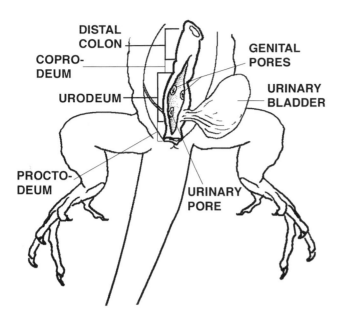

DISTAL COLON

COPRO-DEUM

URODEUM

PROCTO-DEUM

GENITAL PORES

URINARY BLADDER

URINARY PORE

Figure 6.3. Lizard cloaca.

the oviduct may serve a similar function to the non-placental uterus of mammals by providing nutrients for the developing non-shelled embryo (DeNardo 1996). DeNardo (1996) refers to all ovoviviparous reptiles as viviparous. The eggshell is secreted in the oviduct of oviparous lizards and is occasionally referred to as the "shell gland." The eggshell of many lizards (except Gekkonidae) is somewhat pliable, as seen in snakes, rather than rigid, as seen in tortoises and birds.

Male lizards have paired hemipenes that are invaginated into the proximal ventral tail slightly lateral and caudal to the vent. During mating one hemipenis is everted by relaxation of the retractor muscle and the filling of vascular spaces of the hemipenes with blood. Following mating fertilization is internal and occurs within the oviduct. No urinary structures are present within the hemipenes of lizards.

Sexual dimorphism occurs in some species of lizards, while in others determining sex may be difficult. For most juvenile lizards of all species there is no reliable method to determine sex. For adult lizards, the technique of sex determination is determined by species (Table 6.2).

External sex characteristics may be applied to many lizards. These characteristics include the presence of obvious sexual dimorphism such as the horns of *Chamaeleo jacksonii*, preclocal pores of many Gekkonidae, femoral pores of many Iguanidae, and post-cloacal tail bulging of the hemipenes in many species. Researching the anatomy of the species in question is the best method to determine if external sex characteristics are applicable.

Cloacal probing, the primary technique used in sex determination of snakes, may be applied to monitors (Varanidae), but is not 100% accurate in all species. A blunt or ball-tipped smooth metal sexing probe designed exclusively for this purpose is used. The only other acceptable instrument may be a sovereign red rubber urinary catheter or feeding tube. This procedure carries the risk of causing trauma to the patient; therefore, proper restraint and proficiency are required. The probe is inserted into the vent and directed caudally just lateral to the ventral midline in a position parallel to the surface of the tail. In males, the probe enters the inverted sheath of the hemipenis and travel a distance into the tail. This distance is subjective and variable by species. In some female monitors the distance the probe travels is shorter when compared to the male.

Radiographic sex determination is possible in some monitors. This technique is based on the presence of calcifications in the hemipenes of some species. These mineralizations are absent in males of both Nile and savannah monitors.

Surgical or endoscopic sex determination is obviously definitive. Surgical scar tissue formation, difficult visualization, and availability of equipment are potential complications. Sedation is required for either procedure.

Manual eversion of the hemipenes is advocated for some species (*Pogona* spp., *Corucia zebrata*) (de Vosjoli 1993, de Vosjoli et al. 2001). This method is commonly used in juvenile snakes. The procedure involves bending the tail slightly dorsally distal to the cloaca while simultaneously applying light pressure with the thumb in a rolling motion proximally toward the cloaca. This process will evert the hemipenes in some male lizards. Whereas this method definitively identifies males by the presence of the hemipenes, it only identifies females by exclusion. Males that do not evert a hemipene may be mistaken for females.

Hydrostatic eversion of the hemipenes is a definitive method for sexing monitors, but carries moderate to great risk of injury to the lizard. Proper restraint and mastery of technique are paramount. The principle is that injection of sterile saline caudal to the retracted hemipenis everts the organ through its cloacal opening. In female lizards, with proper technique, no hemipenis will evert and the oviductal papillae of the female may be visualized. This technique should be performed in sedated patients and restricted only to those animals in which no other method of sex determination is available.

Table 6.2. Sex Determination in Selected Captive Lizards.

Species	Anatomic	Probe	Manual eversion	Hydrostatic eversion
Bearded dragon, *Pogona* spp.	A		J	
Frilled lizard, *Chlamydosaurus kingi*	A			
Uromastyx, *Uromastyx* spp.	A			
Veiled chameleon, *Chamaeleo calyptratus*	A			
Three-horned chameleon, *Ch. jacksonii*	A,J			
Day geckos, *Phelsuma* spp.	A,j			
Leopard gecko, *Eublepharis macularius*	A,j			
Green iguana, *Iguana iguana*	A,j			
Blue-tongued skinks, *Tiliqua* spp.	a		j	A
Prehensile-tailed skink, *Corucia zebrata*	a		A,j	
Tegus, *Tupinambis* spp.	a	A		
Nile monitor, *Varanus niloticus*		a		A
Savannah monitor, *V. exanthematicus*		a		A

Note: A = preferred method, adult; a = inconsistent method, adult; J = preferred method, juvenile; j = inconsistent method, juvenile.

Nervous System

The central nervous system consists of a cerebrum, cerebellum, brainstem, and spinal cord. The spinal cord extends to the tip of the tail as opposed to mammals, in which the cord terminates proximal to the sacral vertebrae. The peripheral nervous system consists of twelve cranial nerves and numerous peripheral nerves to the viscera, trunk, and limbs.

Pain receptors and pain responses in reptiles are still poorly understood (Bennett 1996a). It is apparent that lizards have a withdrawal response or reflex from traumatic wounds such as punctures, lacerations, or surgical incisions; however, expected withdrawal reflexes and responses from potentially traumatic heat are not observed (Mader 2000b). Captive management of lizards must take into account these apparent behavioral and/or neurologic reflex differences from mammals with regard to cage heating (see Husbandry).

Sense Organs

The majority of lizards have movable eyelids and a nictitating membrane. Those without movable lids (some Gekkonidae, and *Ablepharus* spp.) have a clear spectacle as seen in snakes. The spectacle is a scale-like structure formed by the fusion of the upper and lower eyelids. As with snakes, the spectacle is impermeable to topical medications. True chameleons possess turret-like eyelids and eyes that are capable of independent movement. Glands are present in the eyelids of lizards and may become swollen in cases of hypovitaminosis A.

The muscles of the iris are striated and under conscious control; thus, pupillary light reflexes are not predictable and the use of standard mammalian mydriatics is not possible (Williams 1996). The pupil may be circular or elliptical.

The parietal eye or "third eye" is apparent in some species (Iguanidae; Tuatara, *Sphenodon punctatus*). This structure is located on the dorsal head and is connected via the parietal nerve to the pineal body in the brain. The parietal eye is a photoreceptor that is integral in hormonal production and thermoregulatory behavior (Goin et al. 1978).

The lizard ear consists of an external acoustic meatus, tympanic membrane, middle ear cavity, and inner ear cavity. Within the middle ear cavity is the columella bone that receives vibrations from the tympanic membrane via the extracolumella cartilage (Rossi 1998b). The tympanic membrane of some lizard species is clear and in others it is covered with scales and not visible.

The vomeronasal organ or Jacobson's organ is present in many lizards and located in the dorsal oral cavity ventral to the nasal cavity but not continuous with the nasal cavity (Goin et al. 1978). Scent particles collected on the tongue are transferred to sensory cells when the tongue is retracted into the mouth. This organ is primarily used by lizards to track prey items and possibly to detect mates or enemies by detecting pheromones.

HUSBANDRY

Understanding the natural history (anatomy, physiology, habitat requirements, reproductive habits, behavior, longevity) of the patient in question is the greatest diagnostic tool in differentiating between normal health and disease. Combining this knowledge with the presenting complaint, medical history, physical examination, and laboratory data is necessary for the treatment and rehabilitation of the diseased patient. For instance, understanding the differences in dietary and habitat requirements of two common similarly sized lizard pets, the green iguana (*Iguana iguana*) and savannah monitor (*Varanus exanthematicus*), is essential even to obtain an appropriate history. It is not possible for even the most educated zookeeper to know every aspect of natural history of every lizard, nor is it expected that the veterinary technician can become educated in the feeding habits of every species of lizard kept in captivity. There are, however, several fundamental aspects of knowledge regarding lizards with which to simplify the approach to understanding natural history.

The following are general categories and associated specific questions with which the technician and practitioner should be familiar regarding every lizard patient:

Native habitat and microhabitat: Does the patient inhabit tropical rain forest, desert, mountain slope, estuary, beach, etc.? Is the patient arboreal, terrestrial, aquatic, or subterranean?

Anatomy and physiology: What is normal coloration and can the patient change coloration in response to environmental, seasonal, health, reproductive, or behavioral influences? Are there size or other physical differences based on sex? What is the normal mucous membrane color? Does the patient normally have four limbs and a certain number of digits? Does the patient normally have secretions from the eyes or nostrils? What are the characteristics of normal feces and urates? How long does the patient normally live?

Diet: Is the patient insectivorous, carnivorous, herbivorous, or omnivorous, and does the diet change with respect to life stage or seasonality? If insectivorous, does the patient have a preferred food item or size of food item (i.e. ants, centipedes, spiders, etc.)? How does the patient prehend food and at what time of day does it normally feed? How does the patient normally obtain water?

Behavior: Is the patient diurnal, nocturnal, or crepuscular? Is the patient solitary or communal? Does the patient experience climatic seasonality? Does the patient hibernate or aestivate? Does the patient use different microhabitats during different seasons or life stages? How does the patient reproduce and how often?

These natural history parameters for all species of lizards would require volumes to list and these are questions to which the technician or veterinarian may not always know the answer. There are many similarities among genera, but even within the same genus there are marked differences between species in husbandry requirements.

Looking again at the green iguana and the savannah monitor: the green iguana is a tropical, arboreal, diurnal, somewhat communal (though not in captivity), generally non-seasonal, and non-hibernating lizard (de Vosjoli 1992, Obst et al. 1988), whereas the savannah monitor is a temperate, semi-arid, terrestrial (and burrowing), crepuscular (to diurnal), solitary, somewhat seasonal, and occasionally hibernating lizard (Obst et al. 1988, Balsai 1997). The diet of green iguanas is generally herbivorous, though as with other species, in their native habitat they may be opportunistically insectivorous. For the savannah monitor the diet is carnivorous or insectivorous (depending on the life stage and food availability). Remember, however, that one can only speak of living systems in generalities; adaptation is the key to survival and many captive lizards "adapt" to the captive environment. Thus, behavior observed in nature may not occur in captivity.

Reptile hobbyists who pride themselves on maintaining and breeding common and rare lizards in captivity have learned that recreating the native environment in almost every aspect is the key to success. These achievements are accomplished by observing the animals in their native habitat, corresponding with other hobbyists or zoologic professionals, and logging countless hours of trial and error. Occasionally substantial investment is made in the construction of suitable habitats that far exceeds the monetary value of the lizard in question.

Enclosures and Environment

Cages

There is no way to generalize a basic lizard cage. There are, however, categories of habitats from which the foundation for housing most species can be derived. In general terms lizards are categorized as arboreal or terrestrial. Remember that some arboreal lizards are occasionally both terrestrial and arboreal. Therefore, suitable cage design may not be exclusive for either habitat. Native habitat use is listed in Table 6.1 for common species. Key requirements for all enclosures include security from escape, protection from injury, access for cleaning, and environmental control of light, heat, humidity, ventilation, and water and food availability.

True chameleons (*Chamaeleo* spp.) and day geckos (*Phelsuma* spp.) are good examples of primarily arboreal lizards. Though these species vary greatly in size and in microhabitat distribution, most species benefit from a vertically spacious cage that offers visual security on three sides and from above. Typically enclosures for arboreal lizards contain numerous limbs, branches, or plants in both a vertical and horizontal orientation. The cage is typically rectangular and may range from 0.3 m by 0.3 m by 0.5 m to 1 m by 1 m by 2 m. The primary, if not exclusive, construction material should be plastic screen with metal or plastic frame for chameleons and a glass or plastic aquarium for geckos. Screen allows for good ventilation and is relatively non-abrasive to the lizard. Wire mesh can lead to skin abrasions and may be more difficult to clean. Glass or plastic (plexi-glass) offers no ventilation and may lead to overheating, but allows for maintenance of higher humidity. The cage floor may be solid (wood, glass, or plastic) or mesh. Though a mesh floor with removable tray beneath may be most accessible for cleaning, it potentially allows escape of insect food items or may cause injury to the lizard. A solid floor with removable indoor/outdoor carpet is relatively easy to clean and provides security for chameleons. A well-sealed cage and lid are required for geckos because they are masters of escape. The cage ceiling is typically screen for both chameleons and geckos to allow adequate ventilation and humidity control (Figure 6.4).

Substrate for chameleons should be simple: newspaper or indoor/outdoor carpet is best. Soils, mulches, and shavings are messy and not essential for housing chameleons. Glass enclosures for arboreal lizards requiring higher humidity, such as day geckos, may contain soil in which plants are grown. The great majority of arboreal captive lizards do not use the substrate except to oviposit and this substrate may be provided in the form of a nesting box or potted plant when required. Though aesthetically pleasing, particulate substrates such as soil, sand, gravel, and wood chips pose a great risk to small (<20 cm) lizards because accidental ingestion may result in gastric or intestinal obstruction or impaction.

The leopard gecko (*Eublepharis macularius*) and the savannah monitor (*Varanus exanthematicus*) are good examples of primarily terrestrial lizards. As opposed to the arboreal cage design, terrestrial enclosures are horizontally spacious to accommodate a large cage floor and may contain one or several diagonal or horizontal perches of relatively large diameter. Smaller cages range from 0.2 m by 0.3 m by 0.5 m to many meters in length, width, and height. Because many terrestrial lizards are relatively strong, more durable construction materials may be required for cage design. The glass aquarium is the standard enclo-

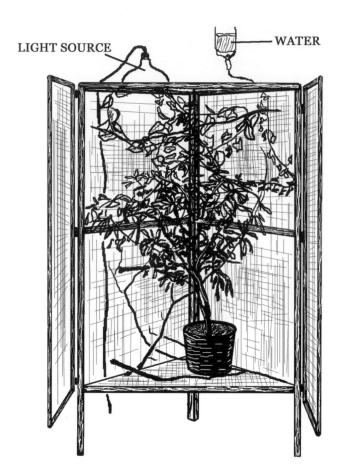

LIGHT SOURCE   WATER

Figure 6.4. Arboreal habitat.

sure for most small terrestrial lizards. Larger lizards, such as monitors, commonly require custom built enclosures made from wood, glass or plastic, or wire mesh. Commonly these larger lizards are housed in outdoor enclosures where climates are favorable (Figures 6.5, 6.6).

Lighting

Lighting requirements vary greatly among species. Some lizards require ultraviolet light (specifically UV-B) for vitamin D_3 (cholecalciferol) synthesis and subsequent calcium absorption from the gastrointestinal tract (Frye 1991, Donoghue and Landenberg 1996, Boyer 1996). A general rule is that primarily insectivorous (Gekkonidae), primarily herbivorous (*Iguana* spp, *Uromastyx* spp.), and omnivorous (*Pogona* spp.) lizards require supplemental UV-B light and most primarily carnivorous lizards (monitors) do not. Many lizard owners provide artificial lighting in the form of various incandescent and fluorescent fixtures.

It is important to understand that ultraviolet light does not penetrate glass or plastic; therefore, sunlight

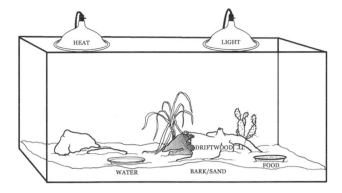

Figure 6.5. Terrestrial habitat.

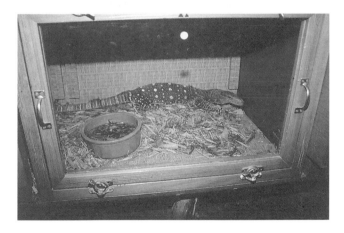

Figure 6.6. An inappropriate size cage for a lizard.

through windows and fluorescent lighting filtered by glass is inadequate to meet ultraviolet light requirements. Direct sunlight is the best source of ultraviolet light for lizards and may be provided periodically (once or twice weekly for fifteen minutes) to lizards which otherwise are maintained indoors (Ritchie 1992). Most if not all lizards become stimulated when exposed to direct sunlight and may become aggressive and very quick, making escape possible. Lizards should never be housed in enclosed or open-top glass or plastic containers when in direct sunlight to avoid life-threatening hyperthermia. Some nocturnal lizards such as leaf-tail and flat-tail geckos (*Phyllurus* spp., *Uroplatus* spp.) avoid bright light and are not active by day when in good health.

Light fixtures for lizards should be mounted outside the enclosure so that the lizard cannot directly contact the light (or heating element). Ultraviolet light sources should be within eighteen to twenty-four inches of the closest basking surface. Many claims made by commercially available UV-B-producing lights are not true and there are no regulations governing the legitimacy of such claims. Recent research (Mitchell 2009) indi-

cates that the newer coiled "screw-in" type fluorescent bulbs manufactured specifically for reptile enclosures provide adequate UV-B radiation for lizards in enclosures. Historically, the long "tube-type" fluorescent bulbs were considered the standard of artificial lighting for reptiles. Additional lighting sources for pet reptiles include mercury vapor lights and possibly compact halogen lights, which are new to the reptile market.

Heating

Most common pet lizards require additional heating during some portion of their captive existence. Because lizards are ectothermic they seek microhabitats that meet their preferred optimal temperature zone (POTZ). The POTZ is the temperature range in which normal physiology is most efficient (Barten 1996a). It is important for the client to understand that a lizard uses a range of temperatures, not a uniform cage temperature, to create the POTZ; in the cage setting this range is commonly referred to as the thermal gradient. It is also important to understand that various physiologic conditions such as pregnancy or disease may change the POTZ for a given animal. Observing the natural history and behavior and the study of lizard physiology is important for deriving the POTZ of each species. These values are available in many books, manuals, and journals for the species in question (Table 6.1). Lizards achieve their POTZ by thermoregulation. By altering their exposure to light, orientation to light, and reflectivity of light (coloration), and by radiating heat (gaping, respiration), lizards are able to regulate body temperature within a few degrees.

Heating a lizard cage is generally not as difficult as providing an adequate thermal gradient. The ideal heat sources should be located outside the cage so that the lizard cannot directly contact the heating element. In-cage heating elements such as hot rocks are poor choices for heating reptiles and should never be recommended by veterinary staff. Similarly, ceramic radiant heating elements and light bulbs, which mount into incandescent fixtures, should not be placed inside the enclosure. All in-cage fixtures may cause thermal burns to lizards through prolonged direct contact (Color Plate 6.7). Lizards have a poor sense of conductive heat and do not necessarily avoid contact with hot surfaces (Mader 2000b). Ideally cage heating should be provided through radiant heat from an overhead light or ceramic heating element. Commonly heating tape or heating blankets are placed outside and beneath the cage. Care must be exercised to avoid regions of the substrate or cage floor where heat is excessive. Additionally, below cage heating may lead to increased evaporation of water sources and increased cage humidity.

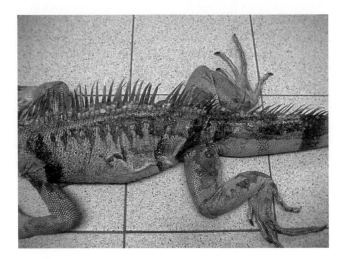

Plate 6.7. Thermal burns. (Photo courtesy of Dr. Stephen J. Hernandez-Divers, University of Georgia.) (See also color plates)

Some desert species such as Uromastyx spp. may require daytime basking temperatures that range from 37°C to 43°C (100°F to 110°F) to nighttime temperatures of 25°C (77°F) (de Vosjoli 1995). Montane forest lizards such as Jackson's chameleon (*Chamaeleo jacksonii*) require daytime temperatures of 25°C (77°F) and night temperatures near 17°C (62°F) (de Vosjoli and Ferguson 1995). Arboreal lizards generally do not benefit from under cage or substrate heating. Certain temperate and some sub-tropical lizards may require cooler temperatures during winter months to induce brumation or hibernation that is essential for successful breeding. Temperature is best measured with thermometers or temperature probes placed inside the enclosure at various locations.

Humidity can be a difficult parameter to regulate in the lizard enclosure. In a smaller enclosure humidity is more difficult to regulate. As with temperature, many lizards benefit from a humidity gradient—another example of microhabitat use by lizards. In larger cages this gradient is created by the interface between substrate and cage ornaments such as rocks or logs. Small covered plastic containers containing moistened substrate such as vermiculite or moss may be provided. These are called humidified shelters (de Vosjoli 1997) and are particularly useful to assist shedding in some desert species such as leopard geckos and juvenile bearded dragons.

Ventilation
In well-ventilated cages, such as those for true chameleons, hand misting or electronic misters, vaporizers,

or nebulizers are useful for increasing humidity. These are easily regulated by automatic timers. Regulating ventilation with screen lids or the addition of small fans is helpful to control humidity for glass aquariums or terrariums. Humidity is an important factor in both the respiratory and epidermal health of some lizards. Hygrometers are used to measure humidity in the lizard cage.

Ventilation is primarily controlled to indirectly regulate heat and humidity. Ventilation can be modified by cage design or may be controlled by external and internal cage accessories. Small fans, such as computer cooling fans, are quiet, and capable of moving large quantities of air. To a lesser extent, moving water such as small waterfalls, misters, and passive evaporation create some air circulation for more humid enclosures. It is important with any electrical devices that all wires be fully insulated from contacting water or metal in or on the cage and that they cannot be altered by cage inhabitants. Also, fans must be housed outside the enclosure so that the lizard cannot contact the turning blades.

Water and Food Availability
Water availability and water quality must be closely controlled. Some desert species such as *Uromastyx* spp. do not require standing water to be available in the cage (de Vosjoli 1995). Instead, these animals may be removed from the cage and soaked in water once weekly or they may be misted in an enclosure separate from their cage once weekly. Some tropical lizards such as true chameleons may drink only dripping water off leaves or other cage ornaments. In time these lizards may learn to drink from containers or from hand misting. The client should be educated that not all lizards readily accept water from containers or they are not physically capable of ingesting standing water. If water is not provided in the form that these lizards typically drink, they will dehydrate rapidly. Water containers for all lizards should be cleaned at least weekly. Soaking with a 10% bleach solution for fifteen minutes is sufficient for disinfection. Because some lizards may defecate or otherwise contaminate larger water containers, more frequent cleaning of water containers may be required.

Feeding stations for lizards are preferred over the random introduction of food items into the enclosure. Carnivorous lizards should be fed pre-killed food items such as small mammals from a container within the cage, or the lizard may be moved to a separate cage for feeding. Most insectivores only eat moving insects and therefore must be fed live food items such as crickets, mealworms, and waxworms. These food items may be introduced into small bowls within the enclosure. Many lizards readily adapt to eating from containers. Invariably some food items will escape into the cage and are usually consumed by the lizard. Presenting food in containers can reduce the risk of accidental substrate ingestion. It also may provide a central location at which the lizard may be observed while feeding to evaluate appetite and health. Feeding live foods such as small mammals and crickets increases the risk of bodily damage to the lizard by the food item. Crickets, just as mice and rats, may feed on the flesh of lizards if deprived of food for more than a day in the enclosure.

Herbivores are generally fed prepared meals in containers. Most healthy herbivorous lizards consume their daily share of food at one feeding, though in nature these animals generally browse throughout the day. Uneaten food should be removed from the cage on the day of feeding to prevent spoiling. Prepared foods such as powdered, frozen, or otherwise processed herbivore foods should be provided with strict attention to the manufacturer's recommendations for rehydration, thawing, and feeding frequency. For herbivorous lizards freshly prepared vegetable diets are preferable over processed diets.

QUARANTINE

The most important consideration often overlooked by the owner of new pet lizards is quarantine. Many clients who own one lizard eventually increase their collections, establish breeding colonies, or expand their interests to other reptiles. In their excitement to introduce new pets to the home, they ignore the potential for contagious infectious diseases that may affect their entire collection of animals.

Acariasis is a significant contagious disease seen In: Reptile collections (see Parasitology). Mite infestations can lead to reduced fertility, multisystemic disease, and death in captive reptile collections, and may be extremely difficult to eradicate once established in large collections (Mader 1996a). Intestinal parasitism is a prime concern in lizards housed together. Other diseases that are generally not contagious but may opportunistically spread are bacterial and fungal dermatitis, pneumonia, and infectious stomatitis (primarily from fighting).

Though recommendations on quarantine vary, a minimum of thirty days of isolation in addition to physical exam and clinical laboratory tests are required. Wild-caught lizards should have the quarantine period extended to sixty to ninety days with serial fecal exams performed monthly. In the absence of fecal parasites, prophylactic deworming may be indicated in wild-caught animals and many herpetoculturists routinely medicate new animals without the diagnosis of parasitism. Clients who prophylactically deworm their pets should be thoroughly informed of the potential side effects of medications and the potential side effects of killing parasites in the patient's body. Prophylactic treatment with antibiotics is not recommended unless clinical signs of bacterial or protozoal infections are observed or clinical disease is diagnosed.

Housing during quarantine should consist of an enclosure that provides comfort and visual security for the lizard, but also provides visualization of every aspect of daily (or nightly) activity. Substrate, when possible, should be paper to visualize and collect feces, urates, and urine. Feedings should be provided at a consistent feeding station and supervised to observe all aspects of feeding behavior and quantify food intake. Impeccable sanitation and cage hygiene is essential.

Ornaments, hide boxes, and water bowls should be simple and either disposable or easily cleaned. Minimizing accessories and having duplicates for each cage aids in cleaning. Safe and effective disinfectants for home use are chlorine bleach at a 1:10 dilution of the commercially available concentration and ammonia at 5% solution (McKeown 1996). **The two products should never be mixed to prevent the release of poisonous chlorine gas.** Soaking surfaces for fifteen minutes is adequate for disinfection with chlorine bleach at a 1:10 dilution (Ritchie 1992). When cryptosporidiosis is a concern, soaking accessories with 5% ammonia and allowing them to dry for a minimum of three days is advised (Bennett 1996c).

Record keeping by the client is essential both for long-term captive lizards and new arrivals. Recording dates of feeding and ecdysis, environmental parameters, and especially weekly or monthly weight (in grams) are all helpful in monitoring for disease. With the exception of hibernation or parturition, lizards rarely lose weight as part of normal physiology. Juvenile lizards that fail to grow or adults that progressively lose weight are usually diseased. Casual observations such as the frequency and consistency of defecation and urination and daily activity patterns should also be recorded.

NUTRITION

One adaptation that has allowed lizards to colonize nearly every terrestrial (and some aquatic) habitat on earth is their variation in dietary preference.

Consequently, their prime vulnerability in captive management becomes nutritional related disease when proper diet is not provided. Lizards are commonly classified as herbivorous, insectivorous, carnivorous, or omnivorous. Though the differentiation between insectivorous and carnivorous may seem subtle, some species are so highly specialized to eat specific arthropods and gastropods that they refuse to eat and fail to thrive in captivity if offered any substitutes. Additionally, when fed proper whole animal meat diets, carnivorous lizards generally do not require supplemental ultraviolet lighting, whereas the great majority of insectivorous lizards do require routine ultraviolet light exposure, even when fed calcium-enriched or supplemented insect diets (Donoghue and Landenberg 1996).

Just as there is no way to describe the basic lizard cage, it is impossible to generalize lizard diets. Each species has specific dietary requirements and variation in food availability in their native habitats that dictate diet preferences on a seasonal or even monthly basis. Carnivorous lizards (monitors, tegus) ingest other vertebrates (fish, reptiles, birds, and mammals) as their primary diet, but remain opportunistic and usually attempt to eat anything that moves and anything that will fit into their mouth. Some carnivorous and omnivorous species may also eat carrion or may be cannibalistic (Balsai 1997, Donoghue and Landenberg 1996). Carnivorous lizards that are not fed whole animal meat products are more likely to develop nutritional disease (Donoghue and Landenberg 1996). Some herbivorous lizards are opportunistically carnivorous or insectivorous, which, with some species in captivity, may cause serious nutritional disease when animal protein is fed in abundance (see Common Disorders).

The ultimate paradox with the cause of some nutritional diseases in lizards, however, is that the causes of disease may have nothing to do with food. Temperature, humidity, landscape, water, infectious organisms (intestinal endoparasites, bacteria), and especially light (specifically ultraviolet light) commonly factor into nutritional health despite the provision of proper diet. Thus, proper husbandry becomes the key to providing proper nutrition.

Nutritional requirements pertain to all lizards. Feeding behavior, digestion, the absorption and assimilation of nutrients, and cellular physiologic activity are all somewhat dependent on temperature for all reptiles (Barten 1996a, Donoghue and Landenberg 1996). The POTZ (preferred optimal temperature zone) and thermal gradient must be provided for each species to optimize nutritional value of foods. Improper humidity also impacts overall patient health and may lead to decreased feeding response. Donoghue and Landenberg (1996) provide excellent discussion of the nutrient requirements and daily energy needs of various reptiles and the nutrient values of various animal, plant, and commercial food items.

The quality and variety of food offered is important for all lizards. Food items should be fresh or provided promptly after thawing if frozen. Foods offered once to lizards should be disposed and not refrozen or preserved and offered again. Protein content and quality is generally met with whole animal diets and insects. For herbivores, the entire protein requirements should be plant origin. Good plant protein sources include: romaine lettuce, spinach, alfalfa sprouts, clover, dandelion, bean sprouts, and bamboo shoots (Donoghue and Landenberg 1996).

Calcium is an essential element for all captive lizards and its deficiency is the cause of metabolic bone disease (MBD) that encompasses a vast syndrome of physiologic disorders. Calcium absorption and excretion is regulated by several factors. Calcium absorption in the small intestine is regulated by an activated metabolite of vitamin D_3, cholecalciferol, which occurs in some animal tissues (Frye 1991). Vitamin D_2, ergocalciferol, occurs in plants and does not apparently facilitate the uptake of calcium in the gut of lizards and does not appear to be beneficial as a dietary supplement for reptiles regarding calcium metabolism. (Boyer 1996). Therefore, supplements claiming to contain vitamin D should be scrutinized as to which form of vitamin D is provided. Vitamin D_3 may be exogenously consumed in the form of dietary animal tissues and some dietary supplements or it may be endogenously produced when the lizard is exposed to appropriate ultraviolet (UV) radiation. Cholecalciferol is synthesized in the skin of lizards, and then is hydroxylated first in the liver and then the kidney to become 1,25 dihydroxycholecalciferol, the active metabolite of vitamin D_3. (Frye 1991). The consequence of this pathway is that in spite of adequate dietary calcium, lizards may be prone to MBD in the absence of adequate vitamin D_3. Clinically this is most commonly the result of insufficient exposure to UV-B radiation.

Ultimate control of blood calcium homeostasis rests with the parathyroid glands and their production of parathyroid hormone (PTH). The occurrence of hypocalcemia or hyperphosphatemia results in increased production of PTH. Calcium is removed from bone (calcium resorption) to increase calcium ions in the blood. Additionally, PTH stimulates the production of the active metabolite of cholecalciferol (vitamin D_3) to increase intestinal calcium absorption. When calcium levels in the blood are adequate, the thyroid hormone calcitonin inhibits the effects of PTH and bone resorption slows or reverses.

Excess phosphorous in the diet is also a nutritional concern. High phosphorous diets can induce nutritional secondary hyperparathyroidism that ultimately depletes calcium stores in bone (Frye 1991, Mader 2002a). In addition to the overall content of calcium in the diet, attention must be given to the calcium to phosphorous ratio (Ca:P). This ratio should be 1:1 to 2:1 for the entire diet (Frye 1991, Donoghue and Landenberg 1996). Whole animal diets (rodents and chicks) provide this ratio. Organ meats such as heart, liver, and muscle without bone are excessively high in phosphorous. Most commonly fed insects have a Ca:P of 1:9 and thus require periodic to routine vitamin and mineral supplementation (Donoghue and Landenberg 1996). Salads containing leafy greens such as beet greens, broccoli leaves, outer green cabbage leaves, collards, dandelion leaves, and mustard greens are calcium-rich (Donoghue and Landenberg 1996, Boyer 1996).

Nutritional supplements abound for reptiles and are required for optimal nutritional health of insectivorous and herbivorous lizards (Donoghue and Landenberg 1996). Calcium with vitamin D_3 (Rep-Cal, Los Gatos, CA) or calcium and phosphorous containing powdered supplements are preferred. Some vitamin and mineral supplements contain no (Nekton-Rep, Clearwater, FL) or very low (Herptivite, Rep-Cal, Los Gatos, CA) calcium and additional calcium must be mixed or given separately. Supplements are applied to insects by "dusting," in which the prey items are placed in a container and the powder added. With gentle swirling of the container the supplement is attached to the insect and then fed to the lizard. For herbivores the supplements are sprinkled over or mixed with the salad. Supplements should be provided once weekly for adult lizards that are fed well balanced diets. Juvenile or growing lizards should be supplemented two to three times weekly. Problems associated with mineral supplements include decreased palatability or refusal of supplemented food items; disproportionate distribution, improper ratio, or decomposition of nutrients within supplements; toxicities from overdosing or ingestion of high levels of certain nutrients; and false claims made by manufacturers. Supplements do not compensate for the feeding of imbalanced or poor quality diets.

Herbivorous Lizards

The dietary requirements of the captive herbivorous lizard diet have been well documented in the literature and the veterinary staff is responsible for informing clients of these requirements (Barten 1996a, de Vosjoli 1993, Rossi 1998b, Donoghue and Landenberg 1996, Boyer 1996, de Vosjoli 1995, de Vosjoli 1993). For years the green iguana has been the standard after which all herbivorous diets have been modeled, but the natural history of various species necessitates modifying the approach to feeding these pets for optimal health. Barten (1996a) presents the best summary of the green iguana diet in the current literature. Several of the primary to exclusive herbivorous lizards seen in practice include green iguanas (*Iguana iguana*), rhinoceros iguanas (*Cyclura* spp.), desert iguanas (*Dipsosaurus* spp.), spiny tailed iguanas (*Ctenosaura* spp.), chuckwallas (*Sauromalus* spp.), prehensile-tailed skinks (*Corucia zebrata*), and spiny-tailed agamids (*Uromastyx* spp.). The green iguana is highly adaptive in its dietary preferences in a captive environment and is known to eat commercial dog and cat foods, rodent diets, insects, fish, mice, and a wide variety of plant materials (de Vosjoli 1992).

Several beliefs regarding the feeding of iguanas have been modified over the past few years. Hatchling and juvenile iguanas do not eat insects as a substantial portion of their diet and then switch to primarily vegetarian diets as adults (Barten 1996a). Contrary to popular belief, leaf lettuce is an acceptable source of protein and calcium for herbivorous reptiles (Donoghue and Landenberg 1996). Iguanas of any age DO NOT require animal protein in the diet; this includes insects; whole animal or organ meat; and commercial pet foods for dogs, cats, primates, and fish. All protein in the diet of the green iguana should be derived from plant sources.

Herbivorous lizards at all life stages are generally fed more often than carnivorous lizards and in many cases daily feeding is indicated. Adult herbivores are commonly fed every other day. Most herbivores conserve water well and obtain the majority of their water needs from plants. Tropical lizards such as green iguanas and particularly juvenile green iguanas should have constant access to water. Desert species are best soaked in water in buckets or other containers once weekly to meet their water requirements. This treatment helps reduce the risk of certain respiratory and skin diseases that may occur from elevated enclosure humidity.

Insectivorous Lizards

Insectivorous lizards, among the most popular pet lizards today, have nutritional and feeding needs similar to herbivorous lizards. The insectivores comprise the majority of all modern lizards and because of their dietary diversity their nutritional needs are the least known of captive lizards. The likely key to understanding insectivorous lizard nutrition is likely not in the food items themselves, but in the food *of* the food items themselves (Donoghue and Landenberg 1996, de Vosjoli 1997). Lizards in nature eat insects that browse on numerous plants, detritus, feces, soil, and other animals. The assimilation of these nutrients may be crucial for the health and survivability of some species. For example, in amphibians, poison dart frogs derive skin toxins secondarily from alkaloids and other chemicals originating in plants through the insects that they ingest in their native habitat. In captivity, when wild-caught frogs are fed similar insects that are not exposed to native plants, the skin toxins are greatly reduced or absent.

Herpetoculturists of insect-eating lizards are becoming aware of the importance of "prey item nutrition" and specialty diets to feed to crickets have appeared on the market (Ziegler, Gardners, PA). Some research suggests that some high calcium diets are inappropriate for crickets and may affect the growth and reproduction of these insects (Donoghue and Landenberg 1996). The diet for captive insectivorous lizards should be varied and supplemented with vitamin and mineral powders. Because most domestically raised insects are low in calcium and have improper Ca:P, calcium supplementation is crucial. Little is known about the dietary needs for amino acids, vitamins, other minerals, and trace elements. Generally these are supplemented in addition to calcium.

Insectivorous lizards as a group have the same light requirements for vitamin D_3 synthesis as do herbivores (Frye 1991, Donoghue and Landenberg 1996, De Vosjoli 1993). This is particularly true of juvenile insectivorous lizards. The author has observed numerous juvenile to young adult *Chamaeleo* spp. present with MBD that are fed a varied diet routinely supplemented with calcium. The deficiency arises from insufficient UV light exposure. Questions must arise, however, regarding the required light exposure of nocturnal insectivorous Gekkonidae such as *Phyllurus* spp. and *Uroplatus* spp. that hide by day.

The patterns by which animals choose their prey are described under the optimal foraging theory (OFT) (Helfman 1990). It is theorized that animals choose between energetic costs and energetic gains when selecting food items. Insectivorous lizards have been observed to choose certain species of insects even when multiple species of a similar size of insect are present or the lizard chooses a certain size of insect when different sizes of the same species of insect are available. For example, the energetic costs involved in prehend-

ing, swallowing, and digesting ten 10-mg crickets may exceed the energetic costs of capturing and eating a single 100-mg cricket for a particular lizard. Therefore, the lizard ignores the smaller food items and searches or waits for a larger item. This behavior is seen in captivity as the refusal of certain size foods. Lizards that are incapable of dismembering or shredding large food items usually avoid catching and eating them. Similarly, large lizards typically ignore small food items that the lizard may have eaten as a juvenile. Both the size and type of food items must be considered when feeding captive lizards.

Some lizards eat only one or two specific prey items and may or may not accept crickets or other domestic insects at the expense of anorexia (*Moloch horridus*, some *Phrynosoma* spp. [ants], *Dracaena* spp. [snails]) (Obst and Jurgen et al. 1988). Most other insectivores accept domestic insects such as crickets, mealworms, waxworms, superworms, and roaches. Field sweepings for wild insects can also be offered to smaller insectivores, though the owner must be cautious of pesticides and potentially venomous or dangerous insects. Insects are offered in an amount that the lizard can consume in one feeding which is typically several hours in a day or overnight in the case of nocturnal lizards.

Insects loose in a cage can be as much a hazard to insectivorous lizards as live rodents are to carnivorous lizards. Adult crickets are capable of chewing through skin, digits, and eyes of lizards that cannot escape from the enclosure. Mealworms are also similarly implicated in trauma or death to otherwise healthy lizards (de Vosjoli 1997). Feeding stations that restrict the movement of these insects can reduce the possibility of health risk to caged lizards. Most insectivorous lizards should be fed daily, though as with adult herbivores, every other day feedings are appropriate (de Vosjoli 1992, de Vosjoli 1997). Dusting with vitamin and mineral supplements is done as with various life stages of herbivorous lizards.

Carnivorous Lizards

Clinically carnivorous lizards typically present less often with nutritional diseases than do herbivorous or insectivorous lizards. Carnivores are generally fed whole animal vertebrates such as small mammals or birds which, when fresh, are generally well balanced with nutrients (Donoghue and Landenberg 1996). These lizards also are more likely to accept a wide variety of food items which allows for more variety in nutrients. Several reasons based on natural history for the nutritional stability of carnivorous lizards in captivity include: a generally wider POTZ than herbivores and insectivores, less specific humidity requirements, and with proper diet less specific light requirements, all of which make habitat management less time consuming and less expensive for the owner. Several intangible reasons for the nutritional stability of carnivorous lizards include: they are less shy about eating in captivity and the availability of food as a whole animal requires less work by the owner to prepare the meal and provide balanced nutrition. Though several of these reasons suggest owner non-compliance, they are unfortunately substantial causes for the prevalence of nutritional disease in many herbivorous reptiles in the pet trade.

Consideration must be given to the quality of the carnivore diet. Live foods should never be fed to carnivorous lizards to prevent rodent bites. Similarly, live wild-caught vertebrates and most purchased "feeder" reptiles and amphibians should not be fed to prevent the transmission of some parasitic, bacterial, and viral diseases. Fresh-killed prey items have equal nutritional value to live prey (Donoghue and Landenberg 1996). Frozen vertebrate food items are commonly offered after complete thawing. These items should have been frozen immediately after death, thawed only once, and disposed if not consumed within hours after feeding. Thawed frozen tissues decompose rapidly after thawing and the author has observed regurgitation by lizards within days after the ingestion of apparently rancid food items. Adult monitors and tegus are fed several adult mice or small rats several times weekly. This feeding schedule may be adjusted for obesity or leanness.

Prepared foods such as poultry meat, beef, and dog and cat foods are not substitutes for whole animal meals and should not be offered. Exceptions may be made for short periods if rodents are unavailable or if assisted feeding is required for health-compromised individuals. In these cases canned cat foods are the better choice for feeding these patients. A variety of prepared diets specifically for lizards are available through pet suppliers. Veterinarians and herpetoculturists should thoroughly research dietary claims and scrutinize research for these products before recommending them as a sole source of nutrition. Lizards fed diets of primarily fish may be susceptible to thiamin and vitamin E deficiencies (Donoghue and Landenberg 1996, Barten 1996a).

Hatchling and juvenile carnivorous lizards can present a few nutritional challenges to their owners. Because of their smaller size, these lizards may not accept whole vertebrate food items early in life. Therefore, insects are commonly offered to smaller lizards and newborn or "pinkie" mice are offered to larger juvenile lizards. Because insects have a relatively poor Ca:P (1:9) ratio, dusting of these insects with calcium powders is recommended. Pinkie mice (1:1) have a lower calcium content than do weanling (1.1:1) or adult mice (1.4:1), though the Ca:P ratio is suitable and due to the relatively short term that these food items are offered, calcium supplementation is not likely required (Donoghue and Landenberg 1996). Hatchling and juvenile carnivorous lizards should be fed at least every two to three days.

FINALLY, NEVER FEED LARGE ADULT CARNIVOROUS OR HERBIVOROUS LIZARDS BY HAND. The potential consequence to fingers and hands is obvious, but more serious is the conditioned response that is created by this behavior. Lizards are wild animals whose behavior is driven by instinct and conditioning, not by reasoning. A lizard cannot discern between the end of the food item and the beginning of the human hand until after the bite occurs. The client should also be instructed to exercise caution when removing uneaten food items from cages.

COMMON DISORDERS

Diseases of lizards include many diseases common to reptiles in general and a few that are unique to particular species or families of lizards. Many disorders are husbandry related. Some diseases are more common in imported lizards than in domestically captive raised lizards; therefore, it is important to inquire or discern the origin of the patient.

Not all disorders require medications. Many diseases require correction of improper husbandry and supportive care. The author advocates increasing quality caloric intake for all traumatic injuries and many infectious diseases to strengthen immune response and speed tissue repair in reptiles. Observation of POTZ and humidity is essential for the healing of all reptilian diseases.

Integument
Rostral abrasions are a common skin disorder of many lizards including *Iguana* spp., *Physignathus* spp., *Chlamydosaurus kingi*, and some *Varanus* spp. Abrasions are less common in Gekkonidae or in deliberate or slow moving species such as *Uromastyx* spp. and *Chamaeleo* spp. The most common cause of rostral abrasions is facial impact with glass walls of aquariums or pacing and rubbing the nose on cage walls. Many larger imported iguanas and water dragons develop these abrasions from handling during the importation and distribution process to pet stores. Animals not adjusted to captivity commonly attempt

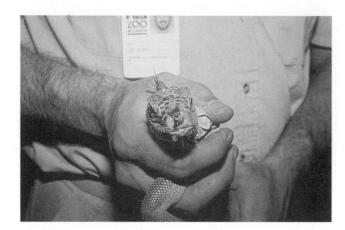

Plate 6.8. Rostrum abrasion. (Photo courtesy of Zoo Atlanta.) (See also color plates)

escape by incessantly rubbing on cage walls or lids or crash into walls when startled by movement in the room around them (Color Plate 6.8).

Recovery from rostral abrasions may be prolonged and the patient may be subject to recurrent injury. Treatment must include altering the enclosure to prevent further injury. Creating visual security such as a paper covering or the painting of glass walls or adding other visual barriers, even if temporary, is mandatory. Various antibiotic ointments may be used if indicated for infection. Note: Inform the client that treatment through habitat or behavioral modification is more important than medicating the lesion.

Traumatic injury may occur from bite wounds, thermal burns, and skin autotomy. Both burns and bite wounds (cage mate or prey item) commonly require surgical debridement of damaged or necrotic tissue and primary or delayed secondary closure. Secondary bacterial and/or fungal infections are common and systemic antibiotics are indicated in most cases. Bacterial culture and sensitivity is indicated for all slow or non-healing wounds that do not respond to empiric therapy. Topical cleansers such as chlorhexidine (Rossi 1996, Barten 1996a) or chloroxylenol (personal observation) (Vet Solutions, Fort Worth, TX) are excellent topical antimicrobial agents. These injuries invariably result in scar tissue formation and occasionally disfiguration. Reptile skin is slow to heal and open wounds require sequential shedding to fully close. Proper nutrition is vital for wound healing and the author recommends increased quality caloric intake for these patients to increase the rate of shedding and repair. Note: Inform the client to expect prolonged (months) healing and to expect permanent scarring to the affected skin.

Bacterial and fungal dermatitis may occur as primary or secondary infections and are typically the result of improper husbandry. It is essential to know if the patient is captive raised or wild-caught and if any cage mates are similarly affected. Clinically these diseases are more common in terrestrial species. Improper hygiene and increased humidity are suspected as the primary causes of infection (Rossi 1996). Other potential causes include acariasis, trauma from cage ornaments or accessories, immunosuppression from a variety of factors (temperature, nutrition, metabolic disease, overcrowding, capture and importation), prolonged exposure to water or sitting in water bowls, and dysecdesis. Histologic microscopy, fungal culture, and bacterial culture are all indicated for diffuse or focally extensive disease. Treatment is based on diagnostic testing and may include enteral or parenteral antibiotics, topical antibiotics or antifungal agents, and most importantly identification and correction of improper husbandry. Note: Inform the client of prognosis based on diagnostic testing and response to treatment. Correcting any existing husbandry is essential for both healing and prevention of reoccurrence.

Dysecdesis is more a clinical sign of disease rather than a disease itself. Shedding problems are most commonly the result of underlying diseases or improper husbandry, particularly low humidity and malnutrition. Low humidity may not be an entire enclosure phenomenon as much as a lack of humidity gradient. Even some desert dwelling lizards benefit from micro-environmental humidified shelters to aid in shedding. Occasional misting for some species is beneficial. Other diseases that may contribute to dysecdesis are external parasitism and possibly thyroid disorders (Rossi 1996).

Complications that arise from dysecdesis are extremity necrosis, particularly toes and tails. This process arises from portions of the extremities that incompletely shed (occasionally more than once in several layers) and form a tourniquet to the distal extremity. Devitalization is quick and necrosis follows slowly over days or weeks. Lizards with thick skin or heavy scales may show no apparent signs of necrosis for weeks. Amputation of the affected extremity to the next proximal viable joint is required. Similar treatment is required for tails (see ascending tail necrosis, below).

Broken tails resulting from tail autotomy and not from traumatic amputation usually do not require medical treatment. In rare cases hemorrhage may be profound or extend beyond one minute. In these cases pressure bandaging may be used. An appropriate size syringe casing packed with gauze is taped to the tail for one day if needed. The lesion should be cleaned if indicated and the patient maintained on a clean surface with no substrate for several days following the injury. Topical or systemic antibiotics are indicated only if wound contamination has occurred and only then for several days. Surgical repair is contraindicated in autotomous species because this inhibits or prevents tail regeneration. Note: Inform the client to maintain a clean environment and report any signs of inflammation; the less manipulation of the wound, the better; and regeneration will occur over months resulting in a smaller and often darker regenerated tail.

Tail amputation in non-autotomous species or ascending tail necrosis in all species may require surgery and antimicrobial therapy. Traumatic tail amputation, though uncommon, may occur in chameleons, prehensile-tailed skinks, and rarely monitors. Also common is ascending tail necrosis that results from trauma to the tail such as bite wounds, handling injuries, enclosure injuries, or dysecdesis. Gradually ascending darkening and devitalization of the tail proximal to the injury characterize this disease. Skin may slough at times, revealing devitalized vertebrae. Surgical tail amputation at a level proximal to the devitalized tissue is required. The gangrenous nature of this disease may lead to sepsis and systemic antibiotics are indicated. For non-autotomous lizards, the tail stump can partially regenerate and is generally not sutured, though hemorrhage control with pressure is essential. Note: Inform the client to observe diligently for any signs of continued ascending devitalization and to be aware of signs of lethargy or anorexia that may result from sepsis.

Skeletal System

Metabolic bone disease (MBD) is a somewhat overwhelming and confusing disorder that might be best described as a syndrome with variable manifestations. The pathophysiology of nutritionally derived MBD is described in the nutrition section. Clinically one of the most common signs of MBD is generalized or hind leg weakness or paralysis; and, therefore, might best be considered a neurologic disorder. MBD is the primary rule-out for lizards presented with this clinical sign. Other common signs include failure to grow, generalized weakness, anorexia, soft or pliable mandible on palpation, palpably swollen or thickened long bone(s), fractures of long bones, and occasionally tremors or fine muscle fasciculations. In profoundly weak lizards the pupils may appear to dilate and constrict erratically, possibly an ocular manifestation of muscle fasciculations (personal observation). Presentation of a lizard with flaccid paralysis is an emergency. These

clinical signs are most common in species of Iguanidae and Varanidae.

In species of Chamaeleontidae clinical signs are commonly generalized weakness, anorexia, inability to grasp or climb, loss of balance, swollen joints, soft mandibular bones, crest deformities (*Chamaeleo calyptratus*), and occasionally flaccid tongue paralysis. Clinically MBD is related to inadequate exposure to UV light. Prognosis for recovery for severely affected juvenile chameleons with MBD is poor at best. Tremendous nutritional support and great care in handling is required for rehabilitation.

A detailed history of diet, dietary supplementation, and lighting are essential. Diagnostic testing includes blood chemistry and radiographs (if fractures are suspected). If hypocalcemia is detected, the patient should be considered critical and intramedullary (via catheter) or intracoelomic calcium gluconate 10% is administered at a dose of 100 mg/kg every six hours until weakness and/or muscle tremors resolve (Boyer 1996). Blood calcium levels are monitored routinely. Advanced cases of hypocalcemia with paresis carry a grave prognosis. Assess hydration and treat as indicated. Non-hypocalcemic patients are treated with oral calcium glubionate (Neo-Calglucon) at a dose of 1 ml/kg PO every twelve hours. This treatment may continue for several weeks to months until normal appetite returns. Nutritional support is required in hypocalcemic patients (see Techniques). Exposure to unfiltered sunlight for fifteen minutes once or twice weekly and oral vitamin D_3 supplementation is indicated. Fracture management is conservative for patients with MBD. Traction and immobilization of forelimb and hind limb fractures with external coaptation is performed (see Techniques).

MBD is physiologically a gradual onset disease. From the client's perspective the clinical signs of MBD are rapid. Note: Educate the client about the basics of MBD pathophysiology with emphasis on the interrelationships among diet, dietary supplements, and UV light exposure. Explain that a deficiency in one of these factors can lead to MBD. Most importantly stress the fact that recovery from MBD may require months and may result in some permanent debilitation or disfiguration in the patient that presents with advanced disease.

Cardiovascular System

Cardiovascular diseases are rarely reported in the literature. The author has observed one case of suspected heart failure in an adult savannah monitor. The patient presented with generalized limb and coelomic swelling. Aspiration of the coelomic cavity revealed straw-colored amber serous fluid that was relatively devoid of cells. Cardiac auscultation revealed a grade III-IV/VI holosystolic murmur. Pulmonary auscultation was unremarkable. Unfortunately, work-up of the case was not permitted and the deceased animal was not available for necropsy.

Respiratory System

The most common true respiratory disease in lizards is pneumonia. In lizards etiologic agents of pneumonia are bacteria, fungi, and parasites (see Parasitology). Clinically pneumonia develops with improper husbandry and rarely as contagious disease and generally presents in the advanced stages of the disease. Pneumonia associated with pulmonary parasitism commonly occurs as a secondary bacterial infection (Murray 1996).

The most prominent clinical sign of pneumonia is dyspnea. The posture may be altered with the neck held in extension and the mouth held open. Occasionally oral and nasal mucoid secretions are observed, though neither of these signs is pathognomonic for respiratory disease. Secretions originating from the mouth or esophagus can appear foamy in lizards with normal respiratory health. Thoracic auscultation may reveal crackles or popping sounds with pneumonia. These sounds in the absence of oral secretions are highly suggestive of pneumonia. The absence of any air sounds may indicate lung consolidation and advanced disease.

Radiographs are the diagnostic test of choice for pneumonia. Transtracheal wash (see Techniques) with cytology and bacterial culture with sensitivity of the wash are diagnostic for the etiology of pneumonia. For seriously compromised patients, a swab of the glottis or aspiration of tracheal exudate without flushing is recommended. Fecal exam is indicated in cases in which tracheal wash is not possible to diagnose lungworm infection.

Treatment is initiated upon diagnosis of pneumonia and modified based on cytology and culture and sensitivity results if indicated. Pneumonia in lizards many times presents as an emergency and treatment must not be delayed. Antibiotics commonly used are broad-spectrum and bactericidal. These include aminoglycosides, beta-lactam antibiotics (cephalosporins), fluoroquinolones, and advanced generation semisynthetic penicillins, all of which should be administered parenterally either IM or SC (Murray 1996).

Recovery from pneumonia is prolonged physiologically by the accumulation of pulmonary exudates in recesses of the lungs (particularly caudally) and an inability of achieving the MIC of antimicrobial agents in these relatively poorly vascularized regions.

Nebulization with bacterial antimicrobial agents may be beneficial. Aerosolized particles must be 3 microns or smaller to reach the lungs (Murray 1996). Treatment periods are ten to thirty minutes at a frequency of every six to twelve hours. Duration of treatment may be several days to one week pending clinical improvement.

Note: Meticulous investigation of all aspects of husbandry and correction of improper husbandry are required to develop a complete treatment plan. Inform the client of the seriousness of the disease and be realistic regarding prognosis. Treatment of pneumonia often requires protracted hospitalization, repeated diagnostic testing, moderate to marked financial investment, and tremendous patience.

Digestive System

Anorexia is the one of most common presenting complaints for digestive disorders, the cause of which can be a challenge to diagnose. Though anorexia is not a disease, it is both a clinical sign of nearly all reptilian diseases and a contributor to several other diseases. Comprehensive history is required because improper husbandry often contributes to the cause of anorexia. If history and physical exam fail to uncover improper husbandry issues or clinical disease, a series of diagnostic tests is indicated, including fecal exam, blood chemistry, complete blood count, and radiography (including positive contrast). Treat the diagnosed underlying disease and provide nutritional support.

Infectious stomatitis occurs as a secondary disease in lizards (Mader 1996d, Barten 2002). This disorder may be unobserved by clients because the patient is presented for anorexia, lethargy, weight loss, or occasionally oral or nasal exudate. Oral exam may reveal focal or diffuse gingival erythema, petechia, swelling, erosion, ulceration, and mucoid or purulent exudate (Figure 6.7).

The glottis mucosa may be involved in diffuse disease. In severe cases, aspiration of infectious exudates may lead to pneumonia (Mader 1996d, Murray 1996). Because the oral cavity communicates with the nasal cavity dorsally through the choana, exudates may be observed bubbling from the nose in the absence of true respiratory disease.

Immunosuppression resulting from a myriad of underlying causes contributes to the development of infectious stomatitis. Improper temperatures, poor nutrition, and trauma from fighting with cage mates or oral cavity manipulation may be implicated. The infectious agent is determined through bacterial culture and sensitivity and is commonly identified as normal oral cavity bacterial flora including *Aeromonas* spp. or

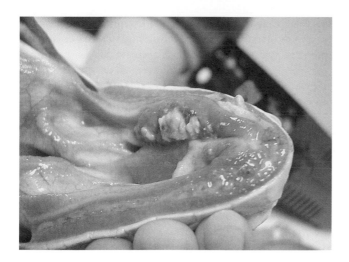

Figure 6.7. Stomatitis in a lizard.

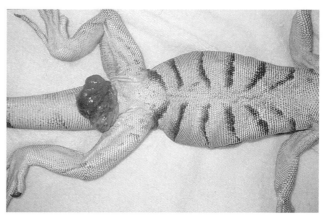

Figure 6.8. Cloacal prolapse in an iguana.

Pseudomonas spp, bacteria which are opportunistic pathogens.

Treatment is based on degree of involved tissues, husbandry parameters, and sensitivity values. Small (2- to 3-mm) focal regions of stomatitis may require only warming the environment and no antibiotic treatment or a single topical antiseptic or antibiotic application. Generalized or deep infections may require sedation, debridement, and a combination of topical and systemic therapy. Aminoglycosides (gentamicin, amikacin) and fluoroquinolones (enrofloxacin) are most commonly administered. Note: Inform the client that recovery may be protracted in severe cases of stomatitis. Routine rechecks are necessary to monitor progress of healing of infection. Correcting improper husbandry is of primary importance.

Obstruction and impaction are common and may present days or weeks after the onset of the actual disease. The usual presenting complaint is anorexia, but bloating, lethargy, weight loss, diarrhea, constipation, and rarely regurgitation may be observed. Diagnosis may be suspected based on history alone. Investigating the patient's enclosure substrate, feeding habits, and normal defecation habits is important. Confirmation of obstruction can occasionally be made on physical exam, but commonly radiographs or exploratory surgery are required for definitive diagnosis. Complete foreign body obstruction commonly results in gas bloating which is evident radiographically; the causative item, however, may not be radiographically visible. Complete obstruction with gas bloating is an emergency.

Impaction is the result of fine particulate substrate, rodent hair, arthropod exoskeleton, or other food item accumulation in the intestines and may develop inde-

pendently, in association with, or secondary to foreign body obstructions. Impactions are commonly palpable and visible on radiographs. If the lizard is alert and marked gas accumulation is not observed on radiographs, enemas and/or oral laxatives are indicated (see Techniques). Soaking in tepid water for ten to fifteen minutes may also stimulate defecation. Assess for dehydration and treat as indicated. Impaction may occur secondary to a number of husbandry issues, dehydration, improper diet, and hypocalcemia. Weak lizards with diagnosed or suspected obstruction should have blood chemistry analyzed. Surgical correction is required when laxatives, enemas, or other conservative therapy fails.

Intestinal parasitism is very common if not ubiquitous in imported lizards (Klingenberg 1993, Lane and Mader 1996). Signs of intestinal parasitism include anorexia, diarrhea, weight loss, failure to gain weight, and weakness. Treatment is based on diagnosis (see Parasitology). Quarantine, fecal screening, and cage hygiene are essential in limiting reinfection. Some parasites are zoonotic (see Zoonoses) (Johnson-Delaney 1996).

Cloacal prolapse may occur as a digestive, reproductive, or excretory disorder. The prolapse may occur secondary to straining from enteritis, egg laying, and uroliths, and may comprise the colon, oviduct, or urinary bladder, or a combination of the three. Treatment is based on which organ is prolapsed and the duration of the prolapse and resultant trauma to involved tissues (Figure 6.8).

The colon is a tubular, smooth structure with a lumen. Fecal material may or may not been seen within the lumen. The oviduct is a thin-walled, longitudinally banded structure with a lumen and no fecal material will be present. The urinary bladder is a globular, thin-walled, smooth structure with no lumen and may be fluid filled. Prolapse of these organs originates from the coelomic cavity cranial to the vent. Paraphimosis, or prolapse of the hemipenes, originates from the proximal aspect of the tail caudal to the vent. The prolapsed hemipenis is a solid, fleshy structure with no lumen. All organs may be darkened in color from devitalization or necrosis. Cloacal prolapse of coelomic structures is an emergency.

In cases in which prolapse is recent, tissues may be cleaned and lubricated with a water-based lubricant and gently reduced through the cloaca (Bennett 1996c). A single transverse cloacal suture is loosely applied to maintain the reduction yet still allow the passage of urates and feces. If swelling of the tissue is present in the absence of necrosis, swelling may be reduced with hypertonic sugar solutions followed by manual reduction. Necrosis of prolapsed tissue requires surgical resection in the case of coelomic structures or amputation of the hemipenis (see Anesthesia and Surgery).

Excretory System

Renal failure is generally a secondary disease caused by either improper nutrition in primarily herbivorous lizards or by aminoglycoside toxicity in all lizards. Clinical signs and diagnostic test results may mimic those seen with MBD with the absence of bony lesions. History may indicate polyuria, anorexia, weakness, and weight loss. Blood chemistry commonly reflects hyperphosphatemia, normo- or hypocalcemia, and normal or elevated uric acid. Radiographs may reflect enlarged kidneys that appear as masses within and slightly cranial to the pelvic canal. Renal enlargement is occasionally palpable.

The dietary etiology is theorized to be a result of excessive dietary animal protein. Aminoglycoside toxicity is well documented as a cause of renal insufficiency in mammals and reptiles. Treatment consists of fluid support and diuresis, though prognosis is typically poor for recovery and long-term survival. Other renal diseases seen in lizards include pyelonephritis and neoplasia.

Reproductive System

Lizards are presented with several reproductive abnormalities. Dystocia in females and paraphimosis in males are most common. Other disorders include cloacal prolapse of oviducts, ectopic eggs, and neoplasia. It is possible for lizards to ovulate and deposit infertile shelled eggs in the absence of a male. When gravid or pregnant, most lizards do not eat but remain alert and active for a period of several days prior to egg laying and many retain eggs until a suitable sub-strate or nest box is provided. Any dystocia accompanied by weakness or non-responsiveness despite the presence of a suitable nesting area is a critical emergency.

Dystocia in lizards can be pre-ovulatory (as follicles on the ovary) or post-ovulatory (as follicles or shelled eggs in the oviduct) (Stahl 2000). Differentiation of the two is made by radiography as the pre-ovulatory eggs are non-shelled and located dorsally in the abdomen and post-ovulatory eggs may be shelled and are more caudo-ventral in the abdomen. Conservative management is advised when the lizard is alert and active with pre-ovulatory or post-ovulatory dystocia. Environmental modification such as providing a suitable nesting area or more visual security may be curative.

Traditional mammalian treatments for post-ovulatory dystocia refractory to conservative management include oxytocin and calcium injections to stimulate smooth muscle contractions. Calcium gluconate at a dose of 100 mg/kg IM or ICe followed in one hour by oxytocin at a dose of 5 to 30 IU/kg IM or ICe are given (Stahl 2000, De Nardo 1996b). Oxytocin may be repeated within thirty minutes of the first injection. Efficacy is unpredictable and may only approach 50% in lizards (De Nardo 1996b). Manual reduction of retained eggs may be attempted for one or two eggs in close proximity to the cloaca and distal to the pelvic canal. Tremendous care must be exercised to avoid prolapse, oviductal rupture, or trauma to the kidneys. If the eggshell is not clearly visible emerging from the cloaca, manual reduction is contraindicated. Lizards with distal oviductal or cloacal dystocias following normal oviposition may be hypocalcemic.

Many cases of dystocia require surgical management. These are weakened and visibly distressed animals or those in which a radiographic diagnosis of obstruction is diagnosed. Obstruction may result from eggs too large to pass through the pelvic canal or from coelomic masses or enlarged kidneys that prohibit the passage of eggs.

Paraphimosis is managed similar to cloacal prolapse (Barten 1996b). The prolapsed hemipenis is assessed for viability and replaced or amputated as indicated. Transverse cloacal suturing is indicated with reduction of paraphimosis.

Nervous System

Diseases of the lizard nervous system are typically secondary to systemic, metabolic, or nutritional disease or trauma. Hypocalcemia from the various forms of MBD is one of the most common causes of neurologic weakness or paralysis in captive lizards (Barten 1996b).

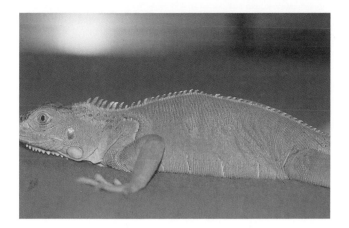

Figure 6.9. Spinal cord injury with vertebral column fracture due to trauma. Note the dorsal displacement caudal to the forelimbs.

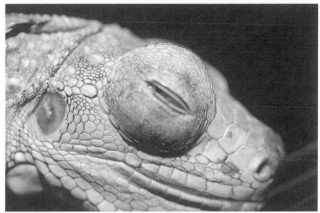

Figure 6.10. Retrobulbar abscess in an iguana.

The pathophysiology of hypocalcemia is described in the nutrition section. All lizards presented with weakness, tetany, or muscle fasciculations should have blood calcium levels assessed immediately.

Trauma is a common cause of neurologic disorders in lizards and is common in lizards that are free-ranging in homes or traveling with the owner (Figure 6.9). Both cerebral and spinal trauma occurs and is treated empirically with corticosteroids and time. Prognosis for even apparently severe injuries may not be grave if the client is able to provide adequate supportive care (see Emergencies).

Ophthalmology

Periocular inflammatory diseases are clinically the most common ophthalmic disorders in lizards. Infectious agents do not cause all periocular diseases. Many inflammatory diseases, however, result from or give rise to secondary bacterial infections. Williams (1996) reports that the majority of ocular diseases are a sign of more generalized infection.

One nutritional disorder that affects the eye is hypovitaminosis A. This disease is not specific to the eye, but also affects glandular mucous membrane epithelium including the respiratory and digestive tract. Clinically hypovitaminosis A is most commonly seen in turtles and occasionally in lizards. Clinical signs include blepharitis, chemosis, and epiphora. Secondary bacterial infection is commonly observed in these cases and topical ophthalmic antibiotics are commonly indicated in addition to weekly vitamin A injections (Williams 1996). Recovery may be prolonged to several months. A thorough review of diet is recommended.

Several species of geckos have spectacles (see Anatomy). Subspectacular abscesses and retained spectacles occur as in snakes. The abscesses may be unilateral or bilateral and often are the result of ascending bacterial infection from the mouth. Treatment consists of surgical drainage and irrigation of the abscess along the ventral margin of the spectacle as well as treatment of associated stomatitis. The surgical incision remains open to drain, but commonly seals in a matter of days. Subsequent shedding of the spectacle results in complete closure of the surgical incision and resolution of the abscess. The spectacle revealed following shed may appear wrinkled and typically requires several shed cycles to return to normal appearance.

Foreign bodies and trauma commonly result in blepharospasm. Evaluation of the globe and periocular tissues may require sedation. Treatment of lesions depends upon thorough examination of the globe, eyelids, and conjunctiva (Figure 6.10).

BEHAVIOR

The primary reported behavior disorder of lizards is aggression and is categorized as dominance or fear aggression, as seen in dogs and cats. Dominance aggression may be conspecific (same species) or intraspecific (different specics) among lizards housed together and it may be difficult to separate from fear aggression in cases of lizard-human interactions. Aggression is most often observed against humans in cases of large lizards such as iguanas, monitors, and tegus, especially during breeding season, and is likely hormonally induced. This behavior is variable and may be directed at only one person in the household (personal observation). The author suspects the possibility of pheromonally induced aggression in iguanas against women who may be in estrous cycle. Aggression in large lizards directed against humans is a serious and dangerous problem (see Zoonoses). Seasonal aggression is treated with ovariectomy or orchiectomy.

TOXICITY AND MISCELLANEOUS NUTRITIONAL DISORDERS

Toxicities occur from a variety of substances including pharmaceuticals, insecticides, dietary supplements, chemicals, and cigarette smoke (Williams 1996). Pharmaceutical toxicities are most commonly seen from injectable aminoglycosides and ivermectin, oral metronidazole, and topical pyrethrin or organophosphate compounds. The author is unaware of Teflon toxicity in lizards as reported in birds, but this possibility should be considered. A thorough history is required for diagnosis of toxic exposure, because there are rarely pathognomonic clinical signs for exposure to any of these compounds. Treatment is supportive depending on the underlying exposure. Mader (1996a) recommends standard atropine, diazepam, and isotonic fluid therapy for lizards with pyrethrin toxicity (see Emergencies).

Nutritional disorders leading to neurologic signs of disease include vitamin B_1, vitamin E, and selenium deficiencies. Thiamine (B_1) deficiency is seen in carnivorous lizards fed raw egg diets in which the compound avidin inhibits vitamin B. Vitamin E deficiency is seen in lizards fed high fatty fish diets (Donoghue and Landenberg 1996). Treatment consists of dietary correction and injectable vitamins as indicated.

Gout is a disease of lizards and other animals with several potential etiologies. In lizards, gout can originate both from improper nutrition or secondary to pharmaceutical toxicity. In vertebrates the pyrimidine amino acids are metabolized into CO_2 and NH_3 and eliminated from the body. Purine amino acids are metabolized into various degradation products of which uric acid is the final product in reptiles (Mader 1996c). Uric acid in high concentrations in the blood becomes insoluble. Simplistically, gout is the result of excessive uric acids in the blood that crystallize and precipitate in tissues prior to elimination from the body via the kidneys. Common sites of this deposition are serosal surfaces of internal organs and synovial membranes. A common presenting complaint of gout is swollen joints or white to yellow nodules of the oral mucous membranes.

Gout is seen in lizards on diets high in purines, most commonly in herbivorous lizards fed a primarily animal rather than plant protein diet. Gout may also be renally induced secondary to dehydration or renal disease most commonly in association with renal tubular toxicity from aminoglycosides or sulfonamides. Even at proper dosages these antibiotics can induce renal disease if the patient is or becomes dehydrated during treatment. Gout is a managed disease and not curable in most cases. Medications to lower blood uric acid concentrations and anti-inflammatory agents are recommended (Mader 1996c). In cases of advanced gout palliative therapy may be insufficient. This disease is best prevented before it occurs with proper client education regarding diet and the judicious use of potentially nephrotoxic medications.

ZOONOSES

Client education regarding zoonotic diseases must be a priority for all veterinary health professionals. Unfortunately, popular literature, television/radio, and the Internet are saturated with misinformation regarding reptile zoonotic diseases. The threats posed to humans, however, should not be underestimated. This information gap is prevalent within human medicine as well, and human physicians fall victim to the lack of education reflected by the popular press regarding disease in many domestic pets.

All veterinary staff should take the following steps to understanding zoonotic disease:

1. Gain a complete understanding of the pathophysiology and method of transmission (direct or indirect and vector) of the disease in question, both in the potential source animal and in humans.
2. Have a complete understanding of risk factors for humans to contract the disease in question, including immunosuppression and human behaviors when handling the pet.
3. Know which pet species are more likely to harbor particular zoonotic pathogens.
4. Gain a thorough knowledge of laws governing the possession and treatment of exotic species in a given jurisdiction.

Human behavior is likely to be a primary cause or facilitator of contracting zoonotic diseases from reptiles. Because many lizards are particularly sociable and exhibit behaviors that are commonly anthropomorphized, their owners form a human-animal bond that is similar to that seen with other domestic animals. Therefore, reasoning regarding the potential for zoonotic diseases is commonly ignored because of emotional considerations.

Behaviors that greatly increase the risk of contracting infectious diseases from lizards include:

- Housing or handling lizards in or near food preparation or storage areas
- Allowing lizards to soak in bathtubs, basins, or containers used for human hygiene
- Allowing any part of the lizard to contact a human mouth or face
- Allowing lizards to roam free in any facility of human habitation
- Allowing young children to handle or have access to pet lizards when not under direct adult supervision
- Handling lizards by any person under treatment of immunosuppressive medication(s) or having contracted any immunosuppressive disease
- Not washing hands and exposed skin following handling of pet lizards

Other risk factors include possessing aggressive or potentially dangerous lizard species, disregarding proper handling techniques of any lizard, feeding pet lizards by hand, and failing to maintain proper cage sanitation.

Bacterial diseases are most commonly implicated among reptilian zoonoses. Of these diseases salmonellosis (*Salmonella* spp.) is most notorious for causing disease in humans. See Johnson-Delaney (1996) for a comprehensive discussion of salmonellosis. Salmonellosis is directly transmitted by a fecal-oral route. Transmission of infective serotypes does not require the direct contact of fecal material by a human. Because lizards are commonly maintained in enclosures where they defecate, invariably bacterial organisms from feces may contact the skin of the pet. Handling the pet can transfer infective organisms to human skin. It is likely that disease transmission will not occur given the combination of a relatively low number of infective organisms and an immunocompetent host; with zoonotic diseases, however, there is no acceptable level of risk.

Other bacterial infections may occur in humans from fecal-oral contamination or from penetrating wounds such as bites or scratches. *Aeromonas* spp., *Pseudomonas* spp., and other Gram-negative bacteria may be normal flora in the mouths of lizards. *Mycobacterium* spp. infections may occur in reptiles and are potentially infectious to humans through direct contact with skin defects and inhalation. This infection in reptiles may appear in any organ. *Chlamydiophila psittaci* has been identified in infec-tions of various species of lizards (Jacobson 2002). Direct transmission of *Chlamydia* from reptiles to humans is unknown. Several fungal infections, mycoses, that have the potential to infect humans have been reported in reptiles.

Reptiles are the definitive host for tongueworms, pentastomids, of various genera that are know to infect humans incidentally (Lane and Mader 1996, Johnson-Delaney 1996). Transmission is direct and fecal-oral by ingesting eggs or larvae. Because humans are incidental "dead-end" hosts, they do not pass infective stages of pentastomids. Larval forms of these worms may migrate and then die in humans, resulting in localized immune response and calcification or granulation of lesions.

There are a variety of indirectly transmitted diseases for which lizards may be reservoirs of disease or carry the vectors of zoonotic disease. A variety of ticks, mites, and biting insects are implicated in transmitting disease such as viral, rickettsial, and bacterial diseases. Lizards have not been implicated in acting as a reservoir host for these diseases, but they may harbor ticks and mites that can bite and infect humans (Johnson-Delaney 1996).

An often overlooked yet significant risk to humans from captive reptiles is trauma from bites and scratches. With all infectious diseases aside, there is no excuse for humans to incur bite wounds from pet lizards. Some species are simply poor choices for the average hobbyist. These include *Heloderma* spp., adult green iguanas, large monitors, and some adult tegus. There is risk of bite wounds or other injuries from these species when simply performing routine maintenance and a minimal amount or even no handling. Generally, however, injuries occur from careless interaction with the animals.

The importance of this issue becomes evident when legal authorities attempt to strip the rights of pet owners to possess these animals because of accidental bites or the irresponsible behavior of a few people. Many local ordinances restrict or prohibit the sale or possession of certain exotic animals, particularly venomous reptiles and large snakes or lizards, because of perceived danger to humans. Accidental bites that occur at zoological parks and large snake escapes that are reported by the media contribute substantially to the hysteria that enables much knee-jerk improper legislation. Veterinary staff have a critical role in educating clients about the proper handling of exotic animals and in advising clients about exotic animals which are unsuitable as pets.

Additionally, however, veterinary staff must be aware of these laws when admitting or treating pets that are illegal to possess. Injuries sustained to staff or clients by these pets (and others) are the responsibility of the practice owners when on the premises. Similarly, advising clients regarding the home treatment of potentially dangerous animals should be approached with great discretion. For a somewhat complete but already outdated overview of laws regarding reptiles in the United States see Levell (1998).

HISTORY, RESTRAINT, AND PHYSICAL EXAM

History

In the practice of exotic animal medicine, as much can be learned about a patient from the history as from any other diagnostic procedure. With lizards, a veterinary technician or receptionist educated with a basic understanding of the patient's husbandry needs can often develop a working diagnosis well before the veterinarian examines the patient. It is the very diversity of husbandry requirements among species of lizards that demands a fundamental knowledge of all natural history aspects of the patient.

It is essential to not dismiss any observation by the client as trivial or inconsequential. The client may be the most educated person in the exam room with regard to the natural history of the patient, and with long-term captive lizards, the client is usually aware of a pattern of "normal" behavior. Discovering the deviations from normal behavior is essential to obtaining a complete history.

These are several fundamental questions for clients to answer regarding their lizard pets:

1. What is the presenting complaint(s), what is the duration of the problem, how rapidly has the problem developed, and does the client believe that the problem is related to any external influence(s) on the lizard?
2. What is the species, age, and sex? How long has the lizard been in the client's possession, and are there any known previous disease or health problems? Has the client or anyone else medicated the lizard or been instructed to medicate the lizard, and if so, by whom and for what reason?
3. Is the lizard captive born or wild-caught? This is not essential to the diagnosis, but can be very helpful in developing a diagnostic plan for infectious disease.
4. In the area of general husbandry, in addition to obtaining a general overview of housing, lighting, temperature and heating, humidity, substrate, water availability, cage cleaning, and cage accessories, it is essential to ask the following: Does the lizard ever roam free in the house or in any area other than the cage or enclosure or has the lizard ever escaped from its enclosure? Does the lizard have any direct or indirect exposure to any other animals presently or in the past and are those animals similarly affected? Is the lizard ever handled or observed by anyone except the client? Where is the cage located in the house? Is it ever moved? What are potential exposures to noxious materials such as cleaning agents, cigarette smoke, fuel exhaust, etc., and are there temperature, light, humidity, or ventilation fluctuations?
5. Regarding nutrition, determine *exactly* what the lizard is fed and the origin of the food (i.e. does the client collect food in the environment to feed or purchase the food at a pet store or grocery store?) How often is food offered, at what time of day is food offered, and in what quantities is food consumed? In cases in which a variety of food items are offered, which portions are usually consumed? Does the client use any commercially available foods or vitamin and mineral supplements and if so, how often and in what quantity? Does the client actually observe the lizard eating the food items or just notice that food is missing after a period of time?

Restraint

Portions of the physical exam, most diagnostic procedures, and many treatments require restraint (Figure 6.11). The veterinary staff must be aware that every species of lizard can bite. Most, however, will not bite or scratch unless restrained and the more firmly they are restrained, the more they will struggle and attempt to bite or scratch the handler. Lizards with delicate skin should not be handled for physical examination unless absolutely necessary. These species include the Malagasy geckos *Geckolepis* spp. (fish-scale geckos) and *Phelsuma* spp. (day geckos) that may autotomize both tails and skin with minimal physical restraint. This behavior rarely results in death of the lizard, but it may cause permanent disfigurement. These patients can be observed through clear enclosures such as plastic pet carriers or they can be placed inside a 5- to 6-cm. diameter clear plastic tube for examination (Barten 1996b).

There are some lizards that **at all times should be considered dangerous** to handle. These include all lizards greater than 1 m length, especially all large species of iguanas and monitors. Large lizards may be calmed by covering the head and eyes with a towel in

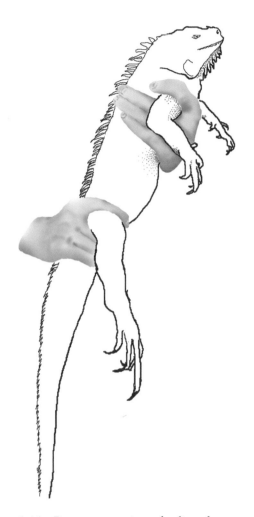

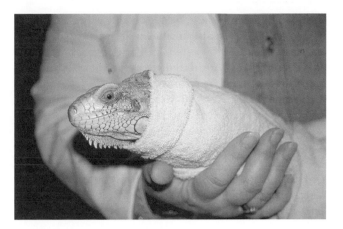

Figure 6.12. Lizard restraint using a towel.

Figure 6.11. Proper restraint of a lizard.

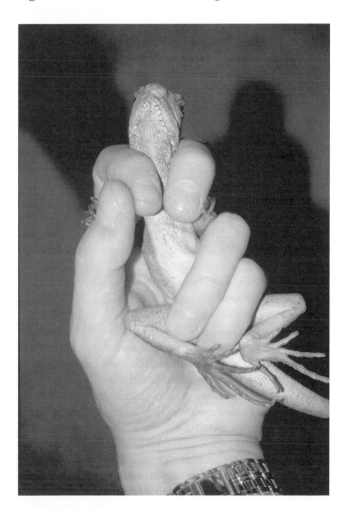

Figure 6.13. Restraint of a small lizard.

addition to wrapping the body in a large towel or blanket to prevent clawing (Figure 6.12). The head, however, must be fully and firmly immobilized at all times. Occasionally these lizards cannot be safely restrained and examined without sedation (see Surgery and Anesthesia). Other species, though smaller and typically docile, are capable of producing digit amputation, disfiguration, or extremely painful bites to humans. These include prehensile-tail skinks (*Corucia zebrata*) and some adult Tegus (*Tupinampis* spp.). Some smaller lizards such as the Tokay gecko (*Gecko gecko*) tend to be aggressive and will attempt to bite without being handled. Even small lizards such as fat-tailed geckos (*Hemitheconyx caudicinctus*) are capable of producing painful bites when handled and may be reluctant to release when biting a hand or finger (Figure 6.13).

The veterinary staff should refrain from inappropriate contact with pet lizards. This includes kissing the

patient, placing the patient near a human face, placing fingers or hands within the mouth of the patient, or allowing the patient to cling to clothing or hair in an unrestrained fashion. This behavior is both irresponsible and unprofessional and may result in serious injury to either the patient or veterinary staff. Clients should also be informed of the potential health risks that may result from these behaviors. The veterinary staff should never allow the client to assist in the restraint of a potentially dangerous patient during examination or when performing a treatment or diagnostic procedure. Though lizards may become somewhat tame, there are no domesticated lizards and their behavior may not be predictable.

Physical Examination

The traditional physical exam for most companion animals is a hands-on affair. More can be learned, however, by simple observation of the lizard patient at rest in a cage while in the exam room or waiting area. These observations can commonly be made during the traditional question-and-answer session and may quickly uncover potential emergencies that have not been realized by the client. First observe the posture (again, the technician must first be familiar with normal posture of a particular species). Quadruped lizards generally hold the head somewhat erect and may have a portion (if not all) of the body held suspended above the ground. For diurnal lizards, assess alertness. Does the lizard follow the observer in the room with eyes or head? Healthy chameleons, for example, are constantly surveying their environment with turret-like eyelids and generally do not sit still except when restrained or confined. For lizards with movable eyelids (all but some geckos), are both eyes open and are they clear?

Observe general body condition, paying particular attention to the muscle mass of the dorsal tail, dorsal pelvis, and dorso-lateral scapular region. Emaciation results in diminished subdermal fat and muscle mass and the skin may have a concave contour to one or all of these body regions. Additionally, the eyes may have a sunken or recessed appearance from diminished retrobulbar fat or from dehydration. Species that routinely present with signs of emaciation include the green iguana, spiny-tailed lizards (*Uromastyx* spp.), prehensile-tailed skinks (*Corucia zebrata*), bearded dragons (*Pogona* spp.), and monitors (*Varanus* spp.). It is important to understand that the physical changes associated with emaciation are chronic and do not occur over several days. Some lizards, which are laterally or dorsally compressed, may appear thin or underweight but they are in fact normal. Some of these species include leaf-tailed geckos (*Uroplatus* spp.), some true chameleons (*Chamaeleo* spp.), and spider geckos (*Agamura* spp.). Observe for symmetry, particularly of skeletal structures. Except for some skin

appendages the external and skeletal anatomy of lizards is bilaterally symmetric.

As with general body condition, the skin can be observed without handling the lizard. There is great structural variation among lizards in skin and scale texture. Lizards such as bearded dragons and horned lizards (*Phrynosoma* spp.) have roughly textured and armored skin. Others, such as some geckos (*Phelsuma* spp.), have relatively small granular scales and thin skin which is delicate. Observe for missing scales, abnormal skin coloration, crusts, dysecdysis (incomplete shed skin), subdermal swellings, and external parasites including mites and ticks. Pay particular attention to skin folds, flaps, nostrils, eyelids, axillae, and ears for mites and ticks. Observe for signs of trauma such as rostral abrasions, necrotic or missing toes, damage to the tail, bite wounds, and signs of thermal or chemical burns that may appear as erythema or tissue necrosis. Inspect for missing, damaged, or discolored toes or toenails. Remember that not all lizards have four legs and five toes per leg. *Ophisaurus* spp. and *Lialis* spp. are two examples of legless lizards. *Chamaeleo* spp. have five toes which are fused into two gripping bundles per foot.

While observing the lizard systematically pay attention to respiration and the respiratory effort. As with caged birds, respiration for most lizards at rest is relatively effortless and nearly imperceptible from a distance. Gaping (holding the mouth open) associated with dyspnea may be the result of upper or lower respiratory disease. Overheating, defensive posturing, and stress or anxiety may also lead to this behavior. Similarly, mucoid oral and nasal secretions are not normal, though crystalline or salt secretions may be normal in some species such as *Uromastyx* spp. and *Iguana* spp. Thoracic auscultation should be performed over the entire dorsal and lateral thoracic regions. When performing auscultation, a moistened paper towel or thin cloth may be wrapped over the diaphragm of the stethoscope to reduce noise from rough skin or scales.

An essential part of the physical exam for most lizards is the oral exam. This examination may require physical or chemical restraint and must be performed with consideration to safety of the veterinary staff and health risk to the patient. Some lizards (*Iguana* spp., *Varanus* spp., *Chamaeleo* spp., *Pogona* spp., some *Gecko* spp.) may voluntarily open the mouth when approached in the cage or when restrained, making oral examination less physically challenging. In these species (excluding *Gecko* spp.) the mouth may be opened with gentle retraction of the dewlap while the maxilla is secured with the other hand. This approach is contraindicated in patients that have normally fragile skin (most species of Gekkonidae) or those with diseased skin as with hypovitaminosis C. The author has observed the dewlap skin easily tear in malnourished *Chamaeleo* spp. suspected of having hypovitaminosis C among other malnourishment-related diseases. The gentle introduction of a rubber spatula into the mouth is useful as a speculum. Metal and wood speculums should be avoided because they may result in damage to gums and teeth as well as damage to or accidental ingestion of the speculum (or portions thereof) with stronger lizards. For very small lizards plastic spoons or plastic credit cards may be used as a speculum. For large lizards or those with dark pigmented oral epithelium an otoscopic or laryngoscopic illuminator is useful to visualize the oral anatomy.

Chemical restraint is required to examine the oral cavity with some species because of strong jaws and a reluctance to open the mouth. These species include spiny-tailed lizards, prehensile-tailed skinks, some monitors, some tegus, and occasionally bearded dragons. Similarly, lizards with metabolic bone disease or those with thin mandibles may suffer traumatic iatrogenic fractures from manipulation of the mouth. Tremendous caution and attention must be used when manipulating the mouth of adult iguanas and monitors. Any distraction or a mistake in handling may result in serious injury or amputation of a digit to the handler. The bodies of larger lizards must be fully immobilized prior to opening the mouth to prevent the patient from exerting any leverage by thrashing or spinning the body, should an accidental bite occur.

Examination of the oral cavity includes observation of the choana, dentition, glottis, and mucous membranes. While manipulating the head, palpate for the firmness and symmetry of the mandible and maxilla. Bones that compress or bend in a lateral fashion may signify metabolic bone disease. The mandibular symphysis is fused in lizards. Abscesses and granulomas may occur in the mandible with no apparent mucous membrane abnormalities. The oral cavity should be bilaterally symmetric. The mucous membranes of the oral cavity are generally uniform in color. Many lizards have a pink to pinkish white color to the oral epithelium with a somewhat glistening surface. Some lizards may have pigmented oral epithelium. The oral mucous membranes of some old world chameleons (*Chamaeleo* spp.) and bearded dragons (*Pogona* spp.) are yellow and should not be interpreted as icteric or jaundiced. In a healthy lizard there is little to no mucus, blood, pus, or other exudates in the mouth. The glottis should be observed through several respiratory cycles of inspiration both to observe normal movement of glottis cartilages and to observe for any exudates from within the glottis. The choana should be clear of any exudate. The dentition and gingiva should be free of erythema or exudate. Similar to snakes, some *Gecko* spp. have a spectacle which covers the eye. Subspectacular abscesses are commonly observed in conjunction with and may arise from infectious stomatitis (Mader 1996d); an oral exam is always warranted with the presence of subspectacular abscesses.

Examination of the external cloaca or vent also requires physical restraint. The vent should have appearance consistent with that of the remaining dermis with the exception of specialized scales that vary among species. Some lizards possess femoral pores that extend laterally from the vent onto the ventral aspect of the hind legs and pre-femoral pores cranial to the vent. The vent and surrounding integument should be bilaterally symmetric. As with the integument, observe for signs of trauma, swelling, exudates, and crusts, and observe for prolapse of cloacal tissue or hemipenes.

Abdominal palpation is a non-invasive method to evaluate gastrointestinal, reproductive, and urinary systems. Palpation is performed gently with the fingertips to create minimal stress and reduce the risk of internal damage to delicate or diseased patients. Caution must be exercised if gastrointestinal obstruction or bloating is suspected to prevent iatrogenic rupture to dilated gastrointestinal structures. In dorsally compressed lizards, such as bearded dragons and uromastyx, the kidneys may be palpable in the dorsal caudal coelom. It is difficult to differentiate the kidneys from other abdominal structures in laterally compressed or very large lizards without forceful palpation. Uroliths may be palpable as in dogs and cats. It is also difficult to impossible to differentiate gastrointestinal structures on palpation other than by extrapolating their location. Paired fat bodies are present in the caudal coelom. These are bilateral and may be confused with kidneys or masses in the coelom. The fat bodies are particularly evident in dorsally compressed lizards such as bearded dragons and *Uromastyx* spp.

Small lizards, particularly many Gekkonidae, have semi-transparent ventral abdominal walls and skin. This allows for visualization of some abdominal structures while the lizard is contained in a clear plastic or glass container. This technique is particularly useful for visualizing eggs in these species. An oviparous lizard carrying eggs is termed gravid and a viviparous lizard carrying embryos is termed pregnant. Both terms are used interchangeably for both conditions.

Eggs are generally visible against the body wall or palpable in many gravid oviparous lizards. Pregnancy in viviparous lizard is suspected with generalized coelomic swelling, though developing embryos may not be palpable.

RADIOLOGY

Radiographic imaging is particularly useful in evaluating skeletal disorders in lizards. Evaluation of respiratory disorders and gastrointestinal disorders is also possible, though gastrointestinal imaging must commonly employ contrast media. Other coelomic structures that are evident on radiographs are kidneys, liver, coelomic masses, fat bodies, and occasionally uroliths. During ovulation, ovaries and shelled or non-shelled eggs as well as developing embryos may be observed; otherwise, gonads are not visible on radiographs in lizards.

Radiographic equipment should have several capabilities. A milliampere (mA) setting of 300 mA and exposure times approaching 1/60 second (5 mAs) with relatively low kVp (45 to 60 kVp) produce excellent exposures using high-detail, rare-earth intensifying screens (Silverman and Janssen 1996). A collimator is essential because multiple exposures are commonly made on a single film for relatively small patients. The radiographic machine should have horizontal beam capabilities, though without this, and through creative positioning of the patient, acceptable imaging is possible. A minimum of two exposures is desired of the coelomic cavity: dorsoventral and laterolateral (lateral). Similarly, extremities should be imaged in at least two planes.

For many lizards a table-top technique is employed without a grid. Exposure techniques vary widely with different radiology units. For most small lizards (5 cm or less in thickness), small animal extremity techniques work well. For lizards larger than 5 cm, small animal thoracic techniques yield good exposure. Remember that the lungs of many lizards, in part, may extend caudally to the pelvis. The author commonly uses small animal extremity techniques even for larger iguanas with satisfactory results. Generally settings of lower kVp are desired because bone density is relatively lower in reptiles than mammals (Silverman and Janssen 1996). Similarly, the coelomic body fat of reptiles is typically lower than that of adult domestic animals, making the contrast of viscera more difficult to obtain with higher kVp. The standard dorsoventral and lateral positioning techniques may not reveal the true nature of coelomic structures or abnormalities.

Therefore, partial rotation of the patient to a 30-degree or 45-degree lateral exposure can be useful as a third exposure when evaluating the coelom.

The difficulty with radiology in lizards is restraint and positioning. Large healthy or aggressive lizards should be sedated without exception. This minimizes bite risk and radiation exposure risk to the handler(s). Small lizards that are slow moving or calm may be allowed to rest unrestrained on the cassette for the dorsoventral vertical beam exposure. Lateral horizontal beam exposures are possible without restraint for some still or chemically restrained lizards. Small fast-moving or delicate lizards may be placed inside a clear plastic container or tube or cloth bag and positioned appropriately for exposure. Though some detail of the image may be lost, this may be the only option to obtain radiographs of these patients. When sedated, gauze ribbons may be used to extend limbs as needed. Tape should be avoided because it may remove scales or otherwise damage skin.

Contrast media is commonly employed when non-skeletal imaging is required. Gastrointestinal contrast studies are not only beneficial for evaluating complete or partial obstructions, but are also particularly useful for evaluating extraintestinal coelomic masses. Barium sulfate is the standard contrast material for gastrointestinal contrast imaging. Frye (1991) recommends the use of 10% barium sulfate at a maximum dose of 20 ml/kg. Barium for gastric and small intestinal imaging is administered via an oral ball tip dosing needle or flexible, non-rigid rubber catheter (see Techniques). Unless the imaging of the esophagus specifically is required, administration of barium via a gastric tube is best. Oral cavity dosing may result in partial aspiration and loss of barium through the mouth or nostrils. In diseased lizards gastric to colonic transit times may be delayed substantially, though the author experiences partial to complete transit of barium within twenty-four hours in non-obstructed patients.

Retrograde or percloacal barium administration is indicated when distal intestinal obstruction or caudal abdominal coelomic masses are suspected. Barium is administered via a flexible, non-rigid rubber catheter. In small lizards (<200 grams) rigid or metal catheters should be avoided to prevent iatrogenic cloacal or colonic perforation (see Techniques). The clinician should approximate the amount of barium required for the desired image. Diseased colon or intestine may rupture with even the slightest pressure; therefore, resistance on the syringe is not a good practice for approximating dosing for administration of oral or percloacal barium.

ANESTHESIA AND SURGERY

Once uncommonly performed, coelomic cavity surgery or celiotomy is now routine for many pet lizards. These include ovariectomy, orchiectomy, salpingotomy, gastrotomy, enterotomy, cystotomy, biopsy, and tumor excision. Other surgeries that do not require celiotomy include amputation (digits, limbs, tails, hemipenis), enucleation, fracture repair, laceration repair, prolapse (intestinal, oviductal) repair, and reconstructive surgeries.

Anesthesia

Injectable and inhalant anesthetics are commonly employed both for surgery and sedation for diagnostic or treatment procedures. The most common injectable anesthetics are the dissociative agents ketamine and telazol (tiletamine plus zolazepam). Ketamine is administered IM or SC at a dose of 22 to 44 mg/kg. A dose of 55 to 88 mg/kg is reported for surgical anesthesia (Bennett 1996a). Telazol is more potent than ketamine and is the author's preferred injectable anesthetic. Telazol is administered IM or SC at a dose of 4 to 5 mg/kg (Bennett 1996a). Its potency allows for the administration of substantially less volume of injection, the effects are rapid, and recovery is typically quicker than with ketamine. Telazol is best used as a pre-intubation anesthetic for surgical procedures or as a sedative for diagnostic or treatment procedures. Intramuscular administration, when possible, is preferred for injectable anesthetics because induction of anesthesia is typically more rapid than with subcutaneous administration. This is likely the result of quicker or more complete venous absorption. For procedures more invasive than cutaneous lacerations inhalant anesthesia should be employed because movement of the anesthetized patient may continue with either ketamine or telazol.

An additional injectable anesthetic, propofol (Diprivan, Rapinovet), is also used in reptiles for anesthetic induction and restraint. Propofol must be administered IV or via intraosseus catheter (IO) at a dose of 3 to 10 mg/kg (Schumacher 2002a). The drug is administered slowly over thirty to sixty seconds or until the desired sedation is achieved. Propofol is eliminated rapidly from the blood and therefore is suitable for short diagnostic procedures or to achieve intubation for inhalant anesthesia. Its anesthetic effects may be extended by slow constant rate or intermittent infusion. Unless an indwelling catheter exists in the patient to be sedated, other injectable or inhalant anesthetics are preferred. Propofol is an ideal anesthetic when repeated, daily sedation is required.

Opioids such as butorphanol (Torbugesic) provide a smoother induction when administered as a premedication for injectable or inhalant induction. Butorphanol is administered IM at a dose of 0.4 to 2 mg/kg (Bennett 1996a). The author uses 1 mg/kg IM routinely for reptile surgical anesthesia.

The benefits of the anticholinergics atropine or glycopyrollate (Robinul) as preanesthetic medications in lizards are questionable. Atropine is administered IM at a dose of 0.01 to 0.04 mg/kg and glycopyrrolate is administered IM or SC at a dose of 0.01 mg/kg (Bennett 1996a). In mammals anticholinergics are administered to decrease salivary and respiratory secretions and for counteracting bradycardia during general anesthesia. These drugs may thicken respiratory secretions in reptiles (Murray 1996), causing tracheal or endotracheal tube occlusion, and their efficacy at reducing the incidence of bradycardia is uncertain.

Inhalant anesthetics are preferred for maintenance of general anesthesia in lizards. The inhalant anesthetic of choice for lizards is isoflurane (Aerrane). Another recently introduced inhalant anesthetic is sevoflurane (Schumacher 2002a). Halothane and methoxyflurane are not recommended. Isoflurane provides relatively rapid induction if used alone for short sedation procedures. Because ventilatory suppression is common during anesthesia, recovery, though smooth, is prolonged (up to fifteen minutes) compared to the typical recovery of mammals of similar size induced and maintained on isoflurane. The author has observed no benefit of quicker induction with sevoflurane in lizard patients. Additionally, recovery is typically as long or longer with sevoflurane compared to isoflurane for both healthy and health-compromised lizards. Based on the dramatic price difference between these inhalants, isoflurane is still the inhalant anesthetic of choice for lizards (Figure 6.14).

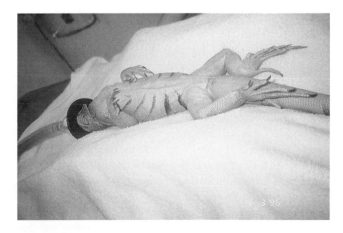

Figure 6.14. Mask anesthetic induction of a lizard.

Lizards should be intubated for inhalant anesthesia whenever possible. Intubation is relatively easy for the sedated lizard. The glottis is visible in the floor of the mouth at the base of the tongue. Minimal lubricant, if any, is applied to avoid obstruction of the small diameter tracheal tube (2 mm to 4 mm). Lizards that are too small for intubation may be maintained on a mask. A cone constructed of appropriate size syringe casing covered by a rubber glove, similar to that used for rodents, is ideal.

Reptilian respiratory physiology differs from that of mammals. In reptiles the spontaneous ventilation rate is directly related to temperature and the partial pressure of oxygen (PO_2) and in mammals respiration is driven by carbon dioxide (PCO_2) (Murray 1996). Thus, in high oxygen environments spontaneous ventilation is suppressed because the demand for oxygen by tissues is met by the oxygen saturation of inhalant anesthesia. As with mammals, control of the airway during anesthesia is helpful for the control of depth of anesthesia and is essential for assisted ventilation. Breath holding is a common problem during the induction phase of inhalant anesthesia in some lizards. Because lizards experience profound respiratory depression during general anesthesia, assisted or intermittent positive pressure ventilation (IPPV) ventilation is commonly required.

IPPV is performed at two to four breaths per minute at a pressure of less than 10 cm water in medium to large lizards and much less in smaller lizards (Bennett 1996a). Ideally the anesthetist should visualize rib expansion for several cycles of IPPV to discern the ideal pressure or ventilatory volume before the patient is draped. To avoid excessive pulmonary pressure and possible pulmonary rupture, the pop-off valve should never be fully closed when ventilating reptile patients. The great majority of lizards are maintained on a non-rebreathing anesthetic circuit. An oxygen flow rate of 300 to 500 ml/kg/minute is indicated. Lizards over 5 kg can be maintained on a closed or circle circuit (Bennett 1996a). Isoflurane is typically maintained at 1.5% to 3% depending on the sedation obtained by injectable anesthetics.

Anesthetic monitoring is essential during reptilian sedation. Unlike snakes, cardiac movement may not be detectable through the chest wall because of the presence of a cartilaginous sternum. Contrary to some reports, the author has found pulse oximetry to be satisfactory in monitoring at least the heart rate of sedated lizards. For small lizards the finger probe may be placed across the dorsal head with the infrared transducer above the head and the receiver in the mouth. For larger lizards, the orientation is reversed on the mandible, or may be placed across the tongue. The advantage of pulse oximetry is the detection of blood flow that is reflective of mechanical cardiac activity as opposed to simply the detection of cardiac electrical activity that may continue after mechanical activity is compromised. Electrocardiography (ECG) is also valuable and is used with a three lead system. A Doppler blood flow probe may be taped to the thorax over the heart for audible blood flow monitoring.

Reptile patients are warmed during surgical anesthesia with water recirculating heating pads. Electrical heating pads put the patient at risk for thermal burns. Surgical temperature should match the POTZ for a given species, but a range of 78°F to 85°F is sufficient for most patients. Supplemental heating is also indicated during the entire phase of anesthetic recovery. Lizards sedated with injectable anesthetics may require hours to recover. In debilitated animals, this time is prolonged. For ketamine and telazol, recovery times from one to ninety-six hours are reported in reptiles.

Surgery

Celiotomy is commonly performed in lizards for the surgical procedures already listed. Surgical preparation for lizards is similar to that of small mammals. The lizard is placed in dorsal recumbency with legs and tail restrained by tape to the surgical table. The surgical site should be scrubbed with mild detergent if necessary to remove dirt or debris. Standard surgical preparation is performed. The author uses or chloroxylenol 2% (Vet Solutions, Fort Worth, TX) as the sole surgical preparation. This agent, similar to chlorhexidine, provides excellent antibacterial and antifungal activity on contact. Surgical draping is required. A fenestrated paper drape or a combination of clear plastic and fenestrated paper drape is used. The benefit of clear plastic drape is visualization of the patient for anesthetic monitoring during the surgical procedure (Bennett and Mader 1996).

Surgical incisions are made with consideration for skin and abdominal musculature lines of force, trauma to tissues, visualization of the desired surgical field, and wound healing. The long accepted standard approach to celiotomy is the ventral paramedian incision in an effort to avoid transection or manipulation of the large ventral abdominal vein (see Anatomy). This incision requires the transection of ventral abdominal muscle, which increases surgical bleeding, may decrease surgical field visibility (both from bleeding and from left versus right coelom access), and may increase post surgical pain when compared to a ventral midline incision through the linea alba. In larger lizards the ventral abdominal vein may be gently retracted during the ventral midline incision.

The most common procedures performed during celiotomy are ovariosalpingectomy or salpingotomy for dystocia, ovariectomy, orchiectomy, and enterotomy. In most cases hemostatic clips are used for ligation of ovarian and oviductal vessels as indicated by surgical procedure. Great care must be exercised when handling all reproductive and mesenteric tissues in lizards, because they are delicate and quite friable. Closure of the celiotomy incision is two layers consisting of abdominal musculature or linea with absorbable suture, followed by the skin. The skin is closed in an everting pattern with absorbable or non-absorbable tissue or skin staples. Reptilian skin heals significantly slower than mammalian skin. Suture removal is delayed until a minimum of four to six weeks post surgery (Bennett and Mader 1996).

A common non-celiotomy surgical procedure is digit or limb amputation. This procedure is indicated when trauma sustained from bites of cage mates, bites from rodents, or fractures result in non-healing wounds or ascending limb infection. Surgical preparation is standard as in celiotomy. Amputation is performed at the most distal non-infected joint for limbs and preferably at the metacarpal or metatarsal-phalangeal joint for digit amputation. General anesthesia is required for limb amputations. Peripheral nerve block may be performed for some digit amputations.

Amputation of the hemipenes is indicated in cases of paraphimosis complicated by trauma, infection, or necrosis. This procedure may be performed with appropriate sedation using only injectable anesthetics such as ketamine, tiletamine/zolazepam, or propofol. Aseptic preparation is standard. Amputation of one hemipene does not sterilize the lizard because the hemipenes are paired. No compromise of urinary function will result from amputation, because there is no incorporation of urinary structures in the hemipenes or penis of reptiles (Barten 1996d).

Percloacal prolapse of colon, oviducts, or urinary bladder may require amputation or resection of the affected tissues. Exposure of affected tissues or severe trauma may result in necrosis if the prolapse is not reduced promptly after occurrence. Necrosis of large portions of these tissues may require celiotomy to evaluate viability and repair the affected organ.

Open reduction and internal fixation of long bone fractures in reptiles are performed following surgical approach and principles applied to mammals. Intramedullary pins, orthopedic wire, external skeletal fixation, and bone plating are employed as indicated.

Orthopedic devices are removed following the principles used in mammals, though healing of fractures in reptiles is slow and hardware may require removal prior to radiographic evidence of complete bone healing (Bennett 1996b).

PARASITOLOGY

Many reptile owners are unaware of the prevalence of parasitism in their animals. It is safe to assume that all wild-caught reptiles are parasitized (Lane and Mader 1996). Commonly many captive-born reptiles are subclinically parasitized. In wild animals internal parasites maintain a homeostasis with the host animal, because the host is essential for the survival of the parasite and a means of transporting future generations of the parasite to suitable areas for transmission to another host. Factors that maintain homeostasis include the host's immune system and the dilution of infective stages of the parasite in the environment that the host occupies. Thus, in many cases the captive environment offers a prime opportunity for imbalances in favor of the parasite through the stress and subsequent immunosuppression of the host and through the increased risk of reinfection of the host due to concentration of infective stages of the parasite.

Based on an awareness of parasites in some reptiles, however, some herpetoculturists advocate the prophylactic treatment of all reptiles with antiparasiticides for the more common intestinal parasites (de Vosjoli and Ferguson 1995). It is interesting, however, that the majority of hobbyists do not prophylactically treat for external parasites. This is perhaps because of an understanding of the potential side effects of pesticides applied to the animals. The side effects of oral deworming are similar. Though some therapeutics may be relatively safe at high doses, the potential effects of killing massive loads of intestinal parasites in an already immunocompromised animal can be severe. The safer alternative to prophylactic treatment of parasites is quarantine, serial parasite screening, and treatment of specific clinically identified diseases.

Techniques for identifying reptilian endoparasites are the same as those for small mammals. Fecal floatation of fresh fecal material in concentrated salt or sugar solutions and wet mount direct smears in saline are essential to screen for reptilian endoparasites. Smaller infective stages of some parasites may only be observed by direct smear. Stains such as Lugol's iodine solution (5 grams iodine crystals and 10 grams potassium iodide in 100 ml distilled water) both kills motile protozoans and stains cysts to make identification easier. Lane (1996) recommends examining both stained and unstained direct smears in addition to the fecal floatation.

External Parasites

External reptilian parasites consist of ticks, mites, chiggers, leeches, and biting flying insects. Acariasis, or mite, tick, or chigger infestation, is a serious disease of reptiles. Clinically tick infestations are most common in imported lizards. Mader (1996a) reports that there are seven genera of ticks and more than 250 species of mites that parasitize reptiles. Chiggers, also called red bugs, are the larval stage of Trombiculid mites and are generally self-limiting in lizards. Reptile mites (*Ophionyssus natricis*) are mobile and highly transmissible between reptiles and are capable of infesting multiple animals in a room or household without direct contact between hosts. These mites may be transmitted between hosts on the skin or clothing of people, though human infestation is supposedly rare.

Reptile skin provides many sites for attachment and protection for both mites and ticks. Ticks are commonly found beneath scales or in crevices such as the junction of the limbs and body or around the eyelids. Mites may be seen crawling freely over the lizard, but commonly concentrate in protected skin folds. It is not uncommon to diagnose mites after handling a lizard and then observing them on the human skin or seeing dead mites in water bowls of lizards that soak themselves routinely. Lizards that increase soaking behavior are commonly infested with mites.

Eradicating mites from individual animals is easier than eradicating them from the premises. Infestation of one animal indicates the possibility and likelihood of widespread infestation. Thus, prevention through quarantine of new animals is imperative (see Husbandry) and treating the cage and cage accessories and maintaining cleanliness of the surrounding environment is imperative.

Treatment consists of physical removal of ticks and inspection for the presence of ticks over several weeks. For mites the best treatment is pyrethroid flea sprays such as flea sprays for dogs and cats. Pyrethroids are synthetic pyrethrins and are less toxic to reptiles than pyrethrins. Allethrin is a common example of a pyrethroid. Note: Sprays containing pyrethrins or organophosphates should be avoided (Mader 1996a). Prior to spray application, mineral oil or ophthalmic lubricant should be placed on the eyes of lizards. The pyrethroid spray is then applied to the entire lizard and rinsed immediately. Avoid spraying in the mouth or onto exposed wounds or mucous membranes. Oral exposure increases the risk of toxicity. The spray must be applied in a well-ventilated area and not into partially enclosed vivaria containing animals. All exposed mites are killed on contact. Pyrethroids are effective against mites in the environment, but not against eggs; therefore, reapplication on a weekly basis for two to three weeks is advised. The author is unable to confirm reports on the safety of fipronil spray as a miticide in lizards.

Ivermectin (Ivomec, Merck; and generics) is reported as both a topical and systemic treatment for mites in reptiles (Klingenberg 1993). The topical formulation is 0.5 cc ivermectin 1% (5 mg) added in 1,000 cc water and applied as a spray. The systemic administration is 0.2 mg/kg ivermectin 1% SC or PO. Clinical experience reflects unpredictable results and variable degrees of toxicity or side effects on a species-to-species basis with the injectable protocol, though no lethality has been observed in lizards by the author. Topical administration is absolutely not reliable. The miscibility and stability of ivermectin in water as a spray is questionable.

Many over-the-counter pet industry products are available for mites. These are generally "soap and water" mixtures designed to reduce the surface tension of water and allow water to penetrate the spiracles or airways of mites that essentially drowns the mite. The active ingredients are generally fatty acids (listed by scientific name) in an aqueous base.

Other home remedies include the use of pest strips, organophosphate-impregnated resins designed to kill flying insects. These products are also quite effective in killing reptiles. Unfortunately, if used in a safe manner (or by sheer luck), these products have been effective in environmental control of mites in large collections. The narrow safety margin, however, prohibits recommendation of these products.

Finally, some insecticidal powders (Sevin dust, Ortho) have been effective in environmental control (Mader 1996a). Their use on the floor of well-ventilated cages of large terrestrial lizards beneath paper or carpet substrate is effective. This treatment is particularly effective against infestations refractory to other topical and environmental treatments. The enclosure is typically treated continuously for a period of one month and possibly repeated in one month if indicated. Note: Prepare the client for a long duration of treatment and for the strong possibility of both the contagious nature and high relapse rate of reptilian mite infestations. Also inform of the potential side effects of treatments both to lizards and humans from pyrethrins, pyrethroids, and organophosphates.

Internal Parasites

Internal parasites comprise many families and induce the majority of parasitic diseases in lizards. It is possible for many parasites to remain latent in the body and manifest disease during host immunosuppression from stress or other concurrent disease. Intestinal parasites consist of protozoa, nematodes, and trematodes.

Protozoans

Many protozoa inhabit the gastrointestinal tract of lizards as nonpathogenic or commensal organisms. The amoeba *Entamoeba invadens*, various species of coccidia, and specifically the coccidia *Cryptosporidium* spp. are responsible for the diseases amoebiasis, coccidiosis, and cryptosporidiosis, respectively.

Amoebiasis is directly transmitted by a fecal-oral route in reptiles and is pathogenic and highly virulent to some snakes and lizards. Amoebiasis is nonpathogenic in turtles and crocodilians, but may be transmitted by both (Lane and Mader 1996). The life cycle of amoebiasis is as follows: the passing of infective cysts from a host, ingestion of cysts by a suitable host, multiplication into trophozoites in the intestinal tract, invasion of trophozoites into host tissues, formation of infective cysts, and shedding of infective cysts.

The pathogenesis of clinical disease is multifactorial and is caused by the tissue invasion of trophozoites and cellular destruction and from secondary bacterial infection. Clinical signs include diarrhea or loose mucoid stools, anorexia, dehydration, and weight loss. Infective trophozoites may spread to other organs hematogenously, causing inflammation and potentially organ failure (Lane and Mader 1996).

Diagnosis is made by fecal examination. Cysts are identified by fecal floatation or direct saline smear and trophozoites are identified only by direct smear. For direct saline smears, a drop of Lugol's iodide is helpful to immobilize and stain the organisms.

Treatment of amoebiasis consists of antibiotics and antiprotozoal medications. Antibiotics are administered to treat potential secondary bacterial infections or potential septicemia. Aminoglycosides such as amikacin at a dose of 2.5 mg/kg IM or SQ every seventy-two hours for three to five treatments are appropriate. Metronidazole is administered at a dose of 50 mg/kg once weekly for two to three weeks while checking fecal samples for cysts or trophozoites (Lane and Mader 1996). Strict hygiene and sanitation are required to prevent horizontal transmission.

Coccidiosis is directly transmitted by fecal-oral route and is caused by protozoans of the genera *Eimeria*, *Isospora*, and *Caryospora*. The life cycle of coccidia is similar to that seen in mammals: oocysts passed in the stool sporulate outside the body and are ingested by a suitable host, sporozoites are released to invade host epithelial cells and mature, and the epithelial cell ruptures and releases merozoites which infect other cells and then can either multiply to infect other cells or form intracellular gametocytes which eventually become infective oocysts to pass in the stool. Clinical disease results from cellular destruction and from secondary bacterial infection. Detection of oocysts is made by fecal floatation or direct smear.

Understanding the pathophysiology is important because infective oocysts are shed intermittently; thus, clinical disease can occur in the absence of a detectable infectious agent. Clinically lizards may be asymptomatic or have diarrhea, anorexia, weight loss, or failure to gain weight. The author has observed a higher incidence of coccidiosis in bearded dragons (*Pogona* spp.) than in other species of lizard with routine fecal examination. This phenomenon is also reported in popular literature (de Vosjoli et al. 2001). Many adult lizards with coccidiosis appear to be asymptomatic carriers, but neonates and juveniles with coccidiosis are usually clinically diseased. Coccidiosis can cause death in small or young lizards if undetected and untreated.

Treatment consists trimethoprim-sulfamethoxazole (Sulfatrim) at a dose of 30 mg/kg PO once daily for fourteen days or sulfadimethoxine (Albon) at a dose of 90 mg/kg on day one, then 45 mg/kg PO once daily for fourteen days (Klingenberg 1996,; Donoghue and Landenberg 1996, Lane and Mader 1996). Strict hygiene and sanitation are required to prevent horizontal transmission. Repeat fecal examinations are imperative.

Cryptosporidiosis is a highly virulent pathogen of snakes and lizards. There is speculation regarding zoonotic potential, but at this point this potential is unknown (Cranfield and Graczyk 1996). Because cryptosporidiosis is considered untreatable in all animals caution should be exercised when handling infected animals. The pathogenesis of cryptosporidium in reptiles is not fully understood. Direct fecal-oral transmission is known to occur and it is speculated that there is a possibility of indirect transmission through an intermediate prey item. Cryptosporidiosis is reported in *Lacerta* spp., *Chamaeleo* spp., *Iguana iguana*, and two species of geckos (Cranfield and Graczyk 1996).

Oocysts are diagnosed by direct smear. Oocysts are 4 to 5 um in size and are best identified by modified acid-fast staining (Cranfield and Graczyk 1996). Serial fecal tests should be performed because of the intermittent shedding of oocysts. Diagnosis may be achieved through histopathology from gastric mucosal biopsy or by cytology of gastric lavage.

Though no treatments are known to be 100% effective, Sulfatrim as dosed for coccidia and the human drugs spiramycin and paromomycin have been used. Suspected or known positive animals are best isolated, not bred, and handled last in the maintenance of a collection of animals. Many traditional disinfectants have proved to be ineffective in environmental control. Ammonia solutions at 5% for a period of three days are effective for disinfection (Cranfield and Graczyk 1996).

Nematodes

Various nematodes infect lizards. Those infecting the gastrointestinal and respiratory tracts include various species of the familiar roundworms and hookworms; pinworms, *Oxyurus* spp.; hepatic worms, *Capillaria* spp.; strongyles, Strongyloides spp.; and lungworms of the genus *Entomelas*. Treatment for all intestinal and respiratory nematodes follows descriptions.

Roundworms in lizards are similar to those in mammals. Transmission is indirect and diagnosis is made by fecal floatation and identification of the typical thick-walled round to ovoid oocysts. Diagnosis may also be made by identification of the adult worm in feces or vomitus. Because they require an indirect life cycle, these parasites are most commonly observed in carnivorous lizards and occasionally in omnivores.

Hookworms (*Oswalsocruzia* spp.) have direct transmission by fecal-oral route or through skin penetration. Diagnosis is made by fecal floatation and identification of the typical thin-walled oval eggs. Hookworms are responsible for more clinical disease in lizards than are roundworms because of the mucosal attachment of adult worms in the intestines. Clinical signs may include diarrhea, anorexia, and weight loss.

Pinworms (*Oxyurus* spp.) have a direct transmission by fecal-oral route and are found as adults in the large intestine of lizards. Diagnosis is made by fecal floatation and identification of the typically embryonated cigar-shaped larvae. Mammal pinworm ova or larvae may be passed in the stool of carnivorous lizards but do not infect the lizards themselves. Typically pinworms are an incidental finding on fecal examination, though diagnosed infections should be treated.

Hepatic worms (*Capillaria* spp.) have both direct and indirect transmission by fecal-oral route or through infected prey ingestion, and the oocysts somewhat resemble those of whipworms (*Trichuris* spp.) of dogs. *Capillaria* spp. typically inhabit the intestinal tract but may also migrate to other organs. Pathology due to these species is unclear. Diagnosis is made by fecal floatation and treatment is indicated on identification.

Strongyloides spp. have a somewhat complex life cycle with direct transmission by a fecal-oral route or through skin penetration. *Strongyloides* spp. inhabit the gastrointestinal tract and greatly resemble the lungworms *Entomelas* spp. on fecal flotation. Diagnosis for either species is made by fecal floatation and identification of larvae (*Strongyloides* spp.) or embryonated eggs (*Entomelas* spp.). Diarrhea, anorexia, or weight loss may be seen with *Strongyloides* infection. Increased respiratory secretions, pneumonia, anorexia, and weight loss may be seen with *Entomelas* infections.

Treatment of all intestinal and respiratory nematodes consists of fenbendazole (Panacur) at a dose of 50 mg/kg PO once daily for three days, then repeated in three weeks followed by repeat fecal flotation (Klingenberg 1996). Because the majority of nematode parasites have direct transmission, proper hygiene and sanitation are imperative.

Cestodes

Tapeworms are infrequently encountered in captive lizards. Transmission is indirect, typically through an arthropod intermediate host as seen in dogs and cats. Diagnosis is made by observations of proglottids in the stool or identification of oocysts on fecal flotation. Treatment consists of praziquantel (Droncit) 5 to 8 mg/kg PO or IM and treatment is repeated in two weeks (Klingenberg 1996).

Treatment of intestinal parasites in lizards is not without potential side effects. Anecdotal reports of sudden deaths in *Chamaeleo* spp. treated with standard single doses of fenbendazole and ivermectin (Stahl 1998) are known and the author has observed this effect on several occasions. Over several years the author has made similar observations of a dramatic decline in health following the deworming of some individuals of wild-caught *Uromastyx* spp., *Varanus* spp., and *Chlamydosaurus* spp. at a reptile wholesale distribution facility. Some of the affected animals had no apparent compromised health prior to treatment, but were housed with conspecifics in relatively small cages, experienced repeated movement of humans around the enclosures, and may not have been on the optimal plane of nutrition (Color Plates 6.9–6.20).

EMERGENCIES

Many health disorders of lizards are potential emergencies simply because of the latency in which they are

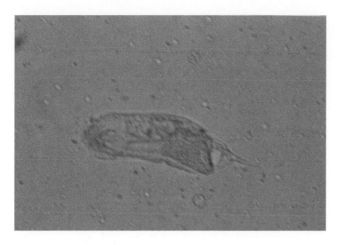

Plate 6.9. *Flagellate, original magnification 40×. (Photo courtesy of Zoo Atlanta.) (See also color plates)*

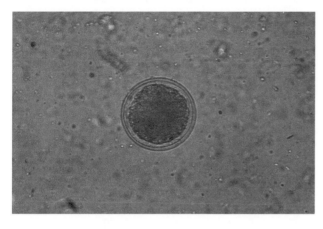

Plate 6.10. *Roundworm, original magnification 40×. (Photo courtesy of Zoo Atlanta.) (See also color plates)*

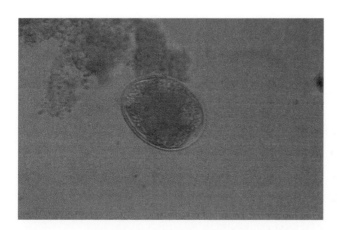

Plate 6.11. *Ascarid, original magnification 40×. (Photo courtesy of Zoo Atlanta.) (See also color plates)*

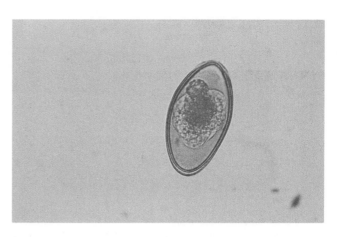

Plate 6.12. *Oxyurid, original magnification 40×. (Photo courtesy of Zoo Atlanta.) (See also color plates)*

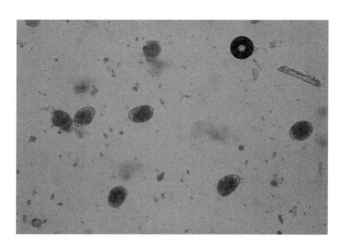

Plate 6.13. *Ascarid, original magnification 40×. (Photo courtesy of Zoo Atlanta.) (See also color plates)*

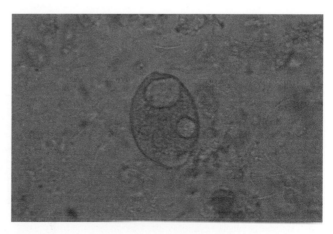

Plate 6.14. *Coccidia, original magnification 40×. (Photo courtesy of Zoo Atlanta.) (See also color plates)*

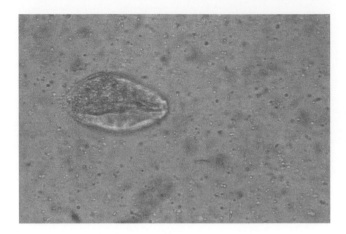

Plate 6.15. Nyctotherus, original magnification 40×. (Photo courtesy of Zoo Atlanta.) (See also color plates)

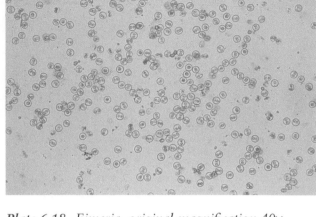

Plate 6.18. Eimeria, original magnification 40×. (Photo courtesy of Zoo Atlanta.) (See also color plates)

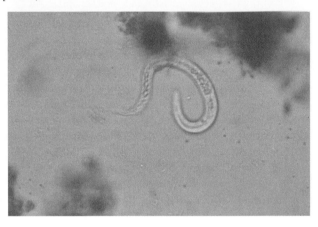

Plate 6.16. Strongyle larva, original magnification 40×. (Photo courtesy of Zoo Atlanta.) (See also color plates)

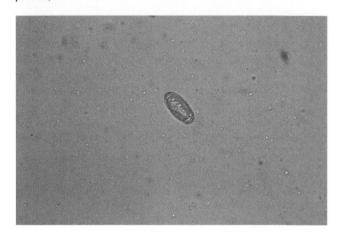

Plate 6.19. Capillaria, original magnification 40×. (Photo courtesy of Zoo Atlanta.) (See also color plates)

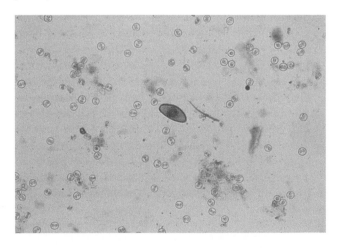

Plate 6.17. Pinworm and eimeria, original magnification 40×. (Photo courtesy of Zoo Atlanta.) (See also color plates)

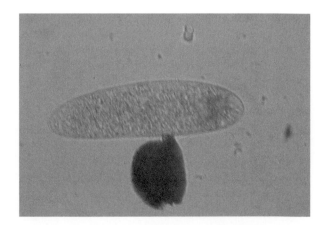

Plate 6.20. Pinworm, original magnification 40 ×. (Photo courtesy of Zoo Atlanta.) (See also color plates)

presented or other related or consequential disorders with which they present. A few diseases or presenting complaints, however, are considered critical and death is imminent without immediate medical care. Some critical cases may present moribund or deceased and may require the same level of diagnostic attention to determine the cause of death.

Trauma

Trauma, as with any animal, may be an emergency. Many cases of trauma present ambiguously because the patient is found in a compromised state and the owner did not observe the inciting cause. Trauma should be suspected whenever the onset of clinical signs is acute; that is, within hours of the patient observed in a normal state and no history of gradual onset of lethargy, anorexia, weight loss, pregnancy, or other abnormal physiology. The presence of a thin or dehydrated animal or any history of anorexia should indicate the presence of another or an additional underlying disease process. Infectious or metabolic diseases rarely show acute clinical signs in lizards.

Diagnosis of trauma may be speculative because no external clinical abnormalities may be apparent. Radiography is the desired diagnostic test to evaluate for abnormal anatomy. Hematocrit and blood profile parameters may be normal, though creatine kinase (CK) values are commonly elevated with skeletal muscle injury. Radiographically suspected intracoelomic fluid may be aspirated for analysis.

With a high degree of suspicion of traumatic injury, empirically derived doses of corticosteroids are indicated in addition to providing proper thermal gradient. Warmed intravenous, intraosseus, or intracoelomic fluids are indicated for hypotension. Stabilization of fractures or luxations is performed following cardiovascular and thermal stabilization.

Toxicity

Unless presented with the known history of chemical toxicity, the veterinary staff must be meticulous at obtaining a history to support this diagnosis. The clinical signs of chemical or pesticide toxicity in reptiles are ambiguous, which leads to a diagnosis by exclusion of other metabolic diseases and delay in appropriate treatment. Generally, chemical toxicities in lizards are relatively acute and have no history of anorexia, paralysis, or weight loss preceding the onset of clinical signs.

The most common exogenous chemical toxicities in lizards are exposure to pesticides containing pyrethrins or organophosphates that are applied to treat mite infestations of the patient or the enclosure. Profound depression, death, or a variety of neurologic abnor-malities including muscle postural abnormalities, tremors or fasciculations, seizures, and paralysis may occur.

With reasonable suspicion of pesticide toxicity treatment is similar to that of mammals, including cleaning or removal of the inciting cause, supportive care, and treatment with anticholinergics (see Common Disorders). Diazepam at 2.5 mg/kg IV or IM is reported for seizures (Rossi 1998a, Schumacher 2002b).

Hypocalcemic Metabolic Bone Disease

This form of metabolic bone disease (MBD) is separated from the classic osteopathic MBD. Diagnosis of hypocalcemic MBD should be suspected of any patient presenting with abnormal neurologic signs and no history of trauma or toxin exposure. Physiologically this disease is gradual in onset, though the onset of clinical signs may be acute or subtle and unnoticed by the owner. Herbivorous or insectivorous lizards are clinically most affected, but all lizards are susceptible to hypocalcemia. History regarding diet and light exposure may help to confirm suspicion of this disease prior to diagnostic testing.

The most common clinical signs include hind limb paresis or paralysis, muscle fasciculations or twitching, and depression. It is not uncommon for the only clinical sign to be hind limb paresis with a normal appetite and no other physical abnormality. The progression of clinical signs from paresis to profound mental depression is usually gradual. Hypocalcemic MBD is a critical emergency when the patient is substantially depressed or stuporous.

Diagnosis is highly suspected and supported by history in herbivorous lizards fed improper diets, no calcium or vitamin D_3 supplements, or little to no exposure to ultraviolet light. Diagnosis is confirmed with blood chemistry. Radiographs may be helpful in excluding other disorders such as trauma or diminished bone density, but they do not confirm hypocalcemia.

Treatment is supportive with warming; IV, IO, or IC fluids; and calcium gluconate at 100 mg/kg SC, IM, or IC. Treatment is long term and prognosis for recovery is grave for the most critical cases.

Gastrointestinal Obstruction

Signs of gastrointestinal obstruction may be vague, though history supports a gradual onset (days) of anorexia, constipation, depression, weight loss, bloating, and rarely regurgitation. All species of lizards are susceptible, but terrestrial lizards are much more likely to ingest foreign materials from their environment. Impaction or constipation may occur in arboreal insectivorous lizards, especially if dehydrated. A diagnosis of obstruction may also be supported by a history of feeding improper foods, such as processed meat products to herbivores.

Diagnosis is based on history, physical exam, and radiographs. The radiographic presence of a foreign body or generalized gas distention of small and/or large intestine is indicative of obstruction. Because large herbivorous lizards have a relatively large distensible gut and relatively narrow pelvic canal, obstruction may occur much lower in the gastrointestinal tract than is classically seen in dogs and cats. Obstructions at the pelvic inlet exhibit marked abdominal bloating and commonly large and small intestinal gas distention. If these signs are observed radiographically in the absence of a detectable foreign body, retrograde percloacal barium is indicated to identify the obstruction. On rare occasions repeated enemas administered by the owner or veterinary staff may result in colonic perforation and stricture that may mimic foreign body obstruction. With the degree of gas distention commonly seen in obstruction, ultrasound may be of little value diagnostically.

With high degree of suspicion of obstruction in the depressed patient, supportive care and surgery are indicated. Trocharization to relieve gas is not indicated because the thin gastrointestinal membranes may rupture and spill their contents into the coelomic cavity. Careful advancement of an oral feeding tube may aid in the reduction of bloating presurgically.

Dystocia

Dystocia, also called egg-binding, in oviparous lizards has varying degrees of presentation in lizards with many similarities to birds. Single or multiple eggs may be retained and the lizard may be in varying degrees of physical health. Those lizards presented with dystocia in a profoundly weakened state must receive immediate supportive care and surgery. Placement of IO catheter and fluid therapy is indicated.

Diagnosis is confirmed with history, physical exam, and radiographs. Ovario-salpingectomy is indicated for lizards with dystocias of more than a few retained eggs because surgery time is greatly extended for multiple salpingotomy incisions that are required for multiple eggs. Lizards retain reproductive ability when ovariosalpingotomy or unilateral ovariosalpingectomy is performed.

Pneumonia

Though generally a straightforward diagnosis, at first appearance pneumonia may be confused with severe cases of stomatitis with no associated respiratory disease in lizards. History usually indicates a gradual onset of disease with a moderate to prolonged period of anorexia, weight loss, and increased respiratory effort. Oral or nasal exudates may or may not be present. Thorough physical exam, including thoracic auscultation and thoracic radiographs, is required for definitive diagnosis of pneumonia. Stomatitis may be concurrent or absent. Profound weakness and depression may be the result of profoundly reduced ventilatory capacity or secondary septicemia. Diagnostics and medical treatment are discussed in Common Disorders.

Oxygen therapy is generally not indicated due to respiratory suppression (see Anesthesia). IO fluid therapy and antibiotics are indicated. Nutritional support may be required for prolonged periods. Asphyxiation is a concern because the lizard may be too weakened to expel pulmonary exudates. Passage of a rubber feeding tube and aspiration of tracheal secretions may be performed with caution. Transtracheal wash procedures are performed only in patients that are not critically compromised.

Cloacal Proplapse

Cloacal prolapse is diagnosed by physical examination alone. This disease is an emergency with respect to potential necrosis and loss of tissue from time delay in presentation and treatment.

First aid of cloacal prolapse is cleaning and hydrating prolapsed tissue with isotonic solution. Following diagnosis of the specific nature of the prolapse, hypertonic solutions such as 50% dextrose may be applied to reduce swelling. Sedation or general anesthesia is often indicated to reduce patient struggling and pain. Reduction of viable tissue is first attempted manually when possible and then approached surgically. Systemic antibiotics are indicated despite the method of reduction. Corticosteroids may be administered empirically. The occurrence of reperfusion injury in reptiles is not known.

TECHNIQUES

Intravenous and Intraosseous Catheter Placement

Intravenous (IV) catheter placement is generally limited to the medium to large species of lizards, approximately 20 cm or larger, in the cephalic vein, though there is no reason not to consider catheterization of smaller lizards with proper equipment and skill (Figure 6.15). Sedation is required for catheterization (Jenkins 1996).

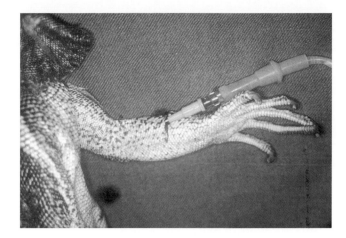

Figure 6.15. Cephalic catheter placement.

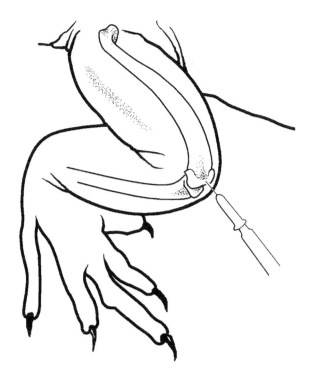

Figure 6.16. IO catheter placement.

Standard sterile preparation of the catheterization site is performed and a transverse skin incision is made across the dorsal distal aspect of the antebrachium, just dorsal to the carpus. The incision in smaller lizards can be made with the sharp angle of a hypodermic needle or with a scalpel blade in the case of larger lizards. Once the vein is identified, standard catheterization technique is used with an appropriate sized intravenous catheter. The catheter is secured with tape or suture.

Intraosseous (IO) catheters are indicated in smaller lizards or those with anatomy or disease that prohibits intravenous catheter placement. The bones of choice for intraosseous catheterization are the femur, tibia, or humerus. Consideration must be given to the location with respect to the ability of the patient to interfere with or manipulate the catheter while hospitalized.

For femoral IO catheterization, standard sterile preparation is performed over the distal femur and a spinal needle of appropriate size is passed through a cutdown in the skin. The needle is advanced through the cortical bone of the distal diaphysis and then directed proximally into the medullary cavity of the bone. The tip of the needle should rest in the medullary cavity approximately one-third the distance from the proximal femur (Jenkins 1996). The catheter is then secured with taping that will also somewhat immobilize the stifle (Figure 6.16).

Sterile hypodermic needles of appropriate size may be used if spinal needles are not available. The tibia is catheterized with a proximal to distal approach. Intravenous and intraosseus fluid therapy is performed with lactated Ringer's solution (LRS) and LRS + 2.5% dextrose at a rate of 0.5 to 1 ml/kg/hour (Jenkins 1996).

Venipuncture

Blood collection in lizards is performed from the caudal tail vein or rarely from the ventral abdominal vein. Small patients are placed in dorsal recumbency and may be wrapped in a towel to ease restraint. Large lizards may remain in ventral recumbency with the tail supported off the edge of a table. Fractious, dangerous, or very small and delicate lizards may require brief anesthesia for blood collection.

A portion of the proximal third of the tail from the vent is selected and aseptically prepared as if for surgery. A needle of appropriate length and gauge is selected for the patient. For lizards greater than 60 cm total length, a 22-gauge 1- to 1.5-inch needle on a 3-cc syringe is appropriate. For lizards less than 60 cm total length, a 22- to 25-gauge 0.5- to 0.75-inch needle on a 1-cc syringe is appropriate. For lizards less than 25 cm total length, a 27-gauge 0.5-inch needle on a 1-cc or smaller syringe is appropriate. Insulin syringes are commonly used for these smallest patients.

Blood collection is performed in a manner similar to that of venipuncture of the tail vein of a cow. The needle is advanced through the skin along the ventral midline in a perpendicular to slightly cranially directed angle until the tip of the needle contacts the vertebral body. Slight vacuum is applied to the syringe as the needle is slowly withdrawn until blood is seen entering the needle hub. Blood collection is slow and may require fifteen to thirty seconds for large lizards and up to forty-five seconds for smaller lizards.

Care is taken to slowly expel blood into the collection tube(s) to prevent hemolysis from narrow-gauge needles. Lithium heparin (green top) tubes are the collection tube of choice for reptile biochemistry and complete blood count (CBC). EDTA may lyse reptilian erythrocytes when used for CBC (Mader and Rosenthal 2000). Whenever possible, the needles of 25 gauge or smaller should be removed from the syringe prior to transferring blood. Most labs that perform reptilian blood chemistries are capable of using samples as small as 25 uL (0.25 cc). CBC may be submitted as a blood smear instead of whole blood when only a small sample is available for serum chemistry.

The ventral abdominal vein may be accessed in very small lizards or in those in which tail autotomy is likely. These patients should be anesthetized. The blood collection site is prepared with the patient in dorsal recumbency and accessed along the ventral midline at a point between the sternum and one-third the distance proximal to the pelvis. The bevel of the needle is directed dorsally and the needle advanced just beneath the skin while applying slight suction (Jenkins 1996). Blood collection may be faster when compared to collection from the ventral tail vein. Cardiocentesis is not recommended for blood collection in lizards because of the risk of trauma and the relative lack of access of the heart in lizards (Figure 6.17).

Transtracheal Wash

Microbiology and cytology specimens may be collected from the lungs in a matter consistent with that of mammals. The glottis is easily visualized in patients that cooperate with opening the mouth. Light sedation

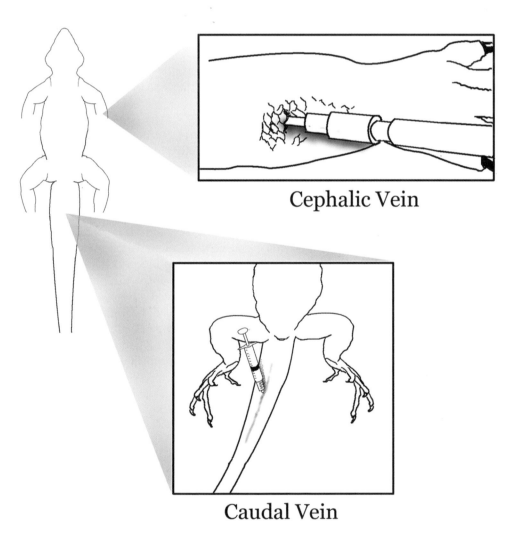

Cephalic Vein

Caudal Vein

Figure 6.17. Lizard venipuncture sites.

may be required for patients that are reluctant to open the mouth. Following a diagnosis of pneumonia a sterile catheter of appropriate diameter and length is advanced through the glottis and directed into the right or left lung as indicated by radiographs. A sterile wire may be inserted into the catheter and molded (using sterile technique) to aid the direction of the tip into the left or right mainstem bronchus (Murray 1996). At no time should the tube be forced if resistance is encountered. A speculum is employed to keep fingers out of the mouth and aid in visualization during the procedure.

Following placement of the catheter, warmed (to ambient temperature of the patient) sterile saline solution is infused at a dose of 1 to 5 ml/kg body weight and then retrieved into the syringe (Murray 1996). Repeated flushing of the saline, gentle coupage, or gentle rolling of the patient following infusion, increases the return of diagnostic material. Following collection the patient is carefully monitored for normal respiration and heart rate. Samples should be submitted for appropriate culture and sensitivity and cytology. Portions of the sample may be preserved in EDTA or fixed on a microscopic slide for cytologic analysis.

When transtracheal wash is contraindicated, bacterial culture and sensitivity may be obtained from pulmonary exudates swabbed from the glottis by culturette. By observing the patient's respiratory cycle, a microtip culturette is carefully inserted into the glottis and then retrieved in a matter not to retrieve oral secretions. This method may not reflect the bacterial population present in the lower respiratory tract.

Cloacal and Colonic Wash and Enema

Techniques for cloacal and colonic wash are applicable for microbiologic and cytologic sample collection, enema, and barium administration for contrast radiography. Colonic wash is performed in the absence of a fresh fecal sample for parasite analysis. Retrograde percloacal colonic catheterization is not as routine and as simple as performed in mammals and improper technique can result in severe health consequences to the patient. Sedation is not commonly required except in fractious patients.

A clean catheter similar to that used for transtracheal wash, a saline-filled syringe, and water-based lubricant are used. Dosage for colonic wash is approximately 10 ml/kg (Schumacher 2002b).

Copious lubrication of the tube is recommended for all procedures. Careful and slow advancement of the catheter in a retrograde fashion through the cloaca will reach the colon. On occasion the urinary bladder may

be accessed accidentally. The urodeum lies ventrally and the coprodeum lies dorsally in the cranial cloaca.

It is imperative not to force the catheter if any resistance is encountered upon advancement. The coelomic tissues may be ruptured easily and the technician or clinician may not perceive a rupture based on the resistance encountered. Occasionally, the slow infusion of fluid upon advancement of the catheter will aid in reducing resistance, especially with constipated animals. Once the catheter has reached the lower intestine, saline solution is infused and retrieved several times and gentle massage of the colon may be applied to maximize return of diagnostic material. A swab and floatation may be performed on the retrieved sample.

Administration of saline or stool softeners such as docusate sodium solution is applied in a similar manner to that of other companion animals. Resistance should never be achieved upon the syringe plunger with the administration of any colonic solutions.

In the event of suspected or confirmed iatrogenic colonic or cloacal rupture, surgery is immediately indicated for primary repair of the defect and copious lavage of the coelom. Most cases of iatrogenic ruptures unfortunately go unnoticed until the animal presents with life-threatening coelomitis and sepsis.

Cloacal swabs for bacterial culture and sensitivity may be obtained in a manner similar to that performed in birds. Washing of the external vent is indicated to reduce contamination of the culturette upon insertion and sample retrieval.

Bandaging

Bandage application and wound care for skin defects are consistent with those of other companion animals with the exception that the healing process is prolonged. Except for deep or extensive wounds or those that may become contaminated, wounds on most lizards are best maintained open in a clean environment rather than bandaged. Bandages may be cumbersome to lizards or may be a source of rubbing or other behaviors that attempt to remove the bandage. Tape is contraindicated on all geckos or other lizards with fragile skin.

Bandage application may be indicated for tail autotomy and amputations temporarily after surgery. Application of antibiotic ointments and gauze-packed syringe casings are ideal to allow hemorrhage control and prevent contamination. Typically these bandages are required for only a few days.

External coaptation of limbs is commonly performed as part of fracture management using materials and techniques applied for other companion animals. The same principles of stabilizing one joint above and below the fracture are followed. A potential splint for larger lizards is their own body. Under sedation forelimbs are secured to the lateral chest wall, with care not to compress the chest cavity, especially in sedated animals. A similar application may be employed with the hind limb to the tail. With this technique, however, proximal humeral and femoral fractures may not receive adequate reduction in motion of the proximal bone fragment, resulting in malalignment.

Spica splints are ideal for both forelimb and hind limb unilateral or bilateral fracture management. Under sedation the rigid splint for forelimb humeral fractures is incorporated into the soft bandage ventrally across the sternum and in the hind limb the splint is applied dorsally across the dorsal pelvis. The soft support bandage of the hind limb is wrapped in a figure-eight pattern incorporating both hind limbs dorsally, creating abduction of both hind limbs. A similar technique is applied forelimb soft bandage. This technique allows for the cloaca to remain free of bandage material and to reduce contamination of bandage material (Bennett 1996b). For more distal fractures of limbs a modified Robert Jones bandage incorporating or encased by a plastic syringe casing and stirrups is ideal.

Carpal, tarsal, and digital fractures may be bandaged with soft bandage material. A ball bandage comprised of a cotton ball applied to the palmar or plantar aspect of the affected foot is wrapped by soft bandage (Bennett 1996b). For all bandage applications, lizards should be maintained on clean non-organic substrate such as paper or carpet, including those lizards requiring a higher humidity environment. Strict attention is given to cage and bandage sanitation and hygiene.

Assist Feeding

One of the most common signs of any disease state in lizards is anorexia. Assist feeding is employed when the normal feeding response is diminished or when the animal is physically incapable of normal prehension or swallowing of food or water.

The technique for assist feeding may also be applied to gastric oral medication administration and diagnostic gastric lavage. Some species of lizards may require sedation to access the oral cavity (*Uromastyx* spp., *Corucia zebrata*, and occasionally *Iguana* spp. and *Varanus* spp.). These species, especially *Uromastyx* and *Corucia*, are candidates for pharyngostomy tube placement when repeated force feeding or oral medication is required.

Assist feeding of lizards is accomplished in several ways. Voluntary feeding for smaller lizards is applied when the patient's normal feeding response or mobility is compromised, but with a little enticement the patient will readily prehend and swallow food. For large or dangerous lizards, tongs or forceps are used to introduce food. Assist feeding is used for patients that can swallow but are otherwise reluctant to prehend prey items; the mouth may be gently opened and the food item placed into the mouth for the patient to swallow. Prepared foods such as vegetarian gruels may be fed by syringe in this matter. Assist feeding is used for patients that are depressed and will not swallow or are incapable of chewing; food is provided by gastric or pharyngostomy feeding tube.

For insectivorous and carnivorous species that are fed only every other day or every few days in normal health, the normal feeding schedule may remain the same. It is important for all lizards to not over feed, especially if assist feeding normal dietary food items. Constipation or obstruction can result from overzealous feeding in these patients. For those species fed specially prepared gruels either by mouth or through a feeding tube, daily feeding is recommended because it is likely that these diets are more rapidly digested and absorbed when compared to the diet of normal health.

The procedures of tube assist feeding are similar to those applied for neonatal companion animals. The stomach of quadruped lizards is measured to the last few ribs. Anguiform lizards are treated as snakes for tube feeding purposes. Rubber catheters or stainless steel ball-tipped dosing needles are appropriate to use as feeding tubes. Because of the stresses imposed on the patient from restraint and opening the mouth by assist and force feeding, feeding frequency is generally no more than once daily for these patients. Alternatively, placement of a pharyngostomy tube accommodates smaller volume multiple daily feedings (Figure 6.18).

Diets are based on identifying the patient as carnivorous (including juvenile omnivorous) or herbivo-

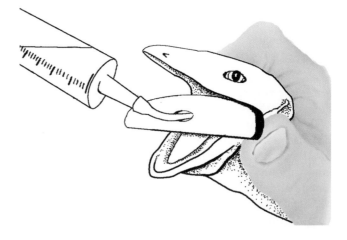

Figure 6.18. Assist-feeding.

rous (including adult omnivorous). The amount of feeding is a calculated daily energy need based on standard metabolic rate (SMR) measured in kcal/day. The formula is SMR = $32*BW^{77}$ where BW = body weight in kg. Alert and relatively non-compromised patients receive 75% to 100% of daily energy needs in the first twenty-four to forty-eight hours. Weak or debilitated patients receive 40% to 75% of their daily energy needs in the first several days (Donoghue and Landenberg 1996). The amount of feeding of the daily energy requirement is gradually increased to 100% as the patient's health and responsiveness improve. And, because the goal of force feeding is to bring the patient back to voluntary feeding, the amount and frequency of force feeding decreases or may abruptly stop pending the patient's recovery.

A variety of enteral diets are available for both human and veterinary use. These include: for omnivores Ensure (Ross Laboratories, Columbus, OH), for herbivores Sustacal Enriched (Ross Laboratories, Columbus, OH), and for carnivores Clinical-Care feline and canine liquids (Pet-Ag, Elgin, IL). The available energy in kcal/ml as well as protein, fat, carbohydrate, and fiber content are available on the packaging.

Therapeutic Administration

Treatment of lizard patients with pharmaceuticals is performed in a manner consistent with that of mammals with several exceptions. First, the oral administration is not always the route of choice: (1) Oral access may be difficult or stressful for some patients receiving daily medications; (2) gastrointestinal transit time and factors affecting absorption of medications varies among species; (3) inexperience or reluctance of the client in administering oral medications may lead to unnecessary trauma to the patient or noncompliance by the owner. When properly counseled, however, most clients enjoy the opportunity to take an active role in restoring the health of their pets.

Examples of antibiotics commonly administered orally in lizards are enrofloxacin injectable and compounded suspensions (Baytril), griseofulvin suspension (Fulvicin), metronidazole injectable and compounded suspensions, sulfamethazine (Albon), trimethoprim-sulfamethoxazole (Bactrim), and compounded tetracyclines. Additionally, many injectable antibiotics or ophthalmic preparations may be applied directly to oral mucous membranes rather than by injectable method to achieve higher drug concentrations at the site of infection. The parasiticides fenbendazole (Panacur) and praziquantel (Droncit) are administered PO. The author does not recommend the application of antibiotics to drinking water or to food items for lizards because of potential drug inactivity and the difficulty in accurate dosing.

Injections are performed using five methods. Subcutaneous (SC) and intramuscular (IM) techniques are most common. Intracoelomic (ICe) technique is used for large volumes of fluids or for drugs that need rapid systemic absorption such as calcium gluconate. Intravenous and intraosseous are typically performed through an indwelling catheter.

It is generally uncommon for clients to administer injectable medications to mammalian patients for routine infections. This practice is relatively common for reptile patients, but it must be approached with great attention to both the client's ability and the patient's cooperation. Considerations include:

1. What is the risk of injury to both the client and patient from the proposed procedure?
2. Is the client capable of adequately restraining the patient while administering the medication?
3. Is the client capable of determining if an undesirable side effect has occurred that prohibits further treatment?
4. Is there risk for abuse of the medication dispensed?

When dispensing injectable medication for the client to administer, adhere to the following:

1. Dispense the medication *premeasured* in syringes for each dose and *only* the amount for the specified number of doses. Administration should be only by the SC or IM route for home administration. If long-term treatment is required, dispense a portion of the amount and only refill the medication with a recheck exam or consultation. Accurately and fully label drug name, concentration, route, frequency, and duration of administration with no abbreviations. Never dispense medications that are potentially dangerous to humans at the prescribed dose (large doses of aminoglycosides, chemotherapeutics, narcotics).
2. Describe, show, and allow the client to practice administration of the medication. Sterile saline may be used for a practice injection.
3. Instruct the client on the appropriate uncapping and capping of needles and handling of the sterile needle.
4. Counsel the client on potential side effects of the drug and potential side effects administration. Describe "what can possibly go wrong" scenarios.
5. Provide the name and number of an employee at the clinic who can be reached at any time if there is a problem.

6. Have the client bring all medical waste products to the hospital or clinic for disposal.

Subcutaneous injections are made in the lateral scapular region. The skin is not drawn or lifted above the body wall as is common practice in mammals. The needle is advanced into the subcuticular space, gentle aspiration is applied to check for incidental venous access, and the injection is administered. Serial injections are alternated between the left and right sides and among different locations within the region. Subcutaneous injections are contraindicated in most *Chamaeleo* spp., all *Phelsuma* spp., and many other Gekkonidae because of skin autotomy, scarring, and skin discoloration caused by the injection. PO administration is indicated in these species.

Intramuscular injections are administered in epaxial muscles or triceps muscles in large lizards. IM injections are generally not possible in smaller lizards. When possible, intramuscular injections are preferred for lizards to decrease the risk of skin inflammation.

Intracoelomic injections are administered in the right lower quadrant of the abdomen slightly cranial dorsal to the rear leg (Klingenberg 1996). Drugs administered in this way are sterile fluids, calcium gluconate, potassium penicillin, and some injectable anesthetics.

It is essential to understand not only the intended use of the medication, but also potential undesired or side effects. Side effects may be the result of a single administration, a series of administrations, a route of administration, or a cumulative dose. Individual variation as seen in mammals may also occur in reptiles. Side effects also involve the restraint or manipulation necessary to administer a particular administration. When considering the use of therapeutics, the old adage "do no harm" must be remembered.

EUTHANASIA

Euthanasia of captive lizards may be required for several reasons. The procedures for lizard euthanasia more closely resemble those of domestic laboratory animals than of dogs and cats. The relative inaccessibility of peripheral veins for injection of euthanasia solution necessitates injection of euthanasia solution directly into the heart (Mader 1996b) or occasionally into the occipital sinus or foramen magnum. Intracoelomic injection of euthanasia solution can be performed, but cardiac arrest may be prolonged and detection of death uncertain. The client must be fully prepared for euthanasia techniques prior to performing the procedures.

Humane euthanasia in the veterinary hospital is best performed under heavy sedation with the dissociative agents ketamine or telazol. Ketamine at a dose of 100 mg/kg IM or telazol at a dose of 25 mg/kg IM will assure adequate sedation (Mader 1996b). Euthanasia solution as specified by the manufacturer for mammals is applied to lizards. Injections may be given intracardially with a sternal or lateral percutaneous approach to the heart. If the patient is dehydrated or severely debilitated and the cardiac approach is not possible, injection into the occipital sinus is indicated.

REFERENCES

Balsai M. 1997. *General Care and Maintenance of Popular Monitors and Tegus*. Escondido: Advanced Vivarium Systems.

Barten SL. 1996a. Biology: Lizards. In: *Reptile Medicine and Surgery*, edited by Mader DR. Philadelphia: W.B. Saunders Co. 47–61.

Barten SL. 1996b. Differential Diagnosis by Symptoms: Lizards. In: *Reptile Medicine and Surgery*, edited by Mader DR. Philadelphia: W.B. Saunders Co. 324–232.

Barten SL. 1996c. Specific Diseases and Conditions: Bites from Prey. In: *Reptile Medicine and Surgery*, edited by Mader DR. Philadelphia: W.B. Saunders Co. 353–355.

Barten SL. 1996d. Specific Diseases and Conditions: Paraphimosis. In: *Reptile Medicine and Surgery*, edited by Mader DR. Philadelphia: W.B. Saunders Co. 395–396.

Barten SL. 2002. Diseases of the Iguana Oral Cavity. In: *Proceedings of the North American Veterinary Conference* (16). Gainesville, FL.

Bennett RA. 1996a. Special Techniques and Procedures: Anesthesia. In: *Reptile Medicine and Surgery*, edited by Mader DR. Philadelphia; W.B. Saunders Co. 241–247.

Bennett RA. 1996b. Special Techniques and Procedures: Fracture Management. In: *Reptile Medicine and Surgery*, edited by Mader DR. Philadelphia: W.B. Saunders Co. 281–287.

Bennett RA. 1996c. Specific Diseases and Conditions: Cryptosporidiosis. In: *Reptile Medicine and Surgery*, edited by Mader DR. Philadelphia: W.B. Saunders Co. 359–363.

Bennett RA, Mader DR. 1996. Special Techniques and Procedures: Soft Tissue Surgery. In: *Reptile Medicine and Surgery*, edited by Mader DR. Philadelphia: W.B. Saunders Co. 287–298.

Boyer TH. 1996. Specific Diseases and Conditions: Metabolic Bone Disease. In: *Reptile Medicine and Surgery*, edited by Mader DR. Philadelphia: W.B. Saunders. 385–392.

Cranfield MR, Graczyk TK. 1996. Specific Diseases and Conditions: Cryptosporidiosis. In: *Reptile Medicine and Surgery*, edited by Mader DR. Philadelphia: W.B. Saunders Co. 359–363.

DeNardo D. 1996a. Special Topics: Reproductive Biology. In: *Reptile Medicine and Surgery*, edited by Mader DR. Philadelphia: W.B. Saunders Co. 212–224.

DeNardo D. 1996b. Specific Diseases and Conditions: Dystocias. In: *Reptile Medicine and Surgery*, edited by Mader DR. Philadelphia: W.B. Saunders Co. 370–374.

de Vosjoli P. 1992. *The Green Iguana Manual*. Lakeside, CA: Advanced Vivarium Systems.

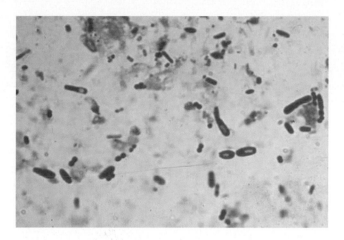

Plate 2.1. *Clostridial overgrowth is apparent in this fecal Gram stain from a parrot. Clostridium shown here is a large Gram-positive rod with no spore, a clear central spore (safety pin shape), or clear end spore (racket shape).*

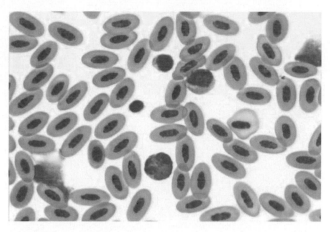

Plate 2.2. *A Diff-Quick stained blood smear from a parrot. Note that birds have nucleated red blood cells. The cell at the twelve o'clock position is a lymphocyte, the two o'clock position is a monocyte, the six o'clock position is a heterophil (like a neutrophil), and the nine o'clock position is a normally occurring nucleated thrombocyte.*

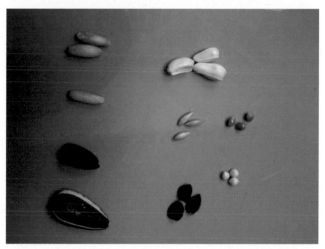

Plate 2.3. *Examples of seeds found in seed diets. The left column, from top to bottom, is oat groats, small black sunflower seed, and large white striped sunflower seed. The right column, from top to bottom, is safflower seeds, red millet, white millet, and rape seeds.*

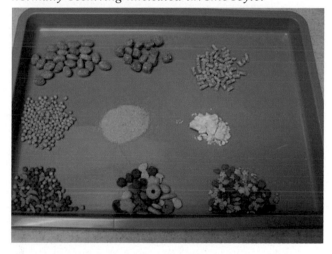

Plate 2.4. *The introduction of pelleted foods for avian species has made it possible to dramatically improve the overall health of companion and caged birds. Various brands of natural and artificially colored pelleted food marketed for birds are shown here. Finely ground formulas are available to mix with water for hand or tube feeding.*

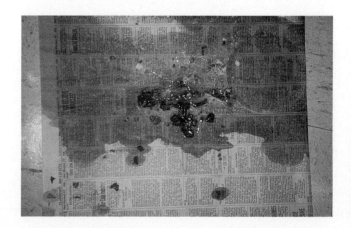

Plate 2.5. *Polyuria.*

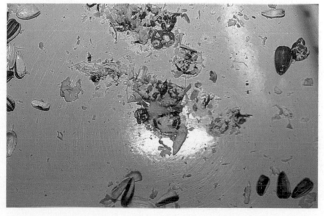

Plate 2.6. *Normal feces.*

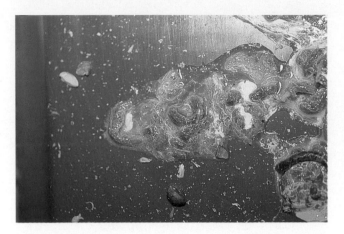

Plate 2.7. Normal feces.

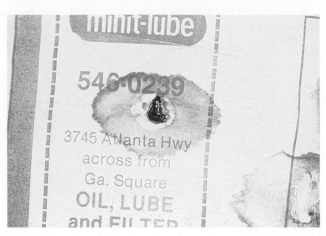

Plate 2.8. Hematuria and melena.

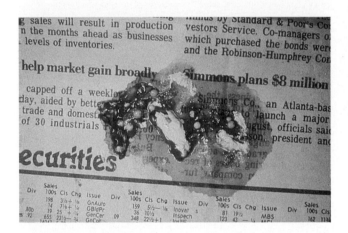

Plate 2.9. Undigested seeds.

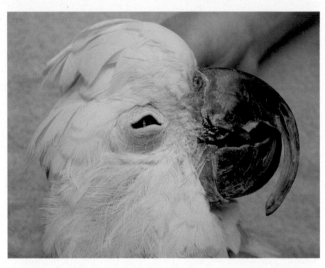

Plate 2.10. Bird with PBFD.

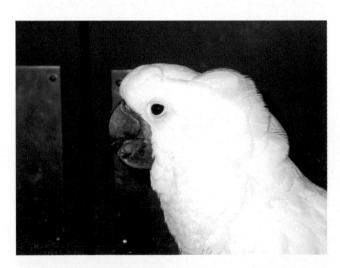

Plate 3.1. Umbrella cockatoo. (Photo courtesy of Dr. Tarah Hadley.)

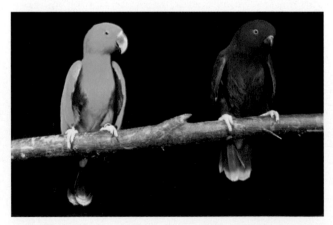

Plate 3.2. Pair of eclectus parrots, one of several sexually dimorphic psittacine species. (Photo courtesy of Dr. April Romagnano.)

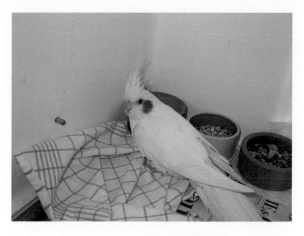

Plate 3.3. *Bright orange cheek patches are often more prevalent in male cockatiels, such as the one pictured here. (Photo courtesy of Dr. Tarah Hadley.)*

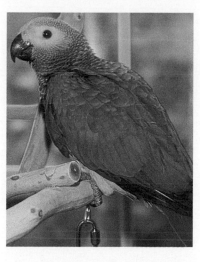

Plate 3.4. *Congo African grey parrot. (Photo courtesy of Cherie Fox.)*

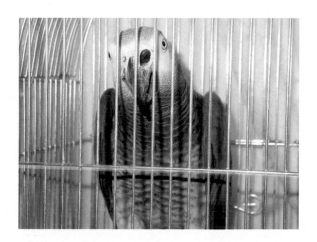

Plate 3.5. *Congo African grey parrot with an enlarged left nare, most likely caused by chronic upper respiratory infections and sinusitis. (Photo courtesy of Dr. Tarah Hadley.)*

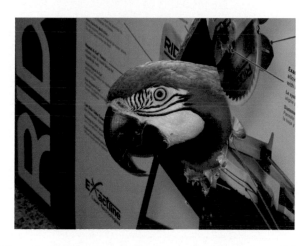

Plate 3.6. *Blue and gold macaw that has chewed its way partly out one side of a cardboard box. (Photo courtesy of Dr. Tarah Hadley.)*

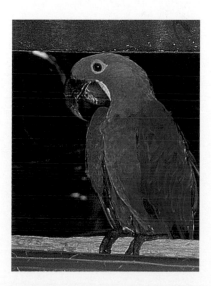

Plate 3.7. *Hyacinth macaws. (Photo courtesy of Cherie Fox.)*

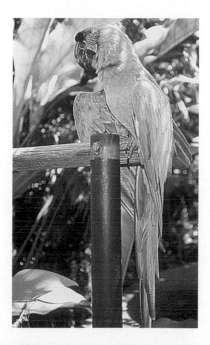

Plate 3.8. *Military macaw. (Photo courtesy of Cherie Fox.)*

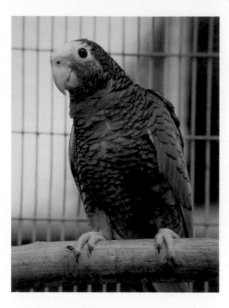

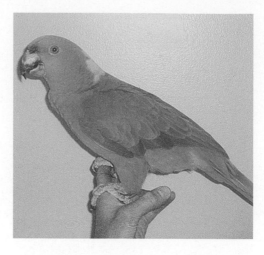

Plate 3.10. Yellow-naped Amazon. (Photo courtesy of Dr. Sam Rivera.)

Plate 3.9. Cuban Amazon in outside aviary on a natural wood perch. (Photo courtesy of Dr. April Romagnano.)

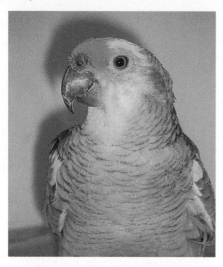

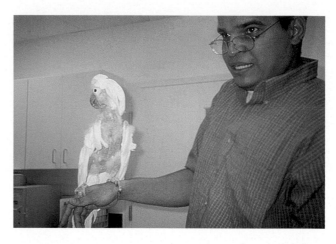

Plate 3.12. A feather picker. (Photo courtesy of Dr. Sam Rivera.)

Plate 3.11. Blue-fronted Amazon. (Photo courtesy of Dr. Sam Rivera.)

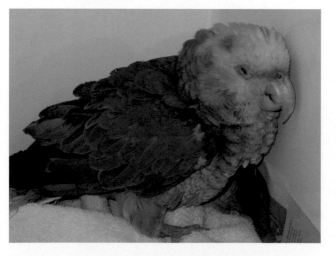

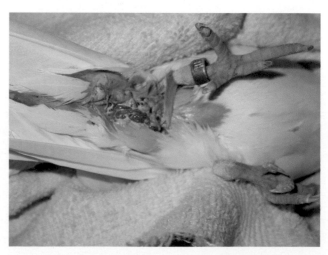

Plate 3.13. Yellow-headed Amazon that presented lethargic with eyes closed and fluffed feathers. (Photo courtesy of Dr. Tarah Hadley.)

Plate 3.14. Cockatiel with fecal staining of vent area secondary to egg binding. (Photo courtesy of Dr. Tarah Hadley.)

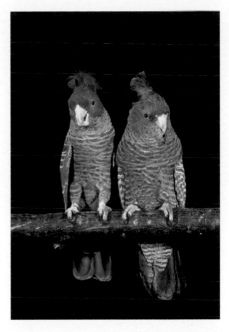

Plate 5.1. Pair of gang gang cockatoos. Note the distinction between the male (left) and the female. (Photo courtesy of Dr. April Romagnano.)

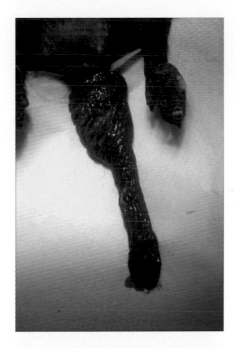

Plate 5.2. Parrot with prolapse of the oviduct. (Photo courtesy of Dr. April Romagnano.)

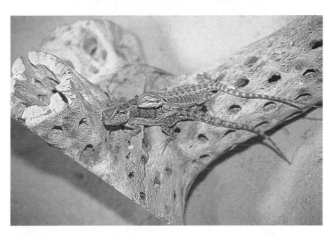

Plate 6.1. Bearded dragon. (Photo courtesy of Ryan Cheek.)

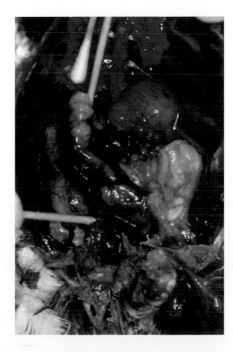

Plate 5.3. Egg yolk peritonitis in a parrot. Note the yellow-tinged coelomic cavity contents caused by a ruptured egg. (Photo courtesy of Dr. April Romagnano.)

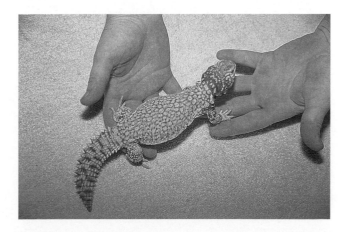

Plate 6.2. Mali uromastyx. (Photo courtesy of Ryan Cheek.)

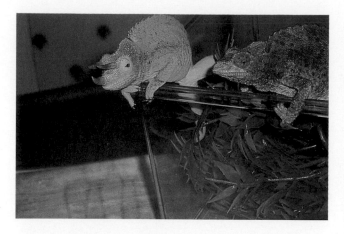

Plate 6.3. *Jackson chameleon. (Photo courtesy of Dr. Sam Rivera.)*

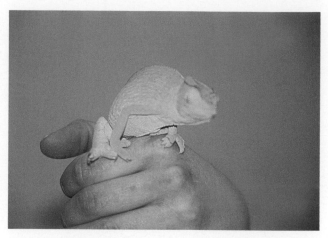

Plate 6.4. *Chameleon. (Photo courtesy of Ryan Cheek.)*

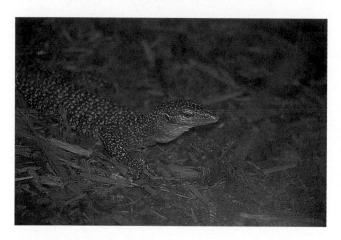

Plate 6.5. *Mangrove monitor. (Photo courtesy of Ryan Cheek.)*

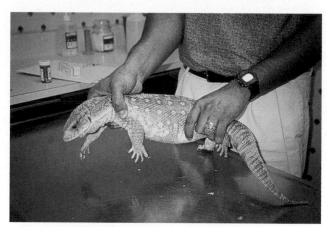

Plate 6.6. *Savannah monitor. (Photo courtesy of Dr. Sam Rivera.)*

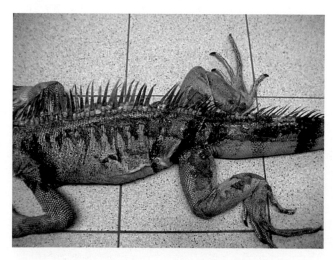

Plate 6.7. *Thermal burns. (Photo courtesy of Dr. Stephen J. Hernandez-Divers, University of Georgia.)*

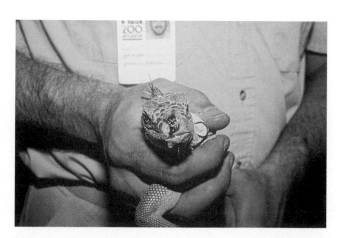

Plate 6.8. *Rostrum abrasion. (Photo courtesy of Zoo Atlanta.)*

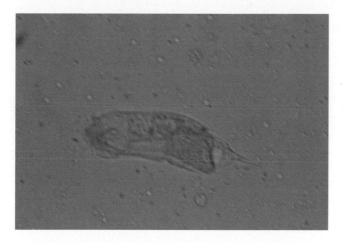

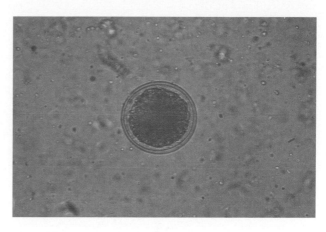

Plate 6.9. Flagellate, original magnification 40 ×. (Photo courtesy of Zoo Atlanta.)

Plate 6.10. Roundworm, original magnification 40×. (Photo courtesy of Zoo Atlanta.)

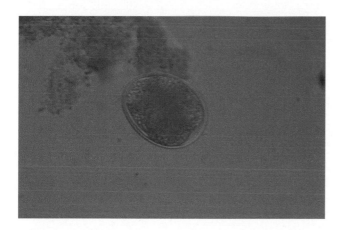

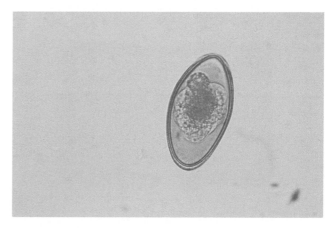

Plate 6.11. Ascarid, original magnification 40 ×. (Photo courtesy of Zoo Atlanta.)

Plate 6.12. Oxyurid, original magnification 40 ×. (Photo courtesy of Zoo Atlanta.)

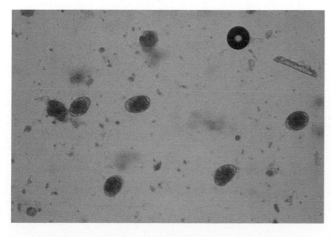

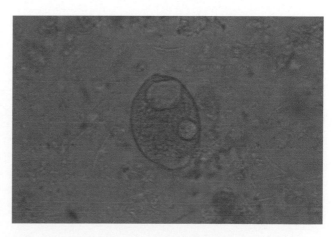

Plate 6.13. Ascarid, original magnification 40 ×. (Photo courtesy of Zoo Atlanta.)

Plate 6.14. Coccidia, original magnification 40 ×. (Photo courtesy of Zoo Atlanta.)

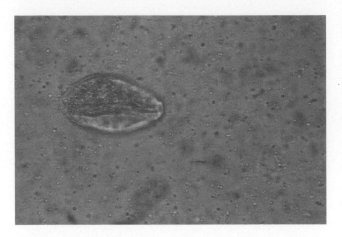

Plate 6.15. Nyctotherus, original magnification 40 ×. (Photo courtesy of Zoo Atlanta.)

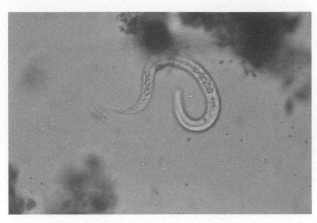

Plate 6.16. Strongyle larva, original magnification 40 ×. (Photo courtesy of Zoo Atlanta.)

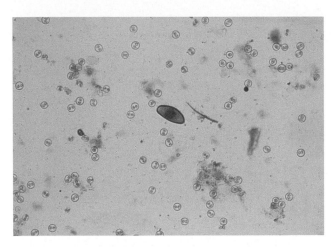

Plate 6.17. Pinworm and eimeria, original magnification 40 ×. (Photo courtesy of Zoo Atlanta.)

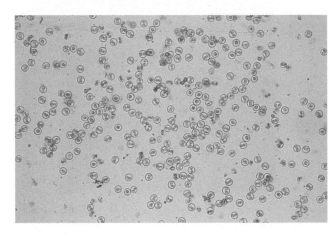

Plate 6.18. Eimeria, original magnification 40 ×. (Photo courtesy of Zoo Atlanta.)

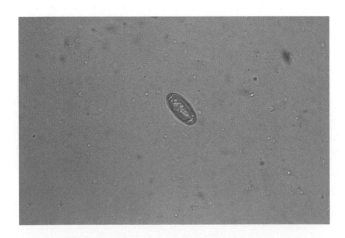

Plate 6.19. Capillaria, original magnification 40 ×. (Photo courtesy of Zoo Atlanta.)

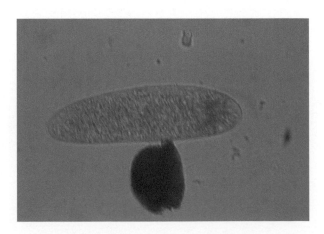

Plate 6.20. Pinworm, original magnification 40 ×. (Photo courtesy of Zoo Atlanta.)

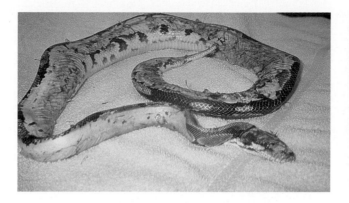

Plate 7.1. A snake suffering from trauma from a prey item. (Photo courtesy of Dr. Sam Rivera.)

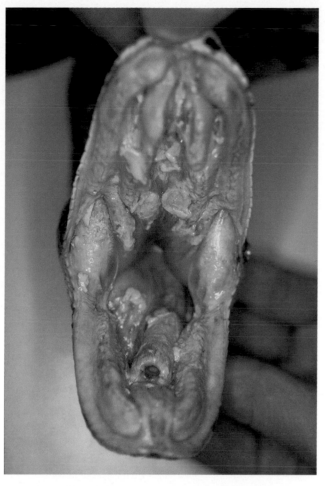

Plate 7.2. Stomatitis in a snake. (Photo courtesy of Dr. Stephen J. Hernandez-Divers, University of Georgia.)

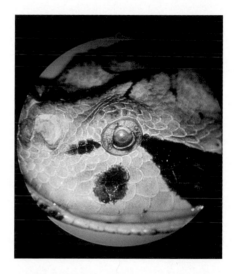

Plate 7.3. Ocular larva migrans in a snake. (Photo courtesy of Zoo Atlanta.)

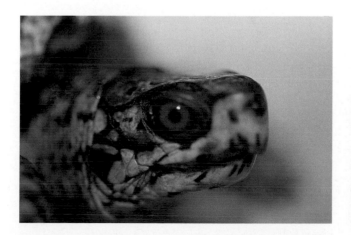

Plate 8.1. Male eastern box turtle showing red eye.

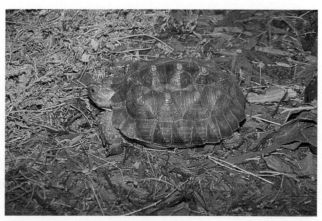

Plate 8.2. Sulcata tortoise.

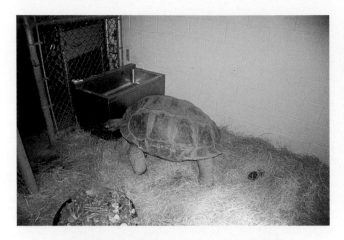

Plate 8.3. Aldabra tortoise.

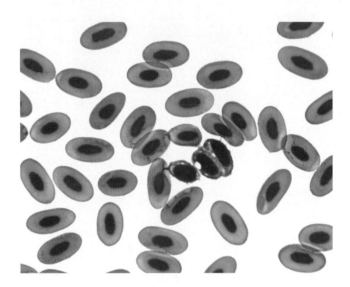

Plate 12.1. Rabbit blood smear showing heterophil. (Photo courtesy of Dondrae Coble.)

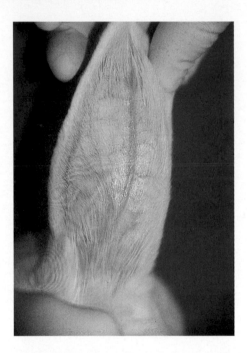

Plate 12.2. Marginal lateral ear vein on the left and the prominent central auricular artery. (Photo courtesy of Ryan Cheek.)

Plate 21.1. Blood smear from an owl: cluster of elongate thrombocytes. (Wright stain, EDTA, original magnification × 100.)

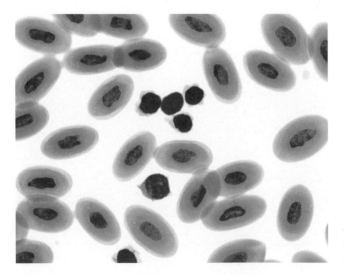

Plate 21.2. Blood smear from a rat snake: cluster of small round thrombocytes, one lymphocyte. (Wright stain, EDTA, original magnification × 100.)

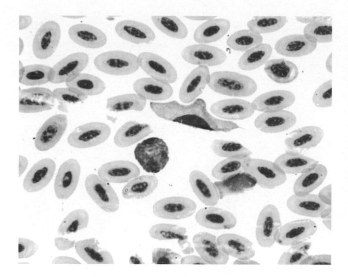

Plate 21.3. Blood smear from a hawk: heterophil, erythrocytes containing hemoparasite, Leucocytozoon. (Wright stain, EDTA, original magnification × 100.)

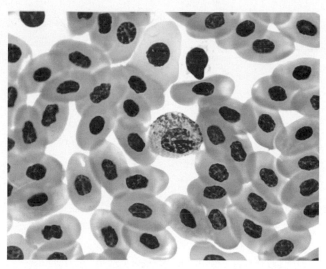

Plate 21.4. Blood smear from a tortoise: heterophil with band-shaped nucleus and area of basophilic cytoplasm. (Wright stain, EDTA, original magnification × 100.)

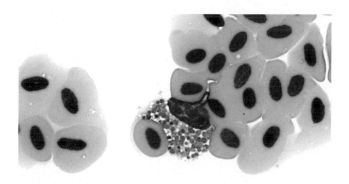

Plate 21.5. Blood smear from an owl: toxic mononuclear heterophil with eccentric nucleus and both basophilic and eosinophilic granules. (Wright stain, EDTA, original magnification × 100.)

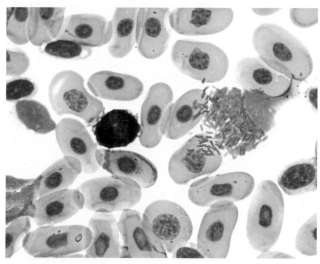

Plate 21.6. Blood smear from a tortoise: basophil with granules obscuring the nucleus, ruptured heterophil with loose granules. (Wright stain, EDTA, original magnification × 100.)

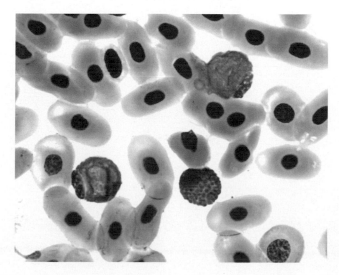

Plate 21.7. Blood smear from a tortoise: heterophil with ill-defined rod-shaped granules, eosinophil with round distinct granules, heterophil. (Wright stain, EDTA, original magnification × 100.)

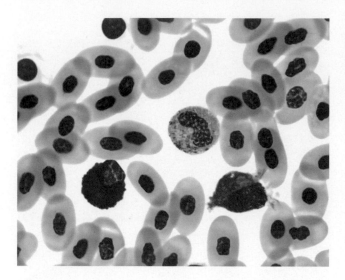

Plate 21.8. *Blood smear from a lizard: basophil, band heterophil, monocyte. (Wright stain, EDTA, original magnification × 100.)*

Plate 21.9. *Blood smear from a lizard: monocyte with gray-blue cytoplasm and oval nucleus. (Wright stain, EDTA, original magnification × 100.)*

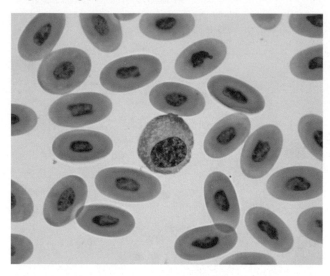

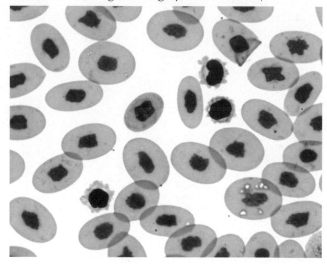

Plate 21.10. *Blood smear from a rat snake: azurophil with granules at cytoplasmic periphery instilling a pinkish-purple hue. (Wright stain, original magnification × 100.)*

Plate 21.11. *Blood smear from a lizard: basophilic erythrocyte in the center, two thrombocytes. Note the irregularly shaped erythrocyte nuclei, tiny cytoplasmic vacuoles in erythrocytes. (Wright stain, EDTA, original magnification × 100.)*

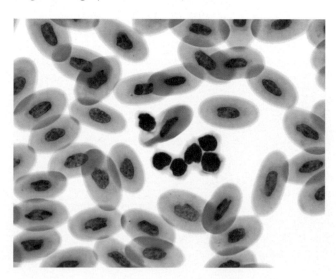

Plate 21.12. *Blood smear from a rat snake: cluster of thrombocytes. (Wright stain, EDTA, original magnification × 100.)*

de Vosjoli P. 1993. The General Care and Maintenance of Prehensile-Tailed Skinks. Lakeside, CA: Advanced Vivarium Systems.

de Vosjoli P. 1995. Basic Care of Uromastyx. Santee, CA: Advanced Vivarium Systems.

de Vosjoli P. 1997. The Lizard Keeper's Handbook. Santee, CA: Advanced Vivarium Systems.

de Vosjoli P, Ferguson G (eds.). 1995. Care and Breeding of Panther, Jackson's, Veiled, and Parson's Chameleons. Santee, CA: Advanced Vivarium Systems.

de Vosjoli P, et al. 1997. The Leopard Gecko Manual. Mission Viejo, CA: Advanced Vivarium Systems.

de Vosjoli P, et al. 2001. The Bearded Dragon Manual. Irvine, CA: Advanced Vivarium Systems.

Donoghue S, Landenberg J. 1996. Special Topics: Nutrition. In: Reptile Medicine and Surgery, edited by Mader DR. Philadelphia: W.B. Saunders Co. 148–174.

Frye FL. 1991. Biomedical and Surgical Aspects of Captive Reptile Husbandry. 2d ed., vol. 1 and 2. Melbourne, FL: Krieger Publishing Co.

Glaw F, Vences M. 1994. A Field Guide to the Amphibians and Reptiles of Madagascar. 2nd ed. Bonn, Germany: Koenig.

Goin CJ, Goin OB, Zug GR. 1978. Introduction to Herpetology. 3rd ed. New York: W.H. Freeman and Co.

Helfman GS. 1990. Mode Selection and Mode Switching in Foraging Animals. *Advances in the Study of Behavior* 19:249.

Innis CJ. 2000. Diagnosis and Treatment of Renal Disease in Tortoises. In: Proceedings of the North American Veterinary Conference (14). Gainesville, FL., 954–955.

Jacobson ER. 2002. Chlamydiosis: An Underreported Disease of Reptiles. In: Proceedings of the North American Veterinary Conference (16). Gainesville, FL., 916–917.

Jenkins JR. 1996. Special Techniques and Procedures: Diagnostic and Clinical Techniques. In: Reptile Medicine and Surgery, edited by Mader DR. Philadelphia: W.B. Saunders Co. 264–276.

Johnson-Delaney CA. 1996. Introduction: Reptile Zoonoses and Threats to Public Health. In: Reptile Medicine and Surgery, edited by Mader DR. Philadelphia: W.B. Saunders Co. 185–203.

Klingenberg RJ. 1993. Understanding Reptile Parasites. Lakeside, CA: Advanced Vivarium Systems.

Klingenberg RJ. 1996. Special Techniques and Procedures: Therapeutics. In: Reptile Medicine and Surgery, edited by Mader DR. Philadelphia: W.B. Saunders Co. 229–321.

Lane TJ, Mader DR. 1996. Reptile Medicine and Surgery. Special Topics: Parasitology. In: Reptile Medicine and Surgery, edited by Mader DR. Philadelphia: W.B. Saunders Co. 185–203.

Levell JP, 1998. A Field Guide to Reptiles and the Law. Melbourne, FL: Krieger Publishing Company.

Mader DR. 1996a. Specific Diseases and Conditions: Acariasis. In: Reptile Medicine and Surgery, edited by Mader DR. Philadelphia: W.B. Saunders Co. 341–346.

Mader DR. 1996b. Special Techniques and Procedures: Euthanasia and Necropsy. In: Reptile Medicine and Surgery, edited by Mader DR. Philadelphia: W.B. Saunders Co. 277–281.

Mader DR. 1996c. Specific Diseases and Conditions: Gout. In: Reptile Medicine and Surgery, edited by Mader DR. Philadelphia: W.B. Saunders Co. 374–379.

Mader DR. 1996d. Specific Diseases and Conditions: Upper Alimentary Tract Disease. In: Reptile Medicine and Surgery, edited by Mader DR. Philadelphia: W.B. Saunders Co. 421–424.

Mader DR. 2000a. Reptilian Microbiology and Antibiotic Therapy. In: Proceedings of the North American Veterinary Conference (14). Gainesville, FL. 961–964.

Mader DR. 2000b. Thermal Burns in Reptiles. In: Proceedings of the North American Veterinary Conference (14). Gainesville, FL. 965–67.

Mader DR. 2002a. Metabolic Bone Diseases in the Green Iguana. In: Proceedings of the North American Veterinary Conference (16). Gainesville, FL. 921–922.

Mader DR. 2002b. Ventral Midline Approach for the Lizard Coeliotomy. In: Proceedings of the North American Veterinary Conference (16). Gainesville, FL.

Mader DR, Rosenthal K. 2000. Proper Collection of Laboratory Samples. Proceedings of the North American Veterinary Conference (14). Gainesville, FL. 958–960.

McKeown S. 1993. The General Care and Maintenance of Day Geckos. Lakeside, CA: Advanced Vivarium Systems.

McKeown S. 1996. Introduction: General Husbandry and Captive Management. In: Reptile Medicine and Surgery, edited by Mader DR. Philadelphia: W.B. Saunders Co. 9–19.

Mitchell MA. Artificial Lighting for Reptiles: What We Know and What you Need to Know. In: Proceedings of the North American Veterinary Conference (23). Gainesville, FL. pp 1783–1785.

Murray MJ. 1996. Specific Diseases and Conditions: Pneumonia and Normal Respiratory Function. In: Reptile Medicine and Surgery, edited by Mader DR. Philadelphia: W.B. Saunders Co. 396–405.

Obst FJ, et al. 1988. The Completely Illustrated Atlas of Reptiles and Amphibians for the Terrarium. Neptune City, NJ: TFH.

Ritchie BW. 1992. Class Notes: Exotic Animal Medicine. University of Georgia College of Veterinary Medicine.

Rossi J. 1998a. Emergency Medicine of Reptiles. Proceedings of the North American Veterinary Conference (12). Gainesville, FL.

Rossi J. 1998b. What's Wrong with My Iguana? Escondido: Advanced Vivarium Systems.

Rossi JV. 1996. Special Topics: Dermatology. In: Reptile Medicine and Surgery, edited by Mader DR. Philadelphia: W.B. Saunders Co. 104–117.

Schumacher J. 2002a. Anesthesia of Reptiles. In: Proceedings of the North American Veterinary Conference (16). Gainesville, FL: ESVA.

Schumacher J. 2002b. Critical and Supportive Care of Reptiles. In: Proceedings of the North American Veterinary Conference (16). Gainesville, FL.

Silverman S, Janssen, DL. 1996. Special Techniques and Procedures: Diagnostic Imaging. In: Reptile Medicine and Surgery, edited by Mader DR. Philadelphia: W.B. Saunders Co. 258–264.

Stahl SJ. 1998. Common Medical Problems of Old World Chameleons. In: Proceedings of the North American Veterinary Conference (12). Gainesville, FL. 814–817.

Stahl SJ. 2000. Reptile Obstetrics. In: Proceedings of the North American Veterinary Conference. Gainesville, FL. 971–974.

Williams DL. 1996. Special Topics: Ophthalmology. In: Reptile Medicine and Surgery, edited by Mader DR. Philadelphia: W.B. Saunders Co. 175–184.

CHAPTER SEVEN

Snakes

Ryan Cheek, Shannon Richards, and Maria Crane

INTRODUCTION

Keeping snakes in captivity has become increasingly popular over the years. With the increase in captive specimens there has is a large demand for veterinarians and veterinary technicians who are educated in proper husbandry and treatment of reptiles. The veterinary staff must be willing to keep up with current treatment protocols (through continuing education courses or literature) because reptile medicine is ever changing and still evolving. One important tool in the diagnosis of any reptile is a thorough history. This is important because most reptiles in captivity become ill due to improper husbandry. Snakes kept in ideal conditions in captivity can live ten to twenty years (depending on the species). This chapter contains general husbandry information on snakes to assist the veterinary staff through the diagnostic process.

CAPTIVE-BRED VERSUS WILD-CAUGHT

It is important to know whether a captive snake has been wild-caught or captive-bred. Wild-caught snakes are those that have been taken from their natural habitats and sold through the pet trade. Unfortunately, this is a common occurrence in the reptile industry. Wild-caught specimens typically have parasites (ticks, mites, and various internal parasites) and can take a long time to adjust to a captive environment, if they do at all. They also can have a host of other illnesses such as respiratory infections that become apparent while in captivity due to stress.

Feeding wild-caught snakes can prove to be challenging as well due to their reluctance to eat in captivity. This reluctance to eat is usually due to the difficulties that a wild-caught snake may have adjusting to a captive environment (especially if husbandry guidelines are not being followed) and not being offered the natural diet to which it is accustomed. For example, a snake feeding primarily on frogs in its natural environment may not be receptive to the white lab mice that are sold commercially as snake feeders. This is not to say that it will never feed on mice in the future, but it will take some time to adjust and may take some trickery.

Captive-bred snakes are those that have been bred and raised in a captive environment. These are obviously better specimens due to their lack of exposure to the diseases and parasites found in wild-caught specimens. Captive-bred snakes also accept commercially available diets better (such as feeder rodents) when offered and are not as finicky about accepting prekilled prey items, which is the recommended method of feeding. Although the temperament of a snake can never be guaranteed, those that are captive-bred tend to be more docile overall and can become more accustomed to handling.

Captive-bred specimens should always be recommended to potential buyers to better ensure the snake's overall health. There are many reputable snake breeders who can provide a more reliable history on the snake. In many cases these snakes are less expensive than those bought from pet retail stores.

BEHAVIOR

Snakes are solitary animals and should be housed separately unless attempting to breed. Some can exhibit territorial behavior and be aggressive to other inhabitants. Signs of aggressive behavior toward other snakes include biting, constricting, and head pinning. The head pinning is a courtship behavior as well. During breeding season, some of these behaviors are observed more often. If these signs of aggression are observed with snakes being housed together, one should be removed immediately. As with any animal, if snakes are fighting, care should be taken if interference is necessary to avoid being bitten while trying to separate the combating snakes. Using hooks or tongs is recommended when human interference is warranted.

Another downside of housing snakes together is that some species (i.e. king snakes) eat other snakes as part of their natural diet. Therefore, all king snakes should be kept separate. Size or gender does not affect the snake's instinctive predatory behavior.

Finally, it is also important to know whether the snake is diurnal (active during day hours) or nocturnal (active during night hours). Knowing when the snake is the most active will aid in making several decisions such as handling and ideal feeding times.

ANATOMY AND PHYSIOLOGY

Integument

As in mammals, the skin of snakes plays several crucial roles. The skin is the cellular protective barrier from the snake's outside environment. It protects the body from microbes and parasites, resists abrasions, and buffers the internal environment from the extremes of the external environment. The skin holds other tissues and organs in place while being elastic enough to allow for respiration, movement, and growth. The skin also serves other roles such as physiological regulation, sensory detection, respiration, and coloration.

The snake's skin consists of two main layers, the dermis and epidermis. The epidermis is covered completely by keratin. This layer of keratinous cells, stratum corneum, shields the living tissue below. The stratum germinativum, the innermost layer of the epidermis, divides continuously to replace the outer layer of dead keratinous cells. As the cells in the stratum germinativum are pushed outward, they slowly flatten, die, and keratinize to form the stratum corneum. The stratum corneum is composed of three layers, the Oberhautchen layer, the beta-keratin layer, and the alpha-keratin layer, from the surface inward, respectively.

The dermis consists of two layers, the stratum compactum and the stratum spongiosum. The stratum compactum is the innermost layer of the dermis. It consists of densely knit connective tissue. The stratum spongiosum consists of connective tissue, blood vessels, glands, nerve endings, and other cellular structures.

Ecdysis, or shedding of the skin, is a normal occurrence for the duration of the snake's life. Young snakes shed much more often and begin to have a longer resting period as they reach adult size. Because the top layer of snake skin consists mostly of keratin, which is dead material, it is incapable of expanding during the snake's growth process. Therefore, it needs to be shed every so often. The cells of the upper stratum germinativum, the outer-generation layer, begin to proliferate and differentiate. The germinative layer begins to divide, producing new layers of cells. These new cells form the inner generation layer, which is the precursor to scales, or the outer-generation layer, for the next ecdysis cycle. At this stage the new epidermal layer is ready. The Oberhautchen then fills with lymph and enzymatic action produces a cleavage zone and the old epidermis is shed (Zug et al. 2001).

Before a snake sheds, it secretes a lubricant underneath the outermost layer of skin to assist with the shedding process. This lubricant is most noticeable on the snake's eyes, which become opaque or blue in color due to this lubricant being secreted. The snake will begin to shed its skin sometime after this optical opacity or dullness in appearance is noticed.

It can take a week or two before the entire shedding process is over and should be repeated at regular intervals. The snake may attempt to use any furnishings in the enclosure to assist in removing the dead skin. The furnishings should be nonabrasive to avoid causing injury. The snake may also attempt to soak in its water bowl to assist in shedding. Water softens the old skin and makes it easier to remove. If the humidity is too low, the snake may have problems shedding.

A snake sheds its entire outer layer of skin all at once. All snakes, with the exception of large boids, should shed in one piece. If there are numerous pieces of the snake's shedded skin or some still present on the snake, the shed is abnormal. Snakes with abnormal shedding may need husbandry changes or may have ectoparasites and should be checked thoroughly. Age, nutrition, species, reproductive status, overall health, and hormonal balance also play a role in frequency of ecdysis.

If some shedding is still present on the snake, soaking or spraying can used to try to assist in the removal of the skin. Infections can occur underneath the old skin if the skin is allowed to build up and not slough off naturally.

Snakes should not be handled or fed while they are in shed. Their senses are dulled (eyes opaque) and because they feel vulnerable, they can also be very defensive. To avoid potential bites, handling is not recommended during this time. It is unlikely that the snake will eat, so feeding should not occur until after it has shed. If offering live prey items, feeding should not occur while the snake is in shed due to the higher potential for rodent bites.

Snakes are either entirely or partially covered by overlapping scales. The surface of each scale is composed of beta-keratin while the interscalar space, or sutures, is composed of alpha-keratin. This distribution of keratin gives a protective covering while allowing for flexibility and expansion. Certain species of colubrids and viperids are nearly scaleless. These species may only have labial and ventral scales. The remainder of the body is covered in a smooth keratinous epidermis. This anomaly is a recessive homozygous trait.

Snakes have paired scent glands at the base of their tails. These glands open at the outer edge of the cloaca. A large amount of semisolid, malodorous fluid is released for defensive behavior in some species and for courting behavior in other species.

Musculoskeletal System

Snakes possess a very complex cranial skeleton. They have a cartilaginous anterior chondrocranium, the portion of the cranium that covers the brain (Zug et al. 2001). This anterior portion of the chondrocranium consists of continuous internasal and interorbital septa and a pair of nasal conchae (Zug et al. 2001). The chondrocranium calcifies between the eyes and ears and forms the basisphenoid. Farther posteriorly, a pair of exoccipitals, the supraoccipital bones, and the basioccipital form just below and behind the brain. These occipital bones encircle the foramen magnum. The exoccipitals and the basioccipitals form a single occipital condyle and the articular surface of the skull and atlas.

The maxilla is loosely connected to the other cranial bones. It connects to a special process on the prefrontal bone. They are connected via a movable articulation. The maxilla is also loosely connected to the cranial bones by the ectopyerygoid (Romer 1997). The snout structures, premaxilla, nasal, septomaxilla, and vomer are movable as a separate series of bones from the maxilla and are also loosely connected to the cranial bones. This adaptation allows snakes to swallow large prey.

The mandible is highly specialized to allow for a large gape when swallowing large prey items. The mandible lacks a mandibular symphysis; an intramandibular hinge allows for the mandible to flex in the middle, and an articulated streptostylic quadrate allows the mandible to move sideways.

The vertebral column in snakes is divided into the atlas and axis, 100 to 300 trunk or precloacal vertebrae, several cloacal vertebrae, and ten to 120 caudal vertebrae (Zug et al. 2001). Each precloacal vertebra has a rib attached. The zygapophyses, the intervertebral articular surfaces, possess a posterior and anterior pair on each vertebra. The anterior zygapophyses flare outward and upward while the posterior zygapophyses flare inward and downward. The angle of the zygapophyses gives reptiles their flexibility or rigidity. Snakes are able to have such great flexibility due to these articular surfaces being angled toward the horizontal plane (Figure 7.1).

The muscular system of snakes consists of several hundred multisegmental muscle chains composed of elongated and interconnecting segmental muscles and tendons. Movement is achieved through individual contraction patterns of the muscle chains. There are six types of locomotion divided into two classes (Pough et al. 2001). Lateral undulation and slide-pushing have no static points of contact with the substrate. Rectilinear, concertina, sidewinding, and saltation do have static points with the substrate.

Lateral undulation is the most widely used method of locomotion in snakes. At fixed points in the snake's environment, force is generated by horizontal waves traveling down alternating sides of the body. These fixed points can be a rock, tree, or any other physical object that the snake contacts. At each point the body generates a force that pushes it posterolaterally. Slide-pushing is similar to lateral undulation but does not use fixed points in the physical environment. Slide-pushing involves very rapid alternating side body waves that generate sliding friction to propel the snake forward.

Concertina locomotion is very slow and consumes large amounts of energy. It is a very complex system of locomotion. First, the anterior portion of the body remains still while the posterior portion draws up in a series of tight curves. The posterior end is then stationary and the anterior end extends forward. The sequence then repeats. Concertina locomotion is most effectively used on the ground where static friction is used to prevent rearward slippage.

Sidewinding is most commonly used on shifting soil such as mud or sand. Most snakes appear to have the

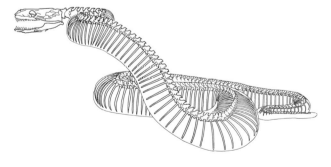

Figure 7.1. Snake skeletal anatomy. (Drawing by Scott Stark.)

ability to sidewind. The forces in sidewinding are directed vertically on the substrate. Sections of the body are alternately lifted, moved forward, and then set down. This produces a series of tracts that are parallel-producing forward motion.

Saltation involves a very rapid straightening of the body from anterior to posterior, lifting the entire body off the ground. This is used only by small species. Rectilinear motion relies on the lateral muscles to work at the same time. The costocutaneous superior muscles pull the skin forward relative to the ribs. The ventral scales then anchor themselves to the ground. The costocutaneous inferior then pulls the ribs and with them the rest of the body forward relative to the stationary ventral scales. This form of locomotion is used by large-body snakes such as boids and vipers.

Cardiovascular System

The Heart

The heart size, shape, structure, and position all depend on the species' anatomy, physiology, and behavior. Heart position has a direct correlation with arboreal, terrestrial, and aquatic habits (Vasse 1994). Terrestrial species have a heart that is close to the head and blood vessels in the distal portion of the body that dilate to receive extra blood. The heart of arboreal species is also located close to the head so that blood can more easily reach the brain when hanging vertically. Marine species have a heart that is found in the middle of the body so the pumping effort is minimal. They do not have blood accumulation in the tail and the low blood pressure is compensated for by the external water pressure (Vasse 1994).

The heart consists of three chambers, a right and left atria and a single ventricle. The ventricle is further divided into the cavum arteriosum, cavum venosum, and cavum pulmonale. Although the ventricle lacks a septum, the snake can still separate oxygenated and deoxygenated blood and can maintain different systemic and pulmonary pressures because the heart is functionally five chambered (Pough et al. 2001). A muscular ridge in the ventricle separates the cavum pulmonale and the cavum venosum. The cavum arteriosum is located dorsal to the other two compartments and communicates with the cavum venosum through an intraventricular canal. There are two inflow routes, the right and left atria, and three outflow routes, the pulmonary artery and the left and right aortic arches. The right atrium receives blood from the sinus venosus. The sinus venosus is a large chamber on the dorsal surface of the atrium. It receives blood from four veins, the right and left precaval vein, the postcaval vein, and the left hepatic vein. The left atrium receives blood from the right and left pulmonary veins.

Blood flow through the heart starts when both atria contract. The atrioventricular valves open and allow blood to flow into the ventricle. When the atria contract, the valve between the right atria and the cavum venosum seals off the intraventricular canal, allowing the oxygenated blood from the left atrium to flow into the cavum arteriosum and the deoxygenated blood from the right atrium to flow into the cavum venosum and then to the cavum pulmonale. When the ventricle contracts, the blood pressure inside the heart increases.

Because resistance is lower in the pulmonary circuit, deoxygenated blood is expelled from the cavum pulmonale through the pulmonary artery. When the ventricle shortens, the muscular ridge that separates the cavum venosum and the cavum pulmonale comes into contact with the wall of the ventricle and closes off the passage between the two compartments. The atrioventricular valves are forced shut as the pressure inside the ventricle increases. When the atrioventricular valves are shut, the oxygenated blood from the cavum arteriosum is pushed through the intraventricular canal into the cavum venosum and out the left and right aortic arches. At this point, the pressure inside the cavum venosum is more than twice that in the cavum pulmonale.

Another remarkable ability of snakes, as well as other squamates and chelonia, is the ability to perform intracardiac shunting. Intracardiac shunts are classified as left-to-right or right-to-left. In a right-to-left shunt, the deoxygenated blood that should normally be flowing out to the pulmonary circuit is being expelled out to the systemic circuit via the aortic arches. This shunt increases the amount of circulating blood and decreases its oxygen content. Primarily, the right-to-left shunt is used to increase the body temperature and bypass the lungs during breath-holding. The left-to-right shunt is used to help stabilize the oxygen content of the blood. The direction and degree of intracardiac shunting depends on the pressure differences between the pulmonary and systemic circuits and the washout of blood remaining in the cavum venosum.

The renal-portal system exists in all fish, reptiles, and birds. It collects blood from the caudal portion of the body and carries it to the kidneys. The blood is then filtered and returned to the heart via the post caval vein. Blood that travels through the renal-portal system only goes through the convoluted tubules and not the glomeruli (Holz 1999).

The location of the heart, being so cranial, has two disadvantages. First, when a snake holds its head down, blood flow to the tail is compromised. Second, and most important, when the head is up or the entire body is in a vertical position, the blood from the tail must travel all the way to the heart against gravity. The veins of snakes do not have valves to prevent back flow so snakes have adapted three ways to ensure that the blood continues to flow toward the heart even while being vertical. The contractions of the smooth muscles that line the vessels help push the blood toward the heart. Snakes undulate or contract their skeletal muscles, massaging the blood toward the heart. The tight skin of arboreal species acts as an antigravity suit, further assisting the blood in traveling toward the heart.

The lymphatic system in snakes, as well as all reptiles, is an elaborate drainage system. Microvessels collect lymph from throughout the body. These microvessels merge into larger vessels that eventually empty into larger lymphatic trunk vessels and then into lymphatic sinuses. All three parts, the trunk, vessels, and sinuses, empty into veins. The lymph can be bidirectional but mostly flows toward the pericardial sinus and into the venous system. Reptiles have a pair of lymph hearts located in the pelvic region but do not possess lymph nodes.

Respiratory System

Snakes have upper respiratory anatomy similar to that of mammals. Air enters and leaves the trachea through the glottis located in the back of the pharynx. The glottis and other cartilage form the larynx. The trachea of snakes has incomplete cartilaginous rings. The ventral portions of the rings are rigid and the dorsal portion is membranous.

Most snakes only have a single right lung and a small nonfunctioning left lung. The right lung is generally one-half or more of the snake's body length. In most species, the posterior one-third is an air sac. In those species that do have a very small functional left lung, it is about 85% smaller than the right. The right bronchi enters the lung and empties into a wall that is lined with faveoli. The faveoli are richly supplied with blood. Most of the gaseous exchange occurs in the faveoli (Zug et al. 2001). Snakes that have only one functioning lung possess a tracheal lung, a vascular sac that contains many faveoli for gas exchange. The tracheal lung extends from the point where the tracheal rings are incomplete dorsally and posteriorly until it touches the right lung. The air sac, or saccular lung, is not used as a site for gas exchange but as a site for air regulation.

All reptiles breathe using a negative-pressure ventilation (Pough et al. 2001). During inspiration, the intercostal muscles expand the ribs the entire length of the body, dropping the pressure inside the lungs to below atmospheric pressure and drawing in air. Then the intercostal muscles relax and the glottis closes, closing the respiratory tract. The snake then pauses for several seconds to several minutes before exhaling. Terrestrial and arboreal species normally have a period of apnea between respiratory cycles. The ribs in the anterior portion of the body are unable to expand for proper inspiration when snakes are swallowing large prey. During ingestion of prey, the posterior ribs expand, causing the saccular lung to inflate and deflate, moving air through the respiratory system (Table 7.1).

Nervous System

The central nervous system is organized the same way in snakes as it is in all reptiles and similar to mammals. The brain of snakes is divided into the forebrain and hindbrain. The forebrain contains the cerebral hemispheres, thalamic segment, and optic tectum, and is further broken down into the telenchephalon, diencephalon, and mesencephalon. The cerebral hemispheres are pear shaped. They contain olfactory lobes that project anteriorly and end in olfactory bulbs (Zug et al. 2001). The thalamic region, which is tube shaped with a thick wall, is hidden by the cerebral lobes and the optic tectum. The dorsal portion of the thalamic region has two dorsal projections. The anterior projection is the parietal body and the posterior projection, the epiphysis, is the pineal organ. The pineal organ is glandular in most snakes. The ventral portion contains the hypothalamus. The optic tectum is located on the dorsal part of the posterior portion of the forebrain and the ventral part contains the optic chiasma. The hindbrain contains the cerebellum and medulla and is also broken down into the metencephalon and myelencephalon. Both are small in extant species of reptiles. Reptiles also have twelve pairs of cranial nerves.

Table 7.1. Approximate Organ Location in Snakes.

First quarter	Trachea, esophagus, heart
Second quarter	Heart, liver, lung, stomach
Third quarter	Stomach, gallbladder, gonads, small intestine, pancreas, spleen, adrenal glands
Fourth quarter	Colon, kidneys, cloaca
Tail	Hemipenes, musk glands

The spinal cord runs the entire length of the vertebral column. Each vertebra contains a bilateral pair of spinal nerves, each of which contains a sensory and motor root that fuse near their origin. The diameter of the spinal cord is uniform all the way down to the end.

Sense Organs

Cutaneous Sense Organs

Boids, pythonids, and viperids have specialized structures in the dermis and epidermis that contain heat receptors (Zug et al. 2001). These pit organs sense infrared heat and are located in different locations in each taxon. In the boids, the pit organs are scattered on unmodified supralabial and infralabial scales. Boids have intraepidermal and intradermal types. Pythonids have a series of pit organs in the labial scales. The heat receptors lay on the floor of each pit. In viperids, the pit organs are located bilaterally between the eyes and the nares. The opening of each pit is forward facing and is overlapped by other receptors. The heat receptors are contained inside a membrane that stretches across the pit, further enhancing its heat-seeking ability.

Ears

The ears of snakes have the same two functions as they do in mammals, hearing and balance. The middle ear in snakes is virtually nonexistent (Platel 1994). It is a very narrow cavity that does not contain a tympanic membrane but does contain one ossicle, the columella, that abuts the quadrate bone for transmission of vibrations. The inner ear of snakes is very similar to that of mammals. The utricle and saccule make up the semicircular canals that ensure balance. Vibrations are received in the inner ear via the columella and pass through the cochlear canal and onto the basilar papilla. Even with the absence of an outer ear and the virtual absence of a middle ear, snakes are adept at hearing (Platel 1994). Snakes pick up vibrations from the substrate on which their head rests because the columella senses vibrations from the quadrate bone that is located on the upper jaw (Funk 1996). It is believed that arboreal snakes can pick up aerial vibrations, enabling them to catch avian prey in midflight.

Smell

It is difficult to determine the amount of olfactory sensation snakes have. Snakes have a large number of olfactory nerves, which leaves no doubt that they are macrosmatic animals. Their olfactory abilities do not work alone; they are closely associated with the vomeronasal sense as well as sight.

Vomeronasal Sense

The vomeronasal organ, or Jacobson's organ, which is connected to the oral cavity by the vomeronasal duct, plays a vital role in predation. It detects nonaerial, nonvolatile particulate odors by the chemoreceptors on the forked tongue. The snake then carries that scent to the vomeronasal organ. The sensory cells inside the vomeronasal organ react with certain molecules that then transfer the scent to the accessory olfactory bulbs, other encephalic centers, and the nucleus globosus. The vomeronasal organ is also used for interspecies relations. Snakes can use the vomeronasal organ to sense a den for hibernating and for reproductive behaviors such as picking up pheromones.

Eyes

The snake has very different eye anatomy than other reptiles. Embryologically, the eyelids of snakes fuse to form a transparent spectacle, which has an extensive vascular network that is optically transparent (Zug et al. 2001). The anterior layer of the spectacle is shed during each ecdysis cycle. The spectacle is separated from the cornea by an epithelial-lined subspectacular space. The globe of the eye is kept moist via secretions made by the harderian glands. The nasolacrimal ducts drain from the medial canthus to the roof of the oral cavity at the base of or just behind the vomeronasal organ. The globe has poorly developed rectus muscles and limited rotational muscles. Snakes lack the scleral ossicles and cartilage of lizards and chelonians. Snakes possess a soft and pliable lens and they focus by the forward movement of the lens by increased pressure of the vitreous applied by the ciliary muscle. The iris contains striated muscle, making dilation and contraction of the pupil voluntary.

The retina, pupil shape, and lens color have gone through evolutionary changes to better fit the species' lifestyle (Platel 1994). Diurnal species usually have a round pupil, yellow lens, and a retina made of all cones. Crepuscular species have a paler lens and the retina contains both rods and cones. Nocturnal species have a vertical slit-shaped pupil, a colorless lens, and a retina consisting of mostly rods with very few cones. These are just generalized statements, with many exceptions. For example, crepuscular or nocturnal pythons have a round pupil and a retina that contains a large quantity of both rods and cones.

Snakes have a very wide range of vision from 125 degrees to 135 degrees for most species. They also can perceive depth and distance using binocular vision. The area that both eyes can see is between 30 degrees and 45 degrees (Platel 1994).

Digestive System

The digestive system in snakes is a linear tract (Funk 1996). It starts with the mouth that opens directly into the buccal cavity. The buccal cavity contains rows of teeth on the upper and lower jaw, the vomeronasal organs, the primary palate, the internal nares, and a highly specialized tongue. Aniliids, the false coral snakes, have developed a partial secondary palate. The morphology of the tongue is variable depending on the feeding behavior of the snake. The buccal cavity contains many glands throughout the entire cavity. Multicellular glands, a component of the epithelial lining of the tongue, produce and secrete mucous that coats the prey, making passage down the esophagus smooth. Snakes also have five types of salivary glands: labial, lingual, sublingual, palatine, and dental. Venom glands are modified salivary glands. The pharynx contains a muscular sphincter that controls the opening of the esophagus (Figure 7.2).

The esophagus is a muscular walled tube that connects the buccal cavity to the stomach. In snakes, the esophagus may be one-quarter to one-half of the body length. The stomach is a very large muscular tube that has the primary role of mechanical digestion and starting the chemical digestion process. The stomach lining has numerous glands that produce secretions to aid in digestion. The pyloric valve controls the food bolus that enters into the small intestine, which is a long, narrow, straight tube. It also has glands to help with the digestion process. At the junction with the large intestine, there is a marked difference in the size. The large intestine has a diameter several times that of the small intestine. Boidea have a small cecum located at the proximal colon. The large intestine is the weakest and most thin-walled structure in the digestive tract. The large intestine ends at the anus and then leads to the dorsal portion of the cloaca, the coprodaeum.

The primary function of the liver in snakes is the same as in mammals. The liver, which is elongated and spindle shaped, produces bile that is stored in the gall bladder and then sent to the duodenum via the common bile duct. Bile aids in the digestion of fat. The pancreas produces digestive fluids into the duodenum. It is usually located in a triad with the spleen and gallbladder, or some species have a splenopancreas (Figure 7.3).

Because the feeding behavior of snakes is not all the same, different physiological and morphological changes occur with different feeding behaviors. Snakes that eat small, frequent meals tend to have a digestive system that is always in an active state. On the other

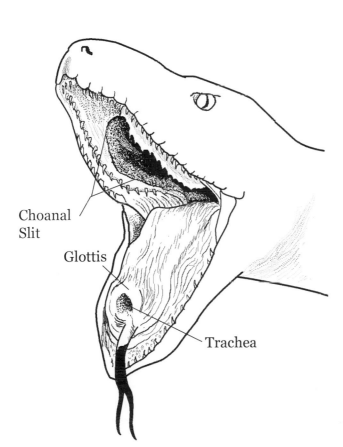

Figure 7.2. *Oral cavity of a snake. (Drawing by Scott Stark.)*

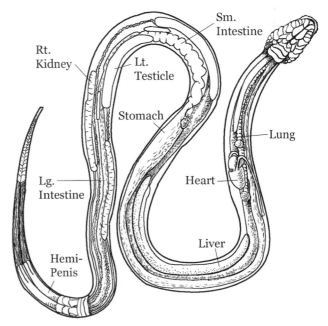

Figure 7.3. *Visceral anatomy. (Drawing by Scott Stark.)*

hand, snakes that eat large, infrequent meals maintain their digestive system in an inactive state until a prey item has been ingested. At that point the gut begins to increase secretions of hydrochloric acid and digestive enzymes. Within one day, the small intestine doubles in size and other organs in the digestive, respiratory, and circulatory system also gain size. When the digestive tract is activated, the metabolic rate increase as much as forty-four times that of the resting metabolic rate. The energy needed to activate the intestinal tract must be received from stored reserves before the digestive process begins for the new prey. Infrequent feeders usually maintain a metabolic rate half that of frequent feeders.

Urinary System

Snakes have a bilateral pair of lobulated and elongated kidneys. They are located in the dorsal caudal coelomic cavity, and the right kidney is located cranial to the left kidney. The kidneys are metanephric in structure and have few nephrons and lack a loop of Henle and a renal pelvis (Divers 2000). The ureters empty into the urodeum in the cloaca. Snakes do not have a urinary bladder.

Snakes excrete nitrogenous waste as uric acid. Uric acid is a purine and is synthesized in several interlocking pathways. It is very insoluble in water. In the kidney tubule, urine stays dilute. Water is reabsorbed when the urine reaches the cloaca, making the urine solution more concentrated and some of the uric acid precipitates. The precipitation of uric acid reduces its concentration, acid allowing more water to be reabsorbed. Again, this leads to more precipitation of uric acid. This process allows nitrogen to be excreted, using very little water. The end product is a white or gray semisolid pasty material containing uric acid.

Endocrine and Exocrine Glands

Pituitary Gland

The pituitary gland is the so-called master gland of the body. It consists of two parts, the neuropophysis and adenopophysis. The neuropophysis produces hormones that stimulate the adenopophysis or act directly on the target organs. The adenopophysis releases six hormones: adrenocorticotropin, follicle-stimulating hormone, luteinizing hormone, prolactin, somatotropin, and thyrotropin.

Pineal Complex

The pineal complex consists of an epiphysis and a parapineal organ. They act as light receptors and are associated with cyclic activities such as circadian rhythms and seasonal cycles. As a gland, both organs release melatonin. All snakes have a pineal gland that lies on the brain but does not exit the skull as in some iguanids.

Thyroid Gland

The thyroid is located in the throat adjacent to the larynx and trachea and is nearly spherical. Snakes can have either a single or paired thyroid gland. The thyroid is responsible for accumulating iodine and producing and regulating hormones that control growth and development as well as ecdysis.

Parathyroid Gland

The parathyroid is located just cranial to the thyroid. It functions as a blood calcium regulator.

Pancreas

The pancreas in snakes, as in mammals, functions as an endocrine and exocrine gland. As an exocrine gland it secretes digestive enzymes, and as an endocrine gland it secretes the hormone insulin via clusters of cells called the islets of Langerhans.

Gonads

The gonads produce the sex hormones. Their function is closely regulated by the brain and the pituitary. Hypothalamohypophyseal hormones and gonadotropins are produced by the brain and the pituitary, respectively, when the gonads are triggered by a hormonal response. Along with stimulating reproductive structures, the sex hormones also produce secondary sexual characteristics and provide a feedback mechanism to the hypothalamic-pituitary complex.

Adrenal Glands

The adrenal glands are a pair of bilateral glands located anterior to the kidneys. They have many functions: produce adrenaline and noradrenaline; affect sodium, potassium, and carbohydrate metabolism; and affect the androgens and the reproductive process.

REPRODUCTIVE BIOLOGY AND HUSBANDRY

The Male Anatomy

All male snakes have a right and left testicle and a pair of hemipenes. The testicles are in the shape of an ovoid mass that consists of seminiferous tubules, interstitial cells, and blood vessels. They are located dorsomedially within the coelomic cavity between the pancreatic triad and the kidneys. The right testis is located just cranial to the left. Snakes do not have an epididymis. The hemipenes are located in the base of the tail and are held in place by a retractor muscle. Sperm is produced in the seminiferous tubules. During copulation, sperm travels to the hemipenis through the Wolffian ducts. The sperm is able to enter the female by means of the sulcus spermaticus located on the outside of the hemipenis. During copulation, only one hemipenis is used. Many snakes, especially boids, have vestigial (pelvic) spurs. These spurs are used in copulation as stimulation and to help position the two cloacae together (Figure 7.4).

The Female Anatomy

The paired ovaries are located similarly to testes. They consist of epithelial cells, connective tissue, nerves, blood vessels, and germinal cell beds encased in an elastic tunic. An inactive ovary is small and granular. Active ovaries are large, lobular sacs filled with spherical vitellogenic follicles. Snakes do not have a true uterus. The oviducts empty directly into the cloaca and have an albumin-secreting and shell-secreting function.

Fertilization

Prior to egg production, fertilization occurs in the upper portion of the oviducts when the sperm and egg unite. Fertilization is usually delayed for a few hours to years after copulation. The sperm storage structures facilitate storage of sperm for long periods of time. This process of delayed fertilization permits females to mate with other males, allowing multiple paternity among the offspring and having a higher fecundity rate, although not all snakes practice this.

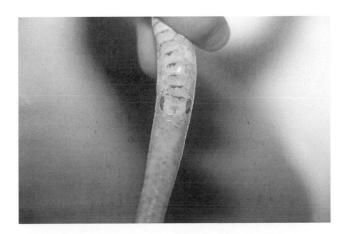

Figure 7.4. Large pelvic spurs. (Photo courtesy of Ryan Cheek.)

Sexual Maturity

Sexual maturity in snakes depends on many factors. Husbandry and nutrition are more important than age. Ultimately, it is the size of the snake that determines sexual maturity. Due to the large difference in care provided to captive snakes, the age of sexual maturity consequently is different as well. With proper husbandry and nutrition, snakes grow quickly and become sexually mature within their first or second year of life.

Follicle Maturation and the Fat Cycle

The female begins to store fat in the months before her reproductive cycle (Ross et al. 1990). This fat plays a major role in the reproductive cycle. Vitellogenesis, the production of yolk, only occurs if enough fat is stored. Furthermore, snakes may not eat at the end stages of gestation, so the fat bodies are used for energy. The follicles mature within the ovaries. When the follicles are mature and palpable, some ova are released into the oviduct while other ova may be released before or after copulation. At this point the snake finds a male and copulates and the female becomes gravid. After the proper gestation period, the female either lays eggs or gives live birth. At this point the female is very thin and weak after using all of her fat deposits during gestation and/or incubation. She cannot stimulate follicular maturation until the fat stores have been built back up. She begins to eat and increases her fat bodies, and after a couple to several months she is back to full weight and can begin the follicular maturation cycle again.

Courtship

It is important to know and observe signs of courtship so proper changes can be made. If communal cages are kept, insubordinate specimens should be separated from the courting pair. Temperature cycling patterns should be started before or at the first signs of copulation. Specimens should be removed or added if either of the specimens seen courting is inappropriate for breeding.

Many courtship behaviors are observed in snakes; most are not species specific. Following is an explanation of four common courtship behaviors that are seen in many taxa (Ross et al. 1990).

1. The tactile chase behavior is characterized by the male pursuing the female in often jerky and erratic movements. The male may flick his tongue over the female's body and begin to crawl over her dorsum, trying to align his body with hers. The female will continue to crawl away if unreceptive to the behavior.

2. In the tail search copulatory attempt the male rotates his tail under the female's tail in an attempt to bring both cloacae together. A receptive female will then lift her tail or allow her tail to be lifted by the male. The male may use his spurs to stimulate the female to lift her tail.

3. Tactile alignment is characterized by the male aligning his tail with the female's, using his spurs as stimulation and to help align the cloacae.

4. Intromission and coitus occurs when a female raises her tail and everts her cloaca to a male. The male then aligns the two cloacae and copulation occurs. This behavior is also known as cloacal gaping.

Oviparous, Ovoviviparous, and Viviparous

Oviparous snakes are those that lay eggs that are protected by a hard shell. Around 70% of snakes are oviparous. Some of the more common oviparous species seen in a veterinary practice are king snakes and milk snakes (*Lampropeltis* spp.), rat and corn snakes (*Elaphe* spp.), and all pythons. Oviparous snakes go to much trouble finding an appropriate place to lay their eggs. Some lay in a natural cavity, hollow stumps, or small mammals' burrows, while others dig their own burrow or make a nest. Most pythons incubate their eggs by hugging them and increasing their own body heat through rhythmic contractions of their abdominal musculature.

Ovoviviparous snakes incubate the eggs inside the oviducts until the eggs hatch. This process ensures proper humidity and temperature levels within the mother's thermoregulative capabilities. Ovoviviparous snakes are found mainly in places where the ground is too cold to incubate eggs (Saint-Girons 1994). There are many disadvantages to ovoviviparous snakes. The gravid female moves very slowly, which opens her up to predation; she is only able to eat very small prey, which are hard to find at times; and she must focus more on thermoregulation. Some examples of ovoviviparous snakes are all boas, all vipers, and garter snakes (*Thamnophis* spp.).

Snakes do not practice true viviparity.

EGG ANATOMY

After fertilization, the embryo begins to develop on the dorsal surface of the yolk. The yolk is then covered by the yolk sac and attached to the embryo by the yolk stalk at the umbilicus. Nourishment is provided by the yolk via the blood vessels of the yolk sac. The amnion is a fluid-filled sac that surrounds and protects the embryo. The allantois is a closed sac that collects waste products. The chorion is a membrane that surrounds and protects the embryo and yolk sac. The shell membranes that cover these three membranes provide gas exchange throughout the shell. The blood vessels in the shell membranes and the yolk stalk combine to form the umbilicus. As the egg passes through the oviducts, the shell and shell membranes are gradually applied by the shell glands.

Timing and Frequency of Reproduction

Environmental factors trigger the breeding season in most species. While some species breed year 'round, breeding season usually begins in the spring after a hibernation period for temperate species. Most equatorial species breed year 'round. There are exceptions to these rules. Some tropical boids reproduce in the cooler part of the year, though temperature changes have a greater diurnal change than seasonal change. Many species in areas where there is a rainy season, such as the monsoons in Southeast Asia and India, time their reproductive cycle with the rainfall.

It is not common for a snake to reproduce more than once in a single year due to the lengthy gestation periods and need to gain back a large amount of fat deposits. The entire reproductive process, starting with follicle maturation and ending with the snake back at full weight, can take several months to more than a year, depending on species.

Maternal Care

Very few snakes show any maternal care. Some pythons coil around the eggs to incubate them and protect them from predators. Some viviparous species show maternal care by helping the newborns out of the amniotic sac and consuming the infertile yolk sac.

EGG INCUBATION AND MANAGEMENT

Artificial Incubation

It is recommended that eggs only be artificially incubated by experienced herpetoculturists. Many herpetoculturists artificially incubate eggs to increase the chance of hatching. In captivity, it is difficult for the female snake to keep the relative humidity high enough to incubate her own eggs. If the decision is made to artificially incubate the eggs, the herpetoculturists must be prepared several days before the female lays the eggs, and the incubator should be ready several days in advance. It should maintain a constant temperature and humidity that is ideal for the species being incubated. For most species, a temperature range of 86°F to 91°F is ideal. Eggs do not benefit from temperature variations so a constant temperature should be maintained. It is not critical to measure the relative humidity, although a high relative humidity should be maintained. As long as condensation appears on the sides of the incubator, the humidity should be high enough.

When the female lays the eggs, herpetoculturists should move quickly to remove them. The eggs become adherent within a few hours after oviposition. It is preferable that the eggs be laid singly in the incubator so they can be properly monitored; the conditions inside the enclosure also may be inadequate for proper incubation, which can be detrimental to the eggs. Eggs can dehydrate within forty-eight to seventy-two hours. Gently remove the eggs and place them in the preheated incubator. The incubator should be checked several times a day for proper temperature and humidity and the eggs should be checked for viability.

Maternal Incubation

Maternal incubation should be performed for several reasons. The eggs should be maternally incubated if the female is too large or aggressive to safely remove the eggs, if she unexpectedly laid eggs and an incubator was not ready, or if normal incubation parameters are not known. The humidity in the cage should not fall below 75%. Because of the high humidity that must be maintained, the cage should be kept in a very clean environment with adequate circulation. The temperature in the cage should be constant. The incubating female should not have to thermoregulate, which requires an excessive amount of energy that many incubating females do not have. The cage should be kept at 88 °F for most python species. If maternal incubation was chosen due to a lack of experience in artificial incubation, extensive research on the natural history of the species should be conducted to determine the proper incubating temperature.

Incubator Design

Incubators can be bought commercially or easily made. The basic requirements of an incubator are: the construction should prevent excessive heat and humidity loss, there must be a constant and reliable heat source, and there must be a thermostat to control the temperature. The actual design of the incubator can vary as long as the above three rules are met.

Some general guidelines should be followed when constructing an incubator. It should be uniformly heated. An easy way to accomplish this is by using heat tape that can be evenly positioned on the bottom of the incubator. Hot water can also be used. An inner container should be installed that does not rest on the bottom of the incubator to allow the heat to be evenly distributed throughout the entire incubator. The thermostat should be sensitive enough to control the temperature fluctuation within one degree, and the temperature should be monitored from the outside of the incubator. To ensure adequate humidity, the incubator and eggs should be sprayed with water that is the same temperature as the incubator every two to three days. The incubator should be lined with Styrofoam to maintain a proper temperature. The best substrates are vermiculite, sphagnum moss, potting soil, sand, shredded newspaper, pea gravel, and paper towels.

Determining Egg Viability

A viable clutch should be uniform in size, have a brilliant white color, and be pliable or elastic (Ross et al. 1990). If an egg is smaller, discolored, or hard or rubbery, it usually is not fertilized. Some female snakes reject an unfertilized egg from the clutch. If an egg does not adhere to the rest of the clutch, it should still be incubated until signs of egg death appear. Wrinkles or depressions at the time of oviposition are not signs of nonviability. A fertilized egg does not show significant change during the incubation period. An unfertilized egg quickly begins to show signs of decomposition.

It can sometimes be very difficult to determine the viability of an egg. If the viability is uncertain, the egg should be incubated until further signs appear. The rest of the clutch will not be in danger. The texture of an egg or irregular calcification should not be used as an indication of nonviability. Another method for determining egg viability is a technique called candling, which uses of a high intensity light to transilluminate the egg. A viable egg should have a network of blood vessels and an embryo during the late stages of incubation. The absence of blood vessels indicates a nonviable egg.

Manual Pipping

Sometimes manual pipping is necessary for the embryo to live. An egg should be manually pipped only if most eggs in the clutch have hatched, no eggs have pipped by the estimated due date, or the due date is unknown. Manual pipping is a very delicate procedure that with time and practice can be a very effective method of saving a clutch. All that is needed to perform this technique is a pair of iris scissors and thumb forceps. A small perforation is made in the shell with the iris scissors. With the scissors pointing up toward the inner surface of the eggshell, a small incision is then made in the shell. Another small incision is made at the site of the puncture creating a V-shaped incision. The wedge can be elevated using the thumb forceps and removed. If done properly, the shell membranes should all still be intact. During this process, one should avoid cutting large blood vessels; small vessels are impossible to avoid. The embryo should not be visible.

The shell membranes should be gently separated from the shell with the thumb forceps, starting at the window that was made and then working outward. More pieces of shell can be removed as the membrane is separated. The embryo can then be stimulated when a large enough window has been made.

To stimulate the embryo, prod it gently with a blunt tip instrument. If it is alive, the embryo will move freely in the egg. The embryo should be intermittently stimulated until the neonate has emerged from the shell. This process usually takes twelve to twenty-four hours.

HOUSING

The following points must be considered when obtaining housing for a snake: (1) the size (length) of the snake to be housed, (2) whether it is a terrestrial or an arboreal species, (3) security of the housing (escape proof), (4) proper ventilation, (5) access for necessary cleaning/disinfecting.

Aquariums are certainly suitable and aesthetically pleasing enclosures for most species of snakes, but can be quite costly to obtain, especially when housing some of the larger species. Ideally, the length of the enclosure should be no less than half of the length of the snake being housed. When housing arboreal species (i.e., green tree python), the enclosure should have more vertical space than horizontal to allow for placement of perches for the snake. If an aquarium is used, it is important that a lid can be secured appropriately. Lids that rest on top of the aquarium without any locking mechanisms are NOT appropriate for snakes because they are escape artists. Aquarium lids should allow proper ventilation (i.e. screen lids) if the aquarium itself does not have any ventilation holes (most do not). The lid must not present a potential fire hazard if heat lamps are used above it. Plastic lids, for instance, will melt (Figure 7.5). Any aquariums with cracks should be avoided due to the potential for the glass to shatter, resulting in injury to the animal.

Building an enclosure for a snake is usually the preferred method of acquiring housing. It is less expensive in most cases and allows for customizing according to the snake's needs. Customizing an enclosure can be enjoyable as long as a couple of guidelines are followed. Obviously, it is not ideal to construct a cage

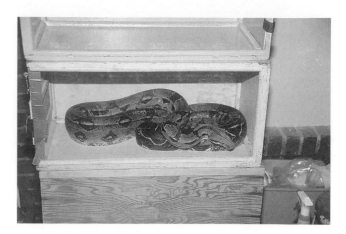

Figure 7.5. Inappropriate housing for a snake. (Photo courtesy of Ryan Cheek.)

solely of wood without any way to view the snake. Glass or Plexiglas should be included when constructing a wooden enclosure. Screen can be used on the sides or even the top of the enclosure to ensure proper ventilation. Without proper ventilation, bacteria accumulate, making the enclosure stagnant. Using screen on the top also allows for proper lighting/heat fixtures to be affixed while preventing the snake from contacting the fixtures. To prevent burns, heat lamps should not be placed inside the enclosure where the snake can contact them.

An enclosure should not be constructed solely of screen, however, because it can become too drafty. The wood used should be sanded and free of abrasive surfaces to prevent potential injuries to the snake. It also must be treated or painted to allow regular cleaning without damaging the wood and so that feces and such do not soak into the porous wood. Priming and painting the inside of the enclosure white can assist in spotting problems such as mites in the caging. The white paint also reflects the light better.

Different locking mechanisms can be chosen, depending on what is preferred to access the inside of the cage. Everything from hinged doors with padlocks to sliding glass doors are suitable for securing the custom enclosure.

Commercially available enclosures such as Neodesha and Visions cages are specifically made for keeping reptiles. These are perfectly suitable for housing snakes if one does not mind the added expense and as long as an appropriately sized enclosure can be obtained.

Substrate
Many different types of substrate are used in snake enclosures (Figure 7.6). There also is a lot of debate about what is appropriate and what can be harmful.

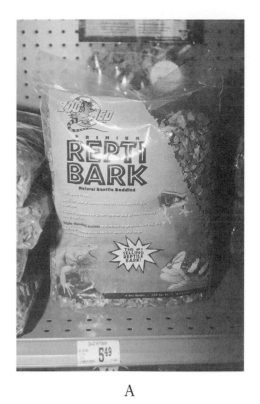

A

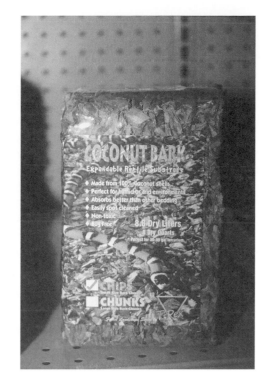

B

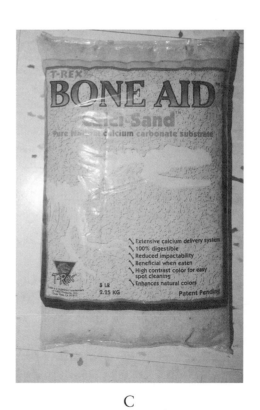

C

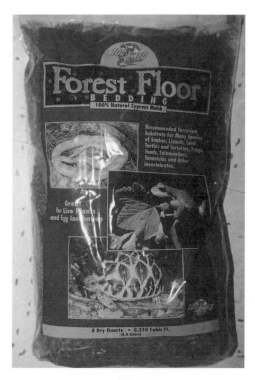

D

Figure 7.6. *Various common commercially available substrates. (A) Repti Bark (fir bark). (B) Ground coconut shell. (C) Calcium carbonate granules. (D.) Cypress mulch. (Photos courtesy of Ryan Cheek.)*

It is necessary to read as much literature about the snake as possible to obtain more information about its natural habitat to better assist in making husbandry-related choices.

Cedar and pine shavings are not recommended as substrate for any reptiles. The oils and natural aroma of these shavings can be toxic to snakes and can even lead to respiratory disorders. Shavings can also lodge in the snake's oral cavity, which could cause stomatitis (mouth rot). Although some companies claim that these shavings are great for snakes because they repel mites and ticks, use of any cedar or pine shavings should be avoided.

Aspen shavings can be used for some of the snake species that require an arid climate. They should not be used for snakes that require high humidity because there are more suitable substrates for maintaining high humidity. The aspen shavings must treated through a baking process, which can help to eliminate any potential for parasites contained in the shavings and to ensure that they are free of toxic oils. Aspen shavings can also become lodged in the snake's mouth so as a precaution, the snake should not be fed on aspen shavings.

Indoor/outdoor carpet or Astroturf is commonly used as substrate. It is aesthetically pleasing and does not present any immediate harm to the snake. It can be purchased by the yard at most local hardware stores. Routine cleaning and disinfecting is more demanding than with other substrates because the carpet needs to be replaced frequently and is more expensive than some options. When a snake defecates or passes urates, the carpet absorbs some of the matter and needs to be washed or replaced or it will become pungent and allow bacterial and/or mold growth. Animals with parasite infections should have the carpet changed completely to avoid recontamination.

Aquarium gravel and corncob should not be used. Some gravel can be abrasive and both can cause impactions if ingested in large amounts.

Sand is used often for desert species, and there are many contradicting statements regarding its use in any reptile enclosure. There is debate about whether it causes digestive problems and obstructions. However, sand is the natural substrate of many desert species. Any loose substrate that is ingested in large amounts could potentially cause these problems as well as stomatitis. The snake should not be fed in the enclosure to reduce the chance of this happening. Some people feed their snakes in plastic tubs or boxes to eliminate the opportunity to ingest substrate while feeding.

Some people buy play sand at the hardware store to use as substrate, while others buy the sand sold at pet stores for reptile substrate. Some of the commercial brands of sand used as substrate for reptiles claim that if it is ingested the sand is less likely to cause impactions than regular play sand due to its calcium contents and fine grain. However, caution should still be used when feeding any reptile on a sand substrate. Furthermore, too much of calcium consumption can be just as harmful as calcium deficiencies. Those who choose to use sand as a substrate can let personal preference dictate their choice. The key is to ensure it is not being ingested, and if that is the case then the substrate should be changed.

Cypress mulch is another good substrate, especially for species that require higher humidity. It can make an enclosure look very natural and it is relatively inexpensive. It is important to make sure that it is actually cypress mulch and not another type of mulch (i.e. eucalyptus) because these can be very aromatic and lead to respiratory problems. The mulch can be mixed with sphagnum moss if the goal is to make a natural appearing environment.

Newspaper is frequently used as substrate, especially when an multiple snakes are kept. Newspaper is plentiful, inexpensive, and easily obtained. It is absorbent and easily replaced during routine cleanings. It is especially good for animals in quarantine, and it is the substrate best suited for feeding because the chances of it being ingested are not as great as loose substrate. Although it is not as aesthetically pleasing as some forms of substrate, it is definitely easier to maintain.

Potting soil should be used with caution. Most potting soils have fertilizers and other chemicals that could be toxic to snakes. If topsoil is used, make sure that it is organic and free of chemicals. Topsoil can be a good substrate to use for snakes that require high humidity because of its ability to retain moisture. This can be used for terrestrial and burrowing species.

Caution should be used if tree limbs, substrate, or any other objects are collected from outside. They can contaminate the enclosure with parasites, molds, fungus, etc. Sterilization can be attempted with these objects via boiling/baking or disinfecting with a diluted bleach solution to minimize contamination. Tree limbs taken from outside should not have any sticky substances such as sap on them.

Good judgment must be used when choosing an appropriate substrate. Knowing the geographic range of the particular snake housed will aid in making husbandry decisions.

Heating and Lighting

Snakes are ectothermic, which means they rely on their surroundings to regulate their body temperature. Unlike mammals, they are unable to do this on their own. Therefore, snakes kept in captivity require heating and lighting supplementation (Table 7.2). Failure to maintain appropriate temperatures for the particular snake can lead to respiratory disorders, food regurgitation, anorexia due to lethargy, and even death.

Whether the snake is desert-dwelling or tropical, it is necessary to maintain an enclosure that mimics its natural surroundings and climate zone. Ideally, snakes need a warm basking area to maintain good health as well as a cooler area to retreat to if they get too warm. Thermometers must be used to ensure that necessary

Table 7.2. *Husbandry Data for Selected Species of Snakes.*

Common name	Scientific name	Average length*	Ambient temperature in Fahrenheit (day)**	Humidity	Geographic range
Boas					
Common boa	*Boa constrictor*	~6'–10'	80–85	50–70%	Central America and South America
Brazilian rainbow boa	*Epicrates cenchria cenchria*	5'–7'	80–85	75–90%	Brazil
Emerald tree boa	*Corallus caninus*	4'–6'	75–82	85–90%	Amazon Basin
Rosy boa	*Lichanura trivirgata*	2'–3'	80–85	20–30%	Southern CA, AZ, Mexico
Pythons					
Ball python	*Python requis*	3'–5'	80–85	60–65%	Central Africa, Western Africa, Borneo
Blood python	*Python curtus*	3'–6'	80–85	70–75%	Borneo Islands, Malaysia, Sumatra
Burmese python	*Python molurus bivittatus*	12'–20'	80–85	70–80%	S.E. Asia
Green tree python	*Morelia chondropython viridis*	4'–6'	75–85	85–90%	Australia, New Guinea
Carpet python	*Morelia spilota*	6'–10'	80–85	60–70%	Australia
Reticulated python	*Python reticulatus*	10'–25'	80–85	65–70%	Thailand, Indonesia, Philippines (S.E. Asia)
African rock python	*Python sebae*	12'–20'	80–85	65–70%	Africa
Colubrids					
Common king snakes	*Lampropeltis getula*	4'–5'	75–85	30–50%	North & South America
Corn snakes	*Elaphe guttata*	4'–5'	75–85	50–60%	Eastern United States, Midwest United States
Rat snake	*Elaphe obsoleta*	5'–7'	75–85	50–60%	North America
Milk snake	*Lampropeltis triangulum*	2'–5'	75–85	50–60%	North & South America
Gopher/Bull/ Pinesnake	*Pituophis* spp.	4'–7'	75–85	30–50%	United States & Mexico
Garter/Ribbon snakes	*Thamnophis* spp.	2'–4'	75–80	60–75%	United States

*Lengths refer to average adult lengths (in feet) not absolute min./max. lengths.
**Temperatures given are average ambient temperatures; basking spots should be 5–10°F higher with a nighttime drop of 5–10°F.

temperatures are being met. These can be bought at most pet stores and have adhesives so they can be easily placed into the enclosure. Ideally, one thermometer should be affixed in the enclosure where the hottest temperature is achieved and one should be affixed in the cool zone. If the snake is a terrestrial species, the thermometer should be placed close to the bottom. With arboreal species, the thermometers should be placed near the areas where the snake can perch (Figure 7.7).

Heat rocks are sold as an artificial heat source for reptiles. These are not reliable heat sources and can in fact injure the snake. The heating element is not on a thermostat and can become extremely hot. The snake can sustain serious burns if it is allowed direct contact with the rock. At other times the rock can be cool to the touch, providing no supplemental heat at all. While the author does not recommend heat rocks, if they are used they should be buried under the substrate so the snake does not have direct contact with them, and they should not be the only source of heat provided.

Heating tape and pads and under-tank heaters are good sources of heat for snakes. They also sold commercially in the pet trade and if used correctly, are safer than heat rocks. The pads and tape can be placed on the outside of the enclosure underneath the tank where the snake cannot have direct contact with the units but still benefit from the heat being emitted. These heating mechanisms distribute the heat more evenly and in some cases cover the entire length of the enclosure. If a heating pad that has a temperature setting control is used, the setting should be kept on low. If the enclosure is made of thick wood or if there is a thick layer of substrate, the pad can be placed on

medium if the low setting is not producing enough heat to benefit the snake. The bottom of the enclosure should always be tested (via touch or thermometers) thoroughly to ensure it does not get too hot. A high setting should never be used. Do not trust that the snake will move if the heating element gets too hot. Thermal burns are easily prevented if caution is used and regular checks are performed on the heating elements.

Heat lamps are acceptable primary heat sources and they also provide the snake with necessary day and night cycles if actual lights are used. These lamps can be used in conjunction with under-tank heaters for snakes that require high temperatures. Clamp light fixtures are relatively inexpensive and can be purchased from a local hardware store (Figure 7.8). These can be placed on top of the enclosure (on a screen, not plastic or flammable material) or clamped to a surface allowing the light to be directed into the enclosure.

Bulbs should be selected based on the snake's temperature needs and the design of the enclosure itself. Incandescent bulbs, ceramic heat emitters, or flood lamps can be used for heating purposes. The wattage of the bulb depends on the dimensions of the enclosure and the snake's temperature needs. In most cases, a 50– to 75-watt bulb is sufficient. Extremely high wattage bulbs or those used for food warming purposes should not be used because they get extremely hot. The heat-emitting bulbs should be sufficiently distant from the snake so that burns do not occur, and the snake should not have direct access to the bulbs. Burns can be sustained from any heat source, including bulbs, if the snake is allowed direct access to them or if they are not placed at a safe distance from the snake.

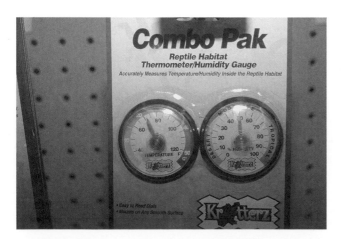

Figure 7.7. Thermometer and hygrometer. (Photo courtesy of Ryan Cheek.)

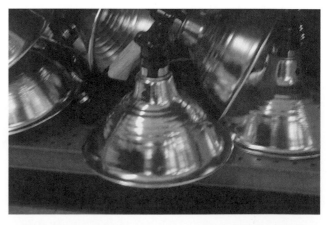

Figure 7.8. Clamp light fixture. (Photo courtesy of Ryan Cheek.)

The snake is allowed a good basking area when the lamp is placed at one end of the enclosure. The other end should be free of any heat sources to provide a cooler zone to retreat to (Figure 7.9).

Lights used as heat sources should not be kept on all the time. Timers can be used to control when the light comes on and turns off. This assists in maintaining natural photoperiods or day/night cycles. Ideally, the snake should have around twelve to thirteen hours of daylight followed by eleven to twelve hours of darkness to mimic nighttime. The timers can be set to mimic the different seasonal day/night cycles by synchronizing them with the different day/night cycles that change slightly from season to season. For example, there are longer daylight hours in the summer than in winter; therefore, daylight should be provided for approximately thirteen hours, whereas in winter eleven hours of daylight is typical.

It is particularly important to follow the photoperiod in snakes if breeding is being considered. Some snakes are only receptive to breeding during certain seasons, so these seasonal changes must be recreated in captivity for successful breeding activity. However, if bulbs are the only source of heat being used, it may be necessary to purchase night bulbs to ensure the snake does not get too cool during the night hours. A slight drop in temperature at night is a natural, but too much can lead to illness. Night bulbs emit heat yet allow darkness. Red, blue, black light, ceramic or commercially available night bulbs can be purchased to achieve this. Reading the temperature gauges in the enclosure assists in deciding whether night bulbs are necessary. Keeping the enclosure in a temperature-controlled room and away from drafty areas (i.e. windows) aids in preventing drastic temperature changes at night when the heat lamps go off.

UV lighting or natural sunlight certainly could be beneficial to the snake, but it is not detrimental to the snake's overall health as with diurnal lizards if it is not provided (Figure 7.10). It should be clear, though, that there no any bulb available that can replace natural sunlight. During the warmer months, if the snake is kept outside, which is not recommended, special precautions are necessary. Glass or Plexiglas enclosures should not be used at all outside because they can get extremely hot in the direct sunlight and prove to be fatal to the snake. The inside of the enclosure can become hot much like in a car with the windows rolled up and no air flow. When other enclosures are used outside a shaded area should always be provided for the animal. Snakes must be able to retreat to an area that is not receiving direct sunlight when they are finished basking or they will become overheated.

Wiring the heating device (bulbs or pads) to a thermostat can assist in more accurately maintaining temperatures and decrease the chance of thermal burns. This is not to say that thermostats are always accurate or 100% dependable, but it certainly helps. Frequent temperature checks should be performed when synchronizing thermostats.

Water and Humidity

Depending on the geographic range the snake derives from, it may be necessary to supplement humidity as well as heat. Tropical species (i.e. emerald tree boas) need relatively high humidity and require some form of supplementation. In some cases, it may be necessary to make husbandry choices to prevent high humidity, as with desert species that require arid environments.

Hygrometers (humidity gauges) can be purchased with thermometers and placed inside the enclosure to provide humidity readings. This provides information about when humidity needs to be increased or decreased so any changes necessary can be made for ideal conditions.

High humidity can be maintained by misting the entire enclosure and even the snake. The mist should be fine and not extremely cold or hot water. It may be necessary to mist multiple times a day for tropical species. Some people even set up misting systems on timers to provide constant and consistent humidity (see Figure 7.7).

Remember that humidity is the presence of moisture in the atmosphere itself. If the enclosure does not allow humidity to stay contained, then it must be modified or a different enclosure should be used. For snakes that require high humidity, enclosures made exclusively of screen are not ideal due to the inability to keep moisture within the enclosure. The moisture will escape. Aquariums are good for maintaining humidity; however, an appropriate lid is necessary. Furthermore, ensure that the enclosure have some sort of ventilation to prevent the air and substrate from becoming stagnant. Typically, if water is added to supplement humidity (via misting, etc.), it should be evaporated at least within twenty-four hours. The enclosure is lacking appropriate ventilation if it does not evaporate. It may take some trial and error to get the humidity right. When obtaining tropical species that require humid environments, appropriate methods should be established before placing the snake in the enclosure. However, most species may not require any supplementation if appropriate enclosures and substrates are used.

A water supply is essential for all snakes and can assist in maintaining humidity as well. The enclosure

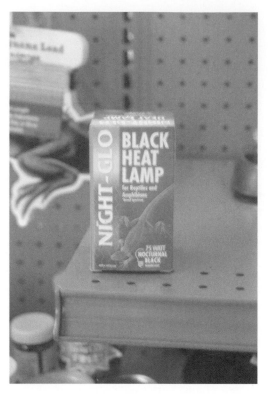

A

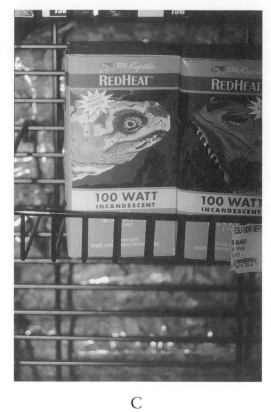

C

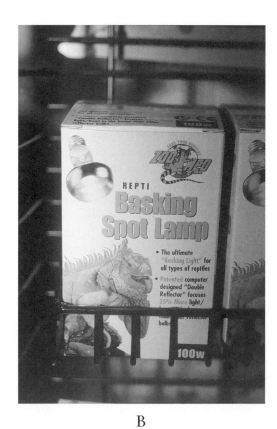

B

Figure 7.9. Various commercially incandescent heat lamps. (A) Night light. (B) Basking day light. (C) Incandescent heat light. (Photos courtesy of Ryan Cheek.)

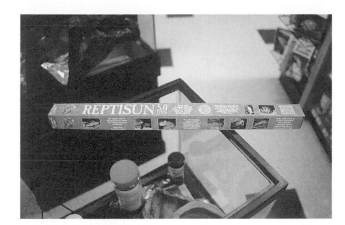

Figure 7.10. UV light bulb. (Photo courtesy of Ryan Cheek.)

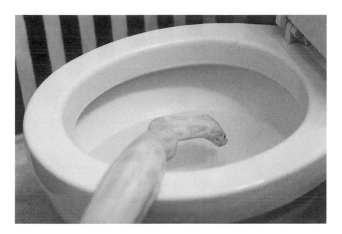

Figure 7.11. This is not an appropriate method of providing water to a snake. (Photo courtesy of Stacy Bailey.)

should contain an appropriately sized water container. Some snakes enjoy soaking in the water prior to shedding, so the snake's size should be considered when choosing an appropriate bowl. Small ceramic bowls work well for smaller snakes (they can not be tipped as easily as lightweight bowls) and plastic tubs work well for larger snakes. Be careful not to overfill because the snake can cause large amounts of water to spill over when submerging. The water should be changed if it becomes soiled or stagnant, and no less than once a week. A water container placed over the heating element (heating pad or tape) creates some humidity and evaporates quickly so the water levels should be watched closely. If the species requires low humidity, obviously the water should not be placed near the heating elements (Figure 7.11).

Substrate can play a vital role in maintaining high humidity. Substrate materials such as topsoil, moss (sphagnum or peat), and mulch are great substrate choices for species that need high humidity. They absorb and hold moisture well unless too much water is added. Regular mistings in conjunction with appropriate substrate are keys in maintaining high humidity. Items such as newspaper, shavings, or rock gravel allow pooling and are not ideal for humid terrestrial environments.

Other Cage Furnishings

Hide boxes are easily constructed and really make a difference in the snake's overall demeanor. A snake that has a place to go where it feels secure is less stressed in its captive environment. This has also been known to assist in the feeding response in some snakes (i.e. ball python). Hide boxes can be constructed from everything from boxes, plastic pots, and Tupperware (not clear), to logs. They also may be purchased from reptile supply stores and dealers. No matter how elaborate or simple they are, hide boxes serve the same purpose and should be provided.

Tree branches or some sort of perching material should be provided for arboreal species. PVC pipe can be used for this purpose as well. The perch should not be any bigger in diameter than the largest part of the snake's body. Anything larger makes perching difficult. Make sure all perching materials are secured properly and free of abrasive surfaces.

Decorative rocks are nice additions to an enclosure but can also injure the snake if there are sharp edges. Snakes often use cage furnishings to assist them when shedding by rubbing against them. Nothing with rough texture should be placed in the enclosure.

QUARANTINE

All reptiles brought into a home or facility should undergo a quarantine period. This is especially necessary in environments where numerous reptiles are housed. There are some diseases in reptiles that can wipe out whole collections if proper quarantine procedures are not used (i.e. inclusive body disease).

A room should be set aside for quarantine purposes and should be absent of other animals, especially other reptiles. During the quarantine period, physical exams and fecal exams should be performed to check for internal and external parasites. Ideally, a fecal culture for salmonella should be performed as well. Salmonella is transmissible to other reptiles and is zoonotic. The quarantine period should be no less than thirty days. Some facilities have a six-month quarantine period for all reptiles. The quarantine period should be extended if the snake becomes ill and continued until the snake is healthy.

Proper cleaning and disinfecting is very important during this time. The enclosures should be set up to meet the snake's individual requirements but also should allow for frequent cleaning. Newspaper is a good substrate to use for quarantined animals due to the ease of cleaning. It is easily changed and is cheap to replace. When the snake defecates or passes urates, the substrate should be changed completely. A dilute bleach solution (one-half cup bleach to 1 gallon of water) should be used to clean surfaces in the enclosure. Make sure the surfaces are dry before placing the snake back in the enclosure. Gloves should be worn when cleaning soiled cages to prevent contamination. Any cage furnishings should be properly disinfected or replaced.

NUTRITION

All snakes are carnivores that feed on whole prey items. Their digestive system is made to digest whole prey and they cast out or defecate the parts of the prey that are not digested, such as fur. Eating whole carcasses provides them with added nutrients such as calcium from bone so that no further supplementation is needed. Feeding packaged meat and poultry products is not an appropriate, balanced diet for snakes. Feeding in this manner may be convenient for some, but it is not as nutritionally beneficial as whole prey items. It should be remembered that just because a snake eats something readily does not mean it is nutritionally sound. It is the responsibility of the person who cares for the captive snake to make sure its nutritional needs are properly met.

Although some commonly kept species feed on invertebrates, most readily feed using commercially bred mice and rats. What to feed the snake depends on multiple factors: (1) availability of prey item, (2) natural diet, (3) whether the snake was captive-bred or wild-caught, and (4) size of the snake.

Prey Items
With the increase in popularity of keeping snakes in captivity, there is a larger and more diverse market for buying varieties of food items. At one point, the most accessible food items were pet rodents at pet stores. Not only was this costly, but the pet rodent's nutritional needs were probably not as closely monitored as those that are sold as food items. It is essential that any prey item is fed a nutritionally sound diet. Those that were starved, fed inappropriately, or otherwise neglected are of little nutritional benefit to the snake that eats them. Just going through the motions of feeding the snake does not ensure nutritional requirements are being met. Remember, you are what you eat.

Today, many companies breed insects and rodents specifically for food items, and they offer every growth stage of rats and mice. Commercially available snake food includes various stages of mice, rats, gerbils, rabbits, guinea pigs, chickens (and other birds such as guinea chicks). For smaller snakes (i.e. garter and ribbon snakes) that feed primarily on invertebrates, there are crickets, various worms, and even small fish available for feeding purposes. In some cases, other reptile and/or amphibian species, such as anoles or frogs, may be used to encourage finicky eaters to feed in captivity. However, most of the commonly kept species feed on rodents. Below are some of the terms used when specifying the stage of feeder rodent desired if standard adult size is not ideal:

- Pinkies: baby mice, no fur present yet
- Fuzzies: baby mice that have just gotten fur
- Hoppers: juvenile mice that have fur and all adult characteristics but are not as large as adult mice
- Pups: usually unweaned or nursing baby rats
- Weanlings: baby rats that are no longer nursing
- Otherwise (for rats): small, medium, large, or jumbo is used to obtain the desired size.

Choose an appropriately sized meal by offering a prey item that is no larger than the biggest part of the snake's body. Some people try to gauge prey size by the size of the snake's head. This can be deceiving because the snake will dislocate its jaw for feeding; therefore, it can feed on prey items that are much larger than its head. Gauging by the actual body itself helps to ensure that the snake is being fed a large enough prey item and yet one that is not so big that could cause an uncomfortable, large, bulging appearance.

Another benefit of easily accessible commercial rodent breeders is the ability to purchase rodents prekilled and/or frozen. Some people find it disheartening and difficult to feed live rodents to snakes. In the wild, the snake feed on live prey, but with the availability of prekilled prey on the market, there is no need for this in captivity. Captive-bred specimens readily feed off prekilled or previously frozen prey items. Offering live prey to snakes causes unnecessary suffering to the rodent, and the snake can endure rodent bites as a result. Significant rodent bites can cause many dermatological problems; some even warrant systemic antibiotics and/or topical treatments of a dilute betadine or chlorhexidine solution. Scars from bite wounds are usually apparent in snakes that are offered live prey items (Color Plate 7.1).

Offering previously frozen prey rather than live prey has many other benefits. It is usually cheaper to and may be purchased in bulk rates if freezer space is available. Another benefit is that a frozen rodent is certainly less likely to introduce parasites to the snake and/or enclosure. Rodents are one of the main sources of parasitic contamination in captive snakes. They can harbor mites, for instance. If a frozen prey item had parasites (endoparasite or ectoparasite), the parasites will most likely be dead due to the freezing process. This is not to say, however, that it is acceptable to knowingly offer parasite-infested animals as food just because they were frozen. Buying snake food from a reputable company helps to make sure the snake's nutritional needs are met.

Do not attempt to feed a frozen rodent to the snake; it must first be thawed out. Putting the rodent in a zip lock bag and submerging it in hot water is an easy way to do thaw it. Some people even place the rodent on a warm surface (under a heat lamp, on a heat pad, etc.) to ensure the rodent is properly thawed. Microwaves are not an option for thawing rodents.

Feedings only need to occur about once a week to every fourteen days for adult snakes due to their slow digestive process. For juveniles, it may be necessary to feed twice a week to ensure that proper nutritional requirements are being met during the growth process. If a snake refuses one meal, do not panic. This occurs occasionally and the snake will not starve in one week's time. If several consecutive meals are skipped, then the snake's inappetence needs to be addressed.

To avoid bites, some reptile hobbyists believe that snakes should not be fed inside their primary enclosure, especially if the only time the enclosure is opened

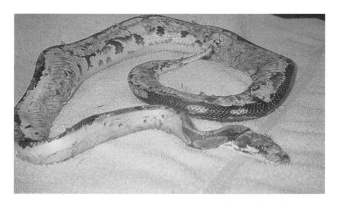

Plate 7.1. A snake suffering from trauma from a prey item. (Photo courtesy of Dr. Sam Rivera.) (See also color plates)

is when the snake is being fed. This creates a feeding response and makes bites more likely to occur. Feeding outside the primary enclosure is safer and also can help to ensure that any loose substrate located inside the primary enclosure is not ingested during feeding.

Why Won't My Snake Eat?

Some people claim that their snake will not take previously frozen prey and will only accept live prey items. Some people have snakes that are reluctant eaters in general. Below are some feeding guidelines and tips to follow for all reluctant eaters.

Some snakes, such as Boidae and pit vipers, have heat-seeking pits that they rely on for locating their warm-blooded prey. Some people confuse these pits for nostrils. These bilateral openings are located on the skin of the upper lip, usually under the nares. If they confront a cold prey item (previously frozen), they are unlikely to show any interest; therefore, make sure that the prey item is warm, using the warming techniques described above, before offering it to the snake.

Motion also can trigger a snake to feed. Tongs should always be used when placing a prekilled rodent into the enclosure. This is especially true when one entices the snake by moving the prey item around. Many snakebites occur during feedings and can be easily avoided if using tongs (not hands) when feeding and keeping a safe distance from the snake.

There are several things to check for if the snake was wild-caught and is not feeding in captivity. Wild-caught specimens are frequently reluctant to eat in captive environments. Remember that they have been taken from their natural habitat and placed in a cage. Furthermore, in most cases they are being offered prey they would have never encountered in their natural habitat. For example, a green tree python feeds primarily on birds, frogs, and occasional small mammals in its natural habitat. Once in captivity, it is offered white mice. This is an unnatural prey item and small mammals are not a large part of the natural diet to begin with. This is not to say that it will never accept commercially bred rodents in captivity, but adjusting to a new captive environment is tough.

Initially at least try to offer a natural diet. Try feeding colored rodents rather than the typical white feeder rodents if the snake is reluctant to eat white rodents. Although more expensive than mice and rats, gerbils are another option to be used for prey. This sometimes helps with wild-caught snakes that are reluctant to eat because gerbils look more like a natural source of prey than white rodents do. Wild-caught specimens will most likely be reluctant to take prekilled prey initially because they are accustomed to live prey items. Therefore, attempting to feed prekilled or frozen prey items to newly acquired wild-caught snakes will most likely be unsuccessful and will take time. Besides the moral issues with keeping wild-caught snakes, this is another reason why they should be avoided as purchases.

Some people attempt to speed up the process of getting a wild-caught snake to accept commercially bred rodents by scenting them. This does work occasionally. Scenting them is achieved by rubbing a natural prey item on the rodent to leave a scent. This works mostly for hobbyists who keep multiple species of reptiles and amphibians. For example, if trying to feed a mouse to a snake that mostly feeds on lizards and frogs naturally, a person can rub the feeder rodent on a lizard or frog that is kept in their collection. This will leave the scent of that animal on the rodent, and possibly trick the snake into eating it.

Another common reason a snake may refuse food is inadequate heat. If a snake is cold, it will most likely refuse food. A snake needs to be warm to properly digest food. Regurgitation occurs frequently in snakes kept too cold. A snake that is too cold spends most of its time in a heat-preserving posture and is not interested in feeding at all. Make sure all heat requirements are being met when dealing with a reluctant eater.

As a rule, when a snake refuses prey, all husbandry requirements should be checked to ensure they are being met properly. Even something as simple as absence of a hide box (a secure place) will cause a snake to refuse prey.

Note: If a snake is about to shed, it will most likely refuse food. Food items should not even be offered until the snake has fully shed to avoid excess stress.

Snakes that are ailing from respiratory disorders or other illnesses most likely stop feeding as well. The onset of illness affects their appetites, just like any other animal. It is extremely important for the snake's owner to read as much literature as possible on the snake being kept. Once again, knowing the natural geographic range of the snake help in making husbandry decisions, which may be the root of many problems. All too often, snakes are impulse buys and the buyer does not bother with reading up on the requirements and responsibilities involved with that particular snake.

TRANSPORTATION

There are several ways to transport a snake. Snake bags are the most commonly used and can be burlap sacks, pillow cases, laundry bags, or other linens that are breathable fabric and can be secured. The snake should be placed in the sack and then the sack should be knot tied at the open end. The bag should then be grabbed above the knot because a bite can still occur through a bag. The bag should be moved using tongs if the snake is venomous. Venomous snakes should be transported in something more durable to safeguard against bites.

Plastic tubs or clean paint buckets with lids can be used as well. This works well for larger species if a large enough bag cannot be obtained. One should ensure that the lid snaps down or can be secured properly in case the snake pushes on it. Breathing holes must be cut in the plastic if tubs or buckets are used taking care not to create abrasive or sharp edges that the snake could contact.

DISEASES AND CLINICAL CONDITIONS

Diseases Affecting the Reproductive Tract

Cloacal prolapse is a common problem seen in snakes. The prolapse can be the colon, hemipenes, uterus, or oviduct. It is usually caused by excessive straining or during copulation. It is important to determine which organ has prolapsed before initiating treatment. The hemipenes are solid and do not have a lumen. The colon is smooth and has a lumen. Feces are normally be seen if the colon is prolapsed. The oviduct or shell gland has longitudinal striations with a lumen. There are no feces present if it is the oviduct or shell gland.

Hemipenile prolapse, or paraphimosishas several causes, including infections from bacteria, fungus, or parasites; swelling secondary to forced probing; forced separation during copulation; constipation; or neurologic dysfunction in the hemipenes retractor apparatus, cloacal vent, or anal sphincter muscles. Treatment should begin immediately after diagnosis. The prolapsed hemipenis should be cleaned, lubed, and replaced. If replacement is unsuccessful or the hemipenis is necrotic, the hemipenis should be amputated. Snakes have two hemipenes, so reproductive ability is not affected.

A prolapsed colon is caused by excessive straining, usually from constipation. The tissue must be moistened and replaced. Most colon prolapses can be replaced through the cloaca, but occasionally surgery is required. When the tissue is replaced it must also be inverted. If replaced properly, a purse string suture is not required. Because this condition is not the primary problem, both conditions must be treated.

Oviductal or shell gland prolapses are most commonly seen during normal oviposition or parturition. They are treated much the same as a colon prolapse.

The prolapsed tissue must be kept moist and replaced through the cloaca. Resection is recommended if a large amount of the oviduct is prolapsed or if the tissue is necrotic.

Dystocia is another common reproductive disorder. There are two types of dystocia in reptiles, obstructive and nonobstructive (Lock 2000). An obstructive dystocia is caused by an anatomic inability to deliver the eggs or live young or by a complication during oviposition. The anatomic defect may be fetal or maternal. Some common maternal anatomic defects that are seen in snakes include misshapen pelvis, oviductal stricture, nonoviductal masses, oviduct scarring from previous infection, or retained eggs or fetuses from previous pregnancy. Fetal defects include an egg that is too large or eggs that have adhered. Diagnosis is made through a physical exam, history, and radiographs or ultrasound. Treatment includes the surgical removal of the eggs or fetuses.

Nonobstructive dystocias are mostly caused by poor husbandry, infection, or poor physical condition (Lock 2000). Improper temperature, humidity, diet, and nesting site can all cause a dystocia. Oviposition requires great strength. Most captive-raised snakes do not have the muscle mass that wild snakes have, which makes it very difficult to deliver eggs or live young. Treatments include massaging the eggs down, percutaneous ovocentesis, posterior pituitary hormones, and, as a last resort, surgery. When massaging, care must be taken to not trap a portion of the oviduct posterior to the egg or live young. If this happens, massage the egg or embryo back to its original position and start over (Ross et al. 1990).

Percutaneous ovocentesis can be performed in oviparous snakes. A needle is inserted into the egg through the ventrum and the contents aspirated. It is important that the coelomic cavity is not contaminated with egg contents. The egg should pass naturally within forty-eight hours. Posterior pituitary hormones such as oxytocin can be used to assist with the oviposition. Surgery must be performed if all attempts have been made and the eggs or embryos are still retained. Successful incubation of eggs after a dystocia is rare. Live fetuses have been raised after a salpingotomy, but it is not common. The prognosis for the female is good following a dystocia. The future reproductive status is also good as long as there were no complications and at least one of the reproductive tracts was left intact. The female is more likely to retain eggs and live young again.

Disorders of the Integument

Dysecdysis, or difficulty in shedding, is the most common disorder affecting the integument. Causes of dysecdysis are numerous but mostly associated with poor husbandry. Some common husbandry problems associated with dysecdysis are too high temperature, too low humidity, no shedding implement such as a rock or log, and malnutrition. Other causes of dysecdysis include systemic disorders, metabolic disorders, stress from excessive handling, loud noises, vibrations, overcrowding, or anything that limits the snake's movements. Treatment includes soaking the snake in tepid water for one to eight hours a day and treating the underlying problem.

Increased ecdysis frequency can occur in snakes. Hyperthyroidism and dermatitis are the main causes of this condition. Frequent ecdysis is also the natural function of healing after a severe trauma.

There are many clinical signs of dermatosis. Abscesses, abrasions, blisters, bullae, discoloration, and nodules are all signs of a diseased integument (Rossi 1996). Abscesses are the most common dermatologic condition seen in captive reptiles. They are commonly caused by bites from prey or cage mates. Most abscesses are filled with a solid exudate. Treatment for abscesses includes surgically removing the abscess, irrigating the area, and using antibiotics pending a culture and sensitivity.

Bacterial dermatoses are also a very common condition. The most common bacterial infection is caused by *Pseudomonas* spp. Other common bacterial pathogens include *Salmonella* spp., staphylococcus, and streptococcus, as well as many other possible bacterial pathogens.

Fungal dermatoses are commonly seen in snakes that live in humid environments. The clinical signs are much the same as in bacterial infections. Clinical signs of both fungal and bacterial infections include a brown to greenish yellow discoloration, blisters, ulcers, nodules, crust, and granulomas.

Vesicular dermatitis, commonly known as blister disease, is common in snakes kept in dirty, very humid enclosures (Rossi 1996). Fluid-filled blisters appear all over the body and are quickly contaminated with bacteria, and septicemia and death quickly follow without treatment.

Another bacterial infection caused by poor cage hygiene is ventral dermal necrosis (Lawton 1991). Snakes kept in dirty enclosures can develop infections underneath their ventral scales. The signs include petechiation, echymosis, and eventual necrosis of the ventral scales. Fluid therapy is often needed due to the fluid loss from the damaged skin.

Contact dermatitis occurs when the snake is exposed to harsh chemicals such as pesticides, cleaners, and harsh aromatic compounds.

The diagnosis for all dermatosis includes a physical examination and history, culture (aerobic, anaerobic, and fungal), and cytology (Rossi 1996). Treatment usually involves topical or systemic antimicrobials and husbandry and nutritional changes. During the treatment of any of these dermatoses the snake should be housed on clean paper. The paper should be changed daily and the cage should be disinfected daily until the condition has resolved.

Disorders of the Cardiovascular System

Cardiovascular disorders are not commonly seen in snakes. The clinical signs are nonspecific, ranging from weight loss to a change in skin color. Nutritional disorders such as hypocalcemia, hypovitaminosis E, and hypercalcemia with hypervitaminosis D_3 have been associated with cardiovascular disease. Infectious diseases affecting the cardiovascular system are usually secondary to a systemic illness. There is potential for endocarditis with any Gram-negative bacterial pathogen. If bacterial sepsis is suspected, a blood culture should be taken. There have been reported cases of congestive heart failure associated with infectious disease and with cardiomyopathy diagnosed.

Disorders of the Nervous System

Spinal osteopathy has been observed in all species of snakes (Bennett 1996b). The exact etiology is unknown. This condition has not been observed in wild populations. There are several possible causes to this disorder. It is suspected that a virus found in mice or a virus of snakes that is spread by mice may be a causative agent. Septicemia is suspected because bacteria are often cultured from the spinal lesions. An immune-mediated disease secondary to septicemia is also suspected. Finally, chronic trauma from excessive handling is thought to be a cause of this disease.

Clinical signs include focal or multifocal swelling along the dorsum, pressure inducing a pain response, hyperflexic cranial to the lesion, motor deficits, trembling, and spinal deformities. The diagnosis is made via clinical signs and radiographs. The snake is still able to function on its own in the early stages of this disease. As the disease progresses, the snake will no longer be able to move, constrict, or swallow prey. Treatment includes blood and local aspirate cultures, antibiotics, and surgical debridement.

Organophosphate and carbamate toxicity have been reported in snakes. Treatment is similar to that of mammals. The snakes should be given atropine and fluid therapy to maintain hydration and renal function. Their temperature should be decreased to slow conduction velocity of nerves to control seizures.

Disorders of the Respiratory Tract

Respiratory infections are the most common illnesses in snakes. They can be caused by bacterial, viral, fungal, or parasitic pathogens (Driggers 2000). Bacterial pneumonia is the most common cause of respiratory illness, and Gram-negative pathogens are the most common. Viral infections are under diagnosed due to the lack of diagnostic assays. Fungal infections are rare but have been reported. Common clinical signs of pneumonia include cyanosis, bubbles coming from the nares or glottis, wheezing or crackles heard during auscultation, and petechiae of the oral cavity. Stomatitis is commonly seen in snakes with pneumonia (Driggers 2000).

The diagnostic plan should include culture and sensitivity, cytology, and radiographs. A transtracheal wash should be performed to obtain samples for the culture and cytology. Antibiotics should be started and changed pending the results of the culture and sensitivity. Fluid therapy should be initiated with dehydrated snakes. The most common cause of pneumonia in snakes is husbandry related. It is crucial to keep the snake within its POTZ and keep proper humidity levels. The cage also must be kept clean at all times.

Other causes of respiratory disease include masses, trauma, aspiration of substrate, and dehydration. Dysecdysis can also compromise the respiratory tract, causing disease (Driggers 2000).

Disorders of the Urinary System

Unfortunately, early detection of renal dysfunction has not been observed in reptiles. Renal diseases are among the most common problems in older snakes.

Gout, though not as common in snakes as it is in other families of reptiles, does occur. It is the result of excessive protein metabolism or catabolism. In this case uric acid production is greater than uric acid excretion. All diseases that lead to renal failure can cause gout (Miller 1998). Gout is found in two forms. In the first, urates are deposited on mesothelial surfaces. Urate deposits commonly occur on the pericardial sac, the peritoneum, the capsule of the liver, and within the parenchyma of the kidneys. In the other form, urate deposits are made in joints, tendon sheaths, ligaments, and periosteum. Both forms of gout can occur simultaneously. Treatment involves diuresis and diet change to a low-purine diet. The prognosis is poor.

Bacterial nephritis is a common disease associated with the urinary system. It is often secondary to other bacterial infections or an immunosuppressive event (Miller 1998). The primary cause should be detected and treated accordingly.

Disorders of the Eye

Retained spectacles are a common reason snakes are brought into the veterinary clinic. Spectacles are retained when dysecdysis occurs. To remove the retained spectacle, place the snake in a very damp environment for twenty-four hours and then wipe the eye with a gauze sponge or damp tissue. The retained spectacle usually will come off easily. If it does not, the snake should be kept in a warm damp environment until the next ecdysis cycle and proper ecdysis occurs.

Surgical intervention should be a last resort. This is a delicate procedure and should be done carefully so the eye is not damaged. Sterile lubricant should be applied to the eye and the spectacle gently removed with forceps. If the old spectacle is still attached firmly, force should not be used to remove it. It may take several days of soaking and/or applying lubricant to fully remove the retained spectacle or any retained piece of shed.

Intraspectacular dermatitis occurs as a localized dermatitis or as part of a more generalized dermatitis. The majority of these cases are caused by retained spectacles. Often, enucleation is the treatment.

Bullous spectaculopathy is caused by obstruction of the nasolacrimal duct (Williams 1996). The obstruction is usually secondary to either infectious stomatitis or a congenital obstruction. The lacrimal fluid is not able to drain from the eye, which causes the distended subspectacular space. Long-term treatment involves surgically removing a 30-degree wedge of the ventral spectacle, allowing for drainage.

Subspectacular abscesses are usually the result of an ascending infection in the oral cavity (Williams 1996). Treatment for these abscesses involves a wedge resection of the spectacle and flushing. The debris should be cultured and the snake should be started on appropriate antibiotics.

Disorders of the Digestive System

Infectious Stomatitis

Infectious stomatitis is a disease that is caused by poor husbandry and nutrition, stress, poor feeding techniques, or trauma. It is crucial that the snake be kept in its POTZ and that proper humidity be maintained. When proper husbandry is not met, the snake's immune system is weakened, allowing for opportunistic bacteria to reproduce. Stress from being in overcrowded cages, excessive handling, or loud noises can also weaken the immune system. Snakes that are fed live prey commonly have small abrasions in their oral cavity that can lead to an infectious stomatitis. Finally, snakes that rub on the sides of the cage have rostral abrasions that lead to an infectious stomatitis (Color Plate 7.2).

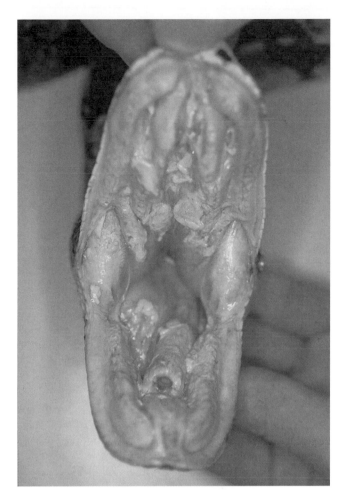

Plate 7.2. Stomatitis in a snake. (Photo courtesy of Dr. Stephen J. Hernandez-Divers, University of Georgia.) (See also color plates)

Vomiting and Regurgitation

Vomiting can occur for many reasons. Stress can make a snake vomit. If disturbed after a meal, a snake may get nervous and vomit its meal. Also, feeding a prey that is too large, feeding a prey that is partially autolyzed, and keeping the snake below its POTZ are all common causes of vomiting. Infectious diseases such as parasitic infections, inclusion body disease, and bacterial infections can also cause vomiting in snakes. Regurgitation is usually associated with lesions in the esophagus, oral cavity, or pharynx.

Diagnosing Lumps and Bumps

Lumps and bumps are a common finding in snakes. They occur on the outside as well as on the inside. When a lump or bump is found on the surface of the snake a fine needle aspirate should be performed. Cytology, culture, and sensitivity should be performed on the sample. If the lump or bump is palpated in the coelomic cavity, a radiograph or ultrasound should be performed to determine the origin. A sample should be obtained and cytology performed. Causes of lumps and bumps in snakes range from parasites to abscesses to neoplasia. Once the diagnosis is made, treatment should begin accordingly.

Viral Diseases

Paramoxyvirus is mainly found in viperids but has been isolated in most taxa of snakes (Schumacher 1996). It is transmitted through secretions of the respiratory tract. Clinical signs are characterized by severe respiratory disease. Neurologic signs such as head tremors, excitement, star gazing, flaccid paralysis, or convulsions can also be seen (Bronson and Cranfield 2006). A presumptive diagnosis of paramoxyvirus should be considered when a pneumonia is unresponsive to antibiotics. A hemagglutination test has been developed and can be used to measure antibodies against ophidian paramoxyvirus. Titers reflect exposure. A rising titer in paired samples is necessary for a diagnosis of active disease (Ritchie 2006). A diagnosis can also be made by histological examination of postmortem lung, liver, kidney, splenopancreas, and brain samples. There is no treatment for paramoxyvirus. Supportive care and antibiotics to treat secondary bacterial infections should be in the treatment plan. The prognosis is grave. If an outbreak of paramoxyvirus occurs in a collection, all sick snakes should immediately be quarantined and strict hygiene procedures must be followed.

Inclusion body disease (IBD) is another serious viral infection that is only found in boids (Figure 7.12). It is believed that this disease is caused by a retrovirus. Species of boa constrictors have been found to harbor species of retroviruses that do not cause disease (Marschang 2001). The route of transmission is unknown. It is suspected that arthropods play a role in the transmission. In boas, the most common first clinical sign seen is regurgitation. In pythons, the first clinical signs may be stomatitis and pneumonia (Ritchie 2006). The disease progresses to severe neurologic signs such as head tremors, disorientation, flaccid muscle paralysis, and the loss of the righting reflex. Secondary bacterial infections are common. Eventually the snake will become anorectic and die. The disease progresses much more rapidly in pythons than boas (Schumacher and Ylen 2006).

Diagnosis can be made by histologic exam of the liver, kidney, stomach, pancreas, and brain. There are no treatments for IBD except for supportive care and treating secondary bacterial infections. The snake will

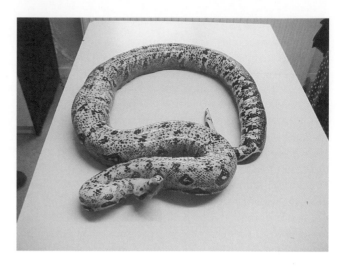

Figure 7.12. Inclusion body disease: note the absence of righting reflex. (Photo courtesy of Dr. Stephen J. Hernandez-Divers, University of Georgia.)

eventually die from this virus. Prevention of this disease involves strict quarantine procedures when introducing new snakes into to an established collection. If confirmed carriers are identified in the collection, euthanasia is recommended to prevent more specimens from becoming infected with the virus.

Zoonotic Diseases

Snakes possess very few zoonotic diseases (Glynn 2001) (Table 7.3). There are two ways in which zoonotic diseases are passed (Siemering 1986). One is by direct contact with the infected animal. The other is by indirect contact, which can be from contaminated feces, urine, secretions, blood, soil, fomites, and aerosols. Zoonotic diseases, for the most part, are easily avoided by following a few simple rules. Do not use the bathtub, sink, or shower as a place to soak a snake. Do not kiss a snake. Wash hands after handling a snake. A physician should be consulted a snake bite occurs and the area should be washed thoroughly. Finally, one should never clean any of the cage furnishings where human food is kept or prepared.

The most talked about zoonotic disease associated with reptiles is salmonellosis. It is believed that most reptiles carry salmonella organisms in their intestinal tract and sporadically shed the organisms in their feces. An estimated 93,000 cases of reptile-associated human salmonellosis is diagnosed each year (Glynn 2001). All clients that either own a reptile or are considering owning a reptile for a pet should be educated about salmonella. Salmonellosis is easily prevented by simply following the guidelines above.

Table 7.3. Common Zoonotic Diseases in Reptiles.

Pathogen	Threat to humans	Mode of transmission
Salmonella spp.	Gastrointestinal	Fecal-oral contact
Campylobacter spp.	Diarrhea and acute gastroenteritis	Fecal-oral contact
Klebsiella spp.	Diarrhea and genitourinary infections	Direct contact
Enterobacter spp.	Diarrhea and genitourinary infections	Direct contact
Yersinia enterocolitica	Gastroenteritis and severe abdominal pain	Environmental contact
Pseudomonas spp.	Cutaneous, respiratory, and digestive	Ingestion, inhalation, or scratches or bites
Mycobacterium spp.	Cutaneous and subcutaneous nodule	Fecal oral contact, inhalation of oral or respiratory mucosa, or bites or scratches
Coxiella burnetii	Q-fever	Inhalation or direct contact

TAKING A HISTORY

Taking a complete history of a snake patient is the first crucial step in diagnosing and treating a sick snake. Such topics as signalment, presenting complaint, husbandry and nutrition information, and any previous medical history are keys to proper diagnosis and treatment.

Signalment

Signalment includes the common and scientific names (ball python, *Python regius*), age, amount of time in owner's possession, whether it was captive-bred or wild-caught, and whether it is kept as a pet or as a breeder. It is important that the common and scientific names of the snake are acquired when the appointment is made. With approximately 2,400 extant species of snake, it is impossible for a single person to know the natural history, husbandry, and nutritional needs of every species. Therefore, it is important that the medical staff be prepared ahead of time to ensure that the owner meets proper husbandry and nutritional needs. Many species of snake also have two or more common names, which can make identification very difficult. For example, most Americans refer to *Python regius* as a ball python, whereas most Europeans refer to *Python regius* as the royal python. By knowing the scientific name of the snake, proper identification can be made, and the appropriate information can be relayed to the owner.

Another key component to signalment is the age of the snake. If the actual age of the snake is unknown, then the amount of time that the owner has had possession of it is important information. The average life span of captive snakes is very short. However, snakes are capable of living to a very geriatric age, with some species known to live more than thirty years. Such short life spans are mostly associated with poor husbandry.

At this point in the history-taking, the origin of the snake should be noted. Wild-caught snakes are often imported in very substandard conditions and arrive at the pet store with a subclinical disease. Internal and external parasites and respiratory infections are most commonly seen with imported specimens. Captive-bred specimens, generally speaking, are much tamer, are free of disease and parasites, and live longer than wild-caught specimens. It is also important to urge owners to buy captive-bred specimens due to the depletion of wild populations caused from the collection of wild animals for the pet trade.

Note whether the snake is kept as a pet or a breeder. Snakes kept solely as pets usually do not need to be hibernated, photoperiods do not need to change throughout the year, and nutritional needs usually do not change throughout the year. Snakes kept for breeding do have nutritional and husbandry changes throughout the year. Temperate species should be hibernated, which takes several weeks of preparation. If hibernation is not done properly, the snake can become very sick and possibly die while hibernating. With regard to nutrition, many female snakes do not eat while gravid. The females normally start eating again when the clutch is laid, the clutch hatches, or the live babies are born. Special nutritional needs must be met before the breeding season starts and when the female snake starts eating again. Also, to ensure a successful breeding season, the photoperiod must be changed to simulate the natural photoperiod.

All snakes that are large enough should be sexed. It is a very simple procedure that should be included in the initial exam.

Presenting Complaint

The presenting complaint is the reason the owner brought the snake to be examined. Some common presenting complaints include wheezing, dysecdysis, anorexia, and lethargy. Approach the presenting complaint as if it were that of a dog or cat. The owner should be asked when the problem started, if there were any husbandry/nutritional changes, if he noticed any other problems, and so on. The medical staff is like a team of detectives that must gather as much evidence as possible to come up with a diagnosis and treatment plan. It is important to get as much information from the owners as possible.

Husbandry and Nutritional Information

The single leading cause of death in captive snakes is poor husbandry and/or nutrition. It is up to the veterinary technician to find out every detail of the husbandry practices and advise the owner if corrections need to be made. This part of the history takes fifteen to twenty minutes. It is crucial to take time and record every detail. Following is a list of questions that should be asked at the initial exam:

- What is the day and night temperature range?
- What is the day/night cycle?
- What light sources are available?
- What are the primary and secondary heat sources available?
- What is the humidity in the enclosure?
- What humidity devices and methods are used?
- How big is the cage?
- Where is the cage located?
- What is the cage made of?
- Is the cage designed for an arboreal or terrestrial species?
- What substrate is used?
- How often is the cage cleaned and disinfected?
- What type of disinfectant is used?
- What cage furnishings are available (rocks, branches, hide box, etc.)?
- How is water offered (drip system, misting, bowl, etc.)?
- What food items are offered and what time of day are they offered?
- Is the snake fed live, frozen-thawed, or fresh-killed prey items?
- How is the prey offered (feeding tongs, set in the bottom of the cage, in a separate cage, etc.)?
- What is the feeding schedule?
- How are the prey items stored?
- Where were the prey items acquired?
- What is the ecdysis/defecation schedule?

- Are there other reptiles or other animals in the same air system?
- Are any of these animals sick or have any died within the past three months?
- Is proper quarantine performed on new and sick specimens?

Previous Medical History

Any previous medical condition or diagnostic tests should be noted in the record. The owner's fecal check and deworming schedule should also be noted in the record.

PREPARING FOR THE PHYSICAL EXAM

The exam room must be prepared ahead of time to ensure a quick and complete physical exam. The exam room needs to be snake proof. The doors must be sealed so the snake cannot escape under the door, large drains in the sink should be covered, air vents should be covered with mesh to prevent the snake from crawling in, and any other holes or cracks that the snake can get into should be covered or sealed to keep the snake from escaping or getting stuck. Appropriate-sized sex probes with lubrication for sexing and a spatula or credit card for oral examination should be in the exam room. Restraining devices such as snake hooks, clear plastic restraining tubes, and capture tongs should be readily accessible for aggressive or venomous species. Large snakes could need two or more people for proper restraint. It may be necessary to have other technicians or assistants close by in the event that more help is needed. Other essential instruments that are needed for a physical exam are a good light source, ophthalmic scope, stethoscope, fecal collection system, and magnifying glass to check for external parasites.

RESTRAINT

As stated previously, snakes can be very unpredictable and should be treated as such to avoid being bitten. Even the most docile of snakes will bite if they feel threatened or cornered. Watch for warning signs such as hissing or an S-shaped striking posture before attempting to handle a snake (Figure 7.13).

Whether restraining or simply holding the snake, it is important to do so properly. If not held properly, not only can one get bitten, but the snake can sustain injuries, too. The body should always be

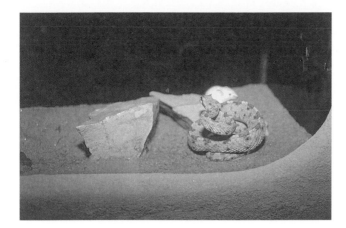

Figure 7.13. A snake in a striking pose. (Photo courtesy of Ryan Cheek.)

supported as much as possible. With larger snakes, it will take more than one person to hold and offer necessary support.

When manually restraining the snake, ensure that someone has control of the head. This should be the first part of the body restrained. The head should be held right at the base and without applying too much pressure around the neck area. This could obstruct the trachea, causing a strangling effect, and the snake could suffocate. In addition, the snake could panic, making it very difficult to manage. The rest of the body can be held with a free hand or by assistants when handling large or aggressive snakes. Do not place a snake (especially large snakes and/or constrictors) around the neck. While this is commonly done, it can be dangerous. If the snake feels threatened and insecure it will begin to constrict around the neck.

Different tools can be used to move snakes or assist in immobilization, including hooks, tubes, and tongs, all of which are discussed below. Snake hooks allow a person to move a snake without having to touch the animal or get too close. This is advantageous when handling aggressive snakes. A hook can be used to get a snake out of an enclosure, as a guide, or as a pinning device. For example, to remove a snake from an enclosure, the hook is used to hook the snake one-third of the way down its body and then gently lift it. The hook can then be used to pin the head to take control of it, but extreme caution must be used because any thrashing by the snake can cause severe spinal cord injury. Only handlers experienced with the hook should use the pinning technique. If the snake is hooked too close to the head or tail, it will usually slide right off. It may be necessary to use more than one hook for larger snakes (Figure 7.14).

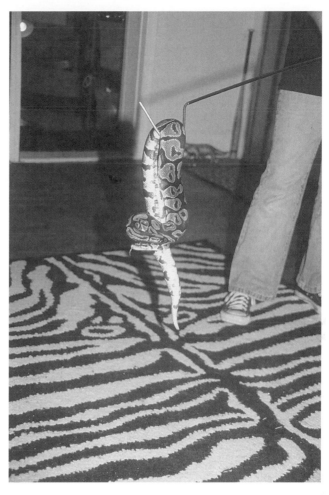

Figure 7.14. Proper use of a snake hook. (Photo courtesy of Ryan Cheek.)

Snake hooks are also used when coercing a snake into a snake tube for physical exam or immobilization. They can be purchased at most reptile supply shops (Figures 7.15, 7.16).

Snake tubes are open-ended, clear, hard plastic or acrylic tubes that are used to hold a snake and view it safely during examination. The tube's diameter must be just large enough for the snake's head to fit into, but not allow the snake to turn around in. One end of the tube should be aimed toward the snake's head and a snake hook used to entice the snake into the tube. Once one-third to one-half of the snake's body is in the tube, the handler should grasp the snake and the base of the tube so it cannot back out. A face mask can be placed on the other end of the tube to administer gas anesthesia and immobilize the snake completely, if necessary. This is the safest way to manage aggressive snakes and venomous species. Most of these tubes are purchased from reptile supply stores or hard-

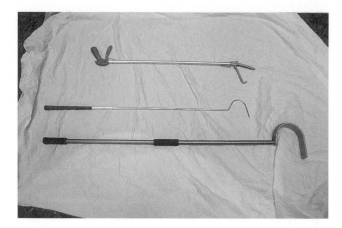

Figure 7.15. *Snake tongs at the top and two snake hooks below. (Photo courtesy of Ryan Cheek.)*

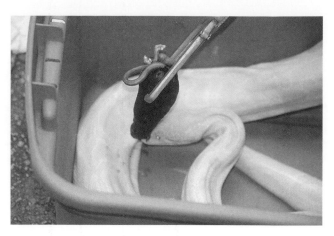

Figure 7.17. *Feeding a python with tongs. (Photo courtesy of Ryan Cheek)*

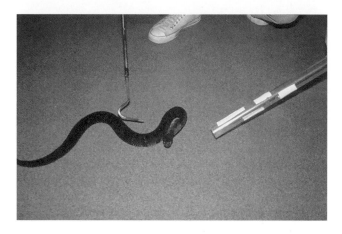

Figure 7.16. *Using a hook to coax a snake into a plastic tube. (Photo courtesy of Zoo Atlanta)*

ware stores (if appropriate materials are found) and come in various sizes.

Another method of capturing an aggressive snake is to place a clear shield over its head. Once the shield is in place, the handler can grasp right behind its head taking control of it.

Snake tongs can be used for many purposes. The most common use is for feeding (Figure 7.17). Offering food items via tongs is obviously safer than using one's hands to offer prey. Tongs allow the feeder to keep a safe distance from the snake and the prey item. Although some people use tongs to assist in restraining snakes, this method is not recommended. Grabbing the snake with tongs can apply too much pressure and, depending on the part of the body that is grasped, the snake can be injured. Snakes can also easily free themselves from tongs if not grasped properly. Tongs can

be used to assist in tubing the snake but not as a primary handling mechanism.

An undesirable method of restraint is to allow a snake to partially swallow prey. This allows the handler time to take control of the head and the body before the snake can strike. However, often the snake regurgitates the prey, making this technique undesirable.

To avoid bites, some reptile hobbyists believe that snakes should not be fed inside their primary enclosure, especially when the only time the enclosure is opened is when the snake is being fed. This creates a feeding response and makes bites more likely to occur. Feeding outside the primary enclosure is therefore a safer practice and also can help to ensure that any loose substrate located inside the primary enclosure is not ingested during feeding.

THE PHYSICAL EXAM

After a very thorough history has been taken and the exam room is prepared, a complete physical exam should be performed. It should begin as soon as the owner brings the snake into the exam room. The snake should be observed as it moves around its environment. Body and muscle tone, proprioception, and mobility should also be observed. Any abnormalities should be noted. An accurate weight in grams or kilograms as well as the snout-to-vent length (SVL) should be measured to determine organ location and monitor growth in juvenile snakes. The cloacal temperature should be recorded to help determine the thermal environment in which the snake lives.

There are several approaches to performing a physical exam. Some clinicians prefer a head-to-tail evaluation, whereas others have a specific order of body systems that are examined. It is important to do the same routine with every physical exam so nothing is left out or overlooked.

Integument

The skin should be checked for parasites, thermal burns, trauma, skin tenting or ridges to assess hydration, dysecdysis, and bacterial or fungal infections. If ecdysis is currently in process, the stage of ecdysis should be recorded.

Respiratory System

The upper and lower airways should be auscultated for any crackles or increased respiratory sounds. Remember that most snakes only have a right lung with the exception of the boids, which have a right lung and a small left lung. The nostrils should be clear of debris and any discharge. The glottis can easily be observed for proper function and for any inflammation. When the glottis opens during respiration, look down the trachea for any swelling, mucous, or foreign material.

Cardiovascular System

Auscultation of the snake's heart can sometimes prove to be difficult. It is crucial that the exam room be silent. Using a damp cloth or gauze sponge can help enhance the heart sounds. The heart is generally around 25% down the body from the snout. A heart rate should be obtained during auscultation. Peripheral pulses should be assessed via the use of a Doppler flow detector. The Doppler can be placed on the ventral tail vein or just cranial to the heart at the base of the glottis.

Neurologic Examination

Neurologic exams are very simple to perform on snakes (Bennett 1996b). The exam starts with the initial presentation of the snake. Watch for any jerking motions, absent or slow righting reflex, or the inability to strike at prey. The site of a spinal cord injury can be found by using the righting reflex. Snakes will right themselves up to the point of the injury. A hypodermic needle may be used to stimulate the panniculus reflex. A neurologically normal snake's skin twitches up to the point of spinal injury. A cranial nerve exam should be performed if a neurologic disorder is suspected. The following methods can be used to examine the twelve cranial nerves in snakes:

CN I: A snake with a properly functioning olfactory nerve recoils from the smell of noxious odors. Alcohol can be placed in front of the snake's nose to see if it reacts to the smell.

CN II: Because reptiles have an iris that is composed of skeletal muscle, pupilary light reflex cannot be used to determine the function of the optic nerve. Carefully watch the eye movements of the snake to assess the function of the optic nerve.

CN III, CN IV, CN VI: This group of cranial nerves is extremely hard to assess in snakes. They are responsible for eye movement coordination.

CN V: Snakes with a malfunctioning trigeminal nerve have abnormal jaw function and a loss of feeling around the face. They cannot thermoregulate or find prey.

CN VIII: The acoustic nerve is difficult to assess. Snakes may show signs of nystagmus, head tilt, rolling, and abnormal righting reflex.

CN IX, CN XI, CN XII: Dysphagia and abnormal tongue movements can be seen in a snake if one or more of these cranial nerves is damaged or malfunctioning.

CN VII and CN X: The facial and vagus nerves are impossible to assess in snakes.

Palpations

The entire length of the snake should be palpated for any abnormalities such as enlarged organs, internal masses, lumps, and bumps. In breeding females, eggs and preovulatory follicles can be felt on palpation. Digital palpation of the cloaca can reveal several abnormalities and should be performed on all snakes that are large enough. An otoscope or endoscope can be used as well.

Ophthalmic Exam

As discussed in the anatomy section, snakes have a transparent spectacle that covers the cornea. The eyes should be clear and smooth. Any retained sheds can easily be seen and removed. Any other abnormalities should be further examined with an ophthalmic scope.

Fecal Exam

All snakes that come in for a physical exam should have a fecal examination performed. This exam should include a fecal floatation and two direct fecal smears, one prepared with a normal saline solution and the other prepared with a Lugol's iodine solution.

Oral Exam

Because most snakes become distressed during the oral exam, it is often best to perform the oral examination last. Gently open the mouth using a spatula or plastic card. Determining the proper mucosa color can be difficult. Most species have a pale mucosa color while others may have a more pink or bluish color. It is important to know the normal color for that species before the physical exam is performed. With all species the oral cavity should be moist without any stringy or tenacious mucus. The clinician should look for any caseous exudates, hemorrhage, and necrosis.

RADIOLOGY

Creating a Technique Chart

A separate technique chart should be made for snakes. A variable kVp or variable mAs technique chart can be made, although a variable mAs technique chart is preferable. The technique chart should start at 2 cm and go to at least 20 cm. Describing the proper method of creating a technique chart is out of the scope of this text. There are numerous texts that describe this process in detail. It is an easy but time-consuming task that if performed correctly will save much time when a radiograph is needed.

Positioning

As with all other animals, two views should be taken, lateral and dorsoventral (DV). Snakes should not be radiographed in the coiled position because this can distort internal organs and decrease detail. The snake should be stretched out over the cassette. If properly collimated, two or more regions of the body can be radiographed on one film. If possible, radiograph both views of the same region on one film to make interpretation much easier. If multiple films are required, the films should be labeled to match the region taken. There are several methods of doing this. The method that this author uses is based on the number of films required to radiograph the snake. If four films are needed, the first film is labeled 1/4, the second film is labeled 2/4, and so on (Figure 7.18).

Restraint

With the exception of very sick snakes, most snakes will not be still enough to radiograph without proper restraint. For docile snakes, manually holding them on the table is sufficient enough restraint for proper technique. For less-docile snakes, placing them in clear plastic tubes allows for proper positioning and technique. If this method is used, the kVp or mAs, depending on the technique chart used, may need to be slightly increased to compensate for the plastic. As a last resort, chemical restraint, either injectable or inhalant anesthesia, can be used. If injectable anesthesia is used, a short-acting drug or one that is reversible is preferred. Some injectable anesthetics can last for hours or even days in reptiles.

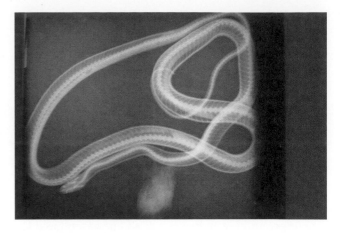

Figure 7.18 *Radiograph of a snake taken while it is in a bag. (Photo courtesy of Ryan Cheek)*

ANESTHESIA

Anatomy and Physiology Considerations

The lungs of reptiles are very fragile. When performing intermittent positive pressure ventilation (IPPV) always stay under 20 cm water to avoid pulmonary rupture (Bennett 1996a). Reptiles do not have a diaphragm, so respiration is accomplished through other muscles throughout the thoracic and abdominal areas. Some of the muscles are paralyzed when the reptile reaches a surgical plane of anesthesia, making IPPV necessary. Keep in mind that many snakes can breath hold and convert to anaerobic metabolism. Many species can live for hours without oxygen. This adaptation makes induction difficult to impossible in some species if inducing with inhalant anesthesia.

Preanesthetic Examination and Considerations

Before placing a snake under anesthesia a very thorough physical examination should be performed. A minimal amount of diagnostics, including a packed cell volume and total solids, also should be recorded to help determine the health status of the snake. More diagnostics may be needed such as a biochemical profile, complete blood count, fecal analysis, radiographs, or cultures if infection is suspected. Any abnormalities on the physical examination or diagnostic testing should be treated or stabilized before the anesthetic episode. The snake should be fasted for one to two weeks for any elective procedures or nonemergency anesthetic procedures. The cardiopulmonary function can be compromised if a large prey is still being digested in the stomach.

Intravenous fluid therapy is needed for any debilitated snake or during long procedures (Bennett 1997). If the snake is dehydrated, rehydration should occur before beginning the anesthetic episode. Any of the crystalloids are appropriate for use in reptiles (Lawton 2001). There is much debate over the use of any fluids containing lactate (Wright 1999). Lactate in reptiles builds to high levels after muscle fatigue and can only be metabolized by the liver. There has been no research performed on this issue as of the date of publication of this text. Until further research has been conducted, it is recommended that fluids containing lactate not be used on a long-term basis in reptile patients. If lactated Ringer's solution is chosen for fluid therapy, potassium chloride must be added to prevent hypokalemia. If fluids are needed interoperatively, an intravenous catheter must be placed in either the jugular vein or directly into the heart. The interoperative fluid rate should be 5 to 10 ml/kg/hour.

Preanesthetic Medications

Preanesthetics are not routinely used in all reptiles. Preanesthetics can be used to provide safer handling of larger snakes to facilitate smoother inductions for general anesthesia. They may also help decrease the amount of drugs needed for induction.

Anticholinergics

Anticholinergics such as atropine sulfate and glycopyrrolate for the most part are unnecessary as a preanesthetic medication. Glycopyrrolate has been shown to help prevent bradycardia; however, bradycardia is usually not a concern in reptile anesthesia.

Injectable Anesthetics

The use of injectable anesthetics in reptiles is very unpredictable. The same dose given to two individuals of the same species can yield completely different levels of sedation (Bennett 1996a). Once the injection is given, the depth of anesthesia cannot be controlled. Reptiles have a very slow metabolism; therefore, recovery time can take from a couple of hours to a week with some anesthetics. Reptiles require a very high dose of narcotics to produce any sedative effects; as a result, narcotics are not recommended in reptiles.

Use of barbiturates is questionable in reptiles. It is unknown how reptiles eliminate barbiturates from their body. It is believed that they rely on metabolism for eliminating barbiturates instead of redistribution to nonnervous tissue (Bennett 1996a). Thiobarbiturates have a recovery time of several days. This can be quickened by increasing the ambient temperature in the cage. The ultra short barbiturates work well in reptiles with a relatively short recovery time of only a few hours. As with all injectables, there is a significant variation in response.

Ketamine is frequently used in snakes for sedation and induction, and can also be used as a surgical anesthetic. Due to metabolic scaling, larger species require the lower end of the recommended dose (Bennett 1997). When used alone, moderate to high doses of ketamine have been associated with increased heart rates, respiratory depression, hypertension, apnea, bradycardia, prolonged recovery times, and death (Bertelsen 2007). However, when ketamine is combined with benzodiazepines or alpha-2-agonists, better muscle relaxation occurs and there is a reduction in the required dose (Bertelsen 2007).

Medetomidine has been used with great success in snakes. When given, it greatly reduces the amount of induction needed and also at higher doses gives enough sedation for quick procedures. Medetomidine is reversible with atipamezole. Medetomidine when given with ketamine shows better anesthetic effects than when given alone.

Telazol, a combination of tiletamine and zolazepam, is recommended as a tranquilizer or induction agent and not the sole anesthetic. Telazol given at a dose of 2 to 5 mg/kg will sedate the snake enough for diagnostic procedures or for intubation. High doses of telazol have been associated with prolonged recovery times (Schumacher and Yelan 2006).

Propofol is a very short-acting nonbarbiturate that can be used as an induction agent or for short surgical or diagnostic procedures. The only disadvantage of propofol is that it must be given intravenously, which can be very difficult in some snakes (Schumacher 2002a). The advantages of propofol are that it produces very rapid induction and recovery times, has minimal accumulation with repeated doses, and produces very little hangover effect after recovery.

Several neuromuscular blocking agents have been used in snakes. Their use should be limited to nonpainful diagnostic procedures because these drugs do not produce unconsciousness or analgesia. Intubation with IPPV is necessary because respiratory paralysis is likely.

Inhalant Anesthetics

Inhalant anesthetics have become the standard of practice for reptiles (Bennett 1997). There are many advantages of inhalant anesthetics versus injectable anesthetics. First, the level of anesthesia is much more precisely controlled. Another significant advantage is that the patient is intubated and receives supplemental oxygen. The recovery time of inhalant anesthetics is much quicker than with injectable anesthetics. Usually the patients are recovered in less than one hour after the anesthetic episode. A nonrebreathing system is recommended for patients that weigh less than 5 kg and an oxygen flow rate of 300 to 500 ml/kg/minute is recommended. Patients that weigh more than 5 kg can use a rebreathing system at an oxygen flow rate of 1 to 2 L/minute. IPPV is recommended in all anesthetized reptiles at a rate of two to four breaths per minute.

Methoxyflurane has been used successfully in snakes. The disadvantage of this inhalant is that it produces slow induction and recovery times, and 50% of the drug is metabolized by the liver, making it inappropriate in patients with any liver problems. Elapids and some pythons have shown sensitivity to methoxyflurane.

Halothane produces a quicker induction and recovery than methoxyflurane. In addition, only 12% of halothane is metabolized by the liver, making this drug a better choice for patients with liver problems. When inducing with halothane, start with a low concentration and slowly increase to prevent irritation. This process can induce breath holding. Venomous species seem to require a higher concentration of halothane, with viperids requiring more than elapids.

Isoflurane is the inhalant anesthetic of choice of this author. It is completely eliminated by the lungs so it causes no metabolic compromise, and can safely be used on debilitated or compromised patients. Induction is quick, taking five to ten minutes, with recovery taking less than thirty minutes on most patients.

The newest inhalant anesthetic on the market is sevoflurane. Sevoflurane gained popularity in the human and veterinary market because of the low blood-gas solubility, which allows for very fast induction and recovery times and improving the control of anesthetic depth (Schumacher 2002b). In humans, cardiovascular stability is better maintained with sevoflurane than with isoflurane. Sevoflurane is also completely eliminated by the lungs. There has been very little research conducted on the effects of sevoflurane in reptiles. Clinical experience shows that species and individuals respond differently to sevoflurane, with some being much more resistant than others (Schumacher 2002b).

Tracheal intubation is easy on snakes (Figures 7.19, 7.20). The trachea sits at the base of their tongue and is easily visible when the mouth is open.

Analgesics

It was once believed that reptiles do not feel pain. However, reptiles have the neurologic components,

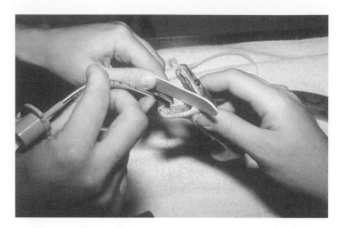

Figure 7.19. Endotracheal intubation of a snake. (Photo courtesy of Zoo Atlanta.)

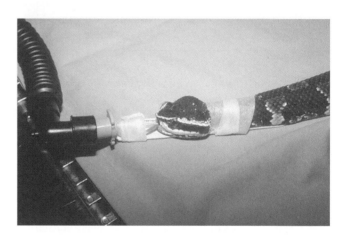

Figure 7.20. Stabilizing the endotracheal tube with a tongue depressor. (Photo courtesy of Zoo Atlanta.)

antinociceptive mechanisms, and behavioral responses to pain that other animals have (Bradley 2001). Reptiles can and do feel pain and therefore analgesics should be provided. Because pain is easier to prevent than treat, analgesics should be given before an anticipated painful procedure. Snakes also share many of the same signs of pain as domestic species. Commonly, snakes shows signs of avoidance of handling, withdrawal, restlessness, agitation, being easily startled, or anorexia when they are in pain. Some more obvious signs of pain are holding the body less coiled at the site of pain, stinting on palpation, and being tucked up and writhing in the affected area.

Recovery

Recovering patients should be placed in an environment that is quiet and within the species' POTZ. Close attention should be paid to the respirations because all anesthetics compromise the respiratory system. Also observe the patient for any pain or discomfort and treat with analgesics accordingly. If the patient received fluids during the procedure, the fluids should be continued until the patient is fully recovered.

Anesthetic Monitoring

The depth of anesthesia in snakes is very difficult to assess. As snakes become anesthetized, relaxation begins cranial and goes caudal and is reversed when recovering. One of the first reflexes a snake loses is the righting reflex. Other reflexes to check are the cloacal reflex and the tail pinch to help determine the depth of anesthesia. At a surgical plane, snakes should still have a tongue withdraw; they will lose this if they are beyond the surgical plane. Each anesthetized snake should be connected to an electrocardiogram as well as a Doppler flow device because the cardiovascular system is very difficult to assess. The heart rate and respiratory rate should be monitored continuously starting when the patient is induced and ending after the patient is fully recovered. Pulse oximetry is only useful in reptiles to monitor trends in arterial oxygen saturation.

SURGERY

The basic principles of surgery are universal. Aseptic techniques should always be used. The patient should be prepared for surgery, induced with anesthesia, intubated, and placed on maintenance inhalant anesthesia. The surgical site should be prepared with an initial scrub with an approved surgical scrub such as chlorhexidine or betadine to remove any dirt or debris from the substrate. When the patient is stable under anesthesia, it can then be moved into the surgical suite. Once inside the surgical suite, all assistants should put on a cap and mask to maintain asepsis. The patient should be properly positioned and taped down to secure it to the table. Snakes can be positioned either in sternal, dorsal, or left or right recumbency. Once the patient is secured to the table, a sterile surgical scrub should be performed. The fluids used to prep the patient should be warmed to prevent cooling the patient. The patient should also be kept at its POTZ during the entire procedure and through recovery. This can be achieved by using a circulating hot water pad or hot water bottles.

Wound Healing

Wound healing in snakes has been studied extensively (Bennett and Lock 2000). When a wound forms, proteinaceous fluid and fibrin fills the space to form a scab. A single layer of epithelial cells grows under the scab and then proliferates to restore the full thickness of the epithelium. Underneath this layer of epithelial cells, macrophages and heterophils move in to clean up any pathogens. Fibroblasts migrate to the area, forming a fibrous scar. Heterophils are present until maturation has occurred. Ecdysis seems to help with the wound healing process (Bennett 1997). It has also been observed that incisions that have a cranial to caudal orientation heal faster than transverse incisions. Furthermore, staying in the upper end of the species' POTZ promotes good wound healing (Bennett and Lock 2000).

The incised skin of reptiles has a tendency to heal inverted. The skin should be closed using an everted suture pattern such as mattress pattern. Skin staples can also be used for skin closure. The sutures should be removed in four to six weeks and preferably after the next ecdysis cycle.

Common Surgical Procedures

Celiotomies are routinely performed on snakes. The incision for a celiotomy should be made between the first two rows of scales dorsolateral to the large ventral scales (Bennett and Lock 2000). This approach is performed to avoid the large midabdominal vein. A zigzag incision is made between the scales in the softer skin. Celiotomies are commonly performed for foreign body removal and exploratory surgery.

The most common surgery of the respiratory tract is removal of granulomas from the trachea. The approach is the same as for a celiotomy. The granuloma is found and removed. The two ends of the trachea are then anastomosed and the incision is closed. The snakes are usually back to breathing normally immediately.

Gastrointestinal surgeries are routinely done to repair abnormalities. These abnormalities may include foreign body removal or resection and anastomosis.

Surgery on the reproductive tract is usually not performed to prevent a reproductive problem (Lock 2000). The most common female reproductive surgical procedure is dystocia and ovariectomy or ovariosalpingohysterectomy. The last two procedures are performed to prevent another dystocia, to remove cysts or tumors, or to prevent another prolapse. The most common surgical procedure on the male reproductive tract is penile amputation. The hemipenis will prolapse and become inflamed and will not be able to be retracted. Often the hemipenis can be replaced, but occasionally it will become necrotic and have to be amputated (Figure 7.21).

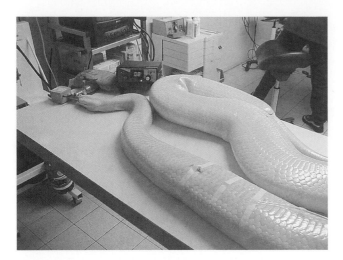

Figure 7.21. A snake in surgery. (Photo courtesy of Dr. Stephen J. Hernandez-Divers, University of Georgia.)

PARASITOLOGY

Diagnosing Parasites

Parasitic infections are relatively easy to diagnose. A fresh stool sample should be obtained, being careful not to collect any urates. When an appointment is made for a snake, the client should be asked to bring in a fresh stool sample. The client can put the stool sample in a plastic sandwich bag and keep it in the refrigerator for up to three days. It is not recommended that the stool sample be stored in a refrigerator that also stores food for human consumption. A double or even triple bag system can be used if the sample is stored with food for human consumption. If a fresh sample is not available, a colonic wash can be performed to obtain a sample. Three diagnostic tests should be performed: a flotation, centrifugation, and saline prepared direct smear. The fecal flotation is used to diagnose nematode ova. The centrifuge helps diagnose protozoan cysts. The direct smear is used to diagnose moving or live parasites. The techniques used to perform these diagnostics are the same techniques used for diagnosing parasites in small animals. Some parasites, like cryptosporidium, require specialized diagnostic testing.

COMMON PARASITES OF SNAKES

External Parasites

Ticks

Ticks are a common finding on snakes. Ticks can be very difficult to find on snakes, especially if the snake has dark skin. Rarely are ticks in such a high number on snakes to cause anemia, but they can transmit blood parasites and viruses. All ticks should be removed with extra care to remove all the mouthparts from the skin.

Mites

Ophionyssus natricis, the snake mite, is a common finding in pet snakes. The mites are small and appear red, gray, or black. Snakes that are infected may spend long periods of time soaking in water or appear to rub or twist their bodies. Visualizing the mite is the only diagnostic method. If mites are suspected, a clean white paper towel or hand towel can be rubbed down the entire length of the snake's body. Often, the mites will come off onto the towel making for easier visualization. Treatment includes cleaning and disinfecting the cage and ivermectin. Ivermectin can be made into a spray or used as an injection. It is also recommended that all wood and porous cage furnishings be removed and paper be used as a substrate until the mites have been eradicated from the area.

Internal Parasites

Protozoa

Amoebiasis Of the many species of amoebae that are found in snakes, *Entamoeba invadens* is the most pathogenic (Lane and Mader 1996). This amoeba causes a very high mortality and morbidity rate in snakes. It is transmitted via the ingestion of infected reptile feces. This parasite has a direct life cycle, making it very difficult to eradicate from snakes. Clinical signs of amoebiasis are anorexia, dehydration, and wasting away. Later stages of the disease show clinical signs of ulcerative gastritis and colitis. This organism can spread to other tissues, causing renal and hepatic necrosis and abscesses. A diagnosis is made through a positive culture. Treatment of this disease includes a broad-spectrum antibiotic, an amoebicide, and supportive care. The snakes can also be kept at a temperature of 95°F.

Coccidia Coccidiosis is a common finding in captive snakes. In wild snakes, coccidiosis is a self-limiting infection, but in captivity, coccidia can cause severe illness and in young or small species it can cause death. Coccidia has a direct life cycle. Sulfonamides are the preferred treatment.

Cryptosporidium is becoming a serious coccidial infection in snakes. The exact source of infection is unknown but it is believed that snakes contract the parasite by either contact with shedding reptiles or from mammalian prey items. Clinical signs for the disease includes midbody swelling, weight loss, and regurgitation. The midbody swelling is a result of chronic gastric hypertrophy caused by the parasite. Cryptosporidiosis is diagnosed by visualization of oocysts on a microscopic exam. A dimethyl sulfoxide (DMSO) acid-fast fecal exam should be performed for proper diagnosis. *Cryptosporidium* spp. oocysts are difficult to find due to their small size of less than 4 microns. The oocysts contain no sporocysts and four sporozoites. There are no safe and effective treatments for cryptosporidiosis. Trimethoprim sulfa, spiramycin, and paromomycin have been shown to reduce clinical signs and reduce or eliminate oocyte shedding. These drugs are given in conjunction with supportive care including fluids, high environmental temperatures, and tube feeding. It is not known if there is a zoonotic potential with this disease, so proper precautions should be taken.

Flagellated Protozoa Many genera of flagellates are found in snakes. Most are nonpathogenic, although there is the potential of *Giardia* spp. to cause disease. Clinical signs include anorexia and weight loss (Barnard 1996). Metronidazole is the treatment of choice for flagellates.

Cestodes

The life cycle of cestodes involves many intermediate hosts. Snakes that are susceptible to cestode infections are those that are fed amphibians, fish, or crustaceans.

Nematodes

Several species of nematodes affect snakes. The life cycle involves one or several intermediate hosts. Nematode infections usually appear subclinical but signs can appear with severe infections. The only species of great concern are the *Rhabdias* spp. and *Strongyloides* spp. (Barnard 1996). *Rhabdias* spp. are known as the lungworm in snakes because these nematodes migrate to the lungs. There are few clinical signs with minimal inflammatory response. Severe infections show signs of dyspnea and mouth gaping. The diagnosis of lungworms can be made by discovering eggs and free-stage larvae in the oral secretions or feces. Strongyles are nematodes that feed on the blood of the host. Clinical signs include anorexia, weight loss, hemorrhagic ulceration, and gastrointestinal obstruction. A fecal exam is performed for diagnosis. Treatment for all nematodes includes any of several anthelmintics and supportive care (Color Plate 7.3.)

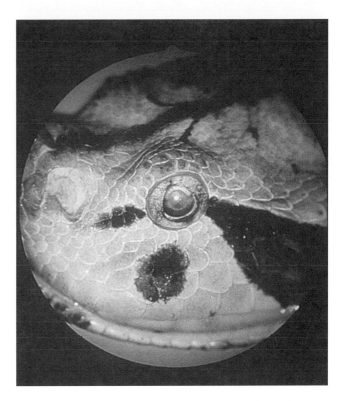

Plate 7.3. Ocular larva migrans in a snake. (Photo courtesy of Zoo Atlanta.) (See also color plates)

Blood Parasites

Extracellular and intracytoplastic blood parasites are commonly seen in snakes. These parasites rarely cause disease and are normally found on routine blood smears. Extreme cases can cause hemolytic anemia. If anemia is found, an antimalarial medication is indicated.

Preventing Parasites

With parasites, like most other diseases, prevention is easier than the cure. A few simple guidelines should be followed. The enclosures should be kept clean and disinfected often. New specimens should follow proper quarantine procedures. Do not feed wild prey items; feed only frozen prey to the snakes. If live prey must be fed, start a breeding colony at home with a parasite-free male and female. Varying the prey offered can help to break any parasite life cycle (Lane and Mader 1996).

EMERGENCY AND CRITICAL CARE

As more and more snakes are kept as pets, the need for proper emergency and critical care is increasing.

The basics of emergency and critical care in snakes are the same as in any other animal. The patient is assessed and diagnostics and treatments are quickly started. An emergency is defined as a sudden, generally unexpected occurrence or set of circumstances demanding urgent action. Unfortunately, the need for urgent care is in the eye of the owner and not trained medical professionals. Many owners wait days to months after first noticing a problem with their snake to seek medical attention, so that the initial problem turns into an emergency situation.

Phone Calls

Many owners call the veterinary hospital seeking advice on their pet snake to determine if emergency medical treatment is necessary. Many problems with snakes that are reported after hours can wait until the morning when the regular veterinarian is available. Most diseases have been developing for weeks to months and initiating treatment can wait another several hours. It is important that the technician screening the phone calls be familiar with snakes. Some clinical signs in dogs could be very serious, while in a snake they are very normal. A common phone call that is not an emergency is an owner worried that his or her ball python (*Python regius*), or any other species, has not eaten in a week or sometimes several months. Obviously, for a snake this is not an emergency. Some of the more common emergencies that do need to be seen immediately are trauma, bite wounds, burns, hypothermia, hyperthermia, dyspnea, and cloacal prolapse. Common nonemergency clinical signs in snakes are lethargy, anorexia, dystocia, and constipation.

Initial Presentation and History

A veterinary technician should make a quick assessment to determine the urgency of care as soon as the patient comes into the veterinary hospital. If the patient is stable, a thorough history should be obtained. If the patient is critical and needs immediate care, the patient should be taken to the attending veterinarian and a quick history should be obtained. This history should include such questions as: What is the ambient temperature in the enclosure? Is the snake eating and drinking normally? Do you feed live or dead prey? What heat sources are used? Has your snake been lethargic? Have you seen any coughing, wheezing, or nasal discharge? Has your snake regurgitated any food? Have there been any other medical problems in the past?

A more complete history can be obtained after the patient is stable and more time can be focused away from the patient. More questions may need to be asked pending the results of the physical examination.

Diagnostics

The clinician will have a diagnostic plan after the physical examination has been performed. This plan may include a fecal analysis, biochemical profile, complete blood count, packed cell volume, total protein, or radiographs.

Treatment

Treatment should begin after the diagnosis is made. For dehydrated or severely ill snakes, fluid therapy should be initiated. Intravenous fluid therapy is preferable but other methods of fluid therapy will suffice. The fluids should be warmed to the preferred body temperature for the species being treated. The snake should be placed in a cage that is heated to the species' POTZ. A full-spectrum UV light should also be provided. Analgesics should be administered to patients that are in pain. Finally, other therapeutics should be started to treat the clinical signs and disease. Nutritional support should be started only after the patient is stable.

EMERGENCY CONDITIONS

Trauma

Trauma of any kind should be treated as an emergency. Bite wounds are common in snakes. Bites normally occur from cage mates and live prey items left in the cage unattended. Lacerations are not as commonly seen in snakes. Most commonly they occur from exposed ends of wire mesh used on cages. Large snakes can easily break through glass cages, causing severe lacerations. Bite wounds and lacerations are treated by either primary closure or secondary intention healing. If the wound is left open, antibiotic ointments rubbed on the wound work well as a barrier. Systemic antibiotics should be used on all bite wounds or lacerations. Analgesics should also be used.

Hypothermia

Occasionally snakes escape from their enclosure and are found in a place that is excessively cold, causing metabolism to cease. Frostbite may be seen on the tip of the snake's tail. If not necrotic, some pigment will be lost. Hypothermic snakes are not able to digest food and often regurgitate prey. It is common to see respiratory disease several days to weeks after an episode of hypothermia. Snakes should be warmed up slowly over several hours and supportive care should be started.

Hyperthermia

Hyperthermia often occurs when the owner lets the snake outside in a glass or plastic enclosure in direct sunlight. Radiant heat quickly warms the snake and it is not able to get into a cooler environment. Treatment for hyperthermia includes subcutaneous or intracoelomic fluids and a quick cool-water bath to decrease the core body temperature. Steroids may also be indicated.

Dyspnea

Snakes do not normally open-mouth breathe. If acute dyspnea occurs the snake should be seen immediately. Dyspnea can be caused by several pathogens or disease processes, but it is most commonly associated with pneumonia.

Thermal Burns

Thermal burns are one of the most common emergencies seen in practice. Often, snakes do not show clinical signs of a burn for several days, making them difficult to treat. Thermal burns are most commonly caused by a malfunctioning heat source or improper use of a heat source. The two most common causes of thermal burns in snakes are hot rocks (or what this author refers to as death rocks) and heat lights that snakes coil around.

Burns are classified as superficial, partial thickness, or full thickness. A superficial burn involves only the epidermis. The snake may appear to be in pain and have some discoloration on its scales. In severe superficial burns some scales may be singed. Snakes with a superficial burn have a good prognosis. Antibiotic therapy should be initiated if any infection is noted. The snake should be housed in its POTZ and should heal by the next ecdysis. Little or no scarring is seen with superficial burns.

Partial-thickness burns involve complete destruction of the epidermis and extend into the underlying layers of skin. These burns appear red, ooze plasma, and will blister. Partial-thickness burns are also very painful. Treatment can take several months to completely heal. Analgesics should be administered immediately because these burns are very painful. The burn should be flushed thoroughly and supportive care should be started. It is not uncommon for these patients to be in shock. After cleansing the burns, a burn cream such as 1% silver sulfadiazine should be applied and a sterile nonstick bandage should be placed. Wet to dry bandages can also be used. The bandages should be replaced every day. The snake should be housed in a glass or Plexiglas container with no substrate until the wound is completely healed. The cage should also be disinfected daily. Antibiotics should be started to prevent infections that are common in burn victims.

Full-thickness burns are characterized by a black eschar. They are not painful because all of the nerves in the skin have been destroyed. Full-thickness burns have a poor to grave prognosis and require very intensive treatment. The wound initially should be treated with a thorough cleansing and fluid therapy to treat for shock. The burn should be debrided to promote healing and a bandage should be placed. Antibiotics should also be started. Daily bandage changes and debridement are necessary for successful treatment. As the skin heals, the wound will become very painful. Analgesics should be started as soon as the patient feels pain. It can take months to a year for full granulation to occur. The owners must be told of the poor prognosis, long-term care, and financial expense of treating a full-thickness burn before treatment begins.

CRITICAL CARE MONITORING

The same principles apply to monitoring a critically ill snake as apply to monitoring a critically ill dog or cat. Neurologic, respiratory, and cardiovascular function all must be monitored and assessed.

The cardiovascular system should be monitored by using a Doppler and electrocardiogram. A heart rate should be obtained from both the Doppler and ECG (Figures 7.22, 7.23). Auscultation should be performed to monitor the respiratory system. The breath sounds should be clear without any wheezing or crackles. A respiratory rate should be obtained and recorded. The patient should also be observed for dyspnea. A neurologic exam should be performed daily. The snake should also be housed in its POTZ.

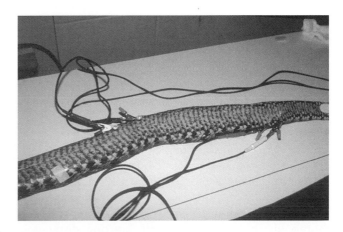

Figure 7.22. ECG lead placement on a snake. The head is to the right. (Photo courtesy of Zoo Atlanta.)

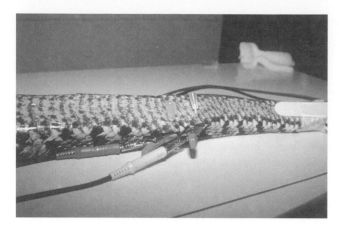

Figure 7.23. *ECG lead placement close-up to show detail. (Photo courtesy of Zoo Atlanta.)*

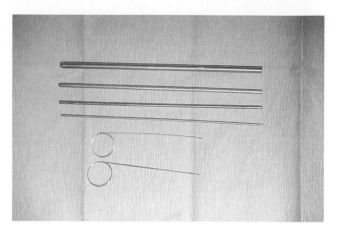

Figure 7.24. *Probes used for sexing snakes. (Photo courtesy of Ryan Cheek.)*

SEX DETERMININATION

Snakes do not possess external genitalia, so determining the sex can sometimes be challenging. There are several acceptable methods used to determine the sex of snakes. Of the methods available, there are various degrees of simplicity and accuracy. It is important to choose a method that best suits the particular snake. For a snake that is kept as a pet, it is best to stick with a more simple method of sex determination. Snakes kept for breeding should be sexed using the most accurate method for that species.

Secondary Sexual Characteristics

With the exception of the boids, most snakes do not show any secondary sexual characteristics. Male boids sometimes have larger cloacal spurs than females. Only technicians that are very familiar with boids will be able to accurately determine the sex by using this method. Another secondary sexual characteristic that can be used to determine the sex is looking for a small bulge in the tail, because the hemipenes are kept inside the tail. Using secondary sexual characteristics is a simple method but is the least accurate.

Manual Eversion

A more accurate method of sex determination is manually everting the hemipenes. This method is best used in juvenile snakes or those that are too small for other methods. This method of sex determination is often referred to as popping. For this process, firmly roll one thumb up the base of the tail, starting distal and working proximal to the cloaca. If it is a male, the hemipenes will pop out. Care must be taken not to

apply too much pressure or the hemipenes can be damaged. This method is unreliable in large snakes and some colubrids in which manual eversion of the hemipenes is not possible.

Cloacal Probing

This is the preferred method of sex determination. It is very simple and accurate if done properly. The probe used can be anything that is straight and has a blunt end. Commercial sex probes are available in sets of various diameters. Insert the lubricated probe into the cloaca and angle it caudally. Position the probe just lateral to the midline. Then gently slide the probe caudally into the base of the tail. If the snake is male, the probe will enter the inverted hemipenis and slide down several millimeters. If the snake is a female, the probe will either not be able to enter the tail base or will go only a couple of millimeters. Female snakes have blind diverticula that are smaller in diameter and shorter in depth than the hemipenes. A major cause of error in sexing is using a probe that is too small. A very small probe can enter the diverticula in females, giving a false diagnosis. The technician must also be careful not to be forceful with the probe. The probe should slide smoothly with very little force needed. Generally, the distance the probe enters the base of the tail is measured in either millimeters or number of subcaudal scales. This number should be recorded in the file with the sex diagnosis (Figures 7.24, 7.25).

Hydrostatic Eversion

Hydrostatic eversion is the most accurate yet difficult method of sex determination. It involves injecting iso-

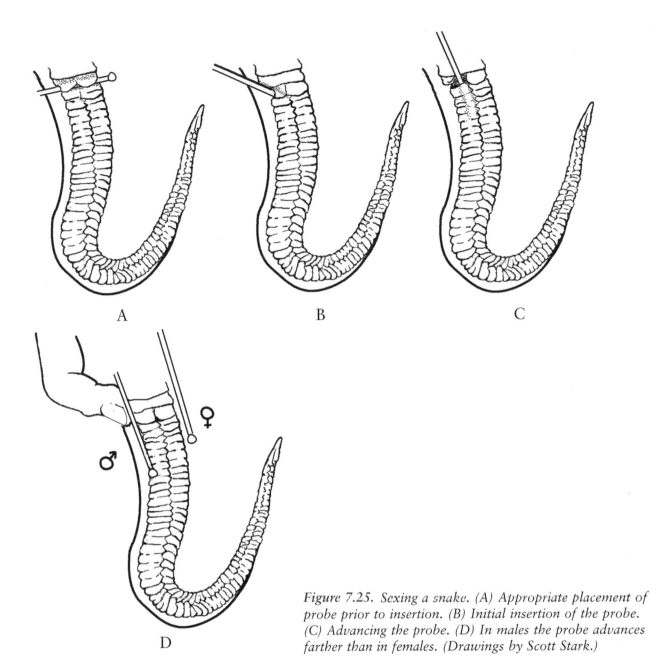

Figure 7.25. Sexing a snake. (A) Appropriate placement of probe prior to insertion. (B) Initial insertion of the probe. (C) Advancing the probe. (D) In males the probe advances farther than in females. (Drawings by Scott Stark.)

tonic saline into the base of the tail just caudal to where the hemipenes would be located. Keep injecting the saline until the hemipenes are everted or resistance is felt on the syringe. A possible danger of this procedure is injecting the saline into the hemipenes instead of caudal. For very large snakes, anesthesia is required to perform this procedure. This method is very accurate because the hemipenes are everted in males, and if the snake is female, the swelling around the cloaca allows for visualization of the oviductal papillae.

CLINICAL TECHNIQUES

Administration of Medications

Intravenous

Intravenous (IV) injections can be given in the tail vein or directly into the heart. Use the same technique used for venipuncture to give the injection. Another vein that can be used for IV injections is the palatine vein. This vein is located in the oral cavity and is best suited for very experienced phlebotomists due to its small size. The palatine vein should only be used in snakes with a healthy oral cavity and no signs of stomatitis.

Subcutaneous

Subcutaneous (SC) injections can easily be given when the snake is coiled and skin folds appear. The needle should be placed between the scales on the lateral coelomic body wall, aspiration applied to the syringe to ensure a blood vessel has not been entered, and then the injection given. If the snake is not coiled, a small piece of skin can be lifted and the injection given.

Intramuscular

Intramuscular (IM) injections can be given in the epaxial and lateral muscle groups. The needle is placed between the scales, aspiration applied to the syringe to ensure a blood vessel has not been entered, and then the injection given.

Intracoelomic

The snake should be restrained in dorsal or lateral recumbency for intracoelomic (ICe) medication administration. The needle is placed between scales in the lower quadrant of the coelomic cavity, being careful to be far enough caudal to avoid the lung. It is very important to aspirate back on the syringe before injecting. If any blood or other questionable fluid is aspirated, the needle should be removed and a new syringe and medication should be prepared. If giving ICe fluids, the fluids should be warmed up to the snake's POTZ before administering.

Oral

Oral (PO) medications are very easy to give to snakes. The medication is drawn up into a syringe and then a red rubber catheter is attached to the end. To prevent the red rubber catheter from passing into the trachea, a catheter should be chosen that is too large to fit into the trachea. The mouth should be opened to ensure that the catheter has gone down the esophagus. After checking for correct placement, administration of the medication can begin. With another syringe filled with water, the medication should be flushed down to ensure that no medicine is left in the catheter. This method can also be used to force feed snakes.

Venipuncture

Tail Vein

The snake can be placed in either dorsal or ventral recumbency (Figure 7.26). With the bevel of the needle

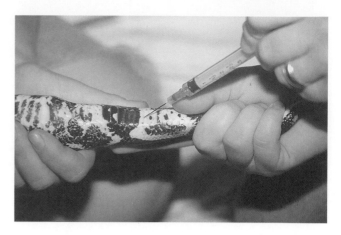

Figure 7.26. Venipuncture using the tail vein. (Photo courtesy of Ryan Cheek.)

facing cranial, the needle is inserted exactly on midline at a 45-degree angle. While maintaining gentle suction, the needle is advanced until a flash of blood is seen. Occasionally the coccygeal vertebrae will be hit first and the flash of blood will be seen as the needle is withdrawn. The needle should be inserted caudal to the hemipenes and scent glands. With smaller snakes, a gentle suction and release may be done to receive enough blood to perform diagnostic testing.

Cardiocentesis

Locate the heart by either manual palpation or Doppler. Apply pressure just caudal and cranial to the heart to stabilize it. After the heart has been stabilized, the needle is inserted at a 45- to 60-degree angle. The needle is advanced until a slight pop is felt and the needle has entered the heart. Aspirate back until enough sample has been taken. Occasionally, pericardial fluid may be aspirated. If this happens, the needle should be withdrawn and the procedure started over with a fresh needle and syringe (Figure 7.27).

Palatine Vein

As stated previously, the palatine vein is only recommended in a snake with a clean oral cavity and no signs of stomatitis. This technique only works on very docile or anesthetized snakes. Restrain the snake with its mouth open. A 25- to 27-gauge needle should be advanced into the vein, and then aspirate gently to prevent the vein from collapsing. Due to the chance of contamination from the saliva, this vein is best used only for IV injections.

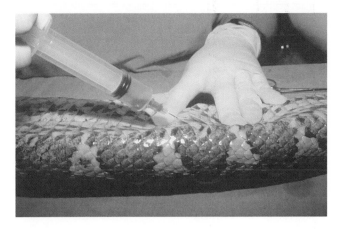

Figure 7.27. Cardiocentesis. (Photo courtesy of Zoo Atlanta.)

Intravenous Catheter Placement

Jugular Vein

A cut-down incision is required for this procedure. The skin should be surgically prepped. The incision should be made at the junction of the ventral scutes and lateral scales just cranial to the heart, about four to seven scutes. It is necessary to bluntly dissect to expose the vein. After the vein has been exposed, the catheter is inserted until a flash is seen in the hub. The catheter is then advanced into the vein. The skin is closed using sutures and with the catheter sutured to the skin. A bandage can be placed to keep the catheter site clean.

Heart

In an extreme emergency, a catheter can be placed in the heart for a short time. The technique used for venipuncture can be used to place the catheter. Once the catheter is placed, it should be secured with suture or tape.

Force Feeding

Properly restrain the snake with its mouth open. An appropriate-sized prey item is grasped with large hemostats and a large amount of lubrication is applied to the entire body of the prey. It is then inserted into the snake's mouth, gently forcing it down. Once the prey is completely inserted, milk the prey down the esophagus until it reaches the stomach. Be very careful that the prey does not scratch the esophagus with its incisors or claws. An easy way to prevent this is to trim the claws and teeth before force feeding.

Snakes can also be force fed by using the same technique for giving oral medications (Figures 7.28, 7.29). Liquefied whole prey or artificially prepared

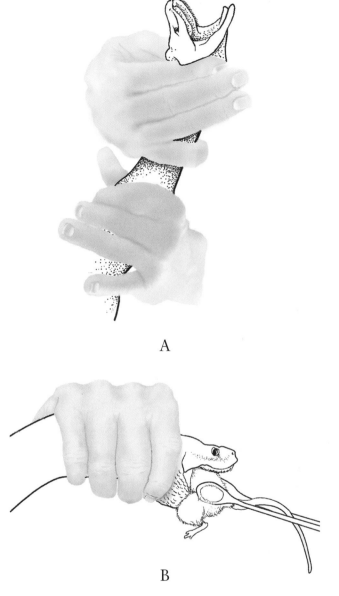

A

B

Figure 7.28. Feeding a snake. (A) Restraint with the mouth open for insertion of prey. A tongue depressor may be used to open the mouth. (B) Using a pair of large hemostats, the prey is gently pushed down into the esophagus. (Drawings by Scott Stark.)

foods can be used. For neonates or smaller snakes a device called a pinkie press can be used.

Tracheal and Lung Wash

Restrain the snake with its mouth open. Pass a sterile red rubber catheter into the trachea. Once the catheter

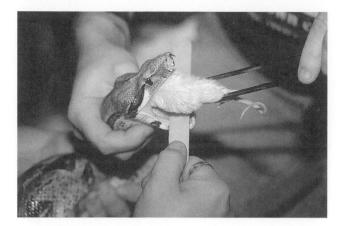

A

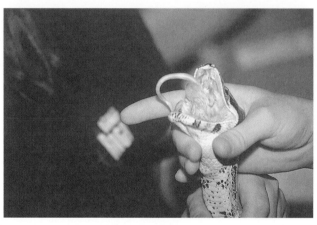

B

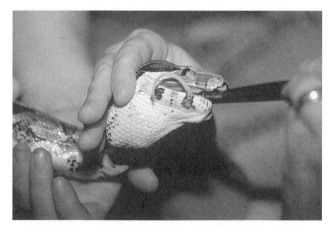

C

Figure 7.29. *Force-feeding a snake. (A) The snake is properly restrained and a tongue depressor is used to open the mouth. The prey is then inserted into the oral cavity. (B) The prey is almost completely into the oral cavity. (C) The prey is then gently pushed down the esophagus. (Photos courtesy of Ryan Cheek.)*

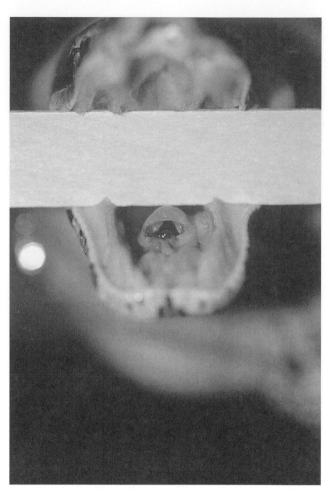

Figure 7.30. *View of the glottis. (Photo courtesy of Ryan Cheek.)*

is in place, infuse sterile saline into the trachea and lung. Do not place more than 5 ml/kg into the lung. After the sterile saline has been administered, aspirate back as much of the saline as possible. The saline can be injected and aspirated as many times as needed to receive a proper amount of sample (Figures 7.30, 7.31).

Colonic Wash and Enema

Insert a well-lubricated red rubber catheter into the colon. To enter the colon, the cloaca should be entered and the catheter aimed ventrally. With a syringe filled with saline, begin flushing the saline into the colon and aspirating it back. This step should be repeated several times to get an adequate sample. This process also helps soften stools in constipated snakes. After aspiration, the sample can then be analyzed for parasites, cytologic examination, and culture (Figure 7.32).

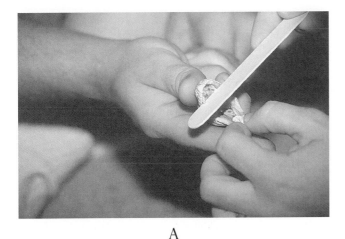

A

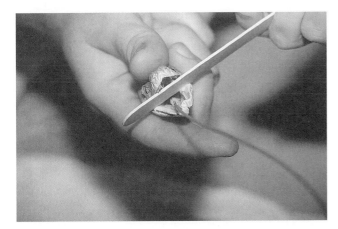

B

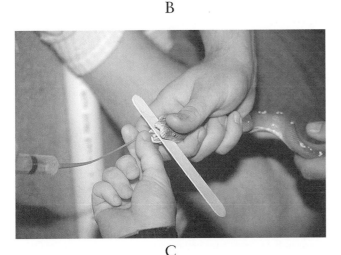

C

Figure 7.31. *Tracheal wash. (A) With the snake properly restrained, the mouth is opened. (B) A tongue depressor is used as a mouth gag, and the red rubber catheter is inserted into the trachea. (C) 0.9% sodium chloride is then gently flushed into the trachea and then aspirated back. (Photos courtesy of Ryan Cheek.)*

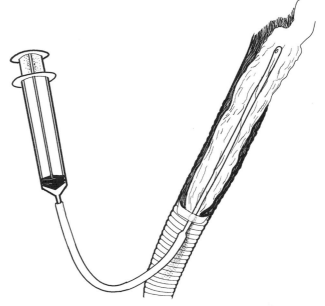

Figure 7.32. *Colonic wash. (Drawing by Scott Stark.)*

VENOMOUS SNAKES

It is not recommended to keep venomous snakes in private collections, especially by novice hobbyists. In some cases, it may be illegal to keep venomous snakes without proper permits. For this reason, it is rare that one would be brought into private practice for medical care. If this occurs, however, proper protocols need to be implemented. Whether a veterinary practice is even equipped for safe handling of venomous snakes needs to be addressed. At the very least, snake tongs, hooks, and tubes are needed for safer handling. Someone trained in handling venomous snakes is also needed. Although tubing and handling techniques can be practiced on nonvenomous snakes, there is obviously more risk involved in dealing with the venomous ones, and others could be put at risk as well.

Most procedures on venomous snakes should be done while the snake is under anesthesia, which involves either tubing or placing the snake in an immobilization chamber. Do not attempt to manually restrain the head of a venomous snake. Those who milk snakes for venom have to do so but it is not a safe method of restraint. Some fangs are long enough to still penetrate a hand while restraining the head.

An envenomation protocol also needs to be in place at the facility. Most human hospitals (if they carry antivenin at all) only have those of indigenous species. Therefore, imported species are riskier to handle due to the lack of accessible antivenin. Most facilities that handle venomous snakes keep the different types of antivenin in stock, not necessarily for self-administration should a bite occur, but to bring to the nearest hospital if the hospital does not have any on hand. This is difficult though, due to both the expenses involved and the lack of accessibility. Expiration dates on the antivenin also must be closely monitored.

Be sure to have a line of communication established with local hospitals to know who is able to handle a venomous snakebite. Contacting the local poison control facility to establish a protocol is helpful as well. Once again, these are all issues that must be addressed before venomous snakes are managed at the facility. Minutes count should a venomous snakebite occur. Time cannot be wasted on calling hospitals to see if they can handle that particular bite. If this seems like too much of a hassle, then handling/treating venomous snakes should not be performed at that facility at all.

EUTHANASIA

Unfortunately, not all patients can be saved. Fortunately, veterinary medicine has the privilege of being able to humanely euthanize suffering animals with terminal illnesses. Euthanizing snakes can prove to be a difficult task. There are several humane methods of euthanasia that are acceptable in snakes. Only the methods that this author feels are humane will be discussed here.

This author's preferred method of euthanasia in snakes starts with an injection of telazol or ketamine HCl. If injectable anesthetics are not available, inhalant anesthesia can be used. Due to the ability of snakes to hold their breath for long periods of time this can be a very lengthy process. After the snake is anesthetized, a cardiac stick is performed and an overdose of a barbiturate is injected. In very small species or very dehydrated snakes, a cardiac stick can be difficult. In that case, a simple IC injection of a barbiturate can be performed. It can take several minutes to several hours before the snake is finally deceased using this method.

The toughest part of euthanizing snakes is determining death. There is not a good answer to the question. Is the snake deceased? An electrocardiograph, auscultation of the heart, or a Doppler can all be used to determine if the snake is deceased. Due to the fact that reptile hearts can still beat for several hours postmortem or can even beat once or twice per minute postmortem, these three tests can prove to be inaccurate. Many reptile clinicians have heard stories of the snake coming back to life twenty-four hours after the

euthanasia. This can be easily avoided if the snake is left in the hospital overnight for observation.

BEING A RESPONSIBLE SNAKE OWNER

As a part of the veterinary team, the technician is responsible for properly informing and educating clients about the needs of particular animals. It is also important to offer guidance when purchases are being considered. Knowing what is involved in snake care and knowing specifics about different species of snakes aids in giving advice to those considering purchasing a snake as a pet. Offering consultations to clients before purchases help to eliminate many of the problems that arise after a snake is purchased. Snakes, in general, do not make good pets. This should be kept in mind when offering advice to potential buyers. Buying a snake that will reach lengths of 20 feet or more is obviously not a choice that should be made by most people, either. These snakes usually become neglected and the owners sometimes begin to fear them due to their size and their predisposition, which may become aggressive.

More and more people are beginning to devise ways to get rid of their snakes when it is no longer convenient to own them. All too often these snakes are impulse buys that are thought of as disposable belongings. The most appalling of these occurrences is when people let them go in their backyards when they don't want to deal with them anymore. Most captive specimens are not even indigenous to the country where their owners set them free. Not only will this most likely kill the animal, but it can upset the natural balance of that particular ecosystem. Some even choose to freeze the snake as their way of humanely euthanizing the animal so they will no longer be burdened. There is nothing humane about freezing a live animal. It is, in fact a slow, painful death.

If an owner no longer wants a snake, then attempts should be made to place it in a home or facility ready and able to meet its needs. Most of the time, this occurs with the larger species of snakes. They can reach astounding lengths and girths and can be extremely dangerous, not to mention the size of the enclosure needed to properly house them. These are obviously not for novice keepers and should be discouraged when an inexperienced individual inquires about obtaining one.

Another point to be made about being a responsible snake owner is understanding that many people fear them. Taking snakes out to public places to show them off is not doing the public any good, and especially not the snake. Being around a lot of commotion can scare the snake and can cause the people to panic as well. This in turn, is doing more injustice to the snake than one would think. The public, as a whole, has a terrible phobia of snakes and forcing the issue by bringing snakes into public places makes it worse. If individuals want to display their snakes, they should offer educational exhibits and lectures. By displaying them in this way they can create a learning environment and offer people the choice of whether to participate or not. A phobia (no matter how silly one thinks it is) is a phobia, and it is not something that can be a forced change.

REFERENCES

Barnard SM. 1996. Reptile Keepers Handbook. Florida: Krieger Publishing Company. 71–73.

Bennett RA. 1997. Reptilian Surgery, Parts 1 and 2. In: Practical Exotic Animal Medicine, edited by Rosenthal KL. New Jersey: Veterinary Learning Systems. 32–38.

Bennett RA. 1996a. Anesthesia. In: Reptile Medicine and Surgery, edited by Mader DR. Philadelphia: W.B. Saunders Co. 30, 243–244.

Bennett RA. 1996b. Neurology. In: Reptile Medicine and Surgery, edited by Mader DR. Philadelphia: W.B. Saunders Co. 142–145.

Bennett RA, Lock BA. 2000. Nonreproductive Surgery in Reptiles. In: Veterinary Clinics of North America: Exotic Animal Practice. Philadelphia: W.B. Saunders Co. 718–721.

Bertelsen MF. 2007. Squamates (Snakes and Lizards. In: Zoo Animal and Wildlife Immobilization and Anesthesia, edited by West G, Heard D, Caulkett N. Iowa: Blackwell Publishing.

Bronson E, Cranfield MR. 2006. Paramyxovirus. In: Reptile Medicine and Surgery 2nd edition, edited by Mader DR. Missouri: Saunders Elsevier.

Bradley T. 2001. Pain Management Considerations and Pain-Associated Behaviors in Reptiles and Amphibians. In: Proceedings of the Association of Reptilian and Amphibian Veterinarians. Eastern State Vet Assn. 45.

Divers SJ. 2000. Reptilian Renal and Reproductive Disease and Diagnosis. In: Laboratory Medicine: Avian and Exotic Pets, edited by Fudge AM. Philadelphia: W.B. Saunders Co. 217.

Driggers T. May 2000. Respiratory Diseases, Diagnostics, and Therapy in Snakes. In: The Veterinary Clinics of North America: Exotic Animal Medicine. Philadelphia: W.B. Saunders Co. 524–528.

Funk RS. 1996. Snakes. In: Reptile Medicine and Surgery, edited by Mader DR. Philadelphia: W.B. Saunders Co. 40–42.

Glynn MK, et al. 2001. Knowledge and Practices of California Veterinarians Concerning the Human Health Threat of Reptile-Associated Salmonellosis. Journal of Herpetological Medicine and Surgery 11(2): 9–13.

Holz PH. 1999. The Reptilian Renal-Portal System: Influence on Therapy. In: Zoo and Wild Animal Medicine: Current Therapy 4th ed., edited by Fowler ME and Miller RE. Philadelphia: W.B. Saunders Co. 249.

Lane TJ, Mader DR. 1996. Parasitology. In: Reptile Medicine and Surgery, edited by Mader DR. Philadelphia: W.B. Saunders Co. 190–202.

Lawton MP. 2001. Fluid Therapy in Reptiles. In: Proceedings of the North American Veterinary Conference. Eastern States Vet Assn. 788.

Lawton MP. 1991. Lizards and Snakes. In: Manual of Exotic Pets, edited by Beymon PH, et al. Ames: Iowa State University Press. 254.

Lock BA. May 2000. Reproductive Surgery in Reptiles. In: Veterinary Clinics of North America: Exotic Animal Practice. Philadelphia: W.B. Saunders Co. 734–737.

Marschang RE. 2001. Isolation of Viruses from Boa Constrictors, Boa constrictor spp., with Inclusion Body Disease. In: Proceedings of the Association of Reptilian and Amphibian Veterinarians. Eastern States Vet Assn. 37.

Miller HA. April 1998. Urinary Diseases of Reptiles: Pathophysiology and Diagnosis. In: Seminars in Avian and Exotic Pet Medicine, edited by Fudge AM. Philadelphia: W.B. Saunders Co. 96–98.

Platel R. 1994. Nervous System and Sensory Organs. In: Snakes: A Natural History, edited by Bauchot R. New York: Sterling Publishing. 51–55.

Pough FH, et al. 2001. Herpetology. 2nd ed. New Jersey: Prentice-Hall Inc. 200–206, 272.

Ritchie B. 2006. Virology. In: Reptile Medicine and Surgery, 2nd ed., edited by Mader DR. Missouri: Saunders Elsevier.

Romer AS. 1997. Osteology of the Reptiles. Reprint. Malabar, FL: Krieger Publishing. 126, 209.

Ross RA, et al. 1990. The Reproductive Husbandry of Pythons and Boas. The Institute for Herpetological Research, Stanford, CA. 55–60, 103.

Rossi JV. 1996. Dermatology. In: Reptile Medicine and Surgery, edited by Mader DR. Philadelphia: W.B. Saunders Co. 106–114.

Saint-Girons H. 1994. Growth and Reproduction. In: Snakes: A Natural History, edited by Bauchot R. New York: Sterling Publishing. 99.

Schumacher J, Yelen, T. 2006. Anesthesia and Analgesia. In: Reptile Medicine and Surgery 2nd ed., edited by Mader DR. Missouri: Saunders Elsevier.

Schumacher J. 2002a. Anesthesia in Reptiles. In: Proceedings of the North American Veterinary Conference. Eastern States Vet Assn. 946.

Schumacher J. 2002b. Sevoflurane in Reptiles. In: Proceedings of the North American Veterinary Conference. Eastern States Vet Assn. 950.

Schumacher J. 1996. Viral Diseases. In: Reptile Medicine and Surgery, edited by Mader DR. Philadelphia: W.B. Saunders Co. 229.

Siemering H. 1986. Zoonoses. In: Zoo and Wild Animal Medicine, 2nd ed., edited by Fowler ME. Philadelphia: W.B. Saunders Co. 64.

Vasse Y. 1994. A Cardiovascular System Working Against the Forces of Gravity. In: Snakes: A Natural History, edited by Bauchot R. New York: Sterling Publishing. 75.

Williams DL. 1996. Ophthalmology. In: Reptile Medicine and Surgery, edited by Mader DR. Philadelphia: W.B. Saunders Co. 181.

Wright K. 1999. Fluid Therapy for Reptiles. In: Proceedings of the North American Veterinary Conference. Eastern States Vet Assn. 817.

Zug GR, et al. 2001. Herpetology: An Introductory Biology of Amphibians and Reptiles. 2nd ed., New York: Academic Press. 49–57, 173.

CHAPTER EIGHT

Chelonians

Samuel Rivera

INTRODUCTION

Turtles belong in the class Reptilia, which is divided into four orders, Chelonia (all turtles), Crocodylia (crocodilians), Squamata (snakes and lizards), and Rhynchocephalia (tuatara). There are approximately 270 species in the order Chelonia. This order contains a primitive group of animals that evolved into a shelled form millions of years ago and is considered the most primitive group of living reptiles. Chelonians include turtles, tortoises, and terrapins. The terms "turtle," "tortoise," and "terrapin" are sometimes confusing because they have different meanings in different parts of the world. In the United States, tortoise refers to terrestrial chelonians; turtles often refer to aquatic or semiaquatic chelonians with the exception of the box turtle, which is terrestrial; and terrapins are semi-aquatic, hard-shelled chelonians. Because of the confusion in terminology, chelonians are often listed by their binomial scientific name, which is uniform around the world.

Hundreds of species of chelonians are kept in captivity (Color Plates 8.1, 8.2, 8.3). Unfortunately, many of the diseases seen in captive chelonians are related to improper husbandry and/or inadequate diet. Accurate identification of chelonian species aids in the evaluation of husbandry and nutritional management. The goal of this chapter is to provide a basic understanding of chelonian husbandry, nutrition, biology,

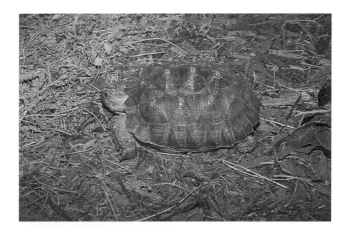

Plate 8.2. Sulcata tortoise. (See also color plates)

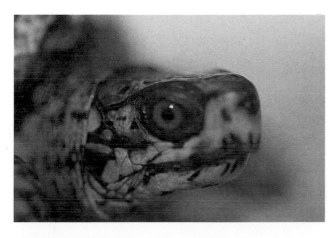

Plate 8.1. Male eastern box turtle showing red eye. (See also color plates)

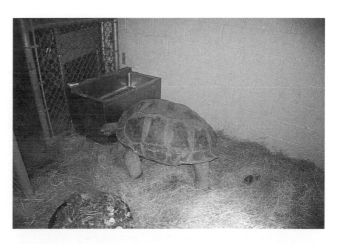

Plate 8.3. Aldabra tortoise. (See also color plates)

167

basic clinical techniques, and common health problems.

ANATOMY AND PHYSIOLOGY

Musculoskeletal System

In this section, the North American eastern box turtle (*Terrapene carolina carolina*) will be described. The most remarkable feature of turtles is their shell, which is divided in two parts. The dorsal part is the carapace and the ventral part is the plastron. The carapace normally consists of approximately fifty bones. The nuchal bone is the most cranial along the dorsal midline. It is followed by seven neural, one suprapygal, and a pygal bone, consecutively. The neural bones are attached to the vertebrae. The costal bones are located on either side of the neural bones. The peripheral bones are located on the lateral aspect of the costal bones and extend from the nuchal to the pygal bones on both sides of the carapace (Figure 8.1).

The plastron consists of nine bones. The cranial part of the plastron is comprised of the entoplastral bone, which is surrounded by the epiplastral bones cranially and two hypoplastral bones caudally. The hypoplastral bones are followed caudally by a second pair of hypoplastral bones and a pair of xiphiplastral bones, consecutively. The bones of a turtle shell articulate with each other by a suture. Box turtles have a movable hinge located transversely between the two pairs of hypoplastral bones.

The bones of the shell are covered with structures made of keratinized epithelium called scutes. The most cranial scute along the dorsal midline is the cervical scute, which is followed caudally by five vertebral scutes. The scutes adjacent to the vertebrals are the pleurals. The scutes outlining the periphery of the plastron are the peripherals. The plastron has six pairs of scutes. The cranial pair is the gular, followed by the humeral, pectoral, abdominal, femoral, and anal scutes, consecutively. The movable hinge is located between the pectoral and abdominal scutes. This hinge allows the plastron to be folded up to enclose the head and forelimbs within the shell. The pelvic and pectoral girdles are contained within the rib cage that is fused to the carapace.

The bones of the limbs of most chelonians are similar to those of other vertebrates.

Respiratory System

Turtles breathe through a pair of nostrils located at the dorsocranial aspect of the premaxilla. The glottis is located at the base of the tongue. The trachea is relatively short and bifurcates into two mainstream bronchi that open into the dorsal aspect of the paired lungs. The lungs are large, compartmentalized structures with a reticular surface containing bands of smooth muscle and connective tissue. The lungs attach dorsally to the ventral aspect of the carapace and ventrally to a membrane that is attached to the stomach, liver, and intestinal tract. Turtles do not have a diaphragm. Respiration is achieved by the contraction of the proximal muscle mass of the pectoral and pelvic limbs (Wood and Lenfant 1976). Aquatic turtles can exchange oxygen through the mucosal surface of the oral cavity and cloaca. Soft-shelled turtles can exchange oxygen through their skin (Girgis 1961).

Gastrointestinal System

The tongue of turtles is large and unable to distend from the oral cavity. They have salivary glands that produce mucus but not digestive enzymes. The esophagus courses along the neck. The stomach lies on the left cranioventral side of the coelomic cavity and has a gastroesophageal and a gastroduodenal valve. The small intestine is relatively short. The pancreas is pale pink and can be located near the spleen or in the mesentery along the duodenum. The liver is large, saddle-shaped, and located ventrally under the lungs. The liver has two lobes and it envelops the gall bladder. It also has indentations for the heart and stomach. The small intestine joins the large intestine at the ileocolic valve. The cecum is not well developed. The large intestine is the primary site of microbial fermentation in herbivorous turtles. The digestive tract empties into the cloaca (Figure 8.2).

Genitourinary System

The paired kidneys are located on the ventrocaudal aspect of the carapace, cranial to the acetabulum. The

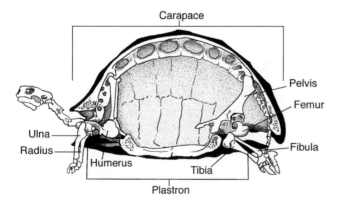

Carapace

Pelvis

Femur

Ulna

Radius

Humerus

Tibia

Fibula

Plastron

Figure 8.1. Skeletal anatomy. (Drawing by Scott Stark.)

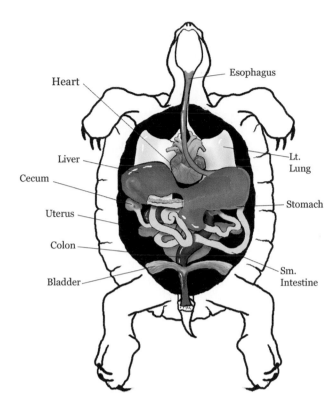

Figure 8.2. *Visceral anatomy. (Drawing by Scott Stark.)*

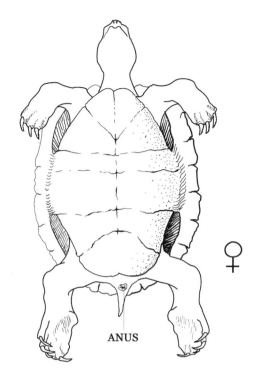

Figure 8.3. *Female reproductive anatomy. (Drawing by Scott Stark.)*

paired gonads are located cranial to the kidneys. The urogenital ducts empty into the neck of the urinary bladder, which is bilobed with a thin membranous wall. Male turtles have a single, large, dark-colored penis. It is located in the floor of the cloaca and it is not used for urination.

Many turtles are sexually dimorphic. The male tortoise has a concave plastron. The males of aquatic turtle species have long nails on their front feet. Generally, the tail is relatively larger in males than in females (Figures 8.3, 8.4).

Circulatory System

Chelonians have a three-chambered heart consisting of two atria and one ventricle. Like other reptiles, turtles have a renoportal circulation system. Its function is to provide an alternate blood supply to the renal tubular cells, and prevent ischemic necrosis when the arterial blood supply to the glomerulus is compromised (Holz 1999).

HUSBANDRY AND NUTRITION

Hundreds of species of turtles are seen in the pet trade, and it is beyond the scope of this chapter to cover turtles by species. A brief overview on the husbandry of aquatic and terrestrial turtles will be discussed. The general public often seeks advice from veterinarians and their support staff about the care and feeding of their newly purchased turtle. It is essential to have a basic understanding of the husbandry and feeding practices of chelonians. Whenever possible, the turtle should be identified so accurate information on its husbandry and eating habits can be obtained.

Aquatic Turtles

Aquatic turtles are one of the most labor intensive reptiles to maintain. Inadequate husbandry often results in health problems. The housing requirements depend on the size and the number of turtles kept. As a rule of thumb, the combined surface area of all the turtles' carapaces should not exceed 25% of the tank's floor surface area (Anonymous 1990). The water should be as deep as the width of the turtle's shell, so that if overturned it will be able to right itself. The simpler the setup, the easier to clean, and clean water is essential to the health of turtles. The best way to keep the water clean is by doing full water changes. The larger the volume, the less the frequency of water changes. The number of animals, the feeding frequency, and the type of food offered also determine

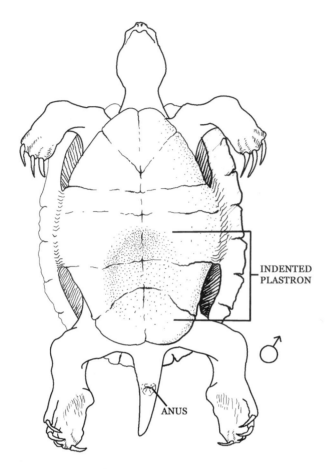

Figure 8.4. Male reproductive anatomy. (Drawing by Scott Stark.)

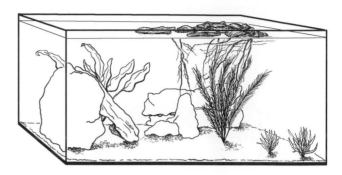

Figure 8.5. Aquatic habitat. (Drawing by Scott Stark.)

the frequency of cleaning. Avoid drastic temperature changes when replacing the water because this can be detrimental to the turtle's health. A filtration system minimizes but does not eliminate the need for complete water changes (Figure 8.5).

Adequate environmental and water temperature are important for good health. Turtles are ectothermic: they rely on the environmental temperature to regulate their body temperature. Turtles have a preferred optimal temperature zone (POTZ), which is the temperature at which they are the most comfortable. The POTZ also allows for normal physiologic functions to occur, such as digestion and fighting disease. Most aquatic turtles have a preferred optimum water temperature of 24°C to 29°C (75°F to 82°F). A dry area should be available so the turtle can dry off and bask, a process by which turtles can regulate their body temperature. An incandescent 50- to 150-watt light bulb with a reflector directed toward the basking area creates a hot spot for basking. Place the basking light approximately twelve to eighteen inches away from the basking area.

An adequate diet is essential for good health. Aquatic turtles are omnivorous with a few exceptions. Younger, rapidly growing animals tend to eat a larger percentage of meat but switch to eating more vegetable matter as they get older (Frye 1991). A varied diet is the key to a healthy turtle. Too much of one food item can often lead to nutritional imbalances. Fish (goldfish, guppies, and bait minnows) is accepted by many turtles. Chopped, skinned adult mice are a good source of vitamins and minerals. Earthworms and a variety of insects can also be fed. Many adult turtles can be fed dark green leafy vegetables and a small amount of fruits. Most pet turtle owners will a commercial pelleted diet. Turtle owners who feed strictly pelleted food should always be encouraged to supplement the diet with other food items to provide the most balanced nutrition possible. Adult turtles can be fed two to three times per week, and young turtles should be fed daily or every other day. Aquatic turtles eat in the water and can be quite messy. Some turtles can be trained to eat in a separate container, which minimizes but does not eliminate the need for frequent water changes.

Some species of chelonians spend the majority of their time in the water but some time on land. The semiaquatic environment, a variation of the aquatic one, is appropriate for these chelonians. This setup involves all the same features of an aquatic setup but includes a land portion for basking (Figure 8.6).

Terrestrial Turtles

Land turtles can be kept in a variety of enclosures, depending on the size and number of animals kept. Where weather permits, tortoises should be kept outside, which allows the animals plenty of room to exercise and graze. Healthy tortoises can be placed outdoors when the temperature is above 18°C (65°F) and the midday temperature reaches 24°C (75°F) or above (Boyer and Boyer 1996). The outdoor enclosure

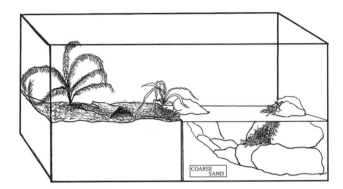

Figure 8.6. Semiaquatic habitat. (Drawing by Scott Stark.)

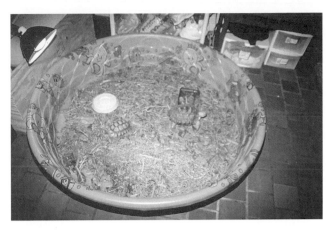

Figure 8.7. Setup for a small tortoise. (Photo courtesy of Ryan Cheek.)

should have a hiding place and a shaded area. The sides of the enclosure should be made of wood or any solid material that can provide a visual barrier. Wire fencing is not recommended because tortoises can injure themselves while trying to climb or push through the fence. The walls should be at least three times the height of the largest tortoise. Some tortoise species like to dig; therefore, wire can be buried around the perimeter, at least ten to twelve inches, to prevent escape.

Tortoises can be kept indoors. Generally they require more space than most reptiles of similar size. As a general rule, the combined size of all the tortoises' carapaces should not exceed 25% of the enclosure's floor (Anonymous 1990). Aquariums, or a wide variety of plastic containers, can be used for small tortoises. Larger species can be kept in enclosures made of wood or cement. A garage or spare room can serve as a holding area for tortoises.

The room temperature should be between 24°C and 32°C (75°F and 90°F). A thermal gradient between 75°F and 90°F is ideal to allow for thermoregulation. This gradient can be created by placing a basking light at one end of the enclosure. The basking light should be placed eighteen to twenty-four inches away from the animals. At night, supplemental heat can be provided with heating pads placed under the enclosure, ceramic heaters with a reflector, or night heat lights. Acceptable substrates include cyprus mulch, large conifer bark nuggets, alfalfa pellets, newspaper, and indoor-outdoor carpeting, among others. Inappropriate substrates include sand, fine gravel, cat litter, crushed corncob, or walnut shells because these can lead to gastrointestinal impactions. Pine and cedar shavings are not recommended because of the presence of oils that can adversely affect the respiratory tract. The cage should be cleaned several times per week. The substrate can be changed as needed.

If the tortoises are kept indoors all year, a source of UV light must be provided. There is a wide variety of UV lights and the manufacturer's instructions must be followed closely. Two points to keep in mind are that most UV bulbs must be kept at a minimum distance from the animals to be effective, and the lifespan of the bulbs is limited and they must be replaced on a regular basis. Natural light is ideal and must be provided whenever possible (Figure 8.7).

Tortoises are mainly herbivores. In the wild, they eat a variety of leaves, stems, flowers, and fruits; in addition, some eat snails, earthworms, and other invertebrates. The ideal diet should be made of 85% vegetables (dark leafy greens, grasses), 10% fruits, and 5% high-protein foods (Boyer and Boyer 1994). The high-protein foods can be provided once or twice weekly. Alternatively, a commercially made pelleted diet can be provided and supplemented with high-fiber food items. Adult animals can be fed two to three times per week, whereas juveniles can be fed daily or every other day.

COMMON DISEASES

Metabolic Bone Disease
This disease is caused by an improper calcium and phosphorus ratio in the diet and/or a vitamin D_3 deficiency. Turtles fed liver, heart, or muscle meat often develop metabolic bone disease. The resulting calcium deficiency often leads to a depletion of calcium from bone, resulting in fibrous osteodystrophy. Clinical signs include anorexia, soft and/or deformed shell, and abnormal scute growth. The treatment involves diet correction and proper vitamin D_3 supplementation.

Vitamin A Deficiency

This is a common presentation in aquatic and terrestrial turtles. It is caused by feeding a diet deficient in vitamin A. The clinical signs include conjunctivitis, blepharitis, swollen eyelids, nasal discharge, dyspnea, and ear abscesses. The condition is treated with parenteral vitamin A and diet correction.

Vitamin A Toxicity

This can be caused by excessive supplementation or administration of parenteral vitamin A. The clinical signs include dry, flaky skin, or sloughing of the skin with secondary bacterial infection. Treatment requires systemic antibiotics if secondary bacterial infection is present, and discontinuation of parenteral vitamin A or any source of over supplementation.

Diseases of the Shell

"Shell rot" is a term used to describe infections of the shell involving loss of scutes. The terms "wet" and "dry" shell rot are used to describe the appearance of the lesions. The wet form is usually associated with a hemorrhagic discharge between the scutes and it is often associated with bacterial infections. The dry form has a dry appearance and is often associated with fungal or bacterial infections. In some mild cases of shell rot, the lesions can be treated topically. Aquatic turtles need to be kept dry for thirty to sixty minutes after topical treatment. Septicemic cutaneous ulcerative disease (SCUD) is a common disease seen in aquatic turtles. The clinical signs include cutaneous ulcerations, anorexia, and lethargy. Treatment of any shell lesion involves debridement and topical antimicrobial treatment. In some cases, systemic antibiotics may be indicated.

Traumatic injuries to the shell are relatively common, especially in wild chelonia. In many cases, radiographs can help determine the extent of the damage. The prognosis is poor if the spinal cord is damaged. Once the animal is relatively stable, the wounds must be cleaned, debrided, and flushed with sterile saline and diluted disinfectant (i.e. chlorhexidine). Be careful when cleaning full-thickness fractures with exposed coelomic cavity. Turtles with full-thickness fractures or severe soft-tissue trauma need systemic antibiotic treatment (Figure 8.8).

Repair of Shell

Superficial cracks on the shell can be repaired using sterile fiberglass cloth impregnated with polymerizing epoxy resin. Contact with the soft tissue should be avoided. Dental acrylic can also be used. Full-thickness fractures where the coelomic cavity has been exposed require surgical repair. In addition to shell repair, these animals require fluid and nutritional support and antibiotic therapy. They often have a prolonged recovery and adequate treatment is needed until the turtle is eating on its own and is free of infection.

Overgrown Beak

Some turtles develop an overgrown beak in captivity. This has been associated with an inadequate diet. The overgrown beak needs to be trimmed on a regular basis. For the most part this can be done without sedation. A Dremel tool works well (Figures 8.9, 8.10).

Respiratory Disease

Respiratory disease is one of the most common presentations in clinical practice. Turtles do not have a

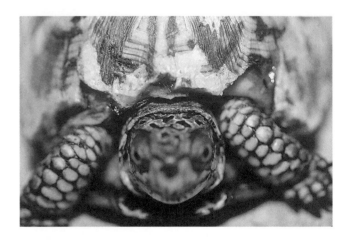

Figure 8.8. Traumatic injury to the shell. (Photo courtesy of Ryan Cheek.)

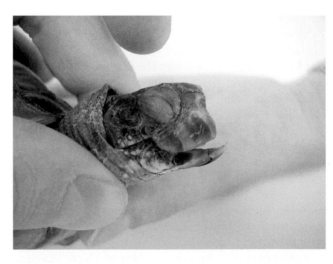

Figure 8.9. Overgrown beak. (Photo courtesy of Dr. Stephen J. Hernandez-Divers, University of Georgia.)

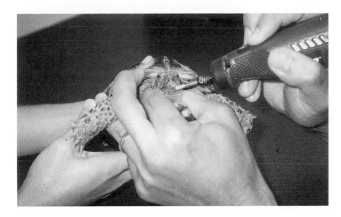

Figure 8.10. Trimming an overgrown beak with a Dremel tool. (Photo courtesy of Stephen J. Hernandez-Divers, University of Georgia.)

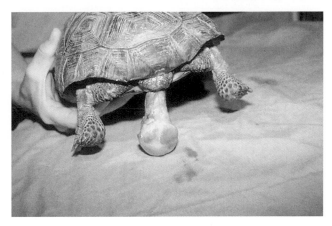

Figure 8.11. Penile prolapse. (Photo courtesy of Zoo Atlanta.)

diaphragm and as a result they cannot clear discharge in their lungs by coughing. Some predisposing factors to respiratory disease include improper diet, inadequate temperature and humidity, unhygienic conditions, and/or inappropriate substrate. Clinical signs of respiratory disease include a mucopurulent nasal discharge, ocular discharge, dyspnea, open-mouth breathing, anorexia, weight loss, and lethargy. Aquatic turtles may show inability to swim normally as they lose control of buoyancy. Pneumonia can be caused by bacteria, viruses, mycoplasma, and certain parasites. The diagnosis is based on the clinical signs, radiographs, transtracheal wash, and culture and sensitivity results. Treatment includes bactericidal antibiotics, nebulization, warmth, fluid therapy, and nutritional support.

Gout

Gout is a condition that involves the deposition of uric acid in the visceral organs and/or joints. It can be caused by kidney disease, dehydration, and diets high in protein. Clinical signs include lethargy, anorexia, lameness, and swollen joints. The diagnosis can be made by measuring serum/plasma uric acid levels, radiographs, and cytological evaluation of the material in the affected joints. The treatment involves the correction of the primary problem, but it is often unrewarding.

Gastrointestinal Tract Disease

A wide range of diseases affects the gastrointestinal tract of chelonians. Stomatitis, parasites, foreign bodies, bacteria and fungal enteritis, and amoebic enterohepatitis are some of the most common conditions encountered in private practice. The clinical

signs of gastrointestinal disease include anorexia, vomiting, weight loss, lethargy, dehydration, and abnormal stools. The diagnosis is based on a complete blood count, plasma biochemistries, fecal examinations, radiographs, endoscopy, and in some cases ultrasonography. The treatment is based on the disease present. Fluids and nutritional support are an important part of the therapy.

Reproductive Disorders

Dystocia is one of the most common reproductive problems seen in chelonians. The clinical signs include anorexia, lethargy, straining, and sometimes bloody discharge from the cloaca. The diagnosis of dystocia is based on radiographs. The predisposing factors include poor environmental conditions, metabolic disease, and improper husbandry.

Cloacal prolapse in females during parturition and penile prolapse in males during copulation are common presentations in chelonians. This can be caused by trauma, infection, or cloacal impaction. Severe cases of penile prolapse often require amputation (Figures 8.11, 8.12).

Aural Abscesses

While relatively common to see, the pathogenesis of aural abscesses isn't completely known. Improper husbandry and malnutrition may be predisposing factors. Treatment involves surgical intervention. The tympanic membrane is incised and exudate removed, followed by debridement and lavage of the wound. An antibiotic ointment may then be applied to the wound. The wound is left open and lavaged daily, followed by ointment application until the wound heals by second intention (Figure 8.13) (Murray 1996).

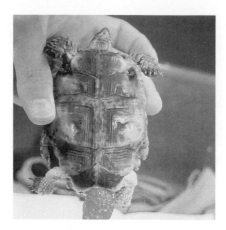

Figure 8.12. Cloacal prolapse. (Photo courtesy of Zoo Atlanta.)

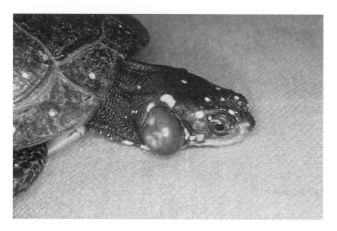

Figure 8.13. Aural abscess. (Photo courtesy of Dr. Stephen J. Hernandez-Divers, University of Georgia.)

ZOONOSES

The greater number of zoonotic diseases associated with keeping turtles involve bacterial pathogens. The most widely recognized disease is salmonellosis. Children, immunosuppressed individuals, and the elderly are at greater risk of contracting salmonellosis. In the 1960s and 1970s, a large number of human cases of salmonellosis were linked to pet turtles as the source of infection. In 1975, laws were enacted banning the sale of baby turtles with a carapace length of 4 inches or less. In 1999, the Centers for Disease Control estimated that of the millions of cases of human salmonellosis reported between 1996 and 1998, only 7% per year was associated with reptile or amphibian contact (CDC 1999). The vast majority of human salmonellosis (approximately 80%) cases was associated with eating contaminated food.

The genus Salmonella contains many species with thousands of different serotypes. Many of theses serotypes have been isolated from healthy turtles and have been associated with human salmonellosis. The symptoms in humans include abdominal pain, diarrhea, nausea, vomiting, and fever. Owners should be made aware of the potential health hazard when keeping turtles as pets.

Proper sanitation is essential to decrease the risk of exposure. There is no effective or practical way to eliminate the bacteria from the intestinal flora of positive animals. The bacterial burden in the environment greatly increases when the feces are allowed to build up in the enclosure. This causes contamination of the turtle's environment and body surface, increasing the risk of transmission to humans, which is why it is so important to practice strict hygiene when keeping turtles. By cleaning frequently, the bacterial contamination in the enclosure will be greatly reduced. Perhaps the decline in percentage of human cases of salmonellosis associated with pet turtles has been due to the increased awareness and practice of adequate hygiene.

Aeromonas, *Campylobacter*, and *Pseudomonas* of reptile origin have been associated with illness in humans. Reptiles can also be affected by several species of *Mycobacterium* that are known to cause disease in humans. *Mycobacterium* can cause a variety of lesions in reptiles. The route of transmission for humans is through direct contact or inhalation of contaminated particles.

The hallmark of disease prevention and decreased risk of exposure to potential zoonoses is adequate hygiene. This goes for both the pet owner and the health care provider. When sick turtles are hospitalized, it is imperative that they be kept in a clean environment and handled carefully to prevent contamination of the hospital environment.

OBTAINING A HISTORY AND PERFORMING A PHYSICAL EXAMINATION

A thorough history is one of the most important aspects of the clinical evaluation. Improper diet, enclosure, temperature, and humidity are often major contributors to illness. Always ask about previous illness. Any change in appetite, behavior, weight, and defecation (consistency and frequency) should be recorded. The origin of the animal (wild-caught versus captive-bred, bought from a pet store versus a private breeder) must be ascertained. Also inquire about other animals in the collection and whether there are other types of turtles and/or other reptiles in the household. Were any animals bought recently? Was the animal quarantined? All these questions will help to formulate a picture of the animal's husbandry and potential exposure to pathogens.

A visual exam should be part of an initial evaluation. Assess motor function if the animal is willing to walk. Check the plastron and carapace for any evidence of trauma or infection. Look at the skin of the legs and nails. Evaluate the head, eyes, nares, oral cavity, and tympanic membrane. Note any discharge, redness, or swelling. The lungs of chelonians can be auscultated by placing a wet hand towel between the carapace and the stethoscope to enhance the surface contact.

RESTRAINT

The neck of most turtles has an S-shaped curve that allows the animal to withdraw the head within the shell. In most turtles the head can be extended by applying gentle pressure with the thumb and index finger behind the mandibles. In many cases the head can be grabbed by reaching from underneath. Turtles quickly withdraw the head when approached from the top. Once you have a hold behind the temporomandibular joints, apply gentle traction to overcome the turtle's resistance; be careful not to be too forceful. It is important to avoid dorsoventral pressure with your fingers because this can cause damage to the soft tissue of the neck and trachea. This technique is limited by the size, physical condition, and disposition of the turtle.

The head of box turtles can be a little harder to exteriorize because a box turtle can move the cranial part of the plastron upward, making the shell an almost impenetrable fort. In this case a tongue depressor or smooth stainless steel speculum can be used to pry the shell open. Insert your tool between the carapace and plastron and apply gentle pressure downward. Once exposed, a limb can be grabbed and an attempt made to restrain the head as described above.

A more gentle approach is to place the turtle in a small amount of warm water. Most turtles will attempt to get out of the water and when they do, an attempt can be made to restrain a limb or the head. If the first attempt to restrain the turtle fails, the animal should be placed in its holding container and tried later. Patience is your best ally.

In aquatic species, with long nails, a towel can be used to wrap the animal and hold the legs within the

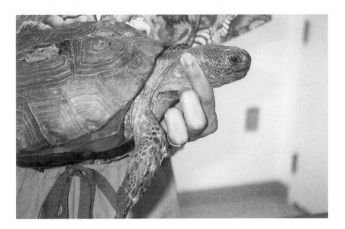

Figure 8.14. Proper restraint. (Photo courtesy of Dr. Sam Rivera.)

shell. Nails can inflict painful scratches to the handler. The towel can also be used to keep the head inside the shell in aggressive species. Remember that turtles, like other animals, stress easily when handled excessively (Figure 8.14).

RADIOLOGY

Radiographs are an important diagnostic tool in the assessment of the musculoskeletal, respiratory, gastrointestinal, and reproductive systems. The dorsoventral (DV), lateral, and anterior-posterior views are recommended. The DV radiograph can be easily taken by placing the turtle on the table. Most often it will stay still long enough to take the radiograph. For the lateral and anterior-posterior views, a horizontal beam is desired. Elevate the turtle by using a round container that fits under the plastron. Make sure the feet do not come in contact with the container. It is desirable to keep the patient in the sternal position. Tilting the turtle on its side is not recommended because this often causes distortion of the lungs and visceral and reproductive organs (Figure 8.15).

ANESTHESIA

The overall health of the patient should be established to assess the anesthetic risk. Turtles should be well hydrated prior to anesthesia. The environmental temperature is also important. When anesthetized, turtles should be kept at their POTZ. Keeping them slightly warmer during recovery is recommended.

There are several techniques for anesthetizing chelonians. The preferred method is the use of parenteral

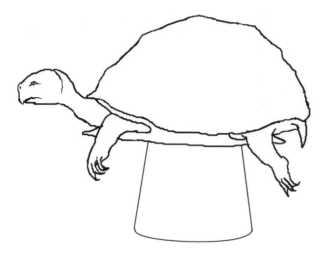

Figure 8.15. Restraint for radiographs. (Drawing by Scott Stark.)

drugs. Chelonians can be anesthetized using inhalation agents via mask or chamber induction but they can hold their breath for a long time, making this technique time-consuming. If gas induction is used, the uptake of the anesthetic agent can be increased by manipulating the limbs in and out. This enhances ventilation of the lungs. The IM and IV routes are frequently used for the administration of induction agents.

Once the turtle is anesthetized it can be maintained using isoflurane or sevoflurane. The animal can be intubated using a proper size endotracheal tube. Alternatively, small red rubber catheters can be modified to serve as endotracheal tubes. In small patients, large-bore intravenous catheters can be used. The laryngeal opening is located near the based of the tongue. A cotton tip applicator can be used to gently move the tongue cranially while inserting the endotracheal tube. It is recommended to use a speculum to keep the mouth open and prevent the animal from biting the endotracheal tube. Keep in mind that large chelonians have a strong jaw tone even if slightly sedated and can cause serious damage to fingers.

Monitoring anesthesia in chelonians can prove challenging. An EKG is ideal to monitor the cardiac function. An ultrasonic Doppler can be used to monitor the peripheral pulse in the limbs. The withdrawal and palpebral reflexes are sometimes helpful but not always reliable. A pulse oximeter with a cloacal probe can often be used to monitor oxygen saturation. It is recommended to use intermittent partial pressure ventilation in chelonians (four to eight breaths per minute), which helps ventilate the lungs and keeps an adequate flow of oxygen and anesthetic agent in the lungs.

PARASITOLOGY

Turtles can be affected by a wide range of parasites. It is important to collect a fresh fecal sample. Dry feces are not recommended for use because many protozoan organisms die as the feces dry. Advise the client to collect the feces at home, place the sample in multiple sealable plastic bags, and keep it refrigerated. Reiterate to the client the dangers of keeping reptile feces where food for human consumption is kept. If the sample is to be kept refrigerated, extreme hygiene is important to prevent cross contamination. The sample can be refrigerated overnight, but longer refrigeration is not recommended. The fecal exams must be done using fecal material and not urates. If a fresh sample is not available, a cloacal wash (see below) can be done to obtain a sample.

Direct fecal exam: Using a small wooden stick, place a small amount of feces on a microscope slide. Place a cover slip on top and examine immediately. The longer the sample sits the more likely motile protozoans will die. Do not use a cotton tip applicator because the cotton can absorb a substantial amount of the sample. Certain cysts can be difficult to identify. The sample can be stained by adding one drop of Lugol's solution. It is ideal to prepare two direct smears, one stained and one unstained. The Lugol's solution kills motile protozoans. Some of the protozoans commonly encountered are *Hexamita*, *Balantidium*, *Nyctotherus*, and coccidia.

Flotation: The flotation technique is done in the same manner as that for small animals. Use as much fecal sample as possible to increase the chances of finding parasite ova.

Cloacal wash: Using a soft rubber catheter, instill a small amount of saline solution in the cloaca. Collect the fluid for examination. This sample can be used for direct exam and flotation.

Turtles can be subclinical carriers of pathogenic amoeba species. *Entamoeba invadens* is an example of an amoeba that causes low morbidity in turtles but can cause severe illness and death in snakes and lizards. Nematodes, trematodes, and cestodes are common in turtles, particularly wild-caught animals. It is important to keep in mind that chelonians are also affected by ectoparasites. Ticks, leeches, and cuterebra larvae can be found in turtles.

EMERGENCY AND CRITICAL CARE

The most common emergency seen in private practice is trauma. Wild turtles hit by cars are unfortunately seen too often. The initial stabilization of the patient requires proper assessment of the injuries, antimicrobial therapy, fluid support, and adequate environmental temperature. When a turtle with severe trauma is presented, the shell as well as the limbs, head, and neck must be evaluated for the presence of blood. Once the wounds are identified, they must be cleaned thoroughly using sterile saline and a disinfectant. Antibiotics may be required to avoid infection of the wounds, which can lead to fatal septicemia. Turtles with massive trauma can become dehydrated quickly. Adequate fluid support is essential for a full recovery. Fluids can be given subcutaneously or in the intracoelomic cavity. Once the patient is stabilized, it should be kept at its preferred optimal temperature zone. This allows for the immune system and other physiologic functions needed for healing to work efficiently. It is also important to provide nutritional support to the patient as soon as possible. Wild chelonians will not eat on their own initially, and need to be force-fed. Adequate nutrition is important for a full recovery. Chelonians with severe trauma take a long time to heal, but if they are handled properly from the time of initial presentation the recovery time can be reduced significantly.

CLINICAL TECHNIQUES

Blood Collection

The sites for blood collection in chelonians are the jugular, brachial, subcarapacial, tail (ventral and dorsal), and femoral veins, as well as the occipital sinus and heart. Chelonians can prove challenging for blood collection. It is always a good idea to be familiar with multiple venipuncture sites. The supplies needed depend on the size of the animal. Prior to blood collection, slides, hematocrit tubes, small-volume (0.5 ml) heparinized tubes, alcohol swabs, needles (22- to 27-gauge), and syringes (0.5- to 3-ml) should be prepared. In patients smaller than 300 g, use a 25- to 27-gauge needle in a 0.5- to 1-cc syringe. In patients greater than 300 g, a 22-gauge needle in a 3-cc syringe can be used. Larger needles (20 g) can be used in turtles weighing more than 5 kg (Figure 8.16).

Jugular Vein

The jugular vein is relatively superficial and located dorsally on the neck. Some turtles may need sedation for jugular venipuncture. In most turtles blood can be collected from this location as long as the head can be exteriorized. The neck should be held in the extended position. In some patients the vein can be visualized by applying digital pressure at the base of the neck; however, this is not always the case. Once the vein is located, the needle should be inserted at a 30-degree angle and negative pressure applied as the needle is advanced. The syringe will fill with blood as soon as the vein is entered. In some cases, the flow is slow. Once blood fills the hub of the needle, stop advancing and release suction on the plunger. Sometimes the vein will collapse. Reapply gentle suction until the desired amount of blood is obtained.

Brachial Vein

The animal should be placed in sternal recumbency. Either forelimb should then be gently pulled to expose the brachial-antibrachial joint. The brachial vein is located deep to the triceps tendon. This tendon can be palpated on the caudal aspect of the extended leg. The needle should be inserted perpendicular to the skin, in the groove located ventral to the distal end of the tendon. Once the skin is entered, negative pressure should be applied and the needle advanced. Redirecting the needle may be necessary to find the vein. Once the vein is entered, the vein blood will flow into the syringe.

Subcarapacial Vein

This vessel is located on the ventral aspect of the carapace along the dorsal midline. The animal should be restrained in sternal recumbency with the front end elevated at a 45-degree angle. With one hand, the head should be held inside the carapace. With the index finger of the other hand, the first vertebrae that is fused to the carapace along the dorsal midline should be palpated. The needle is inserted in the midline position and slowly directed to the space between the carapace and the vertebrae. Negative pressure should be applied as the needle is advanced. Blood will fill the syringe as the vein is entered.

Ventral Tail Vein

The turtle is restrained vertically with the plastron facing the phlebotomist or in dorsal recumbency. Keep in mind that placing the animal in dorsal recumbency is stressful; therefore, this should be done for the shortest amount of time possible. The tail should be extended and held as straight as possible. The needle should then be inserted in the ventral midline, distal to the vent. Keep in mind that the further distal one goes, the smaller the diameter of the vein. The needle is then inserted at a 60-degree angle with the hub directed cranially. The needle should be advanced until the vertebral body is hit. Apply negative pressure and gently move the needle out (1 to 2 mm) until blood flows. This site is generally not

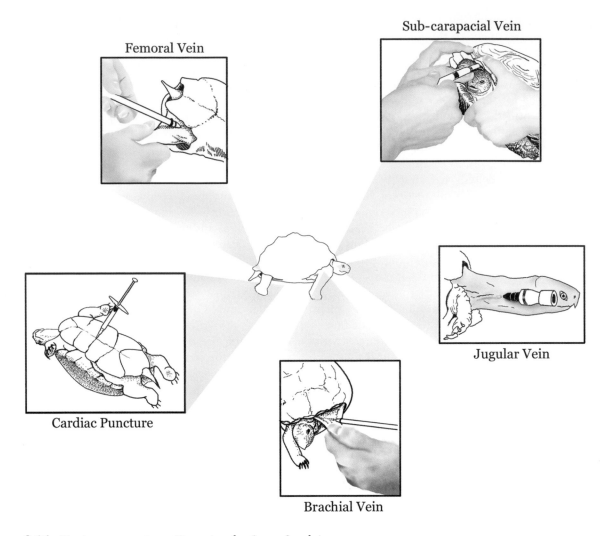

Femoral Vein

Sub-carapacial Vein

Cardiac Puncture

Jugular Vein

Brachial Vein

Figure 8.16. Venipuncture sites. (Drawing by Scott Stark.)

productive because only a small volume can be obtained. Larger turtles in good physical condition can hold the tail close to the body, making the tail very difficult to exteriorize.

Dorsal Tail Vein

The animal should be restrained in sternal recumbency. The tail should be held as straight as possible and the needle inserted in the dorsal tail midline. Insert the needle, at a 30- to 45-degree angle, proximally near the junction between the tail and the caudal margin of the carapace. The needle is then advanced until the vertebral bodies are encountered. Negative pressure should be applied and the needle moved gently out (1 to 2 mm) until blood flows. If the tail cannot be exteriorized, the needle should be inserted in the proximal aspect of the tail midline and the steps followed as described above.

Femoral Vein

The turtle should be restrained vertically with the plastron facing the phlebotomist or in dorsal recumbency. Keep in mind that placing the animal in dorsal recumbency is stressful; therefore, this should be done for the shortest amount of time possible. The femoral vein courses through the femoral triangle (the space through which the femoral vessels run to and from the hindlimb), which is located at the most proximal end of the medial aspect of the hindlimb. With one hand, the hind leg should be extended, and the other hand should be used to withdraw the blood sample. This, like many of the other techniques, is a blind stick. The needle should be inserted at a 45-degree angle and suction applied as the needle is advanced. Blood will fill the syringe as the vein is entered. Repositioning the needle should be minimized because nerves and other vessels located in this area can be damaged.

Occipital Venous Sinus

The animal should be restrained in sternal recumbency and the head extended. The caudal aspect of the skull is then palpated. The sinus is located in the dorsal midline near the cranial cervical region. The needle should be inserted at a 60-degree angle. Negative pressure should be applied once the skin is penetrated as the needle is advanced. The syringe will fill with blood as the sinus is entered. Sometimes the needle can be repositioned to either side of the midline as the sinus can extend laterally. Be careful not to go too deep.

Heart

This technique is relatively invasive because it requires drilling a hole through the plastron. A sterile drill or intramedullary pin can be used to perforate the plastron. The site of entry is where the ventral midline suture intersects the caudal suture of the pectoral scutes. The needle is then inserted perpendicularly as suction is applied. The correct location of the needle can sometimes be corroborated by the slight movement of the syringe caused by the heartbeat. Once blood is collected, the hole must be repaired using dental acrylic or epoxy resin. This is the author's least desirable site for blood collection and it is used rarely.

ADMINISTRATION OF MEDICATIONS

Routes of Administration

Intramuscular Route: Antimicrobial agents and certain anesthesia induction agents are often given intramuscularly. Intramuscular injections are given in the muscle mass of the front legs. Chelonians have a renoportal circulation system. It is believed that medications injected in the caudal half of the body are filtered by the kidneys before entering the general circulation. However, this concept has been challenged in recent studies (Holz 1999). Until more is known about the role renoportal circulation plays in filtering parenteral drugs, these medications should be given in the front half of the body, particularly drugs with potential nephrotoxic side effects.

Subcutaneous Route: Subcutaneous injections can be given in the inguinal and ventral neck skin folds. Fluid replacement can be given at a rate of 20 ml/kg every twenty-four to forty-eight hours.

Intravenous Route: The jugular vein can be used for the administration of fluids. This and the subcarapacial vein can be used for the administration of intravenous anesthetics.

Intracoelomic Route: The coelomic cavity can be accessed through the prefemoral fossa, the space just cranial to the pelvic limb into which the limb is retracted when the animal feels threatened. The intracoelomic route is most commonly used for the administration of fluids. Restrain the turtle in lateral recumbency; this will cause the viscera and reproductive organs to shift away from the injection site. Insert the needle parallel to the plastron and direct it cranially in the ventral aspect of the fossa. If the needle is directed dorsally, there is a risk of injecting the fluids in the lungs. If the needle is directed medially, the fluids can go in the bladder. If the turtle urinates, the needle may be in the bladder; pull and reposition the needle. When injecting fluids into the coelomic cavity, keep in mind that the needle does not have to be inserted very deep. The fluids can be given at a rate of 20 ml/kg every twenty-four to forty-eight hours.

Oral Route: The supplies needed to administer oral medications or force-feeding are round-tip stainless steel tubes or red rubber catheters, speculums, and syringes of various sizes. Many sick turtles are anorexic. Nutritional support is essential for a full recovery. The most challenging part in many cases is opening the mouth. Some turtles will open their mouths when restrained. Take advantage of this and insert a speculum or feeding tube quickly. If this fails, the mouth must be pried open. The upper beak in turtles hangs slightly over the lower beak. A blunt tool can be inserted under the upper beak and inserted in the mouth. Once in the oral cavity, twist the tool to pry the mouth open. Once the mouth is opened, the feeding tube or speculum can be inserted. The tube feeding volume is 1% to 2% of the body weight every twenty-four to forty-eight hours. Hold the head fully extended; measure the distance from the mouth to the mid plastron. Insert the feeding tube to the desired length and administer the feeding formula.

Intraosseous Route: This route is not frequently used but is available when needed. The two most commonly used sites are the tibia and the plastrocarapace bridge that connects the plastron and carapace on the lateral aspect of the body. An intraosseous needle with a stylet is desirable. A 22- to 20-gauge needle with a 25-gauge needle inside to serve as a stylet can be used, which keeps the primary needle from becoming clogged (Figure 8.17).

Cloacal Route: Fluids and deworming medications can be administered via the cloaca. A lubricated red rubber catheter or ball-tipped stainless steel tube can be placed in the cloaca and the desired medication delivered. It is recommended to hold the turtle at an angle, with the cloaca elevated above the turtle's head to improve the absorption rate (Bonner 2000).

Nebulization: One of the most common problems seen in clinical practice is respiratory disease.

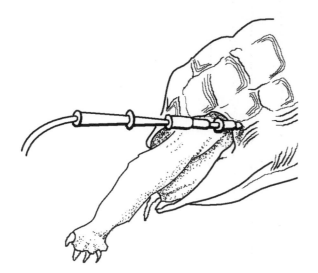

Figure 8.17. Intraosseous catheter. (Drawing by Scott Stark.)

Nebulization is a relatively stress-free method to deliver medications into the respiratory system. Turtles have lower respiratory rates than mammals and birds; therefore, the nebulization time must be extended. In many cases, turtles must be nebulized for an hour or longer to ensure that an adequate amount of medication is administered.

Intravenous Catheter Placement

Jugular catheterization is reserved for patients that are extremely weak and in a very critical condition (Figure 8.18). Patients that are relatively stable make it difficult to maintain and clean the catheter site. The procedure for IV catheter placement in a jugular vein is as follows:

1. Scrub the area of the jugular vein in the anesthetized patient.
2. Make a full-thickness incision on the skin.
3. Identify the jugular vein using blunt dissection.
4. Insert the IV catheter of adequate size, depending on the size of the turtle.
5. Place a butterfly tape over the catheter and cap and suture to the skin.

IV bolus fluids can be given at a rate of 1–2 ml/kg over a fifteen- to thirty-minute period.

EUTHANASIA

In some cases, euthanasia is the most humane course of action. Ill animals with a poor to grave prognosis or

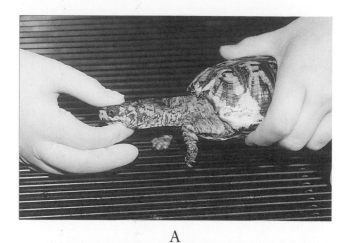

A

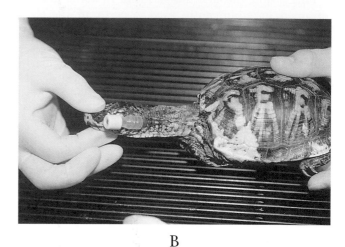

B

Figure 8.18. Jugular catheter placement. (A) Proper restraint for jugular catheterization. (B) Placement of jugular catheter. (Photos courtesy of Ryan Cheek.)

severely injured animals may require humane euthanasia. The hardest part of euthanizing turtles is knowing whether or not they are dead. This can be a tricky question to answer. Some of the signs that help determine if the patient is dead include absence of a heartbeat, no response to pain (i.e. corneal reflex), rigor mortis, cyanotic mucous membranes, and sunken flat eyes. An EKG or ultrasound can be used to assess the heartbeat; however, keep in mind that in turtles the heart can continue to beat several hours after euthanasia.

The author's preferred method of euthanasia in turtles is lethal injection. The euthanasia solution can be given intravenously or intracoelomically. In some cases, it is recommended that the turtle be kept in the clinic overnight to ensure the animal is dead. Several sources have referred to freezing as an alternative method for euthanasia but this is considered inhumane.

REFERENCES

Anonymous. 1990. Guideline for the housing of turtles and tortoises: Minimum standard housing guidelines for pet shops, wholesale animal dealers, and other commercial establishments. New York Turtle and Tortoise Society Newsletter 19(5).

Bonner BB. 2000. Chelonian therapeutics. The Veterinary Clinics of North America, Exotic Animal Practice, edited by Fronefield SA. 3(7): 257–332.

Boyer TH, Boyer DM. 1994. Tortoise care. Bull Assoc Reptil Amphi Vet. 4(1): 16–27.

Boyer TH, Boyer DM. 1996. Turtles, tortoises, and terrapins. In: Reptile Medicine and Surgery, edited by Mader DR. Philadelphia: W.B. Saunders Co.

Centers for Disease Control and Prevention. 1999. Reptile-associated salmonellosis—selected states 1996–1998. MMWR. 48, 1009.

Frye FL. 1991. A practical guide for feeding captive reptiles. Melbourne: Krieger Publishing.

Girgis S. 1961. Aquatic respiration in the common Nile turtle, *Trionyx triunguis*. Comp Biochem Physiol. 3: 206.

Holz PH. 1999. The reptilian renal portal system—a review. Bull Assoc Reptil Amphi Vet. 9(1): 4.

Murray M. 1996. Aural abscesses. In: Reptile Medicine and Surgery, edited by Mader DR. Philadelphia: W.B. Saunders Co.

Wood SC, Lenfant CJM. 1976. Respiration: Mechanics, control, and gas exchange. In: Biology of Reptilians, vol 5, edited by Gans C. San Diego: Academic Press. 225–274.

CHAPTER NINE

Herpetoculture and Reproduction

David Martinez-Jimenez

INTRODUCTION

The reptile pet industry is a growing field with an estimated 13.4 million pet reptiles in more than 4.8 million households in the United States, averaging about 2.8 reptiles per household (APPA 2007/2008). While the number of wild-caught reptile imports has decreased with the establishment of commercial regulations and captive breeding, current reptile imports in the United States are still estimated at about 2 million per year. Captive breeding is therefore a more sustainable and reasonable approach for the pet market.

Proper management and husbandry remain the major obstacles to maintaining a healthy reptile collection. Reptile medicine is still in its infancy. The importance of neonatal care and reptile breeding has a growing significance in the management of these captive reptile collections. Proper captive population management is essential to decrease inbreeding and disease spread, and therefore preserve the health of the collection.

This chapter covers the fundamentals for a healthy reptile collection and the principles behind captive breeding.

CAPTIVE-BRED VERSUS WILD-CAUGHT

Despite the increase in reptile pet ownership, reptile imports remain about the same. This can be explained by the increase of captive-bred reptiles. From 1989 to 1997, 18.3 million reptiles were imported (HSUS 2001). Import of reptiles has seriously harmed many wild populations and, in many cases, continues to occur because captive breeding has not yet been mastered for all species of reptiles, such as chameleons (HSUS 2001) (Table 9.1).

Captive breeding is a more sustainable way of nourishing the growing reptile pet market. Furthermore, it facilitates regulation of the pet market, decreasing the chances of introducing foreign diseases into the environment. For example, the U.S. Department of Agriculture banned the import of some tortoises from Africa because they were carrying ticks, which were vectors of heartwater disease, a highly contagious wasting disease of ruminants (HSUS 2001).

Although reptiles are not domesticated, captive breeding programs promote those individuals that are tame and nonaggressive to reproduce in captivity (high number of offspring and longer reproductive life) and develop resilience to the stress of captivity. Therefore, captive breeding also leads to a type of domestication in itself.

Animal welfare is another important reason for decreasing the import of wild-caught reptiles for pets. Wild-caught reptiles can be captured by means harmful to the animals and environment. They are often kept in substandard conditions without food and water while waiting for transportation, which leads to a high mortality rate. Even with the best care, it is estimated that 90% of all imported reptiles to the United States die within the first year (HSUS 2001).

QUARANTINE

Quarantine is the isolation of animals and people to prevent the spread of infectious diseases. The recommended quarantine period for reptiles is about three months, but up to six months for snakes because of the risk of ophidian paramyxovirus. Quarantine

Table 9.1. Species of reptiles (8,734 species), divided by taxa.

Amphisbaenia (amphisbaenians)	168 species
Sauria (lizards)	5,079 species
Serpentes (snakes)	3,149 species
Chelonia (turtles and tortoises)	313 species
Crocodylia (crocodiles)	23 species
Rhynchocephalia (tuataras)	2 species

should be carried out in a separate room that does not exchange air with other facilities. Individuals in quarantine should be examined at the beginning of the quarantine for evidence of external parasites (e.g. snake mites, *Ophionyssus natricis*) and signs of illness. Body weight, eccdysis (normal skin shedding), behavior, feeding, and urination/defecation should be monitored throughout the quarantine period and recorded appropriately. Accurate record keeping is vital for the assessment of the collection health and disease identification.

Quarantined animals should be handled last, after attending to the animals in the established collection. Cages, furniture, and bowls should be properly identified so they do not leave the quarantine area, and they should not be exchanged among quarantine animals. The quarantine area should have foot baths and foot pump water faucets and soap dispensers to prevent cross contamination. Furthermore, individual cage accessories (bowls, hide boxes, etc.) should be kept to a minimum and should not be cleaned together with other accessories from other cages.

Cages should be maintained in a way to facilitate cleaning and disinfection (e.g. using disposable paper towels as substrate) to minimize the exchange of pathogens between quarantine cages. Commonly used disinfectants include household bleach (sodium hypochlorite) at 1:30 concentration (1 part of bleach per 30 parts of water; in other words, 30 ml/liter of water or 1/2 cup/gallon), 5% ammonia solution (effective against coccidia and *Cryptosporidia*), and quaternary ammonium (effective against common reptile pathogens) at 1:200 to 1:400 for reptile cages and bowls. Other substances commonly used are shown in Table 9.2.

Quarantine is managed according to the "all-in-and-all-out" principle. Once a group of reptiles has started quarantine, those individuals remain as a group and no other reptiles enter the quarantine section or area until the quarantine is over. The introduction of new reptiles implies beginning the quarantine period all over again.

Ideally, three negative fecal tests for gastrointestinal parasites and protozoa are required. Each fecal testing is performed three to four weeks apart. Once parasitism is diagnosed, appropriate treatment is immediately started. Those parasites with direct life cycles (e.g. coccidia) are particularly difficult to eliminate, requiring a regular screening and deworming schedule. Complete blood analysis should be performed at the beginning and end of the quarantine period. In the case of healthy animals, this establishes normal baseline values for future reference in the collection. Individuals

that become sick should be isolated, and any casualty or euthanasia must have a complete necropsy and tissue sampling for histopathology.

Pest control is important not only at quarantine, but also for the collection in itself. Arthropods (insects) can facilitate spread of infectious disease between exhibits, cages, and collections.

MANAGING LARGE COLLECTIONS

Managing large collections of reptiles requires a thorough understanding about each species (natural history, husbandry requirements, etc.), reptile zoonosis, regulations (local, national, and international), and preventive medicine. Preventive medicine includes individual identification, sanitation and disinfection, nutrition, physical examination and quarantine, parasite and disease surveillance, necropsy, and pest control.

A population management plan is required to maintain a large collection of animals. The following questions should be asked: What is the size of the animal collection? How many different species will there be? What is the purpose of the collection (private hobby, captive breeding for commercial purposes, education, zoological, etc.)? How is the surplus of animals managed? How is the genetic pool of the collection monitored? Once the purpose of the collection is established, it is possible to focus on fulfilling the collection's specific requirements to successfully manage it.

Record keeping is fundamental. Data may include feeding details, waste output (fecal/urate), sheddings, weight, reproduction details (number of offspring), and any medical condition. Reproductive data should include temperature and humidity cycling, light cycles, monitoring of time of introduction, courtship behavior, and mating. Gravid females should be monitored throughout the gestation time and oviposition (egg-laying) to maximize offspring and avoid reproductive-related problems such as dystocia. Once the oviposition occurs, it is very important to document the number of live offspring, stillborn, and slugs for viviparous species, and the number of healthy-looking eggs, abnormal eggs, and slugs in the case of oviparous species.

It is important to maintain a proper identification system for the collection so that there is a system of documenting mortality, percentage of viable offspring, compatible breeding pairs, etc. For larger collections of animals, a visual (physical pattern, carapace marking, etc.) and a permanent system (e.g. microchip) is ideal. See Table 9.3 for proper microchip placement in reptiles.

Table 9.2. Disinfectants and their characteristics.

Type	Strength	Effectiveness	Advantages/ Disadvantages	Contact time
Chlorine (e.g. sodium hypochlorite)	2–10%	Fungi, bacteria, algae, enveloped and non-enveloped viruses. Good against tuberculosis microorganism and mycoplasma. Not effective against spores.	Corrosive, irritant to mucous membranes, eyes, and skin in high concentration. Germicidal activity decreases in high water pH (ideally between 6–8) and when temperature is below 65°F. Inactivation in presence of organic material and some soaps	Several minutes for maximal efficacy (10 minutes).
Iodophors (e.g. betadine)	10–100%	Fungi, bacteria, and enveloped and non-enveloped viruses. Good activity against tuberculosis organisms and mycoplasma. Poor sporocidal activity but better than chlorine products.	Inactivated by presence of organic debris and alcohol. Stains skin, fabric, and porous material.	1–5 minutes depending on the concentration.
Biguanides (e.g. chlorhexidine)	90 ml/gal	Fair bactericidal (most Gram-positive and few Gram-negative), viricidal against enveloped viruses, sporocidal and low to moderate fungicidal activity. Good activity against tuberculosis organisms and mycoplasma.	Not an irritant. Maintains effectiveness in presence of organic matter or alcohol, but affected by alkaline pH (precipitation of the active ingredients).	5–10 minutes.
Alcohol (e.g. ethyl alcohol or isopropyl alcohol)	Full strength	Strong bactericidal (both Gram-positive and Gram-negative), slight fungicidal, and viricidal (effective against enveloped viruses). Not effective against bacterial spores and non-enveloped viruses.	Long contact time and inactivated by organic matter. Tissue irritant but noncorrosive. Poses a fire hazard.	20 minutes.

Table 9.2. Continued

Type	Strength	Effectiveness	Advantages/ Disadvantages	Contact time
Oxidizing agents (e.g. hydrogen peroxide)	Full strength	Great for anaerobic bacteria, but not viricidal. Tissue irritant. Blended and/or stabilized peroxides can be used for disinfection of equipment surfaces. Stabilized peroxides may be blended with iodophors or quaternary ammonia. Some products are effective against a much broader range of pathogens including both enveloped and non-enveloped viruses, vegetative bacteria, fungi, and bacterial spores. Examples include: Hyperox, Virkon S.	Inactivated by organic matter. Not effective against bacterial or fungal spores.	1–10 minutes.
Phenol-based compounds (e.g. Lysol, synPhenol-3)	Full strength	Fair bactericidal (especially Gram-positive bacteria) and viricidal (enveloped viruses). Not effective against non-enveloped viruses or spores. Fungicidal.	Not inactivated by presence of organic matter. Skin irritation if prolonged exposure and corrosive to skin. Toxic to cats and reptiles.	10 minutes.
Ammonia Quaternary ammonium compounds (e.g. Roccal, Parvosol, etc.)	5% 1:200 to 1:400	Coccidia and *Cryptosporidia*. Good bactericidal, moderate fungicidal activity, and poor viricidal (effective against enveloped viruses). Poor activity against non-enveloped viruses and not effective against fungi and bacterial spores. Good activity against tuberculosis microorganisms and fair activity against mycoplasma.	Inactivated by organic matter and soaps, and poor activity in hard waters. Low toxicity but prolonged contact can be irritating.	10 minutes.
Aldehydes (e.g. glutaraldehyde)	Full strength	Bactericidal, viricidal, fungicidal and sporocidal. Effective against tuberculosis organisms and *Chlamydophila* spp.	Effective in the presence of moderate organic matter. Corrosive, toxic, and irritant to the eye, skin, and respiratory tract	20 minutes.

Table 9.3. Sites for microchip placement in reptiles. Based on guidelines of the British Veterinary Zoological Society.

Animal	Suggested site
Chelonians (turtles and tortoises)	Subcutaneously in the left hind leg or intramuscularly in thin and small species
Sauria (lizards)	Left quadriceps muscle or subcutaneously in that area. In very small species, subcutaneously on the left side of the body
Ophidia (Snakes)	Subcutaneously on the left side of the neck area at about twice the length of the head
Crocodilians	Cranial to nuchal cluster

Reproducing reptiles in captivity can be complex. Husbandry is very important because reptiles rely entirely on their environment to successfully reproduce. A period of cool temperature is necessary for most species to initiate reproductive behavior. Seasonal cooling is usually referred to as hibernation or brumation (Figure 9.1.); in any case, this is very complex and species specific. Therefore, the author strongly recommends extensive literature research on the species before breeding. Another important factor for reproduction is space availability, which can affect proper copulation and egg deposition. Unfit reptiles are more prone to egg retention or dystocia (Figure 9.2.). Another common cause of dystocia is improper laying conditions such as lack of a nesting box.

Sanitation and disinfection requires a routine schedule. Properly done, it requires a written protocol of cleaning and disinfecting agents used, as well as when and how to use them. Disinfectants can only be used after removal of organic matter and cleaning.

Nutrition should be based on the species maintained. Diet can be complex and it can be almost impossible to reproduce to what would be encountered in the wild. Vitamin and mineral supplements are usually required. Generally, neonates and youngsters require supplementation on a daily basis or every other day and adults require it about once a week. Palatability and composition of invertebrates vary considerably upon stage and species. Certain species of wild insects may contain pollutants and can potentially be toxic (e.g. lightning bugs). Commercial pellet diets are available in the market; however, the nutritional requirements are not completely known and they should not be used as the only food source.

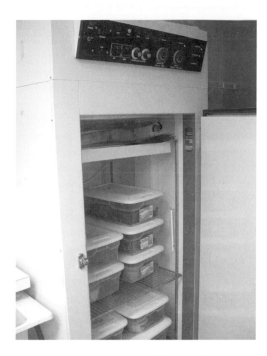

Figure 9.1. A temperature-and humidity-controlled hibernaculum allowing normal reptile hibernation or brumation. (Courtesy of David Perpiñan, LV, MSc, College of Veterinary Medicine, University of Georgia.)

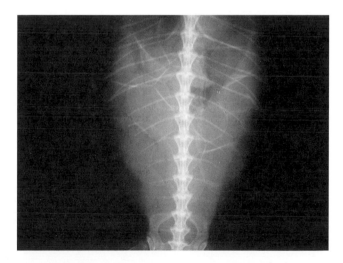

Figure 9.2. Egg retention (dystocia) in a green iguana (Iguana iguana). Notice the distended abdomen full of calcified eggs. (Courtesy of David Perpiñan, LV, MSc, College of Veterinary Medicine, University of Georgia.)

Reptile species should be examined bi-annually or annually depending on age and reproductive stage. The implementation of physical examinations, quarantine, and necropsy aids disease surveillance within the collection. Early detection of an infectious and metabolic disease permits prompt correction and lower morbidity and mortality.

Pest control has important implications for personal safety as well as prevention of disease spread within the collection. Possible pest species should be carefully identified and a control plan instituted. Whatever system is implemented, this must be safe for the species in the collection. The quality of the program must be carefully monitored and recorded. For example, rodent traps should be inspected regularly and the number of animals trapped monitored for control purposes. An increase in the number of rodents trapped may simply correlate with a change in management, such as waste disposal.

MANAGING LARGE COLLECTIONS OF DANGEROUS SPECIES

Dangerous reptile species are those that either can inflict serious injuries from a bite (e.g. crocodile), strangulation (e.g. large boid), or venom (e.g. rattlesnake). The same principles discussed above for keeping a large reptile collection apply for dangerous species. However, these types of species require further safety issues such as proper caging and in most cases, a legal permit. In cases in which multiple people are handling dangerous species, an emergency written protocol is fundamental. An appropriate protocol addresses every danger in the case of injury or escape, minimizing the likelihood of mortality or permanent disability. Every protocol must be specific for the type and number of dangerous reptiles in the collection, and in the case of certain venomous species, maintenance of antivenom may be required. The American Zoo and Aquarium Association and the American Association of Poison Control Centers list the amount and location of available antivenoms for most venomous species. In any case, it is strongly advisable to notify the local hospital about the ownership of venomous species so that medical staff is prepared in the case of a venomous animal bite.

Dangerous species require proper labeling and their handling is restricted to appropriately trained people. Access is restricted by the use of a lock and the cages must be properly secured at all times. This is especially important in the case of venomous species. Venomous reptiles are coded as 1 or 2 depending upon the poten-

tial of a life-threatening injury. Code 1 animals are those capable of causing death, long-term illness, or permanent disability, whereas code 2 animals are unlikely to cause severe or long-lasting effects.

In the event of injury and escape, the victim is responsible for securing the area first and then seeking medical care. A first-aid kit should be available and personnel should be trained in providing first-aid care.

A capture plan should also be part of the protocol. This part of the protocol should include the immediate measures to secure the area, a contact list of people responsible to respond to an escape, equipment necessary for safe capture and handling, etc. If the animal cannot be safely captured, humane killing may be indicated.

METHODS OF SEX DETERMINATION

There are different ways of sexing reptiles but none of them is applicable for all reptile species. The following are methods of sex determination in reptiles:

- Sexual dimorphism
- Probing
- Manual eversion of hemipenes or popping
- Hydrostatic eversion of hemipenes
- Digital palpation (crocodilians)
- Plasma testosterone
- Morphometric measurements
- DNA sexing (karyotyping)
- Ultrasonography
- Laparoscopy

Sexual Dimorphism

Sexual dimorphism is the difference in appearance between males and females of the same species. This is usually apparent in some chelonians (turtles and tortoises) and sauria (lizard) species. Sexual dimorphism is generally apparent in adults, but it can be very difficult in sub-adults and juveniles. General guidelines for the identification of chelonian males are a longer tail with a cloacal opening beyond the rear carapacial shell margin and a plastral concavity (Figure 9.3.). Some other species-specific characteristics are long front leg toenails in slider turtles (*Pseudemys* spp., *Trachemys scripta*), painted turtles (*Chrysemys picta*), and map turtles (*Graptemys* spp.); a red iris in the male eastern box turtles (*Terrapene carolina carolina*); and more prominent mental glands, gular scutes, and body size in male desert tortoises (*Gopherus agassizii*). The female leopard tortoise (*Geochelone pardalis*) has larger toenails in the rear legs than the males and the

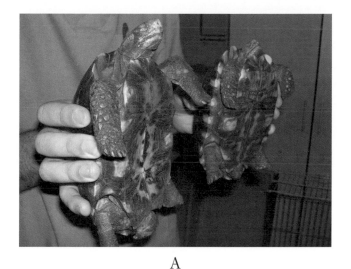

A

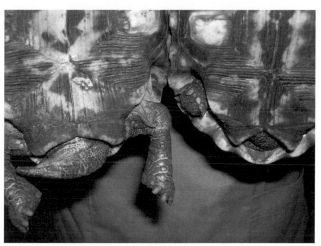

B

Figure 9.3. Sexual dimorphisim in a chelonian species, red-footed tortoise (Geochelone carbonaria). (A) Male chelonians commonly have longer tails with the cloacal opening beyond the rear carapacial shell margin. (B) Plastral concavity is more pronounced in male chelonians than females to facilitate mating. (Courtesy of David Perpiñan, LV, MSc, College of Veterinary Medicine, University of Georgia.)

female map turtles and diamondback terrapins are significantly larger than the males.

Although many lizard species are monomorphic, male lizards have a pair of hemipenes located at the base of the tail. In mature iguanids, geckos, and varanids, a paired bulge from these hemipenes may identify the individual as a male. Some lizards, especially agamids, geckos, and iguanids, also have pores on their ventral thighs (femoral pores) or on the ventral procloacal skin (precloacal pores). The pores are relatively larger in adult males than females (Figure 9.4.). Male monitors have a bone structure in their hemipenes called the hemibaculum. The varanus species reported to have hemibacula are *acantharus, beccarii, caudolineatus, eremius, giganteus, gilleni, gouldi, indicus, karlschmidti, komodoensis, olivaceus, panoptes, salvadorii, storii, tristis,* and *varius.* In these species, the radiography can be used to make apparent the presence of the hemibacula (Funk 2002). Other dimorphism among lizards is based on ornamentation such as the three large rostral horns in male Jackson's chameleon (*Chamaeleo jacksoni*), or more robust appearance (especially of the head) in males such as iguanas and gila monsters (*Heloderma suspectum*).

Sexual dimorphism among snakes is very rare. Among boids, the spurs, located just lateral to the vent, are larger in males than in females. These spurs are used for tactile stimulation of the female during courtship. The spur size is highly reliable in the case of the rosy boa (*Charina trivirgata*) and the sand boas (*Eryx* spp.).

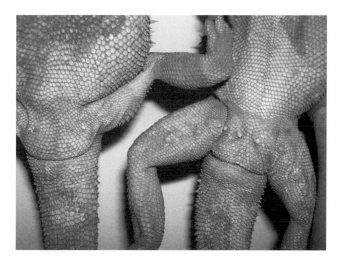

Figure 9.4. Sexual dimorphism in a lizard species, bearded dragon (Pogona vitticeps). The male is on the right and female on the left. Femoral pores and tail bulge from the hemipenes are obvious in the male. (Courtesy of David Perpiñan, LV, MSc, College of Veterinary Medicine, University of Georgia.)

Probing

Probing is a technique in which a lubricated blunt-tipped probe is used for sexing. Only water- or saline-based lubricants should be used because some other lubricants may be spermicidal. This technique is only valid for squamata (lizards and snakes). In males, the sexing probe goes farther down into the tail as it enters the hemipenial pocket. The depth of the hemipenial sac varies among species. In females, probing results in the total inability or limited ability to insert the probe into the tail base. This is the result of probing a pair of blind diverticula, and female lizards may have a tiny homologous structure called hemiclitori. Common species in which these diverticula are well developed, creating difficulty sexing by this method, include the monitors (*Varanus* spp.) and the blood python (*Python curtus*).

Manual Eversion of Hemipenes or Popping

Popping or manual eversion of the hemipenes is a common method for determining the sex of neonatal colubrid snakes. This is accomplished by firmly rolling one's thumb proximally up the tail base toward the cloaca. In females the oviductal papillae can sometimes be identified as two small reddish openings located laterally in the cloaca.

Hydrostatic Eversion of Hemipenes

Hydrostatic eversion of hemipenes consists of the injection of isotonic saline solution (as much as 100 ml) into the tail just distal to where the hemipene is located. If the technique is performed correctly, the hydrostatic pressure created by the saline solution causes the hemipenes to evert (Figure 9.5.). This also causes swelling of the tissue surrounding the cloaca, and may partially evert the cloaca through the vent. For larger

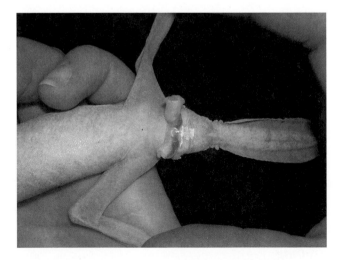

*Figure 9.5. Everted hemipenes in a lineated leaf-tailed gecko (*Uroplatus lineautus*). (Courtesy of David Perpiñan, LV, MSc, College of Veterinary Medicine, University of Georgia.)*

species such as boids, monitors, iguanas, and gila monsters anesthesia may be required because the retractor penis muscle can counteract the hydrostatic pressure created, therefore preventing the eversion of the hemipenes.

Digital Palpation

Digital palpation is the preferred method for crocodilian species. This involves palpating the ventral aspect of the cloaca for the presence of a penis in the otherwise smooth-walled cloaca.

Plasma Testosterone

Plasma testosterone concentration has been used for sexing chelonian juveniles, with or without the use of follicle-stimulating-hormone (FSH) stimulation test (Owens et al. 1978, Lance et al. 1992, Rostal et al. 1994). Males typically have higher levels than females. However, this test also has limitations because older females may have normal elevated testosterone levels and prolonged handling of both sexes has been reported to elevate testosterone levels (Rostal et al. 1994, Innis and Boyer 2002).

Morphometric

Morphometric is the use of body measurements to determine sex. However, this is not a reliable way to differentiate males and females because there are many exceptions among species. It is more common for males to be larger than females in lizards. Female turtles are generally larger in body size than males. However, this may be different in tortoises. The male desert tortoise (*Gopherus agassizii*) is larger than the female.

DNA Sexing

Karyotyping is the use of DNA to determine gender. It can be used for both temperature-dependent sex determination (TSD) species and those that are not TSD species (Demas et al. 1990, Innis and Boyer 2002). Although this technique is feasible, it has received little attention.

Ultrasonography and Laparoscopy

Ultrasonography may be useful identifying males and females by identification of ovaries, follicles, or eggs in the coelomic cavity of females, and testis or the hemipenes in the case of males (Figure 9.6.). Laparoscopy has been also used for sexing. This is a surgical procedure in which an endoscope is guided through their coelom to directly visualize the testis or ovarian tissue (Figure 9.7.). The advantage is that it permits visual evaluation of the reproductive tract and detection of possible abnormalities.

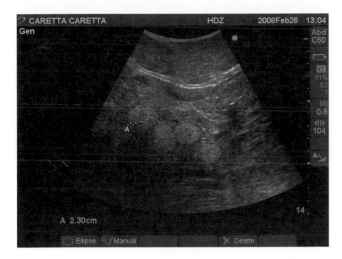

Figure 9.6. Coelomic cavity ultrasound in a gravid female. Note the presence of the follicles (increased round echogenicity) as they lack of the more mineralized egg shell. (Courtesy of David Perpiñan, LV, MSc, College of Veterinary Medicine, University of Georgia.)

REPRODUCTIVE BEHAVIOR

The development of secondary sexual characteristics coupled with courtship behavior is an indication that sexual maturity is approaching (Innis and Boyer 2002). Sexual maturity depends upon the reptile size rather than actual age (Taylor and Denardo 2005). In captivity, reptiles reach sexual maturity at a younger age than their wild counterparts. For instance, captive leopard tortoises (*Geochelone pardalis*) may reproduce successfully in four to six years, whereas their wild-born counterparts do not reach sexual maturity for fifteen years (Innis and Boyer 2002). As a rough generality in captive species, snakes usually mature in two to three years, small lizards in one to two years, large lizards in three to four years, and chelonians in five to seven years (Denardo 2006).

In most reptile studies to date, high plasma levels of testosterone and corticosterone coincide with the mating period. The female estradiol level increases at the onset of the mating season and decreases at the onset of the nesting season. Progesterone levels are high close to ovulation and the beginning of the nesting season, and they decrease during the nesting season (Schramm et al. 1999). Therefore, monitoring the reproductive cycle is possible via plasma chemistry and hormone assays (Innis and Boyer 2002).

The most common stimulus to reproduction in reptiles is a change in temperature. The reproductive cycle

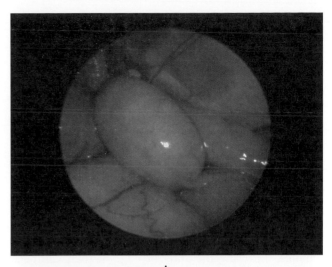

A

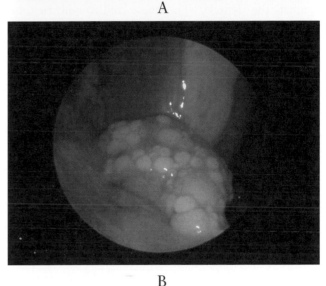

B

Figure 9.7. Endoscopic visualization of (A) a testis in a male green iguana (Iguana iguana) and (B) an ovary in a young female Hermann's tortoise (Testudo hermanni). (Courtesy of Xavier Valls Badia, LV, Clinica Veterinaria Exotics, Barcelona, Spain.)

in chelonians is linked to the temperature and humidity determined by their natural habitats. For species in temperate climates, reproductive activity is restricted to the warmer months of the year when the days are longer. In general, females ovulate and are fertilized in the spring, nest in the late spring and summer, and begin folliculogenesis for the following year's egg in late summer and fall. An exception to this is tropical boids (boas and pythons), which tend to breed during the cooler period (Denardo 2006). In tropical climates, the reproductive cycle follows the rainfall patterns, when temperature and day length fluctuations are minimal (Innis and Boyer 2002).

Light also plays an important role in sexual behavior. Behavioral studies have proven the importance of full-spectrum lighting (UVA, UVB, and visible light; 280 to 700 nm) and its role not only in motion perception and foraging but also intersexual recognition.

Courtship and Mating Behavior

Some degree of courtship behavior is noted in most species. Courtship may last from minutes to hours, and it may even resume on subsequent days. Most terrestrial tortoises such as the Mediterranean tortoises (*Testudo* spp.) display a lunging behavior toward the females, battering the anterior edge of their carapace against the female. The male red-footed tortoise (*Geochelone carbonaria*) may stand in front of the

female with its neck stretched low to the ground, moving it rhythmically side to side while uttering low-pitched, grunting sounds. In some North American aquatic species (e.g. red-eared slider, *Trachemys scripta*), males fibrillate their elongated nails of the forelimbs near the female's face (Innis and Boyer 2002).

Copulation is a short event only lasting for several minutes. Many chelonian and lizard species display biting behavior as the male mounts the female from behind (Innis and Boyer 2002). In snakes, the male of the colubrid neck-banded snakes (*Scaphiodontophis annulatus*) grabs, holds, and bites the female during copulation as part of the mating behaviour (Sasa and Curtis 2006).

During copulation, one hemipenis is everted into the female's cloaca in the case of snakes and lizards (Figure 9.8.). In the case of chelonians and crocodilians, a single penis arising from the floor of the cloaca

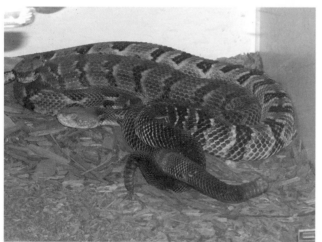

A

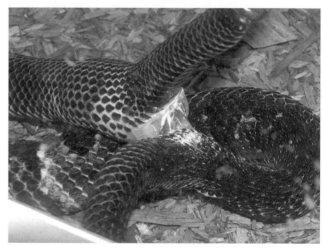

B

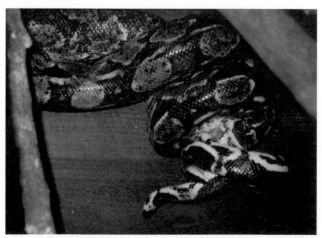

C

*Figure 9.8. Snake copulation. (A and B) Copulation in the timber rattlesnake (*Crotalus horridus*). (Courtesy of BW Smith, Animal South LLC.) (C) Copulation of the common boa constrictor (*Boa constrictor*). (Courtesy of Susana Ringenbach, MVZ, Fauna Silvestre, Merida, Mexico.)*

is everted. In both cases, the sperm flows through a single groove called the seminal groove or sulcus spermaticus from the vas deferens down the penis or hemipenis and down to the anterior portions of the female's cloaca. The spermatozoa travel upward through the oviduct where fertilization occurs. In some species such as iguanids, sperm storage allows the female to lay subsequent clutches (Funk 2002).

Reproduction Without Mating

Amphigonia retardata, or sperm storage, has been described in turtles and snakes. This adaptation allows a female to produce several clutches from a single mating in one season and to reproduce in subsequent seasons. The viability of the storage sperm is not indefinite and varies with the species, ranging from several months to up to six years (Mader 2006).

Another strategy to reproduce without mating is parthenogenesis. In this case, the female becomes gravid in the absence of a male and produces only female offspring (Mader 2006). Interestingly, genetic polymorphism is present to some extent, albeit the lack of genetic recombination.

Studies have shown in true parthenogenetic species, such as the caucasian rock lizard (*Darevskia unisexualis*), that mutations can make a significant contribution to population variability (Badaeva et al. 2008). Parthenogenesis has been reported in more than thirty species of lizards and some snakes. Some common examples include members of genera *Cnemidophorus* (whiptails), *Darevskia* (rock lizards), *Hemidactylus* (geckos), Komodo dragon (*Varanus komodoensis*), and snakes such as the *Rhamphotyphlops braminus* (blind snake) (Table 9.4.).

Table 9.4. Reptile families in which parthenogenesis has been described.

Family Gekkonidae (geckoes)	5 species
Family Agamidae (agamids)	1 species
Family Chamaelonidae (chameleons)	1 species
Family Xantusiidae (night lizards)	1 species
Family Lacertidae (lacertids)	5 species (e.g. Genus *Darevskia*)
Family Teiidae (whiptails and tegus)	15 species (e.g. Genus *Cnemidophorus*)
Family Typhlopidae (blind snakes)	1 species

FOLLICLE AND EGG DEVELOPMENT

Vitellogenesis is the major step of follicle maturation with the accumulation of yolk. Estrogen triggers the liver to convert the lipid from the body's fat stores to vitellogenin, which is selectively absorbed by the follicles. Calcium also accumulates in the yolk during this stage so that the yolk acts as a main calcium reservoir for the embryo. Furthermore, a significant amount of calcium is drawn from the eggshell in oviparous species. The mature ovum is ten-fold to 100-fold larger than its previtellogenic size. In the oviduct, the ovum becomes an egg when albumin and a shell are added for oviparous species. In the case of viviparous species, placentation takes place. This maternal-embryonic relationship varies among viviparous species with the most extreme example being some skinks (*Mabuya* spp.), in which the mother contributes more than 99% of the neonatal mass through a chorioallantoic placenta (Denardo 2006).

CLUTCH DYNAMICS

The frequency with which reptiles reproduce depends on the species, environmental conditions, and health status of the specific individual. Reproduction has detrimental effects for female reptiles because they cease feeding during the latter stages of pregnancy. The length of time during which feeding is reduced varies but it is much shorter in oviparous (weeks) than in viviparous (months) species. This limited amount of energy allocated to reproduction therefore has direct effects on offspring and clutch size. Invariably, the amount of energy is extraordinary, especially in snakes, in which where more than 40% of the female's body mass can be allocated to reproduction (Denardo 2006).

Clutch size is extremely variable in reptiles. For oviparous species, it ranges from one in the case of anoles (*Anolis* spp.) and the pancake tortoise (*Malocochersus tornieri*) to 200 in the green sea turtle (*Chelonia mydas*). In viviparous species, the numbers may be slightly lower with a range from one in the case of shingleback skinks (*Trachysaurus rugosus*) to ninety-two in the garter snake (*Thamnophis radix*) (Denardo 2006).

Many oviparous species can produce more than one clutch per year. This is more common among chelonians and lizards than snakes. Due to the restraints of viviparity, viviparous reptiles are limited to a single clutch per year.

OVIPAROUS, OVOVIVIPAROUS, OR VIVIPAROUS

The oviduct's function in lizards and snakes is fertilization, sperm storage, egg transport and eggshell deposition, maintenance of the early embryo, and expulsion of the egg or fetus. In viviparous species, the oviduct also contributes to the placenta, which is responsible for gas exchange and nutrient provision to the fetus (Blackburn 1998).

Three modes of reptile reproduction have long been recognized: oviparous, ovoviparous, and viviparous. Ovoviparity was applied to those species in which the young are born alive but there was not placental connection between the mother and the offspring. However, more recent investigations have demonstrated some nutrient transfer; therefore, the term ovoviparity may be inappropriate (Funk 2002).

Thus, the term oviparity refers to the condition of laying fertilized eggs and viviparity refers to the condition of giving birth to live offspring regardless of how nutrient exchange may have occurred between the mother and the offspring. Chelonian and crocodilian species are oviparous, while 20% of squamates (some lizard and snake lineages) are viviparous (Funk 2002, Benirschke 2007) (Box 9.1).

Although viviparity has a clear advantage over oviparity, there are several disadvantages worth mentioning. Sustaining the fetuses over an extended period of time limits the female to a single clutch per year. Bearing the offspring also has detrimental effects to the female because viviparous females cease feeding during the latter stages (Denardo 2006) (Figure 9.9.). However, viviparous reptiles have the advantage of regulating incubation temperature and enhancing the fitness of the offspring. Therefore, a phylogenetic transition from oviparity to viviparity has occurred in cold climates (Webb et al. 2006).

EGG INCUBATION VERSUS MATERNAL INCUBATION

A number of factors determine the length of gestation, such as season, ambient temperature, housing, and food supply, among others (Mader 2006). Parental care in reptiles is minimal with few exceptions among crocodilian and pythons. Female pythons are known to brood their eggs during incubation by coiling around them until hatching. Periodic rhythmic contractions of her abdominal musculature is capable of maintaining a mean body temperature of 7.3°C over the mean ambient surface temperature (Mader 2006).

Box 9.1. Oviparity and Viviparity of Commonly Kept Reptiles. (Adapted from Denardo 2006 in Reptile Medicine and Surgery, Mader DR, ed., Elsevier.)

Oviparous
All crocodilians
All chelonians
Most lizards
    All monitors (*Varanus* spp.)
    Most iguanids
        Iguanas (*Iguana* spp.)
        Water dragons (*Physignathus* spp.)
    All geckos
    Most chameleons
        Veiled chameleon (*Chamaeleo calyptratus*)
        Panther chameleon (*Chamaeleo pardalis*)
Some snakes
    All pythons
    Most colubrids
        King snakes and Milk snakes (*Lampropelis* spp.)
        Rat snakes and Corn snakes (*Elaphe* spp.)

Viviparous
Some lizards
    Some skinks
        Blue-tongued skinks (*Tiliqua* spp.)
        Shingle-backed skink (*Trachysaurus rugosus*)
        Prehensile-tailed skink (*Corucia zebrata*)
Some chameleons
    Jackson's chameleon (*Chamaeleo jacksonii*)
Some snakes
    Most boas (except *Charina reinhardti, Eryx jayakari*)
    Most vipers
        All rattlesnakes (*Crotalus* spp.)
Some colubrids
    Garter snakes (*Thamnophis* spp.)

EGG INCUBATION METHODS

Viable eggs are usually firm, dry, and chalky white. Soft-shelled eggs in all snakes, most lizards, and some chelonians are pliable, while the eggs of crocodilians, many chelonians, and some lizards are hard-shelled and therefore rigid (Figure 9.10.).

Artificial incubation is relatively simple. Incubators can be easily designed and maintained by fulfilling three basic requirements: proper regulation of temperature and humidity, even distribution of heat, and a reliable thermostat to control temperature. Although

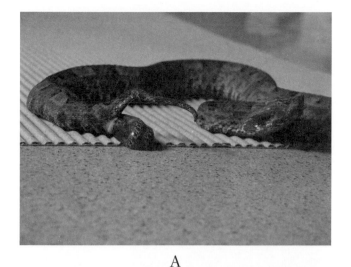

A

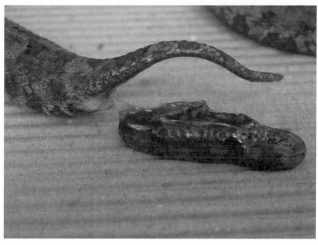

B

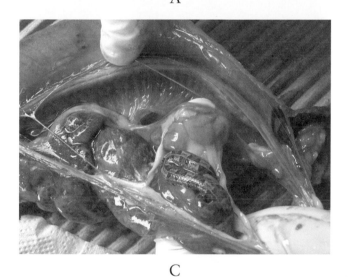

C

Figure 9.9. Viviparity in a rainforest hognose viper (Porthidium nasutum). (A) Hognose viper giving birth. (B) Offspring surrounded by the placenta membrane. (C) Necropsy of a rainforest hognose viper in which several fetuses are contained within a plancenta membrane within the oviduct. (Courtesy of Alejandro Ramirez, student of veterinary medicine and supervisor of the group in Ophidism-Scorpionism University of Antioquia, Colombia.)

insulation prevents the loss of heat and humidity, some degree of ventilation should be permitted (e.g. small holes on the lid of the egg chamber). A study on sea turtle eggs showed that poor ventilation increases incubation time and reduces survival of embryos (Funk 2002). Commercial incubators are available for reptiles, and even chick incubators can be used with minor modifications such as stopping the movement of the egg trays. Most incubators are designed according to a double-chamber principle so that the eggs are located inside a box, which is inside the larger incubator chamber. A Styrofoam cooler can be used as a cheaper alternative for the containment chamber of the nest box. Plastic storage boxes can be used as a nest or inside box. The lid should fit tightly so that the air humidity approaches saturation. The moistened substrate material is filled halfway, and then water is added appropriately so that it is only slightly damp.

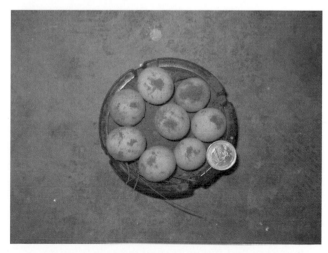

Figure 9.10. Hard-shelled eggs of the Mediterranean spur-thighed tortoise (Testudo graeca). (Courtesy of Jose Luis Crespo Picazo, LV, Nexo CMA Valencia, Spain.)

Heat is provided by heating coils, strips, and pads, and a thermostat assures that the temperature stays constant within the inner chamber with the set-up based on the species' eggs. As long as the three main principles of reptile egg incubation are fulfilled, any container with controlled heat, humidity, and ventilation may be suitable (Figure 9.11.).

Although there is no scientific study indicating otherwise, the eggs should be placed in the incubator in the same orientation as they were laid. A pencil mark on top of the egg may help maintain the orientation when the egg is moved. Soft-shelled eggs are then half-buried within the moist substrate and separated from each other by a small distance (Figure 9.12.). Hard-shelled eggs may be placed in a small depression in the substrate. Maintaining a certain distance between the eggs prevents the spread of disease processes among the eggs. When two or more eggs are strongly adhered to each other, they will have to be half-buried together. Attempting to separate those eggs may lead to permanent damage.

Incubation requirements for most reptilian eggs are similar. Very important factors to remember in reptile reproduction are ambient temperature, humidity, and substrate.

Temperature

Ambient incubation temperature directly affects the length of incubation and, in some species, gender determination (Table 9.5). There are two types of sex determination systems: genotypic sex determination (GSD) determined by the sex chromosomes and temperature-dependent sex determination system (TSD) in which temperature affects sex determination (Wibbels et al. 1991; Delmas et al. 2008). The rele-

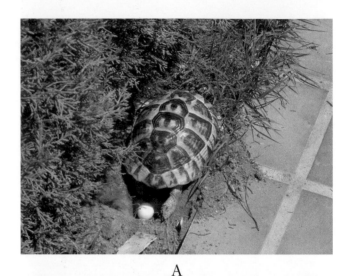

A

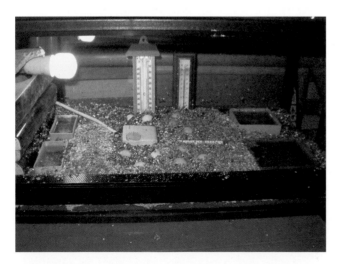

B

*Figure 9.12. After egg deposition, the eggs are removed and placed into the incubator chamber. (A) Egg laying of a Mediterranean spur-thighed tortoise (*Testudo graeca*). (Courtesy of Jose Luis Crespo Picazo, LV, Nexo CMA Valencia, Spain.) (B) The egg chamber contains the half-buried eggs set into the moistened substrate and separated from each other by a small distance. Maintenance of a certain distance between the eggs prevents the spread of disease processes among the eggs. (Courtesy of David Perpiñan LV, MSc, College of Veterinary Medicine, University of Georgia.)*

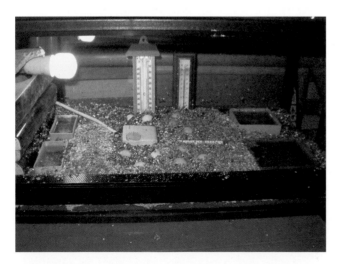

Figure 9.11. A hand-made incubator can be easily designed by creating an environment of controlled temperature and humidity, and even distribution of heat and some degree of ventilation. (Courtesy of Jose Luis Crespo Picazo, LV, Nexo CMA Valencia, Spain.)

Table 9.5. Patterns of temperature sex determination in reptiles.

Sauria (lizards)

Family Geckonidae

African fat-tailed gecko (*Hemitheconyx caudicinctus*) 26°–29°C (78.8°–84.2°F) results in females	Pattern II
30°–32°C (86°–89.6°F) results in males	
34°–35°C (93.2°–95°F) results in females	
Japanese gecko (*Gekko japonicus*)	Pattern IA
Females at higher temperatures, males at lower temperatures	
Leopard gecko (*Eublepharis macularius*)	Pattern IB
26.7°–29.4°C results in 90% females	
>32.2°C results in 90% males	
Rainbow lizard (*Agama agama*)	Pattern IB
26°–27°C (78.8°–80.6°F) results in females	
29°C (84.2°F) results in males	
Jacky dragon (*Amphibolurus muricatus*)	Pattern II
Tuataras (*Sphenodon* sp.)	Pattern IB
Chelonians (turtles and tortoises)	
Some Bataguridae	Pattern IA
Carettochelydae	Pattern IA
Cheloniidae	Pattern IA
Dermochelydae	Pattern IA
Emydidae	Pattern IA
Testudinidae	Pattern IA
Pelomedusidae	Pattern II
Kinosternidae	Pattern II
Macroclemys temminckii (Chelydridae)	Pattern II
Some Bataguridae	Pattern II
All crocodilians	Pattern II is assumed in all crocodilians. Pattern IB is still suggested for some species (*Alligator sinensis, Caimen crocodiles yacare,* and *Paleosuchus trigonatus*) due to the limited available data.

Note: Pattern I-IA: Males produced at low temperatures and females produced at high temperature with a single transition zone. IB: Males produced at high temperatures and females produced at low temperatures with a single transition zone. Pattern II: Females produced at both low and high temperatures with males produced at intermediate temperatures; two transition zones.

Author's disclosure: This table is not intended to represent all reptile species in which gender is determined by temperature (TSD). Not all reptile species have been studied, and in many cases there is not enough scientific data about temperature ranges. Occasionally a reptile species has been reported having TSD pattern IA or IB, and later evidence has proven that it may follow a different pattern, such as pattern II.

vance of TSD over GSD is still unknown but may be related to environmental fitness (Warner and Shine 2008). However sex determination is very complex in reptiles and even both systems can be present in a single species. Sex determination in the montane scincid lizard (*Bassiana duperreyi*) is regulated genetically by sex chromosomes but temperatures can override chromosomal sex generating phenotypically male offspring from XX eggs in cool nests (Radder et al.

2008). TSD occurs in all studied crocodilians and tuataras, it is very common in chelonian, less frequent in lizards and unknown in snakes (Delmas et al. 2008). Although TSD has evolved in several lineages of lizards, there is less information than among the other reptile taxa. The time in which TSD occurs in called the thermosensitive period and is about the middle one-third of the embryonic development (Wibbels et al. 1991; Delmas et al. 2008). TSD may be also evident in viviparous lizards in which sex ratios fluctuate with thermal conditions. In the Spotted skink (*Niveoscincus ocellatus*) there is a higher proportion of male offspring in colder years (Wapstra et al. 2008). There are two distinct patterns of TSD. In Pattern I, there is a single transition zone at which eggs incubated below this temperature zone result predominantly in males and above the temperature zone predominantly in females. Pattern II has two transition zones with males predominating at the intermediate zone and females at both extremes. Pattern I occurs chiefly in turtles in which the adult females are larger than the adult males while Pattern II is primarily present with females being smaller than males or non-dimorphic species (no difference between males and females). Some *Sternotherus* and *Chelydra* are exceptions such that a constant incubation temperature within the transition zone yields 100% males (Eti 2009).

Incubation length is usually reduced by high temperatures, but it increases the risk of congenital defects (Denardo 2006). Furthermore, abnormally high or low temperatures will affect on the health of the hatchlings (Mader 2006). In general, incubation temperature ranges from 26°C to 32°C (80°F to 90°F) (Denardo 2006).

Gestation periods vary. Eggs of most snakes and small lizards hatch in 45 to 70 days, and 90 to 130 days for eggs from larger lizards such as iguanas and monitor lizards. Gestation lengths cannot only vary among species, but also within the same species and within the same clutch. Incubation time of the leopard tortoise (*Geochelone pardalis*) can range from 250 to 540 days and from 30 to 40 days variation within same clutch (Denardo 2006).

Substrate

Commonly used substrates include perlite, vermiculite, potting soil, sand, sphagnum moss, and shredded paper. There is also commercially available substrate for reptile incubators based on a pre-prepared mixture of the already mention substrates. Perlite and vermiculite are preferred by many hobbyists as they are very light, absorbent, siliceous material that naturally resists molding. In any case, the purpose of the substrate is to provide a media that will retain water and maintain humidity within the egg container while preventing excessive fungal growth.

Humidity

The amount of water added to the substrate varies but should be enough to create clumping of the media without dripping of water. Water will be required throughout the incubation period and therefore, more may need to be added. Dampened sphagnum moss can be used to cover the eggs to help prevent desiccation; however it will prevent or make more difficult visual checking of the viability of the eggs.

It is advisable to weigh the incubation box and its eggs periodically so that water can be added to keep the box at its original weight. If water needs to be added, water should be at the same temperature as the incubator.

DIAGNOSING EGG PROBLEMS

In order to diagnose egg problems it is important to understand the basic differences among reptilian eggs. The eggshell in snakes and most lizards is leathery and soft; however the egg of chelonian, crocodilians and geckos is hard as they have a calcareous shell. Both soft-shelled and hard-shelled eggs have three internal membranes (the amnion, the chorion and the allantois) that retard outward water diffusion and allow embryonic respiration. Even the hard-shelled eggs will take water from the environment to some extent and swell in size during embryonic development. All the nutrients will come from the yolk and the white, and any remaining yolk in the egg will be incorporated into the hatchling's coelomic cavity (Mader 2006).

The death of the egg can occur when the environmental conditions for egg development are not fulfilled. Incorrect humidity (high or low), temperature (high or low) and improper ventilation are very common problems that can cause egg death. Other potential causes are excessive handling or trauma. In any case, it may be difficult to determine the cause the embryonic death. Reptiles from temperate zones can stand temperature ranges better than tropical species. For instances, the embryos of the tropical green iguana (*Iguana iguana*) fail to develop at temperatures varying for more than 2°C from the optimum 30°C (86°F) (Funk 2002).

Health assessment of the eggs is based on daily monitoring for color and texture changes. A collapsed egg is a sign of dehydration but not necessarily egg death. Marked changes in color or texture or fungal growth are usually signs of a non-viable egg, either from egg that has died or from a non-fertile egg (Table 9.6.).

Two diagnostic methods of assessing the health of an egg are "candling" and ultrasonography for non-calcified eggs (most squamata). A high-intensity light source (e.g. transilluminator) placed in direct contact with the side of the egg in a dark room can reveal a developing vascular pattern in a viable egg as the

Table 9.6. Common signs encountered during egg incubation, treatment, and prevention.

Problem	Signs	Treatment	Prevention
Diapause	Fails to develop	Correction of environmental conditions	Some eggs enter diapause and resume growth after proper environmental conditions
Egg death	Fails to develop	Proper environmental conditions	Proper environmental conditions, proper monitoring and design of incubator
	Infertile egg	No treatment	Sex determination of individuals, correct level of maturity, and proper pairing
	Fungal growth	Clean fungus gently with cotton tip	Avoid excessive humidity and contact between eggs
Trauma	Depression or deformity	No treatment	Mark egg's orientation with a pencil and avoid trauma or excessive handling
Dessication	Egg shrinkage	Rehydrate with warm spring water	Proper monitoring of humidity and temperature
Fungal growth	Mold on egg surface	Remove growth with a cotton tip, and sprinkle antifungal powder (e.g. athlete's foot powder)	Prevent excessive humidity and avoid contact between eggs. Remove any dead eggs.
Slugs	Waxy yellow deformed and shrink eggs	No treatment	Discard unfertilized ova. It may imply an underlying issue with the female. Seek veterinary attention.

embryo grows or a homogenous diffuse yellow-white luminescence in a death egg. Ultrasonography must be used carefully because the ultrasound gel can potentially damage the eggs by clogging the oxygen exchange pores. Ultrasonography of the developing embryo requires a high-frequency ultrasound transducer (7.5 to 10 MHz) to properly assess development (Mader 2006). In any case, ultrasonography can not only be used to distinguish the general stages of follicle and egg development, but it can also be used to reasonably predict birth by monitoring the loss of yolk, with birth occurring about a week after yolk can no longer be detected (Denardo 2006).

CARING FOR THE NEWBORN

Reptilian neonates are born precocious. In other words, they are fully independent and capable of survival from birth. Adult reptiles rarely provide any care for their offspring. Parental care can be defined as the parental actions after oviposition or parturition that may increases the offspring's chances of survival (Funk 2002). Parental care has been documented in at least 100 species of reptiles but it is limited and nonessential

for survival of the offspring (Denardo 2006). Among lizards, there are few examples of maternal care but this is basic and limited to nesting care against predators in the case of some skinks. Nest guarding has been also documented in chelonians (e.g. Burmese mountain tortoise, *Manouria emys*), snakes (e.g. King cobra, *Ophiophagus Hannah*, and cobras, *Naja* spp.), and virtually all species of crocodilians. In the case of the skink *Eumeces obsoletus*, the female assists during hatching and subsequently licks their cloacas, and supplies them with food up until about the tenth day (Mader 2006). As a part of nest guarding, crocodilians assist the neonates in emerging from the nest and guard them after hatching. Rattlesnakes remain with their offspring until the neonate's first shed (Denardo 2006).

In captivity, neonate care can be divided into three categories: environmental conditions, space, and proper food. The care provided to newborns is minimal and merely a scaled-down version of the care given to adults. Hatching can take from one to four days. In the case of chelonians, the neonate's shell begins to unfold, facilitating yolk absorption. Absorption of the yolk sac may take several days after hatching so neonates should be kept in a clean and moist environment.

In general, hatchlings are maintained at or near the incubation temperature, and many breeders leave them in the incubator for the first few days. A plastic container with clean, moist paper towels is also commonly used for the first few days. Once the yolk sac is fully absorbed and the umbilicus sealed, the neonates can be transferred to a cage with other substrate. Neonates are very prone to dehydration, and thus humidity should be close to 100%. After leaving the incubator, temperature should be close to the adults' temperature range, with slightly higher humidity. Higher humidity can be easily accomplished by using moistened paper towels and a humidity box, a confined box containing moistened paper towels with a small opening that allows the youngsters to get in and out easily. Being such a confined and closed space, this allows a relative humidity of almost 100% as long as the substrate is replaced on a daily basis. Other, more natural substrates can be used as the youngsters grow but paper is generally the preferred option because it is cheap and easily cleaned.

Aggression is very common among neonatal lizards and snakes as part of the survival instinct. Providing enough space is therefore fundamental for them to thrive and decrease stress. The hatchlings should be separated if aggression is obvious. Separating the clutch into smaller groups not only decreases aggression but also helps monitor the health status of the group (weekly weight monitoring) and their appetite.

Feeding the Neonate

Hatchlings usually begin feeding within one and fourteen days of leaving the egg; most neonatal snakes do not eat until their first shed at about one to three weeks after hatching (Mader 2006). Appropriate feeding is critical for proper growth and development. The yolk provides nutrients for the first few days but proper food type and size is fundamental thereafter. A thorough understanding of the dietary requirements of the species is essential. Some species prey on particular species that are not commercially available, requiring "scenting" to train the neonate to eat alternate food items. This is accomplished by rubbing the proper food item (e.g. fish or frog) against the alternate food (e.g. rodent). Herbivore reptiles can be offered a mix of fresh vegetables, which should be finely chopped to the appropriate size. Insectivorous and carnivorous reptiles can be offered insects such as crickets, mealworms, grubs, wingless fruit flies, termites, slugs, small fish (guppies or comets), pinky mice, small lizards (anoles or geckos), small frogs (toads can be toxic), chick legs, hatchling quails, and mouse parts. In any case, the offered food item should never be larger than the width between the reptile's eyes; otherwise, it is potentially too large to be ingested.

The food nutritive value should be enhanced with commercially available vitamin and mineral supplements, and this is especially important for herbivores and insectivores species. There are two basic methods for vitamin/mineral enhancement: dusting and gut loading. Dusting implies sprinkling the supplement over the food item. This technique may decrease the palatability of the food item so careful monitoring is required to assure that the food is completely eaten. In the case of insects, if these are not ingested immediately they can self-groom and remove these powders and therefore decrease the supplement available for the reptile. Alternatively, an enriched media can be offered to these insects for a few days before being fed to the reptiles. This is called gut loading.

Assisted feeding may be required in cases of anorexia. This can be accomplished by the use of an appropriate-size stomach tube to deliver the food into the stomach. Commercially available foods or purees of appropriate food items (rodent parts, eggs, vegetables, etc.) can be used. Assisted feeding is provided by forceful placement of the food into the reptile's mouth. It can potentially damage the back of their mouth (oropharynx) and esophagus, and is stressful. Snakes can be stimulated to eat by using a technique called "slap feeding" by gently tapping the snake's nose with the food item. This tends to initiate a reflex in the snake to strike and grasp the food item (Mader 2006).

REFERENCES

APPA. 2007/2008. APPA's 2007/2008 National Pet Owners Survey.

Badaeva T, Malysheva D, et al. 2008. Genetic variation and de novo mutations in the parthenogenetic Caucasian rock lizard *Darevskia unisexualis*. *PLoS ONE* 3(7): e2730.

Benirschke K. 2007. Jackson's chamaleon *Chamaeleon jacksonii xantholophus*. In: Comparative Placentation, edited by Benirschke K. Ithaca, NY: International Veterinary Information Service.

Blackburn D. 1998. Structure, function, and evolution of the oviducts of squamate reptiles, with special reference to viviparity and placentation. *J Exp Zool* 282(4–5): 560–617.

Delmas V, Prevot-Julliard A-C, et al. 2008. A mechanistic model of temperature-dependent sex determination in a chelonian: the European pond turtle. *Funct Ecol* 22(1): 84–93.

Demas S, Duronslet M, et al. 1990. Sex-specific DNA in reptiles with temperature dependent sex determination. *J Exp Zool* 253: 319–324.

Denardo D. 2006. Reproductive biology. In: Reptile *Medicine and Surgery*, edited by Mader D. St Louis: Saunders Elsevier: 376–390.

Eti, turtles of the world. Temperature dependent sex determination. www.eti.uva.nl/turtles. ETI. Accessed October 8, 2009.

Funk R. 2002. Lizard reproductive medicine and surgery. *Vet Clin Exot Anim* 5(3): 579–613.

HSUS. 2001. The trade in live reptiles: Imports to the United States. Washington DC.

Innis C, Boyer T. 2002. Chelonian reproductive disorders. *Vet Clin Exot Anim* 5(3): 555–578.

Lance V, Valenzuela N, et al. 1992. A hormonal method to determine the sex of hatchling giant river turtles, *Podocnemis expansa*: application to endangered species research. *Amer Zool* 32: 16A.

Mader D. 2006. Perinatology. In: Reptile Medicine and Surgery, edited by Mader D. St. Louis: Saunders Elsevier: 365–375.

Owens D, Hendrickson J, et al. 1978. A technique for determining sex of immature Chelonia mydas using radioimmunoassay. *Herpetologica* 34: 270–273.

Radder R, Quinn A, et al. 2008. Genetic evidence for co-occurrence of chromosomal and thermal sex-determining systems in a lizard. *Biol Lett* 4(2): 176–178.

Rostal D, Grumbles J, et al. 1994. Non-lethal sexing techniques for hatchling and immature desert tortoises (*Gopherus agassizii*). *Herp Mono* 8: 83–87.

Sasa M, Curtis S. 2006. Field observation of mating behavior in the neck-banded snake *Scaphiodontophis annulatus* (Serpentes: Colubridae). *Rev Biol Trop* 54(2): 647–650.

Schramm B, Casares M, et al. 1999. Steroid levels and reproductive cycle of the Galapagos tortoise, *Geochelone nigra*, living under seminatural conditions on Santa Cruz Island (Galapagos). *Gen Comp Endocrinol* 114(1): 108–120.

Taylor E, Denardo D. 2005. Sexual size dimorphism and growth plasticity in snakes: an experiment on the western diamond-backed rattlesnake (*Crotalus atrox*). *J Exp Zool A Comp Exp Biol* 303(7): 598–607.

Wapstra E, Uller T, et al. 2008. Climate effects on offspring sex ration in a viviparous lizard. *J Anim Ecol.* Sep 22.

Warner D, Shine R. 2008. The adaptive significance of temperature-dependent sex determination in a reptile. *Nature* 451: 566–568.

Webb J, Shine R, et al. 2006. The adaptive significance of reptilian viviparity in the tropics: testing maternal manipulation hypothesis. *Evolution* 60(1): 115–160.

Wibbels T, Bull J, et al. 1991. Chronology and morphology of temperature dependent sex determination. *J Exp Zool* 260: 371–381.

Section 4
Amphibians

CHAPTER TEN

Amphibians

Brad Wilson

INTRODUCTION, TAXONOMY, AND NATURAL HISTORY

A fascination with amphibians has gripped mankind since the first recorded history. It continues today through scientific discoveries of remarkable healing and disease resistance properties of amphibian tissues, the discovery of potential therapeutic compounds in amphibian skin, and the understanding of potential human health consequences to environmental alteration. Interest in captive amphibians over the last two decades has increased tremendously and the knowledge gained regarding the husbandry, physiology, and breeding habits of many species has likely exceeded that of any other "exotic pet" group during this time period. Awareness of the demand for health care in these animals and the willingness of many clients to treat these pets has stimulated and necessitated a demand for more education by veterinarians and veterinary technicians.

Taxonomy

The biological saying "ontogeny recapitulates phylogeny" is most appropriately applied to the natural history of amphibians. The life cycle of the amphibian from egg to adult (ontogeny) is the abridged version of the monumental evolutionary adaptations of amphibians (phylogeny) that enabled the vertebrates to leave water and colonize the land 350 million years ago (Wright 2001e; Goin, Goin, and Zug 1978). Modern amphibians comprise more than 4,000 (Wright 2001g) species that are classified into three orders based on anatomic characteristics. The orders are listed with the modern accepted nomenclature followed by commonly used traditional nomenclature in parentheses: the caecilians, Gymnophiona (Apoda); the sirens, salamanders, and newts, Caudata (Meantes and Urodela); and the frogs and toads, Anura (Salientia). See table 10.1 for species commonly kept in captivity.

Amphibians of the order Gymnophiona, Caecilians, are uncommonly kept as pets and even less commonly observed clinically. Originating in the eastern and western tropics, caecilians may be terrestrial (yellow-striped caecilian, *Ichthyophis kohtaoensis*) or totally aquatic (*Typhlonectes compressicauda*) as adults. To many, caecilians resemble snakes or oversized earthworms. All known species are limbless with greatly reduced eyes. Some species are oviparous (egg-laying) and some are viviparous (live-bearing). All known species are carnivorous and consume various arthropods, annelids, or gastropods. Because of their secretive nature, it is likely that many species remain undiscovered. Longevity of captive caecilians is reported at nine years (Goin et al. 1978).

The order Caudata, tailed amphibians, consists of salamanders, newts, sirens, and amphiumas. Sirens were once classified in a separate order, Meantes (Trachystomata). The majority of species inhabit North America, with one species in Africa and no species in Australia or Antarctica (Goin et al. 1978, Duellman and Trueb 1994). Many species of all suborders are maintained as pets, though few are commercially available. Few species venture far from water or moist environs and most species require water for some portion of reproduction or development. Some species are fully aquatic, some facultatively aquatic, some terrestrial, and some American newts (*Notophthalmus viridescens*) are aquatic as larvae, terrestrial as juveniles, and aquatic again as adults. Salamanders are carnivorous as both larvae and adults and consume various arthropods, gastropods, arachnids, annelids, crustaceans, and other vertebrates including mammals. The longevity of salamanders is known to be up to fifty-five years for the Japanese giant salamander (*Adrias japonicus*) (Goin et al. 1978). Generally, the larger species have a longer lifespan than smaller species.

The order Anura, tailless amphibians, consists of frogs and toads. This order represents the great major-

Table 10.1. *Amphibians Commonly Kept in Captivity.*

Common name/ species name	Origin	Habitat	Size (cm)[1]	T/H[2]	Repro[3]	Feed[4]	Care[5]	Handling concerns[6]
Gymnophiona								
Yellow-striped, *Ichthyophis kohtoaensis*[7,13]	SE Asia	fossorial, tropical	50	25/mod	oviparous	an,ar	mod; large	docile, sturdy; escape
Aquatic caecilian, *Typhlonectes* spp.[7,13]	S America	aquatic, tropical	to 50	25	viviparous	an,ar	easy; medium	docile, sturdy; escape
Caudata								
Cryptobranchidae (Giant salamanders)								
Hellbender, *Cryptobranchus alleganiensis*[7]	N America	aquatic, temperate	to 75	15	oviparous	cr,ar,v	diff+; large+#	occas. aggressive, sturdy
Sirenidae (Sirens)								
Greater siren, *Siren lacertina*[7]	e N America	aquatic, temperate	80	20	oviparous	ar,cr,v	mod; large+	occas. aggressive, sturdy
Amphiumidae (Amphiumas)								
Amphiuma, *Amphiuma means*[7]	e N America	aquatic, temperate	to 100	20	oviparous	ar,cr,v	mod; large+	aggressive, sturdy
Proteidae (Neotenic salamanders)								
Mudpuppy, *Necturus maculosus*[7]	e N America	aquatic, temperate	40	15	oviparous	ar,cr,v,g	diff; large#	docile, sturdy
Ambystomatidae (Mole salamanders)								
Axolotl, *Ambystoma mexicanum*[7]	C America	aquatic, tropical	20	20	oviparous	ar,cr,v	easy; medium	aggressive, sturdy
Tiger salamander, *Ambystoma tigrinum*[7]	N America	terrestrial, fossorial	25	22/mod	oviparous	ar,an,v	easy; small	aggressive, sturdy
Waterdog, *Ambystoma tigrinum*[9]	N America	temporary aquatic; terrestrial	20	20	n/a	an,ar,cr,v	easy; small	aggressive, sturdy
Plethodontidae (Lungless salamanders)								
Arboreal salamander, *Aniedes lugubris*[10,11]	w N America	terr/arbor, temperate forest	10	14 to 17/ mod	oviparous	ar	mod; small	occas. aggressive, sturdy
Palm salamander, *Bolitoglossa* spp.[13]	C,S America	terr/arbor, tropical forest	8 to 14	14 to 20/ high	oviparous	t,ar	diff+; medium	docile, fragile
Ensatina, *Ensatina* spp.[10,11]	w N America	terrestrial, temperate forest	7	14 to 17/ mod	oviparous	ar	mod; small	docile, sturdy

Red salamanders, *Pseudotriton* spp.[11]	N America	semiaquatic, streams, forests	15	20/mod	oviparous	an,ar	mod; small	docile, sturdy
Anura								
Pipidae (Clawed frogs)								
Dwarf frog, *Hymenochirus curtipes*[8,13]	Africa	aquatic, tropical	4	25	oviparous	an,ar	easy; small	docile, sturdy
Surinam toad, *Pipa pipa*[8,13]	S America	aquatic, tropical	20	25	oviparous	v,an,ar	mod; large+	docile, sturdy
African clawed frog, *Xenopus laevis*[8,13]	Africa	aquatic, tropical	12	25	oviparous	v,an,ar	easy; medium	docile, sturdy
Pelobatidae (Spadefoot toads)								
Asian leaf frogs, *Megophrys* spp.[13]	SE Asia	terrestrial, tropical	to 15	20–22/mod	oviparous	ar,v	mod; medium	docile, sturdy
Bufonidae (True toads)								
Harlequin toads, *Atelopus* spp.[9]	C,S America	terrestrial, montane tropical	to 5	15–20/high	oviparous	ar,t	diff+; medium	docile, fragile
American toad, *Bufo americanus*[13]	N America	terrestrial, temperate	to 10	20/low	oviparous	ar,g,v	easy; medium	docile, sturdy
Marine toad, *Bufo marinus*[13]	C,S America	terrestrial, temp/tropical	23	22/low	oviparous	ar,g,v	easy; large	occas. aggressive, sturdy
Asian tree toads, *Pedostibes* spp.[13]	SE Asia	terrestrial, tropical	to 10	25 to 27/high	oviparous	t	diff; large	docile, fragile to sturdy
Microhylidae (Narrow mouth toads)								
Tomato frogs, *Dyscophus* spp.[8,13]	Madagascar	semiaquatic, tropical	to 10	25/mod	oviparous	ar	easy; medium	docile, sturdy
Malaysian toad, *Kaloula pulchra*[8,13]	SE Asia	terrestrial/fossorial, tropical	7	25/high	oviparous	ar,t	easy; medium	docile, sturdy
Dendrobatidae (Poison dart frogs)								
Dendrobates, Phyllobates, *Epipedobates* spp.[12,13]	C,S America	terrestrial, tropical	1.5 to 5	22 to 30/high	oviparous	ar,t	easy to diff; varies	occas. aggressive —see below
Hylidae (Tree frogs)								
Red-eyed treefrog, *Agalychnis callidryas*[14]	C America	arboreal, tropical	7	25/high	oviparous	ar	easy; medium	docile, sturdy
Green treefrog, *Hyla cinerea*[13]	N America	arboreal, temperate	6	25/mod	oviparous	ar	easy; medium	docile, sturdy
Monkey frogs, *Phyllomedusa* spp.[14]	C, S America	arboreal, tropical	to 10	25/low to mod	oviparous	ar	mod; med to lg	docile, sturdy

Table 10.1. Continued

Common name/ species name	Origin	Habitat	Size (cm)[1]	T/H[2]	Repro[3]	Feed[4]	Care[5]	Handling concerns[6]
White's treefrog, *Litoria caerulea*[7,14]	Australia	arboreal, desert/ forest	10	25/low to mod	oviparous	ar	easy; medium	docile, sturdy
Ranidae (True frogs)								
Mantellas, *Mantella* spp.[13]	Madagascar	terrestrial, tropical	3	18 to 22/ high	oviparous	ar,t	easy; small+	docile, fragile to sturdy
American bullfrog, *Rana catesbeiana*[13]	N America	semiaquatic, temperate	to 20	22/mod	oviparous	v,ar	easy; large+	aggressive, sturdy
African pyxie frog, *Pyxicephalus adspersus*[13]	Africa	semiaquatic, temperate	to 20	25/mod	oviparous	v,ar	easy; large+	aggressive, sturdy
Eyelash frog, *Ceratobatrachus guentheri*[13]	Solomon Islands	terrestrial, tropical	8	25/mod	oviparous	ar	mod; medium	docile, sturdy
Leptodactylidae (Tropical frogs)								
Surinam horned frog, *Ceratophrys cornuta*[13]	S America	terrestrial, tropical	20	25/mod	oviparous	v,ar	diff; medium	aggressive, sturdy
Ornate horned frog, *Ceratophrys ornata*[13]	S America	terrestrial, tropical	12	25/mod	oviparous	v,ar	easy; medium	aggressive, sturdy

[1] Average maximum adult size.

[2] Average day temperature/relative humidity for adults of species or typical of genus in captivity.

[3] Oviparous (ovi-) = egg laying; viviparous (vivi-) = live birth.

[4] Diet of the adult amphibian *in nature* listed in order of importance for each species: *an* = annelids; *ar* = arthropods; *cr* = crustaceans; *g* = gastropods; *t* = termites and ants; *v* = vertebrates. Many animals will adapt to domestically raised food items.

[5] Difficulty for captive maintenance of wild-caught and some captive-born animals. (Generally, captive-born animals adapt well with proper conditions.) Second value is minimum terrarium size. *Easy* = adapts well to terrarium; *moderate* = specialized feeding, temperature, housing required; *difficult* = only most experienced keepers; *difficult+* = should only be attempted by zoological parks. *Small* = 10 gallon terrarium; *medium* = 15 to 20 gallon terrarium; *large* = 30 gallon terrarium; *large+* = 55 gallon or specially constructed; # = may require chilled water.

[6] Typical response of patient to handling (all animals will resist handling): *Docile* = will not attempt to bite, no special defenses. All caecilians may escape; terrarium must be well sealed. *Occasionally aggressive* = may attempt to bite, but generally will not cause injury to handler. Can bite and seriously damage or kill cage mates. Avoid skin or direct/indirect mucous membrane contact with wild-caught dart frogs and all marine toads. *Aggressive* = species that will routinely bite as defense (Amphiuma) or conditioned feeding response (mole salamanders) or will attempt to eat any cage mates (frogs, mole salamanders). Amphiumas, pyxie frogs, and horned frogs must be approached and handled with caution; bites from adult animals may cut skin and may be painful. *Fragile* = amphibians that may be easily stressed, damaged, or killed by handling. *Sturdy* = amphibians that are not likely damaged from responsible handling.

[7] Wright (2001g, 3–14).

[8] Mattison (1987).

[9] Lotters (1996).

[10] Stebbins (1985).

[11] Petranka (1998).

[12] Walls (1994).

[13] Obst et al. (1988).

[14] de Vosjoli (1996).

ity of all species of modern amphibians and the majority of captive amphibians. A great number of species are available in the pet trade as captive-born animals. Frogs are to amphibians as lizards are to reptiles. Frogs have managed to adapt to and to populate many terrestrial, arboreal, and aquatic (and even several flying or gliding) habitats on earth. Adaptation and specialization of skin, diet, and reproductive strategy have all made this expansion possible. Several species of frogs are totally aquatic and several are adapted to estivate in the driest deserts for months or years. All adult frogs are carnivorous and the majority of their larvae, tadpoles, are herbivorous. Some tadpoles are omnivorous and some are carnivorous. Adult frogs feed on many insects, crustaceans, annelids, and other vertebrates, and some species are specialized to feed primarily on other frogs (*Ceratophrys* spp., *Hemiphractus* spp.). The known longevity for some species is up to thirty-six years (Goin et al. 1978).

Amphibians begin development as fertilized eggs, and with most species the eggs hatch into free-swimming gilled larvae, and then the larvae metamorphose into adults. The post-hatching larvae depend upon a moist environment such as water, inside a gelatinous terrestrial egg (some species undergo direct development and metamorphose to adults inside the eggs), inside a brooding adaptation of the parent (Gastrotheca cornuta and Pipa pipa), or inside a uterus-like oviduct (some amphibians are live-bearing or viviparous). Not all amphibian larvae require standing water to complete development. Similarly, all adult amphibians do not depend on standing water to reproduce, though traditionally most amphibians do return to water both to mate and to disperse eggs. Some amphibians are entirely aquatic and cannot survive out of water for any extended periods of time, whereas others inhabit deserts or may estivate for extended period (years) with no exogenous water. Completely aquatic amphibians are represented in all three families. Some salamanders are neotenic, in which metamorphosis to the typical adult form never occurs yet the larvae develop gonads internally and the larvae are capable of reproduction.

Though most numerous in temperate to tropical environments, amphibians are distributed worldwide. Frogs are found among nearly every habitat on earth except the open ocean and Antarctica. Particularly interesting among the frogs is their colonization of harsh deserts. Adaptation for desert environments is most widespread among the frogs of Australia as seen in both terrestrial (*Arenophryne rotunda*) (Mattison 1987) and arboreal (*Litoria* spp.) species and among the South African terrestrial species (*Breviceps* spp.).

Several South American species (*Atelopus* spp.) are adapted to cool elevations well over 10,000 feet (Lotters 1996) and some species of North American frogs (*Rana sylvatica*) are known to freeze solid during hibernation and then thaw following winter to resume normal physiology (Duellman and Trueb 1994, Mattison 1987, Stebbins 1985).

The veterinary technician should be familiar with herpetological scientific nomenclature and common terminology. It is not uncommon that scientific order, family, or group names of both plants and animals may be modified for use in general conversation or popular and scientific publications. For instance, when speaking of the three orders of amphibians, frogs and toads (Anura) are commonly called anurans. Salamanders (Caudata) are called caudates. In the salamanders and frogs the family names are commonly modified when discussing several of the larger families: the mole salamanders (Ambystomatidae) are ambystomatids, the lungless salamanders (Plethodontidae) are plethodontids, the poison dart frogs (Dendrobatidae) are dendrobatids, the tree frogs (Hylidae) are hylids, the true toads (Bufonidae) are bufonids, and so on.

A great deal of this chapter focuses on frogs. This is due to the fact that frogs are, by far, the most popular and widespread amphibian group in the pet industry. Much of the medicine, anesthesia, and surgery techniques applied to frogs are extrapolated to all amphibians. The general discussion of amphibian medicine focuses on metamorphosed juvenile and adult amphibians with a separate general discussion of larvae. The husbandry and disorders of larvae can differ significantly from the adults of some species.

ANATOMY AND PHYSIOLOGY

General anatomy is similar across all three orders of amphibians and is discussed as applies to all amphibians. Anatomical specializations and clinically significant differences in anatomy are described for the three orders. Physiology varies tremendously, even among genera and species of the same order, and clinically significant differences are noted in the following discussion.

Integument
The evolutionary development of amphibian skin is one of the greatest adaptations that enabled vertebrates to leave the water and exist on land. The epidermal layer of amphibian skin is shed routinely (ecdysis) in a manner consistent with that of lizards and snakes. Ecdysis may occur piecemeal or entirely,

and some caecilians, frogs, and salamanders consume the shed skin—a process called keratophagy or dermatophagy. The dermis layers of skin serve a respiratory function and are highly vascularized. Some caecilians possess small scales that are embedded in the skin (Goin et al. 1978, Duellman and Trueb 1994).

The respiratory function of amphibian skin is particularly important for larvae, adult caecilians, most adult salamanders, and many frogs. Several species of amphibians and one family of salamanders (Plethodontidae) have absent or greatly reduced lungs and rely on cutaneous respiration for the majority of oxygen and carbon dioxide exchange. The hellbenders (*Cryptobranchus* spp.) and giant Asian salamanders (*Adrias* spp.), both of which are aquatic, have well developed lateral skin folds which increase surface area for cutaneous gas exchange. An interesting behavior exhibited by *Cryptobranchus* spp. is a rocking motion in which the salamander sways the body from side to side in slow moving or poorly oxygenated water, presumably to "ventilate" the skin (Duellman and Trueb 1994, Petranka 1998).

The amphibian epidermis is rich with glands. Some epidermal glands produce secretions that moisten the skin to facilitate cutaneous respiration and some frogs (*Phyllomedusa* spp.) secrete waxy substances that protect against dehydration and dessication (Wright 2001b). Poison glands are present in all salamanders and frogs. These are most notable among the poison dart frogs (Dendrobatidae) of Central and South America and toads worldwide. Of all amphibians the skin secretions of *Phyllobates terribilis*, the golden dart frog of Colombia, are the most toxic (Walls 1994). The Chaco Indians of Columbia use skin secretions of three species of *Phyllobates* to coat blow darts used to hunt monkeys, hence the common family name of these frogs. Of the 170 species of Dendrodatidae, only *P. terribilis* is considered lethal to man from simply touching the toxin. Interestingly, wild-caught dart frogs of all species fed domestic diets in captivity and frogs born in captivity lose the majority of their skin toxins (Daly et al. 1994).

Several species of toads and salamanders possess large parotid glands dorsally on the head, just caudal to the skull. These glands are elliptical and commonly the site of profuse toxin excretion. Skin toxins from many frogs and toads are dangerous to domestic animals such as dogs and cats. The author has observed a 20-kg Labrador Retriever suffer violent vomiting, diarrhea, and convulsions following the accidental ingestion of a Cuban treefrog (*Osteopilus septentrionalis*). Anecdotal reports exist of deaths in dogs and cats following exposure to or ingestion of toxic secre-

tions of marine toads (*Bufo marinus*). In general, all terrestrial frogs and toads should be considered potentially dangerous to dogs and cats. Other captive amphibians that should be considered toxic include the European salamander (*Salamandra salamandra*), the American newt (*Notophthalmus viridescens*), and some mole salamanders (*Ambystoma* spp.).

Many of the more toxic amphibians exhibit aposematic coloration and are conspicuous or active by day. Animals that exhibit aposematic or warning colors rely on a learned response of the potential predator to avoid interaction with the particular animal or suffer distasteful or noxious stimuli. Some of the commonly observed aposematically colored amphibians include the European salamander (*Salamandra salamandra*), the red eft phase of the American newt (*Notophthalmus viridescens*), red salamanders (*Pseudotriton* spp.), some poison dart frogs (Dendrobatidae), some harlequin frogs (*Atelopus* spp.), the golden mantella (*Mantella aurantiaca*), and the semi-aquatic fire-bellied toads (*Bombina* spp.). As with some insects and snakes, mimicry in coloration occurs in several "non-toxic" species that co-occur with more toxic species.

Several species of frogs possess unique skin adaptations for raising young. The aquatic female Surinam toad (*Pipa pipa*) carries eggs on her back over several months during which time the eggs invaginate into the skin and undergo direct development into juvenile frogs. Upon hatching the juvenile frogs swim out of the holes in the skin, ending parental care. Another female South American frog, the marsupial frog (*Gastrotheca* spp.), possesses a pouch on the dorsum in which eggs hatch into tadpoles (or undergo direct development in some species) and are then released into a suitable aquatic habitat.

Skeletal System

The skeleton of amphibians is comprised of both an endoskeleton and exoskeleton that is ossified. Exoskeleton is bone formed in the dermis that fuses with underlying endoskeleton and is most notable in the skull of amphibians, particularly in frogs and toads. The amphibian skeletal system has three functions: protection, locomotion, and support for terrestrial existence. A major adaptation for locomotion on land is the development of pelvic and pectoral girdles. These are absent in caecilians, but well developed in most salamanders and all frogs. Great variation of the appendicular skeleton exists among species of frogs and toads. In most frogs and some salamanders the hyoid bones are modified to eject the tongue for prehension of prey (Figures 10.1, 10.2).

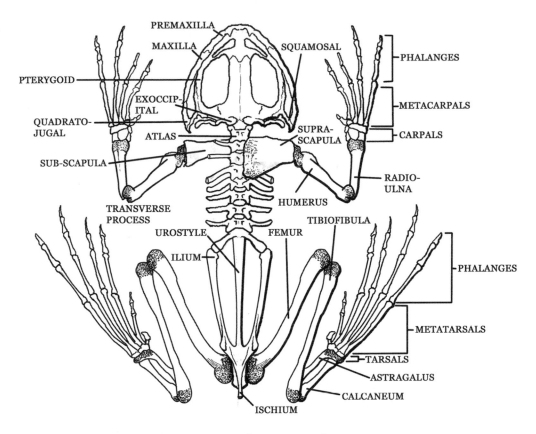

Figure 10.1. Skeletal anatomy of a frog. (Drawing by Scott Stark.)

Digestive System

All adult amphibians are carnivorous and have a digestive tract similar to that of higher carnivorous vertebrates and similar among the three orders of amphibians. The oral cavity of salamanders and frogs is spacious and generally designed for capturing and swallowing whole prey items. A fleshy tongue is present in most species. Aquatic salamanders have a primary fish-like tongue and aquatic frogs (Pipidae) have no tongue (Goin et al. 1978). Amphibian teeth are replaced through life when lost (Goin et al. 1978, Duellman and Trueb 1994).

Prehension of prey may occur by one of several modalities in amphibians: suction, hellbender (*Cryptobranchus* spp.) and Surinam toad (*Pipa pipa*); ambush or direct pounce and capture, mole salamanders (*Ambystoma* spp.) and toads (*Bufo* spp.); luring and capture, horned frogs (*Ceratophrys* spp.); foraging and prehension with tongue, palm salamanders (*Bolitoglossa* spp.) and dart frogs (*Dendrobates* spp.); and scavenging, *Amphiuma* spp., *Siren* spp., and aquatic caecilians (*Typhlonectes* spp.) (Helfman 1990).

The esophagus, stomach, small intestine, and large intestine are similar to those of higher vertebrates. The cloaca is homologous to that of reptiles. The pancreas and gall bladder are present and aid in digestion. The liver serves to convert ammonia into nitrogenous waste products, primarily urea. In at least one frog species, the Australian gastric brooding frogs, *Rheobatrachus* spp., the female ingests the fertilized eggs into the stomach where the eggs hatch into tadpoles and then metamorphose into juvenile frogs. During the brooding period all digestive secretions are stopped in these species (Duellman and Trueb 1994) (Figure 10.3).

Respiratory System

Amphibians exhibit four modalities of respiration: branchial, buccopharyngeal, cutaneous, and pulmonic (Wright 2001c). Adult salamanders use the four modes of respiration; adult caecilians and frogs do not use the branchial mode. In most amphibians the left and right lungs are of equal size. Some caecilians have a greatly reduced or absent left lung, as observed in snakes.

Branchial or gill respiration is present in free-swimming larvae of all amphibians and in neotenic or aquatic salamanders. Those species with external gills may exhibit varying degrees of gill development dependent upon environmental conditions such as dissolved

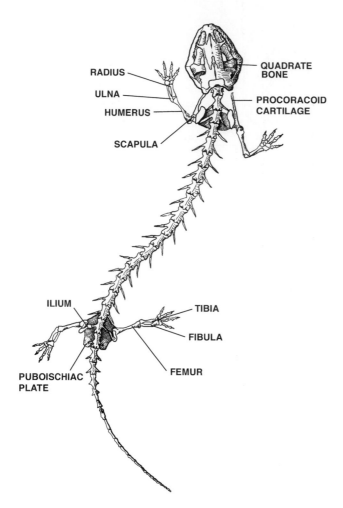

Figure 10.2. Salamander skeletal anatomy. (Drawing by Scott Stark.)

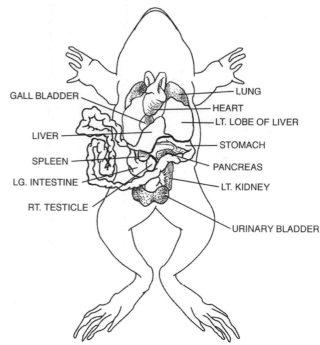

Figure 10.3. Visceral anatomy of a frog. (Drawing by Scott Stark.)

oxygen. In more stagnant oxygen-deprived environments the gills are larger to increase oxygen-absorbing surface area. In well-oxygenated water, the gills are typically smaller. Some aquatic species (Sirenidae, Proteidae, Pipidae) may rely more on buccopharyngeal and pulmonic respiration by gulping air when oxygen content is critically low. Cutaneous respiration is discussed in the Integument section.

Buccopharyngeal respiration is primarily driven by air gulping in aquatic species and gular or buccal pumping in terrestrial species. Atmospheric air is pulled in through the nostrils to the nasopharynx and oral cavity by negative pressure during buccal expansion and then driven out by the collapse of the gular skin. Oxygen exchange occurs through the thin-walled buccopharyngeal capillaries. This pumping action also drives both inspiratory and expiratory pulmonic respiration in terrestrial amphibians. Buccopharyngeal gas exchange in amphibians is analogous to that of

some freshwater air-gulping fishes such as the electric eel (*Electrophorus electricus*) and the lungfishes (*Protopterus* spp. and *Lepidosiren* spp.).

All terrestrial amphibians, except salamanders of Plethodontidae, which do not have lungs, use pulmonic respiration. Amphibian lungs are sac-like, with alveoli most well developed in the Anurans. The lungs of some aquatic amphibians serve as hydrostatic or buoyancy organs in addition to the respiratory function (Wright 2001c).

Vocalization is best developed in frogs, but is also observed in caecilians and salamanders of various species. Frogs are the only order of amphibians in which anatomic vocal structures are well developed and in which vocalization is known to serve as communication for mating, territorial defense, and escape from predators (Duellman and Trueb 1994). Vocalization is unique for every species and is also present in aquatic species. Males are the most vocal of the sexes, but females of some species have "distress calls" which are used when escaping predators or "release calls" to signal males when the female is unreceptive during opportunistic breeding congregations.

Excretory System

The kidney of amphibians is mesonephric and empties into a urinary bladder. The urinary bladder of some amphibians may be bilobate. As in reptiles, urine is collected by the Wolffian duct (mesonephric duct in amphibians, metanephric duct in reptiles) and then routed to the cloaca and not the urinary bladder. Urine passes retrograde from the cloaca into the urinary bladder (Goin et al. 1978).

Nitrogenous wastes of primarily aquatic amphibians are excreted as ammonia, whereas many terrestrial amphibians secrete urinary wastes as urea or uric acid. This conversion of ammonia to urea and uric acid conserves water for terrestrial amphibians and reduces the toxicity of ammonia in the blood. Frogs of the genus Phyllomedusa are uricotelic, being able to convert urea to uric acid for excretion (Wright 2001c).

Reproductive System

Amphibians have paired internal gonads that are hormonally regulated. Collecting ducts (oviducts in female) transport gametes to the cloaca where they are expelled from the body. Viviparous species are present in all three orders and the larvae undergo metamorphosis in the oviduct of the female and are born as fully functional juveniles. Fat bodies are located adjacent to the gonads of all amphibians and are presumed to provide nutrient stores for developing gametes. These bodies enlarge during non-breeding season and are greatly diminished at the end of breeding season.

The testes of frogs are collection of seminiferous tubules connected to the mesonephric ducts by collecting ducts. Frogs exhibit the greatest organizational structure of seminiferous tubules among the amphibians. The testes (and ovaries) enlarge dramatically in response to breeding season. Copulation is observed in all caecilians but only one species of frog, and fertilization is internal in these species. Fertilization for all other frogs is external. Interestingly, fertilization for all but two families of salamanders (Hynobiidae and Cryptobranchidae) is internal with no copulation. Male salamanders secrete a jellylike substance in the cloaca that encases the sperm, the spermatophore, and expel this structure during breeding. The female salamander collects the spermatophore in the cloaca and fertilization occurs internally. Fertilization is internal in only a few frogs.

The amphibian ovaries are located in proximity to the kidneys as seen in higher vertebrates. Following ovulation ova are contained within a thin membrane, the ovisac, which ruptures and releases eggs into the coelom. Eggs are funneled into the ostium of the oviduct by cilia lining the coelomic mesentery and then passed to the cloaca to be expelled into the environment. The lining of the oviduct of viviparous caecilians is consumed by developing larvae as nourishment during development. In oviparous species the oviducts serve to store or hold eggs until spawning occurs. In salamanders a diverticulum of the dorsal wall of the cloaca forms the spermatheca, which stores collected sperm to fertilize eggs upon spawning.

Amphibians, especially frogs, exhibit tremendous adaptation in parental care of developing eggs and larvae. These adaptations are discussed throughout the various sections and more specifically in the Behavior section.

Cardiovascular System

The cardiovascular system is comprised of a three-chambered heart, arteries, veins, and lymphatics. The heart of Siren intermedia and Necturus maculosus contains an interventricular septum, making a four-chambered heart (Goin et al. 1978). As with reptiles, oxygenated and deoxygenated blood mixes minimally in the common ventricle.

The three orders of amphibians exhibit great variation in the development of aortic arch vasculature. A prominent ventral abdominal vein is present in amphibians as in reptiles. This is the vein of choice for blood collection in large frogs or toads. In salamanders not capable of tail autotomy (release of the tail when stressed), blood can be sampled from the ventral tail vein as described for snakes and lizards. Many frogs can also be sampled from the ventral lingual plexus in the mouth (see Techniques).

Lymphatics and lymphatic circulation is well developed in amphibians. All blood cells and proteins except erythrocytes are found in amphibian lymph. Lymph hearts that beat synchronously and independently of the cardia control lymph circulation. Diagnostic samples may be retrieved lymph sacs, which are found in various locations of the body. Most notable of these are paired lymphatic sacs in the skin dorsal and caudal to the pelvis in frogs.

Amphibian blood and tissue fluids have a lower osmolality (200 to 250 mOsm) than mammals (300 mOsm) (Wright 2001c). Thus, isotonic fluids used for mammals are hypertonic to amphibians and result in dehydration of the amphibian patient with long-term exposure. Mammalian saline is 0.9% NaCl. A 0.6% NaCl solution is most appropriate for use with amphibians.

Nervous System

The amphibian nervous system is modified from that of fish with the enlargement of the cerebral hemispheres and the development of more complex neural networks in the spinal cord for the innervation pectoral and pelvic limbs. A withdrawal response is observed in amphibians as a result of trauma such as damage to limbs and toes.

Sense Organs

Amphibian eyes, though not as highly adapted as those of reptiles for complete terrestrial existence, are greatly modified from the eyes of most fish. Movable eyelids and lacrimal glands to moisten the eye are among the most notable adaptations. The eyelids are not present in amphibian larvae, most aquatic amphibians, and the neotenic axolotl. A third eyelid or nictitating membrane is present in many terrestrial frogs. It is similar to the same membrane of dogs and cats and its closure is passive, being achieved by contraction of the retractor bulbi muscle followed by withdrawal of the eye into the eye socket. A portion of the levator bulbi muscle actively controls retraction of the third eyelid back to its resting position.

The amphibian auditory system, while anatomically and physiologically interesting, has relatively little clinical significance. Jacobson's organ, the vomeronasal organ, is present in amphibians, but is much less developed than in snakes and lizards. This sense organ is suspected to function in food recognition and in plethodontid salamanders (and possibly other genera) is thought to function for pheromone detection during courtship and mating.

HUSBANDRY

A basic understanding of the life history requirements of the amphibian species in question (or extrapolated from a closely related species) is needed to gain a thorough history and develop a diagnostic and treatment plan for amphibians. Even among different related species of amphibians, however, there may be dramatic diversity of environmental needs within a single genus. These differences are particularly evident among the genera of Dendrobatidae (*Dendrobates*, *Ameerga*, *Ranitomeya*, *Excitobates*, *Phyllobates*, *Epipedobates*) and the genera *Atelopus* and *Mantella*. The Dendrobatids are a diverse and geographically widespread group occurring from sea level to 2,600 m elevation; some species are terrestrial, some are entirely arboreal; some are 1.5 cm as adults, some are more than 5 cm (Walls 1994). Similarly, the Atelopids have species groups that are termed highland (2,600 to 4,500 m) or lowland (<1,000 m) (Lotters 1996). If a highland species is maintained as a lowland species or vice-versa, the frog will fail to thrive and typically perish within days. Similar though less extreme environmental diversity is seen among *Mantella* spp. (Staniszewski 1997).

Many of the natural history related criteria for evaluating lizards (see Chapter 3) apply to amphibians. The following list highlights the more pertinent information with which the technician and clinician should be familiar for a given species:

1. Origin of the captive patient: Is the patient captive-born or wild-caught? For the more common species in captivity, know which of these are more likely caught in the wild or propagated in captivity.
2. Preferred microhabitat: Is the patient fossorial, terrestrial, arboreal, aquatic, or semi-aquatic? What is the preferred air and/or water temperature of the patient? What is the preferred humidity of the patient?
3. Behavior: At what time of day is the patient active in normal health? Does the patient exhibit seasonal behavioral patterns such as hibernation? Does the patient exhibit certain defensive postures or behaviors when stressed or threatened?
4. Diet: What is the patient's preferred food in nature and what food items is it known to consume in captivity? What is the preferred size of food item? Is the patient an aggressive feeder that may attack or consume cage mates? At what time of day or night does the patient feed in habitat? What is the normal feeding behavior of the species in question?
5. Anatomy and physiology: What is the anatomy of the normal healthy patient, including size or coloration differences between sexes of a given species? Are certain physical characteristics seasonally variable? Is the patient potentially toxic to cage mates?

The diversity of species' environmental adaptations necessitates this knowledge of amphibians even more than among the lizards, snakes, tortoises, and terrapins. Unfortunately, the majority of amphibian diseases progress rapidly or have a narrow window of treatment, making the speed of diagnosis and treatment critical.

The greatest progress in successfully maintaining amphibians in captivity, particularly with the frogs, may be attributed to an understanding of the captive environment for each species. As with many reptiles, success with captive maintenance and breeding of amphibians has improved dramatically in the last ten to fifteen years through the research and experimentation of zookeepers and private hobbyists.

Enclosures and Environment

The four basic generalized amphibian cage designs are arboreal, terrestrial, semi-aquatic, and aquatic. On occasion a mix of these designs is appropriate for some animals and each design may be slightly modified to house a particular species. With each of these habitats, there may be dramatic variation between species with regard to temperature and humidity in any given environment. With many species in their permanent enclosure, effort is made to somewhat reproduce the natural environment to reduce stress and increase adaptability. Once again, having fundamental natural history knowledge of the patient is essential.

The health of the captive amphibian may be directly proportional to the "health" of the terrarium. Certain characteristics apply to all amphibian enclosures. These include security from escape; visual and noise security; refuges for hiding; substrate; and the environmental parameters of lighting, temperature, humidity, ventilation, and water quality.

Security to prevent escape is of primary importance. The most elaborate climate-controlled naturalistic enclosure is of no help to the dried out carcass of an amphibian on the floor of a room. The evolutionary development of legs has greatly improved the ability for escape by amphibians when compared to fish; some of the most escape-prone amphibians, however, are the legless caecilians and the sirens and amphiumas, both of which have reduced limbs. Many fish enthusiasts can attest to similar escapes with eels, ropefish, lungfish, and other anguiform fish species. Though many aquatic and semi-aquatic amphibians perish in the dry environment of a climate controlled room, some, if they find suitable moist habitat elsewhere in the room, can survive quite well outside their intended enclosure. Barnett et al. (2001) mentions the placement of "moist oases" along the walls of such rooms to prevent dessication in case an escape occurs. These may be plastic containers lined with moistened moss and an adequate opening for entry.

Visual, noise, and vibration security is essential for many species. With the exception of the most dominant or aggressive species (*Ceratophrys* spp., *Pyxicephalus* spp., large *Bufo* spp., large Ranidae spp., some *Ambystoma* spp., *Amphiuma* spp.), many amphibians rely on camouflage or escape as the first defense. Thus, when threatened, many frogs attempt escape by jumping. Most enclosures are not of adequate size to prevent collision with the cage walls and the collisions may stimulate further escape behavior. Similar evasion may be seen with some salamanders and many aquatic amphibians, though salamanders typically seek retreats or subterranean refuge. Physical trauma, however, may not be as significant as the stress created and the resultant maladaptation to a captive environment without adequate cover.

Visual security is provided by both internal and external cage design. Painting the external surfaces of the terrarium or applying other external visual barriers is helpful to prevent incessant escape attempts through the cage walls and to reduce sudden visual stimulation from movements outside the enclosure. Certain cage ornaments, accessories, and artificial or live plants are applied inside the cage for refuge and visual security. Clean plastic pots, sections of PVC pipe, the bases of plastic soda bottles, cork bark, sticks or logs, and rocks are all valuable as refuges. Though less natural, the benefit of plastic refuges is that they are easily cleaned or sterilized for reuse. Cork bark may be autoclaved (if an autoclave is available), though it is not recommended to use certain detergents, ammonia, or bleach on any natural or porous cage accessories for amphibians. Soaking organic items in clean, fresh water for several hours may be required to remove cleaning agent residues. Dried hardwood leaves are an excellent renewable refuge for salamanders and smaller frogs. It is also possible to clean these items with diluted bleach solution prior to use.

Understanding the behavior of a species in nature is helpful to proper cage design. Many arboreal frogs, for example, will not use substrate-interfaced or many horizontally oriented refuges but instead require vertically suspended flat leaves (*Agalychnis* spp., *Hyla* spp.) or horizontal branches (*Phyllomedusa* spp.) for resting. Similarly, terrestrial salamanders typically do not benefit from vertically spacious, heavily planted terrariums, though the terrestrial cover provided by such plantings may be beneficial for reducing ground lighting. Larger terrestrial amphibians such as marine toads and mole salamanders seem particularly fond of artificial refuges in a terrarium and regularly return to these areas when inactive. Aquatic caudates such as *Cryptobranchus* spp. and *Necturus* spp. occur in fast moving coldwater streams and require large rocks, logs, or other submerged refuges to escape the currents. Often these animals also forage for food in these microhabitats because many food items similarly use the refuges to avoid strong currents.

Certain plants provide ideal refuges for some caudates and anurans. Bromeliads are an ideal tropical enclosure plant for smaller hylids, some dendrobatids, and the tropical *Bolitoglossa* spp. Some bromeliads, however, may have sharp defensive spines that can prove perilous to many amphibians and their owners. Many smaller aroids (peace lilies, *Spathiphyllum* spp.) are ideal for treefrogs. (Gagliardo, personal communication). Large terrestrial amphibians are best maintained in terrariums that are sparsely planted or contain large sturdy plants. Marine toads, horned frogs, tiger salamanders, and large ranids are quite capable of trampling and eventually killing all but the sturdiest plants in a terrarium. In similar fashion, larger aquatic amphibians (all aquatics except dwarf aquatic frogs and newts) uproot or damage planted aquatic terrariums in a matter of minutes to hours, though these species typically benefit from copious floating or suspended aquatic vegetation.

Plants for the terrarium are selected based on utility and aesthetic quality. Consideration must be given to the possibility for introduction of harmful pesticides, fertilizers, detergents, and potential pathogens. All plants, regardless of their origin, should be cleaned of all soil and thoroughly washed before planting. Furthermore, plants from one established amphibian enclosure should never be moved to another amphibian enclosure to reduce the risk of parasite or other disease transmission to uninfected or otherwise unexposed animals. This must be strictly observed for plants originating from any enclosures containing wild-caught amphibians. Avoid using plants that originate in regions where there are known frog populations inhabiting or contacting the plants.

Basic requirements of an ideal soil-type substrate are a slowly degradable, well drained, well aerated, slightly moisture retentive soil that is free of pesticides, fertilizers, or other potentially toxic chemicals. These soils, though all organic, contain many non-traditional components which include horticultural grade charcoal, orchid bark, tree fern or palm trunk fiber, milled sphagnum, and some peat. Generally this substrate is adapted from epiphytic orchid or tropical pitcher plant (*Nepenthes* spp.) soil mixes that are designed to be well drained and aerated (Gagliardo, personal communication). The author has maintained several larger well-planted terrariums of dart frogs with these soil mixes for more than years with no soil changing. This soil type is best used for dart frogs, harlequin toads, mantellas, hylids, and other arboreal species requiring a well-planted enclosure.

The major benefit derived of this soil type is for the maintenance of plants in the enclosure. An invariable outcome of most peat based or ready-made houseplant soil mixes in terrariums is rapid decomposition, compaction, and inadequate aeration. As this process progresses, the roots of plants die and the plants fail to thrive. Eventually the health of the entire terrarium deteriorates and animals fail to thrive. The bark/charcoal/peat mix requires a longer time period (two to three years) for decomposition and rarely, if ever, compacts in the terrarium. A disadvantage to the "*Nepenthes* mix", however, is that it cannot be used for burrowing species of amphibians. The bark, char-

coal, and tree fern are all potentially abrasive to amphibian skin. This does not appear to create a problem for most small (<5 cm) terrestrial frogs or toads, but can be irritating to larger frogs and some salamanders.

Another soil suitable for substrate is composted leaf litter that is free of fertilizers, pesticides, or other chemicals. This is particularly useful for salamanders and burrowing frogs. Commercially available topsoil preparations must be used with caution because they may contain chemical additives.

Proper lighting of a terrarium raises many questions regarding the light needs of amphibians. Generally, the specific requirements of ultraviolet light (particularly UV-B required for the synthesis of vitamin D_3) are unknown for amphibians (Barnett 1996). Histopathology studies of several Panamanian amphibians (*Gastrotheca cornuta*, *Hemiphractus fasciatus*) indicate that metabolic bone disease occurs in these species (personal observation). Certainly, questions arise regarding the requirements of nocturnal, fossorial, or fully aquatic amphibians. For terrariums containing live plants, attempts are made to simulate natural sunlight so that the plants will thrive. The incidental effects of this lighting scheme on amphibians may be beneficial. As with most terrestrial vertebrates some light is required for vision and photoperiodic behavior.

The amphibian owner should attempt to recreate the lighting scheme of the amphibian in nature. In general, most terrestrial salamanders and nocturnal frogs do not require bright lighting and may avoid it altogether. A natural method to reduce lighting on the cage floor is a well-planted terrarium with full spectrum lighting. It is not unusual for some nocturnal hylids to rest on leaves or branches that are exposed to full sun during some part of the day (White's treefrog, *Litoria caerulea*; green treefrog, *Hyla cinerea*). Therefore, suitable basking sites should be provided for these species. Light fixtures are suitably placed above the enclosure, preferably within 46 cm (18 inches) of the cage floor (Barnett et al. 2001). It is important to note that ultraviolet radiation does not penetrate plastic and glass; thus, any lids that may shield the light should be replaced with screen. Unfortunately, screen also diffuses the penetration of UV radiation into an enclosure (author, personal observation). Also, when a full aquarium hood is used as lid and light source for the enclosure, a tight fit is essential to prevent escape of the inhabitants.

Commercially available full-spectrum lights for terrariums are available as fluorescent tube, coiled compact fluorescent, mercury vapor, and compact halogen. Most, if not all, of the incandescent lights available for aquariums and terrariums do not produce adequate UV-B radiation despite packaging claims. Additionally, because most incandescent bulbs produce copious heat, they should be used with caution for amphibian enclosures. Many brands of full-spectrum lights are available for both plants and animals, each with their own claims of benefits. To date, coiled compact fluorescent, mercury vapor, and compact halogen lights are the best producers of UV-B radiation.

Temperature, humidity, and ventilation for the terrarium are all interrelated and their control and management often dictates cage design more than any other environmental parameter. As many fish hobbyists can attest, the larger the aquarium the easier it is to manage temperature. The same is true for terrariums. This is particularly true for humidity and ventilation. Surprising to many, amphibians as a group inhabit a wide variety of climates from the equator to the Arctic Circle. Caecilians and salamanders are somewhat less adapted to extreme climates than are frogs. Thus, discussion of the more extreme temperature and humidity requirements primarily pertain to certain species of anurans. Some species of amphibians require seasonal cooling to stimulate ovulation and spermatogenesis for breeding. Knowledge of the specific patient's natural history with regard to environmental parameters is essential.

Enclosure temperature for many amphibian patients is controlled by room temperature. The great majority of amphibians can adapt to normal household room temperature of 25°C to 30°C (75°F to 85°F), though there are some exceptions. Most highland tropical frogs (*Atelopus* spp. and some *Mantella* spp.) as well as most North American salamanders fail to thrive for extended periods at temperatures above 21°C to 24°C (70°F to 75°F) (Lotters 1996, Staniszewski 1997, Obst et al. 1988). The Pacific giant salamander (*Dicamptodon ensatus*), the hellbender (*Cryptobranchus alleganiensis*), and the mudpuppy (*Necturus maculosus*) may all require refrigerated water or air conditioning throughout the year. Aquatic species such as the Surinam toad (*Pipa pipa*) and the African dwarf frog (*Hymenochirus* spp.) require heated water with protected submersible aquarium heaters.

Supplemental heating the terrestrial amphibian enclosure is generally not required, though some species of frogs and toads benefit from basking lights or heat sources such as incandescent lights or ceramic heaters. These species include some toads, monkey frogs (*Phyllomedusa* spp.), and White's treefrogs (*Litoria* spp.). Most diurnal frogs (Dendrobatids,

Atelopids, Mantellids) typically do not require basking areas in the terrarium. Avoid heating enclosures with hot rocks or heating elements with which amphibians can make direct contact to prevent dessication and thermal burns.

Enclosure humidity and ventilation are somewhat inversely proportional. Though other factors such as temperature and amount of water in the enclosure contribute to humidity, ventilation has the greatest and most rapid effect on increasing or decreasing humidity. Ideally the amphibian enclosure should be well ventilated with appropriate humidity. A partial or full screen terrarium lid or cover is ideal for allowing evaporation and creating ventilation. Partially occluding the screen lid increases or decreases ventilation and inversely raises or lowers humidity. For large or tall terrariums, small ventilation holes may be drilled in the cage wall and covered with screen to allow ventilation of the otherwise stagnant lower reaches of the enclosure. A small fan may be placed outside the roof of the enclosure to create cross ventilation from these lower air intake ports.

Most terrestrial amphibians benefit from a humidity gradient in the terrarium. This gradient is created by shelters in the terrarium, additional ventilation to portions of the terrarium, and with basking sites as described with lighting. Small depressions, pools, or streams of water may be created in the terrarium with pond liner or plant watering trays. For small frogs, particularly for dendrobatids and mantellids, it is imperative that even the smallest water reservoir have multiple escape routes. Many small frogs are incapable of swimming and will drown in even one centimeter of water. Many salamanders are capable of semi-aquatic life and generally can withstand submersion for longer periods. Placement of limbs, plants, raised gravel, or other cage accessories within or around the water ensures the ability for escape. Similarly, the sides of water enclosures for terrestrial amphibians should have tapered ramps in all directions for small amphibians to escape the water.

Moving water in the enclosure is also helpful to increase both humidity and to a lesser extent ventilation. Small waterfalls, humidifiers, or vaporizers may be used for this purpose. Transfer of vaporized air is achieved by connecting an appropriate size PVC pipe from the vaporizer outflow into the enclosure at the desired location. Connecting the vaporizer to an automatic timer is helpful to create several periodic mistings per day. The misting effect in the terrarium can be quite dramatic. Humidifiers and vaporizers must be cleaned weekly to prevent the growth of potential pathogenic organisms in the water reservoir. Soaking with a dilute bleach solution (1 fl oz or 30 ml in 1 qt or 946 ml water) for 15 minutes and then thorough rinsing is sufficient for disinfecting (Barnett et al. 2001).

Water for the amphibian enclosure should be free of potential pathogens and all treatment chemicals. Aged tap water (allowed to ventilate in a container for twenty-four hours) in many cases is the best water for the terrarium (Barnett et al. 2001). Alternatively, carbon filtered water may be used, though this water treatment may result in developmental abnormalities of tadpoles. Water moving in the terrarium over soil, gravel, or charcoal will generally be filtered biologically. Water that is stationary in containers should be changed as often as possible. Many terrestrial amphibians defecate in these water bowls and bacterial or fungal growth in these containers may be rapid. Cleaning the water bowls in a dilute bleach solution as described for vaporizer reservoirs is recommended at least weekly.

ENCLOSURE DESIGN

The Terrestrial Enclosure

By employing the general principles of security and environmental parameters, design of the amphibian enclosure, based on the species, is relatively straightforward and dictated by practicality. With the exception of temporary housing or quarantine, the smallest recommended amphibian enclosure is a 10-gallon aquarium. Though there is no maximum size limit of a terrarium, access for cleaning, visualization, and environmental control must all be considered.

An appropriate substrate is most important for establishing a well-balanced naturalistic arboreal, terrestrial, or semi-aquatic terrarium and the soil composition is quite variable depending upon the species of amphibians and plants contained within. The type of soil or gravel, however, is only one part of establishing a suitable amphibian substrate. Proper design of the cage floor-substrate interface is crucial for maintaining a long lasting planted or naturalistic terrarium. Ideally the soil mix should be elevated above the cage floor to allow for water and airflow through the soil and the development of a moisture gradient within the soil and terrarium.

Elevation of the soil above the cage floor is achieved by one of several methods. Wright (2001e) uses a standard cage design at National Aquarium in Baltimore (NAIB) by creating a raised platform or false floor of overhead fluorescent light panels (egg crate) cut to fit the tank floor and then raised 2 cm above the true cage floor by pilings cut from PVC pipe (Barnett et al. 2001). This false floor is then overlaid with window screen or horticultural shade cloth and then covered by 1 to 2 cm of gravel and then the sheet moss directly above the gravel. In one corner of the enclosure a 2.5-cm diameter clear plastic tube is placed vertically through the false floor extending to just below the roof of the cage. This tube allows siphoning of the cage floor with a separate smaller siphon tube passed to the bottom of the cage. An optional but highly recommended bulkhead and spigot may be placed through a drilled hole in the cage floor to allow drainage and replace the siphon tube.

The author has used a modified version of this design developed by Ron Gagliardo at Atlanta Botanical Garden with great success. The egg crate false floor is typically inexpensive, but when using standard fish aquariums, prefabricated under-gravel filters (the economy models) are made to fit the size of the tank and come complete with siphon tubes. One or more of these siphon tubes may be used as access for siphon drainage of the cage floor. Additionally, an alternative to the use of aquarium gravel between the filter plate and the soil is to use washed large or medium horticultural grade charcoal that is commonly available for orchids or other special planting mixes. The benefits of the charcoal are lighter weight (especially for large enclosures) and the gradual filtration of organic and inorganic compounds from the water and soil. The benefit of gravel is the large surface area for biologic filtration that likely also occurs with the charcoal. Charcoal has been used as both an enclosure base layer and as a component of custom mixed terrarium soils by the Atlanta Botanical Garden for more than years with no known adverse effects on various species of frogs.

For a planted terrarium a soil depth of at least 5 cm is recommended. Over time some settling of the soil will occur. Plants are added bare root (no soil on the roots) to the soil mix and lightly watered to settle the surrounding soil. Generally plants smaller than the eventual desired size are planted and allowed to grow in the terrarium. Plants in an amphibian terrarium should never be fertilized. Theoretically, soil decomposition, animal feces, and microbes provide all the nutrients necessary for the growth terrarium plants. It is common that many suitable plants soon outgrow the enclosure and require routine trimming.

The water level of the terrestrial terrarium is maintained to achieve desired humidity and fill pools or streams contained within. Plumbing for water accessories may be achieved through drilled holes or siphon tubes through the lid of the terrarium. Water pumps, moving part mechanical devices, and electrical cords should never be inside the terrarium proper. These may be routed through sealed conduits or contained outside the terrarium entirely. Similarly, outflow siphon hoses must be fully protected from cage inhabitants and preferably are located beneath the false floor of the enclosure.

The Aquatic Enclosure

The aquatic enclosure for many obligate aquatic or facultative aquatic amphibians is somewhat similar to the basic tropical fish or goldfish aquarium. Large aquatic amphibians such as *Amphiuma* spp., large sirens, and *Cryptobranchus* spp. are best housed in a 55-gallon or larger aquarium. *Cryptobranchus* and *Necturus* spp. both require chilled water with very high filtration. These animals should not be kept in captivity without properly providing for exact water quality conditions. One requirement for aquatic amphibians is sufficient access to the water surface to breathe air. Because a majority of aquatic amphibians are relatively large and somewhat active, all refuges and ornaments must be secure in their placement. Aquarium heaters (if required) should be contained within a shroud such as PVC or other durable plastic into which numerous holes or slits are drilled to allow water movement over the element and proper heat dissipation. This is to prevent the accidental breaking of glass or ceramic heating elements. The lid must be tight fitting and preferably are latched to prevent escape. With a swimming start, many larger aquatic amphibians are capable of opening lids to a standard aquarium hood.

Some form of water flow is desired for most aquatic amphibians, though frogs such as *Pipa* spp., *Xenopus* spp., and *Hymenochirus* spp. adapt well to still water. Cleanliness of the terrarium is essential and necessitates some type of filtration system. Under-gravel filtration as provided for a fish aquarium is ideal for most aquatic amphibians. Those species requiring high water flow typically require a canister filter or other high flow rate external water pump and/or filter. Most temperate aquatic amphibians require no supplemental heating and adapt well to room temperatures during the entire year. Tropical species are likely to require some supplemental heating if room temperatures fall below 72 °F to 75 °F.

AMPHIBIAN-ENVIRONMENT INTERACTION

Several common problems can be avoided in captive amphibians with a practical approach to cage design. First, the substrate and cage accessories should be appropriate so they do not physically injure the animal. This includes even "natural" elements such as plants. Sharp spines on certain bromeliads or other plants can be lethal to frogs. Certain plants are toxic to amphibians. The toxicity is not necessarily from direct contact, but occurs secondary to ingestion by food items such as crickets or other insects. This is mostly a concern with the introduction of field-collected insects. For example, some plant-sucking insects such as aphids can feed on toxic plants (such as milkweeds, *Asclepias* spp.) and not become distasteful to the smaller amphibians. In the case of milkweeds, the toxicity usually results in death of the animal.

Substrate ingestion is a major problem for captive amphibians. The substrate should be either too large to ingest or small enough that ingested particles are passed through the digestive tract. This may require modifying the substrate in a particular enclosure as the amphibian pet grows.

Almost paradoxically, water in the terrestrial enclosure can result in fatalities of some amphibians. Small terrestrial frogs (mantellids, dendrobatids, and atelopids) are incapable of swimming or will exhaust very easily in water. If a water enclosure is located in the corner of a terrestrial terrarium with no escape possibility against the glass, death of some cage inhabitants from drowning is a certainty. To adequately maintain these species in captivity, standing water is optional or can be provided in the form of a petri dish or other shallow container. Unfortunately, to successfully breed both *Mantella* and *Atelopus* spp., some form of moving or standing water is usually required in the enclosure.

Assume that any opening to the outside of the cage will be used for escape. The lid or covering for the enclosure must be tight fitting or completely sealed. Even strictly terrestrial frogs are capable of limited climbing and jumping to reach the top of the cage. Some salamanders are also capable of climbing glass or plastic.

AMPHIBIAN-AMPHIBIAN INTERACTION

A common question of many amphibian enthusiasts is "Can different species be housed together?" The safe answer to the question is "No." Nevertheless, with experience and thorough knowledge of the species in question, many species that co-occur in nature may be housed communally with proper cage design.

The ultimate rule of housing multiple species (or even the same species from different sources) is that wild-caught individuals from different sources should never, ever be housed together. Clinically, amphibians (particularly frogs) appear to be more commonly parasitized than reptiles, even among captive-born individuals. Exposure of naive animals to certain parasites or bacteria and fungi can result in disaster for an entire collection. An emerging disease concern for terrestrial amphibian owners is the chytrid (Chytridiomycosis) fungus. This pathogenic fungus is suspected to be at least one of the causes of worldwide mortality among wild populations of amphibians and it has been identified as widespread and easily transmitted among captive amphibians (see Common Disorders) (Berger et al. 1998, Daszak et al. 2000, Morell 1999).

Aside from contagious disease is the question of compatibility. For the average amphibian owner, large frogs and salamanders (*Ceratophrys*, *Pyxicephalus*, large *Rana*, large *Bufo*, and *Ambystoma*) are best housed singly in an enclosure. All large amphibians are typically conditioned to feed on anything that is small enough to fit in their mouth. Ambystomatids in captivity are particularly conditioned to bite anything that touches the flanks, even animals larger than they are. The author has witnessed numerous leg amputations and lacerations of frogs and other salamanders that were temporarily housed with a tiger salamander of equal size. Frogs such as *Ceratobatrachus guentheri*, *Ceratophrys*, *Hemiphractus*, *Megophrys*, and *Pyxicephalus* spp. prey on other frog species and other vertebrates as a substantial part of their diet and therefore are generally unsuited for cohabitation with any other amphibians.

Toxicity between different species of amphibians is also a concern, even among the same family of frogs. Many anecdotal reports exist and the author has witnessed that other amphibians (and other *Rana* spp.) enclosed with wood frogs (*Rana sylvatica*) die rapidly, leaving only the wood frogs alive (Duellman and Trueb 1994, Mattison 1987). The exact nature of this suspected toxicity is not fully known. It is possible that similar toxicity exists between different species of wild-collected dart frogs, though there is no observed toxicity among captive individuals.

QUARANTINE

The role of quarantine for new amphibians in a collection cannot be overemphasized. Segregation of new arrivals is most important for those animals that will be introduced into multi-species displays. The quarantine procedure for amphibians, however, is more designed to protect the individual animal from occult disease that may manifest itself some time after arrival into the new enclosure.

The quarantine enclosure is quite basic. A 10-gallon glass aquarium or plastic sweater box with ventilation holes is ideal for quarantine of most terrestrial amphibians. Larger aquatic amphibians should be maintained in an appropriately sized enclosure. For terrestrial amphibians the cage substrate should be non-bleached paper towel and possibly a hide box or other disposable cage ornament to provide security. The quarantine enclosure should be located in a low traffic area of the room where the inhabitants may be monitored for activity from a distance. If necessary the sides of the enclosure may be painted or covered with paper to provide visual security. If possible a feeding station should be provided in the form of a petri dish or shallow dish so that the feeding response can be monitored. Arboreal frogs and salamanders can be quarantined similarly with the addition of horizontal branches for perching. If forced to remain on the cage floor, arboreal frogs may become stressed and fail to acclimate.

A fundamental purpose of quarantine is the collection of fecal material for analysis. This should be performed as soon as the first sample is available. Subsequent fecal samples should be examined every three to five days, depending on availability, and then rechecked every two weeks following a negative or "clean" sample. A final recheck two months after a negative sample is also advised (Wright and Whitaker 2001c).

The quarantine period should be at least thirty days following a negative fecal sample for apparently healthy individuals (Wright and Whitaker 2001c). Wild-collected amphibians, despite the status of fecal testing, should be quarantined for sixty days. Under no circumstances should wild-collected amphibians be introduced into an enclosure with any other animals. Despite antiparasiticide, antibiotic, and antifungal treatment it is possible for these individuals to carry undetected infectious diseases and later transmit them to other naive animals.

It is not uncommon to prophylactically treat new amphibian arrivals for gastrointestinal parasites and some cutaneous fungi. Though this practice is no substitute for fecal examination, it can be effective in eliminating or reducing the burden of some infectious diseases. Unfortunately, there is a risk of adverse side effects with this practice. The author has observed the death of long-term captive imported frogs following deworming with fenbendazole at recommended doses. The animals were four green and black poison dart frogs, *Dendrobates auratus*, which were confirmed infected with various nematodes including great numbers of lungworms, *Rhabdias* spp. None of the animals had exhibited clinical disease and were breeding in captivity. Following a single oral treatment with fenbendazole at 100 mg/kg two of the four frogs immediately stopped eating and subsequently died within five days. A third stopped feeding and then resumed feeding and survived. The fourth frog was not adversely affected. Both surviving frogs continued to shed *Rhabdias* spp. larvae in the feces following treatment, yet the numbers of larvae were reduced. The author has not observed this phenomenon in other similarly infected *Dendrobates* spp. or *Mantella* spp.

A common prophylactic antiparasite regimen includes administering fenbendazole orally at 100 mg/kg followed by ivermectin topically at 0.2 mg/kg (Wright and Whitaker 2001c). Repeating the treatment in three weeks is recommended, along with rechecking a fecal sample prior to treatment. The author has observed that ivermectin treatment may be fatal is some species including Central American glass frogs (Centrolenidae) and the lemur leaf frog (*Hylomantis lemur*). The frog deaths were observed in frogs that were infected with *Rhabdias* spp. Ongoing research and personal observations on the treatment of *Rhabdias* spp. infections in multiple Central American amphibian species indicates that a complete "cure" or elimination of *Rhabidias* spp. infection may not be possible in captive amphibians.

Record keeping of feeding and treatments is essential. The client should record all observations of activity, feeding response, food items consumed, and other pertinent behavior. Weekly weights are also beneficial for healthy individuals when this can be performed accurately and in a stress-free manner.

NUTRITION

If the nutritional needs for amphibians were as simple as tossing a few crickets into the enclosure from time to time, they would all be more popular pets. Instead, the nutritional maintenance for many captive amphibians is as labor intensive (or more so) as that of insectivorous lizards and the nutritional demands of amphibians are more a consequence of the animals being such generalists rather than being specialists on one food item. The variety of food items consumed in the wild likely results in a tremendously varied vitamin, mineral, amino acid, and fatty acid intake that is not duplicated with captive diets. Very little scientific data exists regarding the exact diet and its nutritional composition for amphibians in the wild. Unfortunately,

much is learned about the proper or improper nutrition of amphibians through histopathology.

There is great variability in the feeding preferences of different life stages of metamorphosed amphibians, and this variability has been observed in those animals that have been successfully bred over several generations. For instance, froglets of the golden mantella (*Mantella aurantiaca*) are no more than 8 mm in length at metamorphosis. To a frog this small, even the smallest of domestic fruit flies is too large to eat. These froglets must be raised for several weeks on small insects called springtails (order Collembola) until they may be fed small fruitflies. Adult mantellas, however, are quite ravenous and will eat crickets that are nearly 20% of their body size.

The feeding method of amphibians is also somewhat important when selecting food items. All frogs should be considered food gulpers; after capturing the prey item it is swallowed whole with little to no chewing. In contrast, large salamanders and especially aquatic amphibians (Necturus, Amphiuma, Siren, and *Cryptobranchus spp.*) all exhibit some chewing motions when feeding. This is especially observed in sirens and amphiumas that may repeatedly move food items in and out of the mouth while crushing them. Choosing appropriate food items, or more importantly, avoiding improper food items for certain species, is important.

Another important point to remember regarding most terrestrial amphibians is that they are sight feeders. Generally moving food is preferred over stationary food. Some larger frogs, toads, and salamanders may be conditioned to feed on stationary pre-killed or frozen and thawed food items, but this is more the exception than the rule. Thus, when approaching the dilemma of a non-feeding amphibian, always consider the type and size of food offered.

Perhaps the most important consideration when feeding amphibians is the timing of feeding. The client must be fully informed of the feeding habits of the species in question. Nearly all terrestrial salamanders and many tree frogs are nocturnal and will only feed at night. Many of the larger nocturnal frogs and toads, being opportunists, will feed any time in captivity. The tiger salamander, *Ambystoma tigrinum*, though nocturnal in its native habitat, will readily adapt to daylight feeding. Night feeing may make the monitoring of food consumption difficult with some amphibians. For newly established pets, encourage the client to observe the feeding habits with a flashlight or red light illumination if necessary.

To compensate for the known vitamin and mineral imbalances in food items and for suspected deficiencies in amino acids, many hobbyists apply several commercially available vitamin/mineral powders (called dusting) to the food items prior to feeding. The process of dusting food items is discussed in Nutrition of the chapter on lizards. Additionally, food products specifically for the prey items to consume are designed to enrich the prey item prior to feeding to the amphibian pet. This process is called "gut-loading."

Based on known dietary disorders, several basic provisions must be made for captive amphibians. Calcium and phosphorous (Ca:P) should be provided in a ratio of 1:1 to 2:1 to prevent several nutritional diseases (Wright 2001d, Wright and Whitaker 2001a, Donoghue and Langenberg 1996). Additionally, vitamin D_3 is supplemented in the diet or produced endogenously by the amphibian when exposed to the appropriate quality and quantity of ultraviolet light. A ratio that is too low in calcium or too high in phosphorous may result in metabolic bone disease (MBD). A ratio too high in calcium or vitamin D_3 may contribute to hypervitaminosis D and secondary renal failure (Wright and Whitaker 2001b). Powdered supplements are available from Rep-Cal (Los Gatos, CA; www.repcal.com) and Nekton (Clearwater, FL; www.nekton.de).

Neonatal and young amphibians appear to be most affected by MBD because of increased calcium demand by growing bones. The frequency for calcium supplementation of these animals is increased compared to that of adults. Neonatal or young, growing amphibians may receive calcium and vitamin D_3 supplementation twice weekly when fed daily and most adult amphibians should receive calcium supplemented food items once weekly or less often. Larger amphibians fed whole animal vertebrate diets such as thawed frozen rats or mice likely do not require supplemental calcium in the diet.

Aquatic or semi-aquatic amphibians fed diets comprised solely of fish may develop thiamine (vitamin B_1) deficiency (Wright and Whitaker 2001b, Donoghue and Langenberg 1996). This disorder is the result of high levels of thiaminase in the food items that inactivates dietary and endogenously produced thiamine in the amphibian. Several susceptible species include aquatic salamanders, aquatic caecilians, horned frogs (*Ceratophrys* spp.), African bullfrogs (*Pyxicephalus* spp.), and other semi-aquatic frogs.

FOOD ITEMS

Most clients who maintain breeding colonies or large colonies of amphibians are required to raise their own food items because the expense of purchasing food items can be excessive. The simplest factor dictating the feeding of captive amphibians is the size of the animal and the size of the food item. The standard diet for most larger salamanders and frogs is crickets and the diet of choice for smaller amphibians is fruit flies. Some wild-collected insects such as termites may be available seasonally or throughout the year in warmer climates.

Domestic or gray crickets (*Acheta domestica*) of various sizes are the standard diet for most medium to large terrestrial amphibians. Crickets are commercially available in sizes ranging from 1/16 inch (pinheads) in length to 1 inch (adults) from pet shops and mail order from a variety of sources. The Ca:P for crickets is 0.2:2.6 (Donoghue and Langenberg 1996). Periodic dusting of crickets with calcium and vitamin D_3 powders is recommended for all amphibians.

A variety of specialized cricket diets are available to enrich crickets with nutrients. The efficacy of these products is debatable. Generations of frogs that have been fed crickets raised on fresh vegetables and fruits such as squash, greens, and oranges have reproduced and lived for five or more years with no apparent health abnormalities to themselves or offspring.

Another cultured food item for medium to large amphibians is mealworms. The mealworm is actually larvae of the beetle, *Tenebrio molitor*, which may be cultured easily in one of several different grain meals supplemented with cut pieces of apple or vegetable for moisture. Because the adult beetles are required to reproduce for new mealworms, a tight fitting, ventilated lid is required to maintain the culture. Mealworms are generally a poor food choice for amphibians because of the hard exoskeleton. Though the softer-bodied, newly molted larvae are acceptable, the author has witnessed the unexplained deaths of several frogs and lizards following the feeding of mealworms. Necropsy on several lizards has revealed peritoneal abscessation that was attributed to gastrointestinal perforation from the hard body parts or possibly chewing of the larvae. Because mealworms do not provide an improved Ca:P ratio (0.1:1.2) (Donoghue and Langenberg 1996) as compared to crickets, their use as a primary food item for most amphibians is not recommended.

Similarly, most beetles and other large insects with hard exoskeletons are not a good food source for amphibians. An exception might be made for large frogs and especially toads, which may be observed to nearly consume their weight in beetles while feeding in habitat during summer months. Large terrestrial salamanders and aquatic amphiumas and sirens are generally capable of crushing these insects following capture and therefore may adequately digest them and have minimal risk of gastrointestinal injury.

The flour beetle, *Trilobium* spp., which is a relative of the larger *Tenebrio* spp., is a smaller beetle that can safely be fed to small frogs. These beetles are approximately 5 mm in length as adults with comparable small larvae. They are raised and harvested similar to *Tenebrio* spp., though the adult beetle is fed as commonly as the larvae.

Wingless or flightless fruit flies are the standard diet for smaller frogs and salamanders, particularly for poison dart frogs, mantellas, harlequin frogs, and neonatal amphibians. Two species of flies, *Drosophila melanogaster* (the small vestigial or wingless fruit fly) and *Drosophila hydei* (the larger flightless fruit fly), are commercially available. Fruit flies are easily cultured by the client and may be the sole food source for many captive amphibians. They are cultured in reusable canning jars or disposable plastic cups, both of which are sealed with a permeable (but escape-proof) ventilated lid. Fruit fly growing media is available from Carolina Biological Supply Co. (Burlington, NC; www.carolina.com) or can be made from instant potato flakes, brewer's yeast, and a mold inhibitor. Fruit flies are typically dusted with powdered supplements as with crickets.

Another small food item that is relished by nearly all amphibians is the termite. In warmer climates, such as the southeastern U.S. coastal plain, termites can be collected any time of year. There are methods of "culturing" termites in the wild that involve burying coffee cans punctured with drain holes in the ground and filling them with rolled cardboard. Unfortunately, the risk of infestation to homes and other wooden structures is great, so this practice should not be recommended to clients. Nevertheless, wild collected termites do not appear to cause harm to captive amphibians and certain nutrients not otherwise available to these animals may be provided. Similarly, parasites or other toxins ingested by the termites could put captive animals at risk for disease.

An important but often overlooked food item for small frogs is springtails or leafhoppers, of the insect order Collembola. These very small (<1 mm) white to gray insects that are commonly seen in most terrariums containing soil. They feed on detritus and decaying plant material and can be easily cultured to feed neonatal or very small frogs and salamanders. A plastic container such as a margarine container or plastic shoebox filled with approximately 1 to 2 inches of potting soil is ideal. The soil is slightly moistened and a few pinches of fish food flakes are sprinkled on the surface of the soil. The springtails may be introduced from a decaying leaf from outdoors or from a previously existing culture. A method for easily removing the springtails is to place a small block (10 cm × 5 cm x × cm) of horticultural tree fern fiber on the soil surface, then remove and gently tap the block to remove springtails when feeding is desired.

The only acceptable vertebrate food sources for captive amphibians are fish and thawed frozen pink mice or rats. Large frogs, toads, and salamanders with conditioned feeding responses usually accept these items when offered by forceps, or in the case of fish when offered in a shallow dish. These larger amphibians generally accept other vertebrate prey such as other amphibians, reptiles, large beetles, and grasshoppers. The client should carefully consider the health risk to the amphibian before feeding such items. The risk of parasitism with endoparasites or bacterial or fungal infections is great. Of paramount concern must be the Chytridiomycosis fungus when offering any amphibians. This disease is extremely serious for amphibians and should be viewed on the level of the immunodeficiency viruses that affect cats and humans when considering prevention.

Aquatic amphibians consume a wide variety of food items. Earthworms and fish are the standard diets with other arthropods and some frozen foods occasionally accepted. Ideally the food should be cultured or purchased as cultured rather than collected from the wild. This reduces the risk of introducing infectious diseases into the enclosure.

Certain amphibians, particularly several frog species, are specialists in their feeding choices and may be difficult to feed in captivity. The bizarre casque-headed tree frogs, *Hemiphractus* spp., of South America and several species of horned frogs, *Ceratophrys* spp., are known frog-eating specialists (Mattison 1987, Obst et al. 1988). It may be necessary to feed live frogs to these species while trying to train them to eat various invertebrate or vertebrate prey items. Another finicky large frog (8 to 10 cm) is the climbing toad, *Pedostibes hosei*, of southeast Asia. This frog is known to specialize in ants and termites and may not accept crickets or other large invertebrates in captivity (Obst et al. 1988). This frog may be transitioned to a cricket-only diet by feeding smaller size crickets or beetles. Among aquatic amphibians the hellbenders, *Cryptobranchus* spp., as adults typically feed only on crayfish and must be coaxed to accept other aquatic food items if captive.

Finally, many clients may be misinformed regarding the feeding of manufactured pelleted diets. It is unreasonable to expect any terrestrial amphibians to eat non-moving prepared foods. It is more likely, though not common, that aquatic amphibians will readily accept these diets. Salamanders and newts, more than frogs, will adapt to these diets, but they are rarely substitutes for live foods. Clients should be informed about this fact prior to purchasing amphibian pets. For some the cost of live foods or the time to culture them may not meet their expectations for proper maintenance of amphibian pets. One exception of note is the fact that marine toads (*Bufo marinus*) have been observed and videotaped eating dry dog food from outdoor food bowls in south Florida. So, one can never underestimate the resourcefulness of these animals when it comes to adaptation.

COMMON DISORDERS

Amphibian health disorders arise from infectious bacterial, fungal, and parasitic etiologies to trauma, nutritional, and toxic diseases. Several diseases such as metabolic bone disease (MBD) and cutaneous bacterial infection (red leg) are well documented in veterinary scientific and popular literature. Many specific infectious and metabolic diseases, however, are relatively unknown.

Integument

As with snakes and lizards a very common skin disorder seen in frogs is rostral abrasion. This is particularly common in wild-collected animals, but is just as possible to develop in any species transported in small containers. The common etiology is trauma from escape attempts through clear plastic lids, screens, or glass enclosures. Prevention of this disorder is enhanced with opaque transport containers and packing of the amphibian with moss or another soft substrate to reduce movement within the container.

The primary concern with rostral abrasions is secondary infections from opportunistic or pathogenic bacteria and fungus. If the abrasion is clean and showing no signs of erosion, then no treatment is indicated. For chronic or more extensive abrasions in which active erosion of the skin or exposure of underlying bone is present, treatment with topical antibiotics, including ophthalmic solutions, is indicated. Gentamicin or triple antibiotic solutions are applied once or twice daily. Silver sulfadiazine cream is also efficacious to treat fungal elements in addition to bacteria.

Active lesions associated with erosive dermatitis or osteolysis require aggressive diagnostic and therapeutic intervention. Bacterial culture and sensitivity, and cytology if possible, from an impression smear or tissue sample in formalin may be submitted. In addition to topical therapy systemic antibiotics are indicated. Enrofloxacin at a dose of 5 to 10 mg/kg PO or TO every twenty-four hours for seven days (Taylor 2001) is recommended pending culture results. The client must be vigilant of the patient with regard to healing of these lesions. Amphibians with substantial rostral abrasions should be maintained in a quarantine enclosure for cleanliness and close observation.

Traumatic injuries to limbs are similar to rostral abrasions. Trauma may occur secondary to accidents with enclosure lids closing on legs, and bite wounds from cage mates are possible with some species. These wounds typically require aggressive antibiotic therapy initially rather than just observation. If severe trauma to underlying bone is suspected, amputation is recommended early in treatment to prevent the development of systemic disease.

Bacterial skin infections are common in amphibians and may present as discolorations, erosions, abscesses, and ulcerations. Bacterial dermatitis may be difficult to diagnose on visual inspection alone. Many infections are the result of immunosuppression from a number of factors including improper husbandry, inadequate diet, or the stress of shipping. The resultant infectious agent may arise from the patient's environment or from an apparently unaffected cage mate.

The diagnostic test of choice for any cutaneous lesion is bacterial culture and sensitivity followed by histopathology of affected tissue if possible. Pending the response to empiric antibiotic therapy, biopsy may be required. Unfortunately, the risk of septicemia from a number of bacterial etiologic agents necessitates the initiation of treatment prior to receiving test results. The commonly referenced "red-leg disease" of frogs is actually the result of hyperemia secondary to septicemia rather than simply cutaneous disease. If not treated rapidly and appropriately this syndrome carries a poor prognosis for recovery.

Systemic enrofloxacin is initiated for seven days for the non-septicemic cutaneous disease. For the septicemic patient, a water bath of 0.6% saline to achieve hydration is the initial therapy (Taylor 2001). Antibiotic baths with tetracyclines, semisynthetic penicillins (SSP), and aminoglycosides may be indicated.

Many bacteria are implicated in amphibian skin disease and septicemia. A large number of these are Gram-negative rods including the widely reported and well known *Aeromonas* spp. and *Pseudomonas* spp. *Mycobacterium* spp. are also implicated in various disease syndromes in amphibians, particularly skin disease. Diagnosis is very difficult pre-mortem because the bacteria is difficult to culture. Isolation and neutralization of affected individuals is recommended because there is no known treatment for *Mycobacterium* infection.

Fungal infections are a concern for amphibians. Most notable among these is Chytridiomycosis, "chytrid," caused by *Batrachochytrium dendrobatidis*. The initial clinical sign of this fungal dermatitis is an increased rate of skin shedding with possible associated dermal lesions such as pale skin. It is not known how many different species of amphibians are susceptible to this fungus, but confirmed cases of chytrid have been reported from all continents containing amphibians.

Patients are diagnosed with chytridiomycosis by presence of the organism in shed skin or in formalin fixed skin. Diagnosed cases or prophylactic treatment of suspected infected animals is performed with a bath of itraconazole. A 1% itraconazole stock solution in methylcellulose is diluted to 0.01% in 0.6% NaCl. Treatment consists of a five-minute bath once daily for ten days (Taylor 2001). Resolution of clinical signs is rapid if treatment is initiated early.

Ectoparasites are uncommon among amphibians and are clinically most prevalent among toads. Treatment consists of ivermectin at 0.4 mg/kg PO or TO given once weekly for at least four weeks (Poynton and Whitaker 2001). Some amphibian species have shown sensitivity to higher doses of ivermectin (2 mg/kg) (Poynton and Whitaker 2001, Klingenberg 1993).

Finally, a multisystemic disease most notable in the skin is bloating or edema syndrome. This disease process has several possible etiologies, the most notable of which is osmotic imbalance secondary to sepsis or toxemia. Other possible causes include renal disease or failure, heart disease, metabolic bone disease, and environmental factors. Cases in which an individual animal is affected may be challenging to diagnose. For cases in which multiple animals in an enclosure are affected, environmental causes and infectious disease are most likely. Prognosis may be fair with a diagnosis and rapid treatment. Often, the inciting cause remains unnoticed for some time prior to the onset of clinical signs and the underlying disease progresses beyond the possibility of recovery.

Skeletal System

Though not as common as in lizards, MBD follows the same clinical course as in reptiles. Juvenile or rapidly growing individuals are most susceptible. The pathophysiology of MBD is discussed in the chapter on lizards. An unknown factor regarding MBD in amphibians is the role of ultraviolet light (UV-B) in the development of clinical disease. Because most amphibians are either nocturnal, fossoreal, or otherwise found in shaded forests it is possible that oral cholecalciferol (vitamin D_3) plays more of a role in calcium absorption and metabolism than does that of endogenous vitamin D_3. However, recent studies of juvenile captive-born *Gastrotheca cornuta* at the Atlanta Botanical Garden and El Valle Amphibian Conservation Center, Panama, are highly suggestive that a lack of adequate UV-B radiation contributes to both clinical signs and histopathologic changes consistent with MBD (author, personal observation).

An occasional suspected clinical sign of MBD in amphibians is gastrointestinal bloating. If this sign is observed and there is suspicion of MBD based on history or other physical exam findings, a radiographic study should be initiated to confirm the presence of the disease syndrome. Cloacal prolapse may be an additional sign of MBD in juvenile frogs of some species (*Hylomantis lemur*, *Agalychnis callidryas*). The demonstration of decreased bone density is diagnostic for MBD, though in severe cases, especially among young, growing animals, soft pliable bones are highly suggestive of MBD. Blood calcium testing is not a reliable method for diagnosing MBD because the blood remains normocalcemic until the body stores of calcium are depleted.

Treatment of MBD in amphibians is supportive. Oral calcium glubionate at a dose of 1 ml/kg/day (Wright and Whitaker 2001b) and dietary correction is essential. Oral vitamin D_3 is recommended to enhance the absorption of calcium from the gastrointestinal tract (Wright and Whitaker 2001b, Donoghue and Langenberg 1996). Patients with neurologic disease secondary to MBD may require calcium gluconate 10% at 100 mg/kg ICe every four to six hours until signs resolve. Prognosis for the hypocalcemic state of MBD in amphibians as seen in lizards is poor.

A mysterious disease of newly metamorphosed frogs is called spindly leg disease or syndrome. With this abnormality tadpoles develop normal or nearly normal hind legs, yet the forelimbs either fail to erupt from the skin or are extremely thin and weak, almost as if there were only skin and bone with no muscle. This syndrome has been reported extensively among dendrobatid frogs. This high rate of occurrence may be due to the fact that these frogs are bred in captivity in such great numbers and therefore the chance for occurrence is greater. Frogs that metamorphose and leave the water usually fail to eat and die within days.

The potential causes for this syndrome are diet of the tadpole or parents, improper environmental conditions (temperature, lighting, etc.), genetics, toxins, and possibly chytridiomycosis. Presently a dietary cause is most likely because there are several anecdotal reports of dietary variation in clutches of tadpoles from the same parents raised on different foods that may exhibit the disease. There is no treatment for this disease process.

Respiratory System

Clinical respiratory disease is uncommon among amphibians. It is more likely that respiratory infections in amphibians are under diagnosed rather than less frequent than those seen in reptiles. A common respiratory pathogen is lungworms (*Rhabdias* spp.). Though this nematode is diagnosed with moderate frequency among terrestrial frogs, clinical disease associated with the organism is infrequent. It is likely that the migration of larvae through host tissues and secondary invasion of bacteria with or without septicemia contributes greatly to debilitation of the patient.

Rhabdias spp. infection is diagnosed by demonstrating larvae on direct fecal examination or floatation or by cytology of tracheal wash. Patients exhibiting apparent respiratory distress in association with *Rhabdias* spp. infection are best treated with anthelminthics concurrent with antibiotics such as enrofloxacin for secondary bacterial infection. Those patients that exhibit no active clinical disease are treated only with anthelminthics such as fenbendazole 100 mg/kg PO every fourteen days for three treatments or ivermectin at 0.2 to 0.4 mg/kg PO or TO at the same rate of administration (Poynton and Whitaker 2001). Because the life cycle of this infection (as well as other amphibian nematodal infections) is direct, isolation and strict hygiene is essential to reducing parasite burdens.

Though not an infectious disease, drowning is a common fatal respiratory disease of captive amphibians. It is mentioned only because it is a disease of prevention as described in the section on Husbandry. This avoidable disease results in the deaths of many valuable amphibian pets.

Digestive System

Another rather common though avoidable non-infectious disease in amphibians is foreign body obstruction. Typically the result of inappropriate substrate or feeding practices, this problem often goes unnoticed for some time. The primary presenting complaint is anorexia or occasionally regurgitation. Gravel, soil particles, or rarely invertebrate exoskeleton may cause obstruction. Diagnosis may be presumptive based on history and husbandry practices or definitive with abdominal palpation and radiographic study.

The degree of obstruction, size of patient, and nature of the foreign body dictate treatment. For organic foreign materials, oral laxatives such as psyllium and mineral oil may aid in passage of the obstruction. For larger amphibians, surgery may be indicated.

Intestinal parasitism is clinically widespread among terrestrial amphibians and somewhat less common among arboreal species. Amphibians are infected with a wide variety of protozoa and metazoa parasites. It is common that routine fecal exams of amphibians reveal these organisms in otherwise healthy patients. Some protozoans may not be pathogenic and may not require treatment. Some protozoan and many metazoan (nematodes, trematodes, cestodes) parasites may inhabit amphibian tissues and remain in "balance" with the host with a competent immune system.

The onset of stress and subsequent immunosuppression that results from transport, poor diet, or inappropriate husbandry can rapidly lead to accelerated reproduction, migration, and infestation of these parasites. Similarly, the direct life cycle of many parasites only compounds the reinfection rate when the patient is subject to confinement in a terrarium. This is the likely cause for the apparent higher clinical prevalence of these parasites in terrestrial rather than arboreal species because there is greater likelihood for contact with the infective oocysts or larvae.

Intestinal parasites are best treated when diagnosed. Nevertheless, the client must be educated regarding the potential side effects of treatment. More commonly there is greater risk of death or debilitation from the host's immune response to sudden parasite death than from side effects of appropriately dosed medications. For very valuable animals, treatment of apparently healthy animals should be carefully weighed against the potential loss of the patient. When groups of animals are to be medicated, treatment of a few animals in the group is preferable to medicating the entire group at once.

The most important factor in breaking the life cycle of direct parasites is maintenance of the patient in an immaculately clean, well maintained enclosure. Removal of all feces immediately after passage is imperative. Feeding of the patient should only be performed in an enclosure with no fecal contamination because food items may browse on contaminated surfaces and reinfect the host. Prophylactic treatment for intestinal parasites is discussed in the Quarantine section of Husbandry.

Protozoan parasites present both a diagnostic and treatment challenge. For suspected pathogenic *Trichomonas* spp. and *Entamoeba* spp. Infections, metronidazole is indicated. Dose ranges for adults vary from 10 mg/kg PO every twenty-four hours for seven to ten days for Trichomonas to 100 mg/kg PO every fourteen days for Entamoeba (Poynton and Whitaker 2001). Metronidazole baths at 250 mg to 500 mg/L fresh water for six to eight hours once weekly are indicated for larval amphibians (Poynton and Whitaker 2001).

Coccidiosis is not uncommon in amphibians, yet its diagnosis is complicated by the fact that oocysts are intermittently shed in the feces. Thus, repeated fecal exams over protracted periods are required in some cases for definitive diagnosis. As seen in mammals, coccidiosis is primarily a clinical disease to the very young, very old, or immunosuppressed animal. Nevertheless, treatment is indicated on diagnosis and consists of trimethoprim-sulfamethoxazole at 15 mg/kg PO daily for fourteen days (Poynton and Whitaker 2001). The dosage of TMS in exotic animals is based on the combined concentration of both the trimethoprim and sulfa medications.

Nematodes are treated as described for lungworms (*Rhabdias* spp.) in the section on Respiratory System and Quarantine for prophylactic treatment. It may be difficult to specifically diagnose each species of nematode parasite on fecal exam, though the treatment for each is similar.

Trematodes and cestodes have indirect life cycles in amphibians and interruption of the vector for reinfection is essential for treatment. Treatment consists of praziquantel at 8 to 14 mg/kg PO every fourteen days for three or more treatments (Poynton and Whitaker 2001).

Excretory System

There are no significant renal diseases of amphibians that are not observed in reptiles, birds, or mammals. Renal disease secondary to toxicosis (medications or environmental), mineral imbalances, or gout is possible.

Reproductive System

Failure to lay eggs or "egg binding" is the most common reproductive disorder of amphibians. Potential causes are categorized as environmental, in which certain a suitable oviposition site is not available, unsuitable mate, or other stress that prevents the release of eggs. Other causes include physical inability to lay eggs that may result from environmental factors. If an egg or eggs becomes lodged in the ostium of the oviduct or within the oviduct proper, all retrograde eggs will be retained. Some cases may require surgery when possible.

Ophthalmology

Superficial ocular disease in amphibians is commonly associated with skin disease or arises from a common etiology such as bacterial, fungal, protozoal, or viral disease. Cataracts, corneal lipidosis, and glaucoma have all been diagnosed. Systemic disease or sepsis such as red leg syndrome may account for uveitis in amphibians, as does similar systemic disease in other animals. Diagnosis and treatment of ophthalmic diseases in amphibians is approached as in other animals.

Corneal lipidosis may be commonly confused with infectious or traumatic inflammatory disease and typically slowly progresses to eventually involve the cornea of one or both eyes. Treatment is supportive and should be directed at reduction of dietary fat or cholesterol by altering prey item selection and reducing frequency of feeding (Wright 2009).

Toxicity

Amphibians are quite sensitive to environmental contamination from both naturally occurring and synthetic toxins. These include ammonia, nitrites, nitrates, excessive salts, chlorine, organophosphates, pyrethrins and pyrethroids, and many solvents used in glues and sealants. It is imperative that any cleaning compounds used to disinfect enclosures or enclosure accessories be thoroughly rinsed, soaked, and dried prior to reintroduction into the enclosure. Diana et al. (2001) reports toxicosis among dendrobatid frogs within enclosures that were misted by a newly constructed system composed of PVC pipes. Organic solvents from the pipe cement were found to be the cause of toxicosis. Similar attention must be observed with aquarium glass sealants.

Metabolic Disorders

Hypovitaminosis A is a recently recognized and described disease of captive amphibians (Pessier et al. 2002). This disease progresses in amphibians similar to that observed in reptiles with the hallmark histopathologic change of squamous metaplasia. Multiple organ systems may be affected and clinical signs may vary widely. Wright (2009) recommends vitamin A treatment for any clinically ill captive amphibian for which there is no clear diagnosis or clinical sign of disease. Treatment consists of Aquasol A 1 IU vitamin A/g body weight once daily for two weeks or until clinical signs resolve (Wright 2009).

Zoonoses

Amphibians are known to carry several bacteria which are potentially pathogenic to man and other animals. Though not infectious, certain amphibian toxins are potentially dangerous to man and domestic animals.

Bacteria such as *Listeria monocytogenes*, *Salmonella* spp., and *Yersinia enterocolitica* are all reported as isolated from the feces or digestive tracts of some amphibians (Taylor 2001). There is no link to clinical disease in man from these bacteria arising from amphibians. Care and common sense, however, must be exercised when handling amphibians regarding zoonotic potential. Human carelessness is often a contributing factor to zoonoses when related to exotic animals.

It is the responsibility of the veterinary clinician and technician to educate the client regarding proper handling of the amphibian pet to reduce the risk of potential exposure. The following are several guidelines that should be followed:

1. Do not handle amphibians unless absolutely necessary. Most (if not all) amphibians show no apparent health or quality of life benefit from human contact. In fact, stress may be increased as well as tissue trauma that may lead to an increased incidence of disease to the animal.
2. Never handle or clean amphibians, amphibian foods or food containers, or amphibian enclosures near a human food preparation area or human sanitation area such as a kitchen sink, kitchen table or countertop, bathroom sink, or bathtub.
3. Never allow children to handle amphibians without direct adult supervision and make sure that hands are washed immediately after handling.
4. Do not allow amphibians to remain loose or uncontained in a building intended for human occupation, sanitation, or food preparation.

Unfortunately, the above suggestions may seem to be common sense, but the breakthroughs in common sense are always reported in the popular press by relatively uneducated media professionals, implicating exotic animals in zoonotic disease. Without the responsible education of pet owners there is great risk of continued legislation prohibiting private possession of these animals.

LARVAL AMPHIBIANS

Tadpoles and larval salamanders face a variety of disorders that, for the most part, are never diagnosed or treated. Under controlled conditions with captive breeding the incidence of disease is relatively low, yet many may be susceptible to disease when stressed with substandard environmental conditions. There is tremendous variability in natural and cultural conditions

of larval amphibians and some species demand exacting environmental parameters, while other are adapted to what might be considered nearly unsurvivable conditions.

For practical purposes all larval caecilians and salamanders are carnivorous. Some caeclians are viviparous and consume oviductal secretions while developing in the adult female and are then born as juveniles. For salamanders, carnivory leads to cannibalism in crowded conditions, particularly as metamorphosis approaches. It is possible that the survival strategy of some communal pond-breeding salamanders depends on this strategy for a few animals to survive. In contrast, most frog larvae, tadpoles, are herbivorous. There are, however, a few notable exceptions. Though not commonly bred by hobbyists in captivity, horned frogs (*Ceratophrys* spp. and some other Leptodactylidae) have carnivorous, or more reputedly cannibalistic, tadpoles. Successful rearing of these tadpoles and larvae of other carnivorous species necessitates isolation into individual enclosures for each larva.

The most critical husbandry issue for larval amphibians is water quality. Understanding the natural history and reproductive strategy for a particular species is important for proper care of the tadpoles. Most dart frogs, for example, lay eggs out of water on leaves, in leaf axils, or on flat surfaces near the ground. After hatching, the tadpoles are then transferred to a suitable water area that is generally a small plant with water supplied only from rain. For these species in captivity, elaborate filtration and moving or constantly filtered water is not essential for survival and metamorphosis. Aged tap water or spring water changed periodically generally yields success.

Species that lay eggs above streams or have tadpoles which inhabit moving water usually require some water oxygenation or filtration for survival. Some of these species, such as many larger Central and South American hylids, feed on particulates suspended in the water and require the water movement to supply a constant source of food. Many of these species rapidly perish if maintained in still or stagnant water.

Feeding of larval amphibians, particularly tadpoles, is not difficult in most cases. An exceptional food for larval herbivorous dendrobatids is spirulina powder (Earthrise Co., Petaluma, CA) that is available from most health food stores. The author has raised many generations of various species of dendrobatids and *Mantella* spp. tadpoles on this diet with absolutely no developmental abnormalities. Overfeeding must be avoided, however. Water quality deteriorates rapidly without filtration and death is rapid. Many dendrobatids and possibly other frog species give parental care to tadpoles in the form of "feeder eggs." Information on these species is available in many hobbyist texts.

Larval salamanders can be problematic in that many species in early development require live foods. Daphnia, gammarus (fairy shrimp), and other small crustaceans must be cultured or readily available. Wild collection of these food items is not recommended, because this is commonly a source for infection with the trematode *Gyrodactylus spp.*, the body fluke. These microscopic parasites can be rapidly fatal to larvae, and may be the inciting cause of cutaneous ulcers on adults. Treatment may be accomplished with dilute salt or formaldehyde baths (1.5 ml of 10% formalin in 1 liter water for ten minutes) and survivability is good with early diagnosis. The amphibians undergoing treatment must be watched very closely and removed to freshwater at the first sign of distress in formalin. Dipping the infected animals into the treatment solution within a net is the most practical method for rapid removal.

Larval amphibians are subject to bacterial and fungal infections as adults. Treatment is with medicated baths rather than by individual dosing. Diagnosis of a specific infection is usually obtained by sacrificing one or more larvae from a group for bacteriologic or microscopic analysis.

HISTORY AND PHYSICAL EXAM

History

A complete and accurate history of the amphibian patient may be the most important procedure in developing a diagnosis of disease (or health). Unfortunately, amphibian patients are commonly presented moribund or altered from the original onset of clinical signs, making it difficult to diagnose the underlying etiology based on physical exam. Similarly, the clinician may be presented with a deceased patient from a group of animals and a diagnosis may be required to develop a treatment plan for the remaining group of apparently healthy individuals. Additionally, when gaining new clients who own amphibians (and reptiles), much time is spent in phone conversations with clients who are reluctant to bring the patient into the clinic. Though there is little substitute for physical exam of the patient, there is even less substitute for not having patience with a potential first time client.

The first step in obtaining an accurate history is identification of the correct scientific name of the patient to *at least* the genus (and preferably to species) level. It may be difficult to obtain natural history information based on common or colloquial names.

Identification to the subspecies level (many salamanders) or the variety level (many Dendrobatidae) is not important for developing a history and diagnosis.

Establish the origin of the patient; is it captive-born or wild-caught and imported? This information is particularly important for amphibians because the likelihood of acclimation to a captive environment and the potential pathogens in wild-caught animals must be considered. The client may not know this history, particularly if the animal was purchased at a pet store or reptile and amphibian trade show or swap meet. One characteristic of captive-born amphibians includes juvenile age or relatively young animals when obtained by the client. Imported animals are usually adults because they are more frequently captured in the wild and more likely to survive shipping. Today certain species of frogs are almost exclusively captive-born. Many salamanders and most caecilians are wild-caught.

A particularly important question of the client is the medical history of the patient; has the patient been treated at home prior to or following the client's possession of the patient? Has the patient received treatment from another veterinarian? Home treatment of exotic pets, particularly reptiles and amphibians, is common. Occasionally results are favorable with home treatment, but more commonly the clinical condition fails to respond or deteriorates.

All husbandry parameters should be fully investigated. Descriptions of the enclosure, substrate, accessories, cage mates, feeding schedule, and environmental conditions of both the enclosure and the room housing the enclosure are important. When multiple individuals or species of amphibians are housed together, the client should be questioned regarding the health of these animals as well as any quarantine procedures that were performed.

The exact nutrition (which food items are consumed) of the captive amphibian is generally not as much of a clinical concern as whether or not the patient is actually eating. With respect to food items offered, particularly insects, it is important to learn the size of insect that is fed and the timing of the feedings. Also, ask the client if the patient is observed to actually eat the food items or if the food simply disappears from the cage. Many times insects may escape or hide beneath cage ornaments, leading the client to believe that the insects were consumed. This is particularly true of nocturnal amphibians. Question the client regarding food supplements such as vitamin mineral powders and frequency of application. For aquatic amphibians it is important to know the exact food items offered (live or processed). Many captive amphibians refuse prepared diets such as pellets initially and must be fed live food.

Restraint

The primary consideration when restraining an amphibian is stress on the patient and the potential health consequences of handling. The patient should be touched or restrained only when absolutely necessary. All diagnostic tests or treatments should be prepared prior to handling to consolidate procedures into the fewest episodes of physical manipulation of the patient. Consideration must also be given to the safety of the handler. Some species are capable of producing toxic skin secretions that are irritating and noxious, but rarely lethal to humans.

The following species when known to be wild-collected should be handled with extreme caution: golden poison frog (*Phyllobates terribilis*), black-legged poison frog (*Phyllobates bicolor*), Colorado River toad (*Bufo alvarius*), and marine toad (*Bufo marinus*). It is unlikely that either of the poison frogs listed will ever be seen in practice as wild caught individuals because they are relatively inaccessible for collection and exportation from Colombia, and both species are now widely available as captive-born juveniles and adults. Captive-born dart frogs have greatly reduced skin toxins and are generally not toxic to humans (Daly et al. 1994). Nevertheless, an imported *Phyllobates terribilis* should be considered lethal to humans. The toxins of *P. bicolor* are only 1/50 the strength of *P. terribilis*, yet a wild-caught frog should be considered dangerous (Walls 1994).

The *Bufo* spp. are a concern not as much for their degree of toxicity, which is significant, but for the manner in which the toxin may be secreted. Both species are capable of ejecting copious amounts of toxin from the parotid glands. Reports exist of this toxin spraying six feet or more from the animal (Wright and Whitaker 2001d). Entry of the toxin into an unprotected eye can be serious, not just from the standpoint of direct physical irritation, but also from absorption and systemic effects. All larger *Bufo* spp. and all wild-caught dart frogs are best handled with powder-free latex gloves. Additionally, protective eyewear is recommended when handling or manipulating larger toad species.

When possible, amphibians are best observed in a clear enclosure such as a plastic shoebox, deli cup, plastic bag, or other small enclosure. Handling of all amphibians is performed with a powder-free exam glove that has been cleaned, rinsed, or moistened with distilled water. Small frogs are best restrained with the hind legs extended and held securely between the thumb and index finger. This frees the head, body, and front legs for examination or treatment, yet adequately prevents jumping or escape attempt. Larger frogs and toads may require support by two hands to the body between the front and hind legs. Medium to large salamanders are restrained with a delicate grip of the fist, allowing the head to protrude between thumb and index finger and the tail exiting at the little finger. As in lizards, tail autotomy is possible for many species of salamanders. Most adult anguiform amphibians (caecilians, amphiumas, sirens) are nearly impossible to restrain manually and are best examined in an aquarium or chemically restrained (see Anesthesia).

Physical Examination

As with all exotic animals, the most important physical observations of the patient are made without handling. With the exception of some frogs and in contrast to most turtles, lizards, and snakes, the posture of amphibians is not as significant in revealing clinical disease. This is due to the fact that many species are nocturnal and cryptic, preferring to remain inactive or burrowed during the day. Species in which posture is generally significant are the dendrobatids, atelopids, mantellids, perching hylids such as *Phyllomedusa* spp., and most newts. Activity of the patient may be significant for some species. During a daytime examination all of the previously mentioned species (with the exception of hylids) should be bright, alert, and responsive. In contrast, nocturnal species such as hylids, some toads, ranids, and salamanders are generally inactive. A common indication of poor health in hylids, typically nocturnal, is activity during daylight hours. Red-eyed treefrogs, for example, generally rest on the sides of the enclosure with eyelids shut in daylight. Aquatic amphibians, though generally nocturnal, are generally active in the enclosure on presentation. Exceptions may include some aquatic or large semiaquatic frogs that, by nature, typically are not very active foragers and prefer to wait and ambush prey.

Observing the feeding response of diurnally active amphibians is a practical method to assess overall health. A failure to respond to the proper food item is generally a sign of illness or stress. Nocturnal or shy animals, however, rarely feed upon observation in daylight hours.

With a basic understanding of normal anatomy and body condition of the species in question, the visual exam should first focus on body condition. Is the patient normal weight, underweight, overweight, or bloated? It is important to remember that some frogs will inflate with air as a defense mechanism and may appear bloated, but suffer from no abnormal physiology. Air inflation is not a physiologic adaptation of salamanders and caecilians. As with other animals, emaciation does not occur in hours or days, but in weeks or months. Even the smallest frogs have distinct muscle groups that reveal weight loss. Poison dart frogs, for example, exhibit emaciation particularly on the back, scapulas, and pelvis.

Observe the cloaca for prolapse. This abnormality may remain unnoticed by the client. Also observe a fresh stool sample. For most terrestrial amphibians the feces are ejected as a pellet and should be somewhat moist and dark brown in color. Abnormalities in color and consistency may be significant. A microscopic fecal exam is essential for all captive-born and imported amphibians.

Abnormalities in respiratory effort can be difficult to detect in terrestrial amphibians. Normal respiration is driven primarily by buccal or gular pumping rather than by diaphragmatic or intercostal muscle contraction. There is rarely noticeable variation in this rhythmic pumping motion, even in diseased animals. Bubbling from the mouth or nostrils in terrestrial amphibians, however, is abnormal and a possible clinical sign of respiratory disease.

Abnormality of the integument is one of the more common abnormal physical findings and a common presenting complaint for diseased amphibians. Understanding the natural history and normal characteristics of the integument for a given species is essential. Most toads, terrestrial newts, and some tree frogs have relatively dry skin. Many larger tree frogs such as *Phyllomedusa* spp. and *Litoria* spp. can produce waxy secretions to prevent dessication. Amphibians slough skin, ecdysis, throughout their lives, and this process should not be confused with disease. Coloration varies widely, particularly in frogs, and with many this coloration is bilaterally symmetric. Even cryptic amphibians exhibit some color and pattern symmetry; therefore, observe closely for abnormalities in symmetry of color, texture, and morphology. Amphibians typically do not exhibit color-changing ability as seen in some lizards, though variation will occur from day to night in many hylids. Ulcers, erosions, plaques, and crusts are not normal. Newly acquired or recently imported frogs are susceptible to rostral abrasions that may rapidly progress into necrotizing ulcerations.

Most salamanders and terrestrial frogs have closable eyelids and frogs possess a nictitating membrane that is semitransparent. When awake and alert the amphibian eye should have eyelids open and clear corneas. Iris coloration is variable among amphibians, but is always bilaterally symmetric. As with mammals, unilateral ocular changes are most suggestive of trauma or focal disease and bilateral ophthalmic abnormalities are more suggestive of systemic disease. Iris vasculature may be apparent in the normal amphibian eye. There is great variation in pupil structure from circular to horizontally and vertically elliptic. An ophthalmoscope illuminator or slit lamp is helpful for examination of the eye. Commonly used mammalian mydriatics such as atropine and proparacaine are not effective in dilating the amphibian eye. Wright (2001b) recommends the combination of D-tubocurarine and benzalkonium chloride applied topically for mydriasis (Whitaker 2001).

Oral exam requires physical or chemical restraint in most species. Some species of frog, *Ceratophrys* and *Hemiphractus* spp., are known to gape as a defensive tactic, making oral examination possible without restraint on occasion. Similarly, some larger terrestrial salamanders (*Ambystoma* spp., *Dicamptodon* spp.), particularly those maintained long term in captivity, may exhibit a conditioned feeding response and can be coaxed into biting a soft speculum to examine the mouth. Though it is not recommended as normal practice, these animals, when routinely hand fed, will bite fingers waved in front of the face. It is unlikely that any injury will result to a human from the bite of an ambystomatid salamander. Large frogs (Ceratophrys, Pyxicephalus) and large aquatic salamanders (Amphiuma, Siren, Cryptobranchus) are capable of painful bites to humans. These species generally require chemical restraint for both physical restraint and oral examination.

The clinician and technician should be aware that mandibular bones of many small amphibians are easily fractured with improper or forceful techniques to open the mouth. When properly restrained the mouth of many smaller amphibians may be opened with a variety of apparatus such as plastic cards, laminated paper, coverslips, and small rubber spatulas. Nearly all amphibians will resist the oral exam if not sedated. Observe for uniformity and symmetry in shape and coloration of the oral mucosa and the tongue. Occasionally parasites such as flukes and leeches may be observed attached to the oral mucosa.

Palpation is easily accomplished for larger amphibians, but should generally be avoided in smaller species to prevent iatrogenic trauma. Internal organs of the smallest species may be evaluated by transillumination of the patient through a clear plastic container. This process is ineffective for large or dark pigmented patients. The heart, liver, spleen, gonads, and some vasculature may be observed in this manner. Palpation of larger species may reveal abnormalities such as foreign bodies and calculi, though normal structures may be difficult to assess or identify.

The heartbeat may be visible as pulsations of the skin in the region of the xiphoid on the ventral thorax in some amphibians. Similarly, in some frogs, pulsation of the lymphatic hearts is occasionally observed lateral to the urostyle. Cardiac auscultation is possible in larger amphibians, though the clinical significance of this procedure during wellness exams is question.

RADIOLOGY

As with reptiles, radiology is valuable in the diagnosis of some amphibian disease. This imaging is particularly useful for the diagnosis of skeletal disorders, urinary tract calculi, tissue mineralization, pulmonary disease, gastrointestinal foreign bodies, and other gastrointestinal disease with the aid of contrast materials. Unless abnormality is present, it is generally not possible to clearly differentiate coelomic cavity structures radiographically in amphibians.

Techniques for radiographic exposure are similar to those described for reptiles. Because of the small size of most amphibians, a table-top exposure with detail cassettes yields the best quality image. Generally, an exposure setting consistent with the lowest mammalian extremity setting is sufficient, though with smaller patients overexposure is still possible. For technician safety the use of a collimator to achieve the smallest exposure field is essential. With this technique, multiple exposures are possible on a single cassette.

Restraint of the amphibian patient during radiology is a hands-off affair. Many frogs will sit briefly directly on the cassette for exposure. For those that are reluctant to remain still, placement of the patient in a plastic bag facilitates restraint and manipulation for proper exposure (Stetter 2001a). When possible, a lateral and dorsoventral exposure should be made of every patient imaged. This typically requires the movement of the radiographic beam into a horizontal beam projection as the patient sits on the tabletop or platform.

Contrast studies are easily performed in amphibians. Barium sulfate is the contrast medium of choice and is given orally via a rubber catheter or feeding tube. The dosage varies greatly based on the size of amphibian. A range of 10 to 15 ml/kg PO is generally sufficient, though the technician should approximate the volume of the calculated dose to the patient's body size and adjust accordingly. Percloacal barium administration is also performed for suspected colonic foreign bodies, strictures, or other disease. Great care must be used when manipulating catheters with these tissues to prevent iatrogenic trauma.

ANESTHESIA AND SURGERY

Anesthesia

Anesthesia for amphibians is useful for physical examination of aggressive or reluctantly restrained patients, certain diagnostic and therapeutic procedures, and surgery. Reports exist for the use of injectable anesthetics in amphibians, though current consensus regards these medications as impractical and ineffective for safe chemical restraint. The anesthetic of choice for amphibians is tricaine methanesulfonate (MS-222, tricaine, FINQUEL, Argent Chemical Laboratories, Redmond, WA) (Wright 2001f). It is a white crystalline powder that may be mixed with water to anesthetize fish and amphibians. Amphibians are immersed in a bath of tricaine methanesulfonate until anesthesia is achieved and then maintained in fresh water for the particular procedure to be performed. For longer procedures, the patient may be immersed in a 50% dilution of the original induction solution or intubated and maintained on isoflurane.

Preparation of tricaine solution requires dissolving the powder into clean distilled water. The standard solution is 0.1% concentration: 1 g MS-222 in 1 liter distilled water. Because tricaine is quite acidic, the solution must be buffered to a pH of 7 to 7.4, which is the physiologic range of amphibian tissue. This is accomplished with either sodium biphosphate (Na_2HPO_4) or sodium bicarbonate (Na_2CO_3). Wright (2001f) reports the use of 34 to 50 ml of a 0.5 M Na_2HPO_4 solution to the 1 liter stock solution of MS-222. Stetter (2001b) applies Na_2CO_3 powder (common baking soda) to the stock solution until no more dissolves, yielding the preferred pH range. Ideally pH should be tested with a pH meter.

Tricaine is not stable in water when exposed to light. Therefore, unless multiple anesthesia episodes are planned, it should be mixed only in the quantity desired for a single anesthetic episode. Generally a 1-liter solution is adequate. All dissolved tricaine should be discarded after use and not reused for other patients.

Amphibians are induced in a bath of 1 g/L tricaine methanesulfonate in a suitable induction chamber that may be a plastic bag or other sealable plastic container. Induction time may vary, but usually thirty minutes exposure achieves surgical anesthesia (Wright 2001f; Stetter 2001b). Loss of the righting reflex and lack of voluntary movement is indication of adequate induction. Loss of the withdrawal or deep pain reflex indicates surgical anesthesia.

The patient is then transferred out of the induction chamber onto a treatment pan or receptacle and maintained in clean fresh distilled water or a 50% dilution of tricaine (0.05%) for the duration of the procedure (Wright 2001f). The patient's nostrils and mouth must be maintained above the water level to prevent aspiration. At this time, for longer surgical procedures, large amphibians may be intubated and maintained on oxygen (with or without isoflurane) with intermittent positive pressure ventilation (IPPV). Continued exposure to the 0.05% tricaine bath maintains adequate anesthesia in the absence of isoflurane.

The patient should be monitored for heartbeat throughout the anesthetic procedure. Respiration is reduced or nearly absent and oxygenation of the tricaine bath with oxygen is recommended to enhance oxygen absorption through the skin. The patient is recovered from tricaine anesthesia in clean distilled water, making sure that the nostrils and mouth are not under water to prevent aspiration. The recovery period may range from thirty to sixty minutes.

An additional anesthetic protocol is the topical application of liquid isoflurane. A mixture of 3 cc liquid isoflurane with 1.5 cc water and 3.5 cc KY-Jelly is made in a 10-cc syringe and shaken. The resulting liquid is then applied to the back of the patient at a dose of 0.025 cc to 0.035 cc/g body weight. The lower dose is applied to frogs and salamanders and the higher dose is for toads. The patient is induced in a sealed container over five to fifteen minutes. Following induction the remaining gel is wiped from the skin and anesthesia will last for forty-five to eighty minutes.

Surgery

Though surgical procedures on amphibians are not routine, several pathologic conditions may require surgical treatment. Celiotomy, mass removal, and limb amputation are the most commonly performed procedures. Other procedures include enucleation and orthopedic surgery. All invasive surgical procedures are performed with general anesthesia using tricaine or isoflurane. Pre- and post-surgical administration of antibiotics are recommended for invasive procedures.

The amphibian skin is prepped using 0.2% chlorhexidine (Wright 2001f) or 0.2% chloroxylenol diluted to 0.75% with water. Isopropyl alcohol and iodine compounds are potentially toxic to amphibians and should be avoided. The surgical prep should have as long a contact time as possible prior to surgery, preferably ten minutes. The surgical site should be moistened with saline prior to draping and surgery. Depending on the procedure, draping may not be performed. For celiotomy, sterile clear plastic drape is applied. Peripheral to the plastic drape a sterile cloth drape may be used to maintain a sterile field for surgical instruments.

As with lizards, a paramedian ventral midline incision is recommended to avoid the large ventral abdominal vein that lies on the ventral serosal surface of the coelomic cavity. Closure of surgical incisions is accomplished with non-absorbable monofilament sutures of appropriate size.

TECHNIQUES

Venipuncture

Blood collection in amphibians can be a challenge, yet in some species, with proper technique and anatomical knowledge, the task is routine. Prior to sampling the skin should be prepped with diluted 2% chlorhexidine or 2% chloroxylenol at a 1:40 dilution (Wright 2001f). Alcohol should not be used because of irritation and dessication to the patient. Sampling from salamanders is performed from the ventral tail vein as described for snakes and lizards. A 1-cc or smaller syringe with a 25- or 27-gauge needle is ideal for most amphibians and the sample is preserved in lithium heparin.

Phlebotomy in frogs and toads is performed from a variety of locations. In larger frogs and toads the ventral abdominal vein is the best choice for both quality and quantity of the blood sample. Sampling from this vein is performed in the same manner as described for lizards. (Figures 10.4, 10.5). Because the lymphatic system of amphibians courses parallel to the blood vessels, it is not uncommon to collect lymphatic fluids with peripheral blood. Other sites of blood collection that are generally accessible in large frogs include the femoral vein and the lingual vein located on the ventral surface of the tongue. The volume of blood collected should be no more than 1% of the patient's body weight or 0.5% from a debilitated patient (Wright 2001f).

Celiocentesis

This technique is performed to analyze fluid retained in the coelomic cavity of amphibians. It may be both diagnostic and therapeutic. Fluid may accumulate in the coelom secondary to cardiac, renal, hepatic, or other osmotic imbalances. Similar to phlebotomy, a 25- or 27-gauge needle on a 1- to 3-cc syringe is ideal. The sample site is prepped with a 1:40 dilution of 2% chlorhexidine or chloroxylenol. The preferred collection site is from the mid lateral flank or mid ventral coelomic cavity. The syringe should fill with fluid on gentle aspiration and forceful aspiration should be

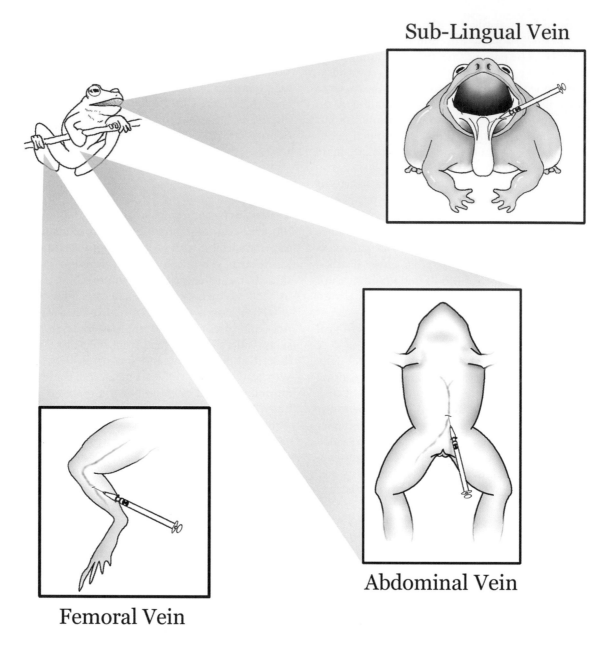

Sub-Lingual Vein

Femoral Vein

Abdominal Vein

Figure 10.4. Venipuncture sites in a frog. (Drawing by Scott Stark.)

avoided to prevent damage to delicate internal organs. Fluid may be smeared immediately or submitted in lithium heparin for cellular and chemical analysis.

Fecal Examination

Fecal exam is one diagnostic test that can be performed in all terrestrial amphibians and nearly all aquatic amphibians with relative ease. Collection of feces is facilitated particularly well during quarantine. The amphibian is maintained on paper towel in a clean cage such as a plastic shoebox or storage container that is adequately ventilated and a sample is collected.

The sample should be examined directly in 0.9% saline and by fecal floatation with standard commercially available fecal floatation solutions. Common parasite ova include nematodes, trematodes, coccidia, various protozoans, and lungworm larvae (see Parasitology).

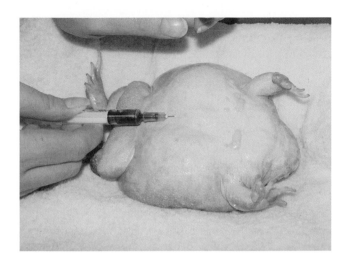

Figure 10.5. Venipuncture of the midabdominal vein (ventral abdominal vein) in a frog. (Photo courtesy of Dr. Stephen J. Hernandez-Divers, University of Georgia.)

Cloacal Wash

Cloacal wash is performed in larger amphibians (>5 cm) to collect fecal material for microscopic analysis when a fresh stool sample is unavailable for analysis. A lubricated semi-rigid plastic or rubber catheter attached to a 1-ml syringe is gently inserted into the cloaca and isotonic saline (0.6%) is infused from and retrieved into the syringe. The fluid volume may be between 0.5 and 1 ml and not all fluid will be retrieved. A portion of the sample is then viewed with a microscope for pathogens. For smaller amphibians (<5 cm) cloacal wash is generally too traumatic to attempt. Examination of fecal samples is recommended for these species.

Transtracheal Wash

The techniques for tracheal wash are identical to those in other vertebrates. The patient must be anesthetized (see Anesthesia and Surgery) and delicate handling of the tissues and apparatus must be performed. A sterile tomcat or small gauge mammalian intravenous catheter may be inserted into the glottis in the floor of the mouth. Depending on patient size, 0.25 to 0.5 cc sterile isotonic (0.6%) saline is infused and gently retrieved.

The sample may then be smeared and stained for microscopic analysis.

Skin Scrape and Impression Smear

These processes are designed to identify fungal, bacterial, and protozoal elements to the skin or wounds on the skin. An impression smear is performed when tissue is damaged or ulcerated and a scraping will only create further trauma. Shed skins are particularly helpful for microscopic analysis and may be fixed in formalin for histopathologic staining to identify certain bacterial and fungal pathogens. A skin scraping is performed with the edge of a coverslip and wetmount examination.

Assist Feeding

Assist feeding is required for amphibians that are diseased and unable or unwilling to voluntarily feed. It is important that the owner understand that this procedure may be stressful on the patient and debilitated patients may not survive repeated handling; nevertheless, this may also be a life saving procedure designed to return the patient to a normal feeding response. Wright and Whitaker (2001d) list the standard metabolic rates (SMR) for caecilians, salamanders, and frogs at temperatures ranging from 5 °C to 25 °C and they recommend that caloric intake for diseased animals should exceed the SMR by 50% on a daily basis.

An ideal feeding formula for amphibians is Clinical Care Feline Liquid (Pet-Ag, Elgin, IL), which provides 0.92 kcal/ml and has a well balanced protein-to-fat-to-carbohydrate ratio for amphibians (Wright 2001d). This liquid product is easy to administer through a small bore tube and provides nutrients and calories evenly in suspension. The patient's normal food items are provided daily under observation to assess for a return to normal feeding. Force feedings are not made daily to reduce handling. Instead, the calculated daily dose may be multiplied by the number of days between feedings (three, five, etc.) and the total dose for those days is administered at one time. Wright and Whitaker recommend that the volume of feeding should not exceed 10% of the patient's body weight in a twenty-four hour period.

The feeding procedure is accomplished in a matter similar to that of reptiles. A red rubber catheter, intravenous catheter, tomcat catheter, or ball tipped feeding needle is passed into the stomach and the food preparation is infused. The technician should be aware that the stomach of most amphibians (especially frogs) is relatively proximal in the coelom; thus, passage of the tube no more than one-third to one-half of the patient's body length (excluding the tail) is recommended.

An alternative to Clinical Care Liquid is a mashed or ground mixture of invertebrates such as fruit flies or crickets administered in the same manner. The author has had great success with anorectic dart frogs using this technique on an every seventy-two hours basis. Several patients have required two weeks or more of assist feeding before feeding voluntarily.

Therapeutic Administration

Amphibians present fewer problems than one may expect with medications. The semipermeable skin enables the clinician to apply some medications topically (TO) for systemic absorption, a technique not applicable to reptiles. Additionally, medicated baths may be used to treat both cutaneous and systemic diseases. Oral (PO) administration is possible and standard for some medications such as deworming agents and antibiotics. Finally, injections may be given intramuscularly (IM) or intracoelomically (ICe) in large amphibians or subcutaneously (SC) in frogs and some salamanders. Intravenous (IV) administration is rare and difficult at best in all but the largest amphibians. Physical restraint of the patient is required for all but the topical route of therapeutic administration.

The application of injectable medications in a topical manner is very practical for amphibians with permeable skin. This method likely results in lower percutaneous absorption rates in toads or in species that produce a waxy skin coating. Antibiotics such as enrofloxacin and ivermectin have been applied topically with great success for various bacterial and parasitic diseases. Baths with medications such as gentamicin, nitrofurazone, itraconazole, sulfamethazine, mettronidazole, and other medications have shown success and safety in combating various diseases.

Oral administration is possible in nearly all sizes of amphibians and is the preferred route of treatment when possible to achieve maximum systemic absorption. This route is contraindicated in those species that are refractory to handling or physical manipulation. Metal feeding tubes or rubber catheters are used in large animals and microliter pipettes are used for small patients. Dilution of the commercially available preparations or compounding of medications is required for smaller amphibians. Dosing for most oral medications is daily or less often depending on the drug.

Injections are possible in amphibians, but carry moderate risk of trauma to muscles or internal organs and may result in chemical trauma or excessive pain and disability at the injection site. Many injectable medications applied orally in amphibians show good systemic absorption. This is particularly true of enrofloxacin that may be otherwise irritating to amphibian skin and may cause skin irritation, discoloration, or sloughing from topical administration or injection. The intracoelomic route is preferred for fluid administration in critically ill or dehydrated amphibians. The method of injection is similar to that of celiocentesis.

A considerable benefit to choosing the topical route for medicating the patient is allowing the client to treat at home for non-critical cases. All other routes of administration require hospitalization or repeated visits to the clinic for treatment by the technician or clinician. Medications should be dispensed in individual syringes with the appropriate amount for each dose drawn up and ready to apply. This negates the possibility of inappropriate dosing by the client. The client should return the used syringes for disposal at the end of the treatment period to allow both a recheck of the patient and to assess compliance of therapeutic administration.

An important fact regarding amphibian disease is that pharmaceuticals are not required to treat or cure every disease. It cannot be overemphasized that diseases resulting from improper husbandry comprise a substantial percentage of presenting complaints with amphibians and reptiles. The number one consideration when choosing pharmaceuticals for disease management is side effects. Though it may be difficult for the client to appreciate that environmental manipulation alone can correct improper health, it is even more difficult to understand further debilitation caused by unnecessary treatment.

EUTHANASIA

Invariably treatments fail to gain response or patients are too debilitated to withstand treatment and the client elects euthanasia. Amphibians and reptiles can pose some problems with euthanasia in that the heart may continue to beat for some time after neurologic incapacitation or death has occurred.

Reducing patient suffering and pain and client discomfort with the euthanasia process may be difficult. If possible the patient may be sedated with one of several anesthetic agents prior to administering euthanasia injections. Ketamine at a dose of 100 mg/kg IM or telazol (tiletamine–zolazepam) at a dose of 10 mg/kg IM (Wright 2001f) is sufficient to achieve sedation for euthanasia. The clinician and technician should understand that both of these injections are likely to cause pain and discomfort to the patient at the injection site. Alternatively, tricaine (MS-222) may be used as a pre-euthanasia sedative or if overdosed as a euthanasia solution (Wright and Whitaker 2001b).

Administration of a barbiturate euthanasia solution such as pentobarbital at a dose of 100 mg/kg intracardiac (if possible) results in instant death. Alternatively, the injection may be given intracoelomically or intracranially through the foramen magnum, though cardiac death may be delayed.

If histopathology is required of the patient, then minimizing trauma to vital organs is essential. In this case, an overdose of tricaine given intracoelomically or immersion of the sedated patient in 20% ethanol will result in death (Wright and Whitaker 2001d). Most importantly, clients should be informed of the euthanasia alternatives and fully understand the procedure to be performed if they wish to be present during the euthanasia process.

REFERENCES

Barnett SL. 1996. The Husbandry of Poison-Dart Frogs (Family Dendrobatidae). *Proceed. Assoc. Amphibian and Rept. Veterinarians*, 1–6.

Barnett SL, et al. 2001. Amphibian Husbandry and Housing. In: Amphibian Medicine and Captive Husbandry. Edited by Wright KM, Whitaker BR. Malabar, FL: Krieger Publishing Co.

Berger L, et al. 1998. Chytridiomycosis Causes Amphibian Mortality Associated with Population Declines in the Rain Forests of Australia and Central America. *Proc. Nat Acad. Sci.* 95: 9031–9036.

Daly JW, et al. 1994. Dietary Source for Skin Alkaloids of Poison Frogs (Dendrobatidae)? *Journal of Chemical Ecology* 20 (4): 943–98.

Daszak P, et al. 2000. Emerging Infectious Diseases of Wildlife—Threats to Biodiversity and Human Health. *Am Assoc. for the Advancement of Science* 287: 443–449.

de Vosjoli P. 1996. Care and Breeding of Popular Tree Frogs. Santee, CA: Advanced Vivarium Systems, Inc.

Diana SG, et al. 2001. Clinical Toxicology. In: Amphibian Medicine and Captive Husbandry. Edited by Wright KM, Whitaker BR. Malabar, FL: Krieger Publishing Co.

Donoghue S, Langenberg J. 1996. Special Topics: Nutrition. In: Reptile Medicine and Surgery. Edited by Mader DR. Philadelphia: W.B. Saunders Co.

Duellman WE, Trueb L. 1994. Biology of Amphibians. Baltimore: Johns Hopkins University Press.

Gagliardo R. Atlanta Botanical Garden. Personal communication.

Goin CJ, Goin OB, Zug GR. 1978. Introduction to Herpetology, 3rd ed. New York: W.H. Freeman and Co.

Helfman GS. 1990. Mode Selection and Mode Switching in Foraging Animals. *Advances in the Study of Behavior* 19: 249.

Klingenberg RJ. 1993. Understanding Reptile Parasites. Lakeside, CA: Advanced Vivarium Systems.

Lotters S. 1996. The Neotropical Toad Genus Atelopus. Koln, Germany: M. Vences and F. Glaw Verlags GbR.

Mattison C. 1987. Frogs and Toads of the World. New York: Facts on File Publications.

Morell V. 1999. Are Pathogens Felling Frogs? *Science* 284: 728–731.

Obst FJ, et al. 1988. The Completely Illustrated Atlas of Reptiles and Amphibians for the Terrarium. Neptune City, NJ: TFH.

Pessier AP, Roberts DR, Linn M, et al. 2002. "Short tongue syndrome", lingual squamous Metaplasia and suspected hypovitaminosis A in captive Wyoming toads. *Proceedings, Association of Reptilian and Amphibian Veterinarians*, pp 151–153.

Petranka JW. 1998. Salamanders of the United States and Canada. Washington, DC: Smithsonian Institution Press.

Poynton SL, Whitaker BR. 2001. Protozoa and Metazoa Infecting Amphibians. In: Amphibian Medicine and Captive Husbandry. Edited by Wright KM, Whitaker BR. Malabar, FL: Krieger Publishing Co.

Stebbins RC. 1985. Peterson Field Guide to Western Reptiles and Amphibians. Boston: Houghton Mifflin Co.

Stetter MD. 2001a. Diagnostic Imaging of Amphibians. In: Amphibian Medicine and Captive Husbandry. Edited by Wright KM, Whitaker BR. Malabar, FL: Krieger Publishing Co.

Stetter MD. 2001b. Fish and Amphibian Anesthesia. *Veterinary Clinics of North America: Exotic Animal Practice.* 4(1): 69–82.

Taylor SK. 2001. Mycoses. In: Amphibian Medicine and Captive Husbandry. Edited by Wright KM, Whitaker BR. Malabar, FL: Krieger Publishing Co.

Walls JG. 1994. Jewels of the Rain Forest—Poison Dart Frogs of the World. Neptune City, NJ: TFH Publications.

Whitaker BR. 2001. The Amphibian Eye. In: Amphibian Medicine and Captive Husbandry. Edited by Wright KM, Whitaker BR. Malabar, FL: Krieger Publishing Co.

Wright KM. 2001a. Amphibian Hematology. In: Amphibian Medicine and Captive Husbandry. Edited by Wright KM, Whitaker BR. Malabar, FL: Krieger Publishing Co.

Wright KM. 2001b. Anatomy for the Clinician. In: Amphibian Medicine and Captive Husbandry. Edited by Wright KM, Whitaker BR. Malabar, FL: Krieger Publishing Co.

Wright KM. 2001c. Applied Physiology. In: Amphibian Medicine and Captive Husbandry. Edited by Wright KM, Whitaker BR. Malabar, FL: Krieger Publishing Co.

Wright KM. 2001d. Diets for Captive Amphibians. In: Amphibian Medicine and Captive Husbandry. Edited by Wright KM, Whitaker BR. Malabar, FL: Krieger Publishing Co.

Wright KM. 2001e. Evolution of the Amphibia. In: Amphibian Medicine and Captive Husbandry. Edited by Wright KM, Whitaker BR. Malabar, FL: Krieger Publishing Co.

Wright KM. 2001f. Surgical Techniques. In: Amphibian Medicine and Captive Husbandry. Edited by Wright KM, Whitaker BR. Malabar, FL: Krieger Publishing Co.

Wright KM. 2001g. Taxonomy of Amphibians Kept in Captivity. In: Amphibian Medicine and Captive Husbandry. Edited by Wright KM, Whitaker BR. Malabar, FL: Krieger Publishing Co. pp. 3–14.

Wright KM, Whitaker BR. 2001a. Nutritional Disorders. In: Amphibian Medicine and Captive Husbandry. Edited by Wright KM, Whitaker BR. Malabar, FL: Krieger Publishing Co.

Wright KM, Whitaker BR. 2001b. Pharmacotherapeutics. In: Amphibian Medicine and Captive Husbandry. Edited by Wright KM, Whitaker BR. Malabar, FL: Krieger Publishing Co.

Wright KM, Whitaker BR. 2001c. Quarantine. In: Amphibian Medicine and Captive Husbandry. Edited by Wright KM, Whitaker BR. Malabar, FL: Krieger Publishing Co.

Wright KM, Whitaker BR. 2001d. Restraint Techniques and Euthanasia. In: Amphibian Medicine and Captive Husbandry. Edited by Wright KM, Whitaker BR. Malabar, FL: Krieger Publishing Co.

Wright KM. 2009. Three things you must know to see amphibians. *Proceedings of the North American Veterinary Conference* (23). Gainesville, FL, 1822–1825.

Section 5
Mammals

CHAPTER ELEVEN

Ferrets

James R. McClearen, Julie Mays, and Tarah Hadley

INTRODUCTION

The art of veterinary medicine has extended into many families of creatures. Among small mammals, also known as "pocket pets," the ferret has become one of the more popular pets in today's society. Although the practice of medicine in ferrets is still viewed as being different from the traditional feline and canine practice, the same techniques that are used in small animal practice may be easily applied to small mammal practice. It is important for the veterinary team to recognize that there are similarities and differences in the application of these techniques compared to small animal practice. Other novel medical approaches may also be used to provide solutions to problems.

The domesticated ferret found in the United States is commercially raised for the pet industry and medical research. It is conjectured that domesticated ferrets arrived in North America as pets from early English settlers more than 300 years ago. They are most likely a domesticated variety of the European ferret (*Mustela putorius furo*). The black-footed ferret (*Mustela nigripes*) is an indigenous species of the southwestern United States. There are strict fish and wildlife regulations that vary from state to state regarding the possession of these animals. Veterinary facilities, which often serve as the first point of contact for the pet-owning public, must be acutely aware of these requirements.

ANATOMY

Conformation

The ferret has an elongated body that allows it to enter small areas and holes for to pursue prey. This feature provides challenges for both owner and veterinary staff in caging and handling. Remember: wherever the head goes so follows the rest of the body. The males are larger than females and their weight fluctuations vary according to season, similar to dogs and cats (Hillyer and Quesenberry 1997).

Skin and Hair Coat

There are three naturally occurring coat color patterns. Sable is the most commonly observed but albino and cinnamon are also seen. The sable ferret, known also as "fitch," has been reported as a cross between the European polecat and ferret. They typically have black-tipped guard hair, a cream undercoat, black feet and tail, and a black mask. In the United States, enthusiasts have developed more than thirty color combinations, including silver, chocolate, panda, and Siamese.

One of the first observations that handlers of ferrets notice about this animal is that there is a distinct odor. This odor is primarily from oil glands and not from the anal glands, as many people tend to think. The odor may become more obvious when the ferrets are excited or during breeding season. There are numerous commercial bathing products that help to make these creatures more "house friendly." Descenting at a young age is a popular procedure performed at breeding farms but unfortunately it has limited effects in preventing the odor.

Ferrets have no sweat glands in their skin. As a result, the veterinary staff must be aware of the possibility of hyperthermia.

Skeletal

The vertebral formula for the ferret is C7, T15, L5 (6), S3, Cd18 (Hillyer and Quesenberry 1997). The anatomical considerations of interest include a small sternum and thoracic inlet, nonretractable claws, and a J-shaped os penis. Skeletal anatomy is depicted in Figure 11.1.

Digestive Tract

The ferret has thirty deciduous teeth and thirty-four permanent teeth. The permanent teeth erupt between fifty and seventy-four days. The upper teeth are as follows: six incisors, two canine, six premolars, and

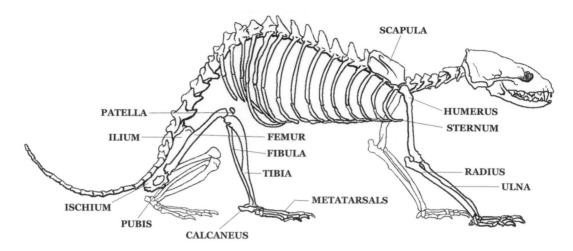

Figure 11.1. Ferret skeletal anatomy. (Drawing by Scott Stark.)

two molars. The bottom arcade has six incisors, two canine, six premolars, and four molars (Fox 1998).

Ferrets have five pairs of salivary glands. Care must be taken not to confuse the mandibular salivary gland with the lymph nodes in that area. The stomach of the ferret is simple and can expand to accommodate large amounts of food (Figure 11.2). The small intestine is short in length and has an average transit time of three to four hours (Fox 1998).

Heart and Lungs
The heart lies approximately between the sixth and eighth ribs. In comparison to other mammals such as cats and dogs, the location of the heart in ferrets is relatively more caudal than expected for auscultation. The lungs consist of six lobes. The left lung has two lobes and the right has four (Fox 1998).

Spleen
The ferret spleen varies greatly in size, depending on the animal's age and state of health. When enlarged, the spleen extends in a diagonal fashion from the upper left to the lower right quadrant of the abdominal cavity. An enlarged spleen tends to be a very distinct finding during physical examination (Hillyer and Quesenberry 1997).

Urogenital Tract
The right kidney is cranial to the left kidney and is covered by the caudate lobe of the liver. The bladder holds approximately 10 cc of urine. In the male the prostate is found at the base of the bladder.

Gender is easily determined in males, which have a ventral abdominal preputial opening similar to dogs.

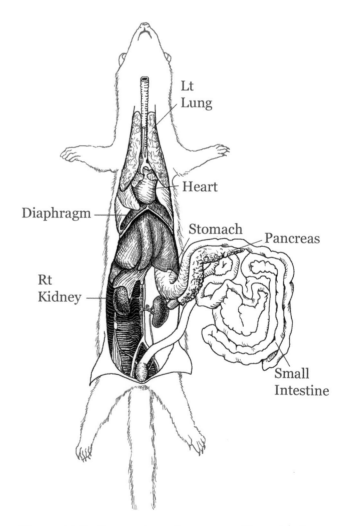

Figure 11.2. Ferret visceral anatomy. (Drawing by Scott Stark.)

In females the urogenital opening has the appearance of a small slit (Figure 11.3). During estrus, the vulva becomes enlarged. The natural breeding season is from March to August.

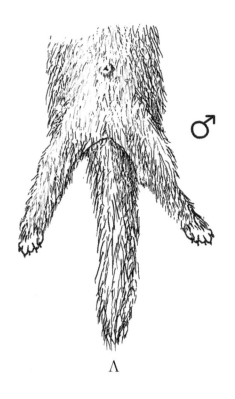

Λ

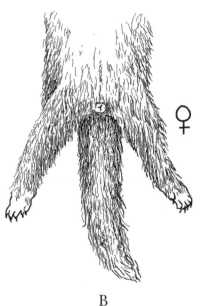

B

Figure 11.3. (A) Male reproductive anatomy. (B) Female reproductive anatomy. (Drawings by Scott Stark.)

Fertility in both genders depends on the photoperiod. Females are seasonally polyestrous and induced ovulators. Ovulation occurs thirty to forty hours after copulation. Gestation typically lasts forty-one to forty-two days. If fertilization does not occur, pseudopregnancy often occurs and that will last forty-one to forty-three days. If these females are not bred, a large percentage of these individuals will remain in estrus with the potential for developing bone marrow suppression secondary to elevated estrogen levels (Hillyer and Quesenberry 1997).

Adrenal Glands
Both adrenal glands lie in the fatty tissue anterior to the cranial pole of the kidneys. The left gland is located medial to the kidney and is approximately 6 to 8 mm in length. The right adrenal gland is more dorsal than the left. It is covered by the caudate lobe of the liver and is attached to the caudal vena cava. It is larger than the left with an overall length of 8 to 11 mm. This knowledge is important when assessment of adrenal gland disease is attempted either surgically or ultrasonographically.

Biological and Reproductive Data
Table 11.1 provides basic biological and reproductive data necessary for proper examination of a ferret or answering common client questions.

BEHAVIOR

Ferrets are active little animals and the trouble that they can get into is limited only by the size of their head. The adult males are called hobs, intact females are called jills, spayed females are sprites, and juveniles are called kits. The ferret has been and still is used for hunting, biomedical research, and most recently as a pet. The domesticated ferret does not fear humans or unfamiliar environments unlike its counterpart, the European polecat (Fox 1998). In pairs they constantly play fight, expelling sounds from a low growl to a high-pitched scream when challenged or in pain. They continuously roll and bite their opponent on the face and feet, with their favorite spot being the nape of the neck.

Many times in the heat of play with humans or companions, ferrets back up across the room chattering and hissing at the same time. They are attracted to quick movements, an instinct developed primarily for hunting prey. Their eyesight is only good up to short distances and they depend upon their excellent sense of smell and acute hearing to help them maneuver in

Table 11.1. Physiologic values for domestic ferrets.

Adult weight	
Male	1–2 kg
Female	600–950 g
Life span	5–8 years average in the United States. Some may reach 12 years of age
Sexual maturity	4–8 months of age (usually reached in first spring after birth)
Gestation period	41–42 days
Normal weight at birth	8–10 g
Eyes and ears open	21–37 days of age (usually 30–35 days)
Weaning age	6–8 weeks
Rectal temperature	37.8°C–40°C (100°F–104°F)
Average blood volume	Mature male, 60 mL; Mature female, 40 mL
Heart rate	180–250 beats per minute
Urine volume	26–28 mL/24 hours

Source: Hillyer and Quesenberry (1997).

their environment. Due to their sense of smell, ferrets constantly keep their noses close to the ground. This predisposes them to loud sneezing, which often alerts their owners as to their location. Ferrets are active about 25% to 30% of the day and asleep the remaining 70% to 75% (Hillyer and Quesenberry 1997).

HUSBANDRY

The word "ferret" means to search out something, to ferret it out, or to find something. This is a pet ferret's whole existence and an extremely important factor in providing a safe and an environmentally rich habitat for these animals. Assume that ferrets can go anywhere. The limiting hole diameter for escape is usually less than 1 inch; anything over that they can easily explore. Cages in the home setting and the veterinary hospital must reflect this attitude. All potential openings to the outside such as heating and air conditioning vents and tubing, dryer vents, doors, and windows are all possible routes of escape.

Ferrets do not fare well outdoors because of their domestication. Inside the house, reclining and other furniture, bedding, appliances, and electrical cords offer potential injury and even death as a possibility. Owners must be acutely aware of the dangers of inges-

tion of household items such as insulation for wiring and pipes, packing material, rubber bands, soft rubber material for shoes, or other pet toys. These latter items are particularly dangerous because ferrets seem to have an affinity for materials made out of rubber. Gastrointestinal obstruction is a common problem seen in young ferrets.

Caging should be of adequate size with minimum dimensions of 24 inches × 24 inches × 18 inches (Hillyer and Quesenberry 1997). Ideal caging should provide multiple levels and a hiding or den area, sufficient area for a litter box, and space for food and water. However, some owners may also set aside an entire room as living quarters for their ferrets. Food bowls should be made of a nontoxic product and safe water bottles are available commercially. Litter pans in a household setting may consist of a small plastic litter box similar to cat pans but may require lowering one side of the pan for entry. In a veterinary hospital, small, low cardboard boxes are useful with debilitated or postsurgery animals. They are also conveniently disposable.

Toys should be "ferret" approved; hard, nonchipping rubber balls, metal toys that make noise, and "ferret" jungle gyms made of PVC pipes provide good entertainment.

NUTRITION

The domestic ferret, European polecat, and black-footed ferret are predatory animals that feed primarily on small mammals and birds. Early ferreters fed their animals bread or corn meal soaked with milk. They survived on this diet as long as it was supplemented with fresh meat.

Most ranch ferrets are fed commercial pelleted foods. Initially, mink diets were fed but they lacked important nutritional components due to their protein base of fish (Bell 1999).

The ferret is an obligate carnivore with a very short intestinal tract. Compared to a cat, the ferret has relatively about one-half the intestinal length. They are spontaneous secretors of hydrochloric acid, like humans and unlike dogs, cats, and many other predators. These animals often hide food in various locations in their environment for future consumption. Because of the inefficiency of the ferret's digestive tract, ferret diets must be high in protein and fat and low in fiber. Traditional ferret diets include 30% to 40% protein and 15% to 30% fat. The type of diet depends on the ferret's health status and life stage, such as if they are growing kits or lactating jills (Bell 1999).

It is important to feed a high-quality domestic ferret food in dry form. Dry food is preferred over moist due to the health benefit for the mouth, teeth, and gums. Young kits require some moistening of the kibble foods until they get their adult teeth. At about ten weeks of age they should begin to handle dry kibble. There are numerous commercial foods available either from pet stores, veterinary clinics, or the Internet. If food availability is difficult, a high quality dry kitten food may be substituted. Some ferret food manufacturers also have senior diets available.

Supplements may be warranted in some situations, such as medical problems, surgery recovery, or cold environmental conditions. Products such as Linatone (Lambert Kay) and Nutrical (Evsco Pharmaceuticals; Division of IGI Inc.) are available through veterinary offices. A common over-the-counter product, Ferretone (8-in-1 Pet Products), is also a good choice. Snacks and treats should be held to a minimum because ferrets will over indulge on their favorite foods and run the long-term risk of malnutrition. Commercial meat or liver snacks for cats or ferrets are acceptable, and an occasional raisin may add a little variety to a ferret's diet. In some medical conditions, such as insulinoma, treats or supplements that are high in sugar may need to be avoided except at the direction of a veterinarian.

Water should be fresh and available at all times.

COMMON AND ZOONOTIC DISEASES

Influenza (orthomyxovirus) is the only documented zoonotic disease of ferrets. In most cases the transmissibility from humans to ferrets is much higher than ferrets to humans. Owners should be aware of that risk to their pets when they have upper respiratory problems. Other potential zoonotic diseases include leptospirosis, listeriosis, salmonellosis, campylobacteriosis, tuberculosis, and rabies. There are no known cases of transmission of rabies to humans from ferrets. Cryptosporidiosis has the potential of transmissibility to immunosuppressed individuals (Hillyer and Quesenberry 1997).

Many disease syndromes are found in ferrets. Upper-respiratory infections are common with ferrets as well as with their owners. Canine distemper is occasionally found manifesting itself in various forms. Early signs include mucopurulent ocular nasal discharge, crusty facial and eyelid lesions, and hyperkeratosis of the footpads. In some individuals there is an orange color change to the skin. These animals are often anorexic, and in advanced cases may show

central nervous signs such as ataxia, torticollis, and nystagmus.

Intestinal obstructions are very common in young inquisitive ferrets. These individuals present with or without vomiting, they may have diarrhea, they are lethargic, and in most situations there is a palpable abdominal mass. Bruxism, which is when a ferret gnashes its teeth from side to side and may froth at the mouth, is a common sign of pain.

Epizootic catarrhal enteritis (ECE) or green slime disease is a debilitating disease of young and old ferrets. ECE is usually brought into the house via introduction of a new young ferret. It is a highly contagious disease of ferrets characterized by profuse green diarrhea, dehydration, anorexia, and progressive wasting.

Tumors present themselves in many ways with ferrets. The most common tumors involve the adrenal gland (Figure 11.4). These tumors may be benign or malignant. Adrenal gland disease most often presents as a dermatological concern. Hair loss on the tail, bilateral hair loss along the abdomen, and vulvar enlargement in spayed females are consistent findings with adrenal gland involvement. Adrenal tumors can also cause behavior change and generalized muscle wasting. Secondary complications of the disease found in male ferrets involve the prostate in the form of prostatic hyperplasia or cysts and they commonly

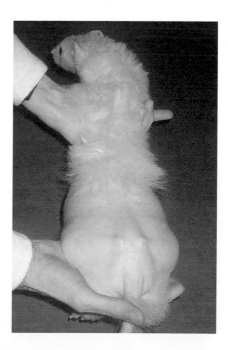

Figure 11.4. Adrenal gland disease in a ferret. (Photo courtesy of Dr. Sam Rivera.)

present with dysuria. Bacterial or fungal bladder infections can be a sequela to prostatic disease in males with adrenal disease. This problem may be extremely challenging to treat.

Lymphoma is found in the ferret in numerous forms. It may involve the lymph nodes, spleen, liver, intestines, kidneys, lung, and bone marrow. Squamous cell, mast cell, basal cell, and sebaceous gland tumors are the most common tumors of the skin.

Insulinoma, a type of pancreatic cancer, is very challenging to manage. Ferrets present very weak and sometimes with seizures. Due to the excessive insulin produced by this pancreatic tumor, blood glucose levels in affected ferrets are very low. These animals often present with significant weight loss, dehydration, moderate to severe depression, anorexia, or in a comatose state.

Renal cysts are found in many ferrets and often are only coincidental findings.

Ectoparasites such as fleas, ear mites, sarcoptic mites, and ticks are common in ferrets and are easily treated. Endoparasites are uncommon but coccidia and giardiasis are occasionally found. There is some geographic prevalence to ringworm (mycotic) in some individuals.

Posterior weakness is a frequent observation in sick or debilitated ferrets. This is also a common sign seen in hypoglycemic animals.

Myofaciitis is a new emerging disease that has been documented in at least a dozen ferrets. This disease is characterized by severe inflammation of muscles and surrounding fascia. Ferrets with this condition tend to be young (six to eighteen months of age) and have multiple clinical signs including pain, high fever, a reluctance to move, diarrhea, vomiting, and anorexia. Individuals also develop a neutrophilic leukocytosis. None of these symptoms typically respond to antibiotics or anti-inflammatories. The cause of this disease, which is rapidly progressive and fatal, is unknown (Garner 2007).

HISTORY AND PHYSICAL EXAMINATION

The procedure for taking a history and performing a physical examination on ferrets should follow routine small animal veterinary protocol. Questions should include: Has your ferret been coughing, sneezing, vomiting, or having diarrhea? Has there been any discharge from the eyes, nose, or any other body orifice? What is your pet's diet and how is its appetite? Does your ferret drink water excessively, have increased urina-

tion, or is it straining to urinate? Is your ferret active and alert?

Physical examination should also be consistent. Begin at the facial region and work caudally. Make sure that all areas are searched. Look for discharge from the eyes, nose, or ears. Examine the ears for masses or signs of mites. Remember, dirty ears do not necessarily need to be cleaned. A certain amount of discharge is normal and is present for protection. Are the eyes uniform in appearance and are there any signs of cataracts? Are all adult teeth present or are there remaining deciduous teeth? Does the rest of the oral cavity appear normal? Gingivitis and tartar are common findings in the oral cavity that should be noted if present. Often the best way to evaluate the oral cavity is by gently scruffing the nape of the neck and waiting for the ferret's characteristic yawn reflex.

Are there any signs of lymph node enlargement? Heart and lung fields are evaluated in the same respect as with other small animals with one slight change. Due to the more caudal location of the heart, auscultation of the heart in ferrets typically occurs at the caudal chest area as opposed to the mid chest area. Are the lung sounds normal and is there any indication of a heart murmur? Does the animal appear normal and of good conformation? Muscle and skeletal systems should be symmetric and show no sign of dysfunction. Do the limbs move in a normal manner? How is the appearance of the skin and hair coat? Canine distemper may cause crusty lesions on the skin or an orange color change. Hydration is also measured by skin turgor. Always be aware of masses of the skin and subcutaneous tissue.

Abdominal palpation is best accomplished by elevating the ferret above the examination table by the nape of the neck or by gently holding it around the neck. Most of these individuals accommodate the examination without too much struggle. Keep in mind that the spleen in many ferrets may be enlarged with no other indication of disease or illness. Examination of the prepuce and penile region in the male and vulvar area of the female is important to look for infection or any indication of endocrine problems.

For neurologic problems consider the overall behavior of the ferret. Is it aware, alert, and curious, or does it appear to be stargazing and unconcerned with its surroundings? Is the ferret having trouble standing? Ferrets with evidence of neurologic disorders, depending on the clinical signs, may have a life-threatening illness that requires immediate medical intervention.

PREVENTIVE MEDICINE

The primary focus for preventive care in ferrets should be centered on annual or bi-annual physical examination. An early vaccination program is imperative in young ferrets. These individuals should be vaccinated at six to eight weeks, ten to twelve weeks, and thirteen to fourteen weeks for distemper (Purevax Ferret Distemper; Merial, Inc., Athens, GA). Rabies vaccination is strongly recommended in environments with risk of infection and may also be required by law in individual states or municipalities. A rabies vaccine (Imrab3, Rhone Merieux Inc., Athens, GA) may be given as early as three months of age. Both canine distemper and rabies boosters are given yearly along with a physical examination.

Despite the creation of safer ferret vaccines, vaccine reactions still commonly occur in some ferrets. Vaccine reactions seen include lethargy, depression, seizures, and cardiac arrhythmias. Veterinary hospitals have adopted various protocols for dealing with newly vaccinated ferrets. Some hospitals monitor these ferrets at least thirty minutes after vaccination. Other hospitals may provide premedication with an antihistamine prior to vaccination. Whatever the protocol, be aware that vaccine reactions have been known to occur at least twenty-four hours post vaccination. Owners should be alerted to the clinical signs and take appropriate measures to seek veterinary care should these signs appear after discharge from the hospital.

Heartworm disease is found in ferrets. Prevention of heartworm disease may be accomplished by off-label use of Heartgard 68 μg (Heartgard-30, Merck Agvet Division, Rahway, NJ). Give one-fourth tablet once monthly. The remainder of the tablet should be discarded because the remaining preparation will deteriorate. A liquid ivermectin preparation may also be used by mixing 0.3 ml of injectable ivermectin (Ivomec 1% injection for cattle, Merck Agvet Division, Rathway, NJ) in 28 ml (1 oz) of propylene glycol. Administer 0.2 ml/kg PO (0.02 mg/kg) once per month. This preparation is light sensitive and should be stored in a light-blocking container. The expiration date is two years as long as the time period falls within the expiration date of the stock bottle (Hillyer and Quesenberry 1997).

Internal parasites are not commonly seen in ferrets; however, an annual fecal examination is strongly recommended.

RESTRAINT

As with any animal, proper restraint involves the humane handling of the patient with consideration for

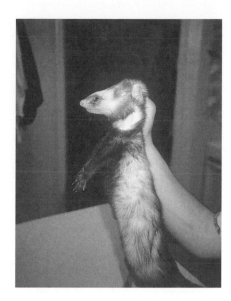

Figure 11.5. Ferret restraint using the scruffing method. (Photo courtesy of Dr. Sam Rivera.)

the safety of the assistant. Although ferrets are usually active creatures, they are easily managed in the clinic setting. Young ferrets and occasionally adults that are less frequently handled may have a tendency to nip. Some of these individuals may latch onto a finger and require a gentle extraction.

The preferred methods for injections and examination are scruffing the neck or forming a ring around the neck using the index finger and thumb (Figure 11.5). The rear legs and rear quarters are firmly pulled caudally but not at full extension. Another method involves wrapping the ferret in a towel "burrito" style (Figure 11.6). This is very effective for jugular venipuncture. Many ferrets may be vaccinated or treated without any physical restraint other than using a treat as a distraction.

A few individuals may require restraint with light sedation prior to the performance of any procedures. Chamber or mask induction with gas anesthesia is usually all that is needed. Besides the risks of anesthesia, minor changes may occur in the results from blood drawn in the anesthetized patient. The advantages are that procedures may be performed quickly and with less stress and struggling on the part of the patient and handler.

RADIOLOGY AND ULTRASOUND

As with many small animals, it is difficult to radiograph a part without radiographing the whole indi-

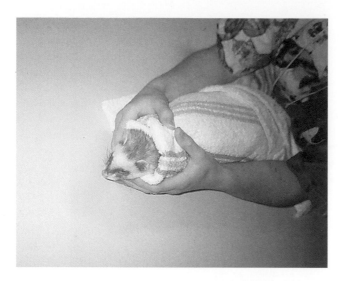

Figure 11.6. Ferret restraint using a towel. (Photo courtesy of Dr. Sam Rivera.)

vidual. Obviously, one should measure the body part of interest and set the machine according to the thickness and the machine's technique chart. Small mammal technique charts must be tailored to each clinic's equipment. Contrast radiography is employed as a diagnostic tool in ferrets. The most common use is in gastrointestinal studies. The protocol, though similar to the cat, should keep in mind the fast gastrointestinal transit time of the ferret.

Ultrasound studies are easily performed and readily tolerated by ferrets with only light restraint. Whole body scans are performed, often with special attention to the stomach, pancreas, lymph nodes, liver, kidneys, adrenal glands, and bladder, and the prostate in males.

ANESTHESIA AND SURGERY

Inhalation anesthesia is the recommended product for induction of ferrets. Isoflurane is the most common product in use. Sevoflurane has more recently been used and lacks the irritating taste of isoflurane. The main disadvantage is the cost of sevoflurane. Intubation may be a challenge with ferrets but is similar to that of cats. The technique may require the use of a stylet. Gas anesthesia is then continued for the duration of the procedure. Use of a forced-air patient warming system (Bair Hugger, Arizant, Eden Prairie, MN) helps to prevent hypothermia. Pulse oximeters, respiratory monitors, and cardiac monitors work well with ferrets.

Analgesia is an important element in the recovery of postsurgical ferret patients. Butorphanol (0.1 to 0.5 mg/ kg IM or SC every twelve hours) is effective in ferrets.

Common procedures in ferrets include gastrotomies, enterotomies, adrenalectomies, cystotomies, partial pancreatectomies, lymph node biopsies, and mass excisions of the dermis. Most orchiectomies and ovariohysterectomies are performed at the breeding farms prior to entry of the ferret into the pet population. Every state has its own regulations regarding breeding, spaying, and neutering. Hepatic and splenic biopsies are employed as diagnostic tools and may be performed surgically or through the use of ultrasound-guided biopsy forceps. Ferrets often have enlarged spleens that may or may not be the origin of disease. Many orthopedic problems common in dogs and cats are not found in the ferret. However, fractures and dislocations do occur in pet ferrets.

PARASITOLOGY

Fecal examinations are routinely performed in young ferrets and in ferrets presenting with clinical signs of illness. Intestinal parasites are uncommon compared to dogs and cats. Coccidiosis (*Isospora* spp.), when found, occurs in young animals. The oocysts are shed between six and sixteen weeks of age and can be demonstrated in fecal examination. The *Isospora* spp. that affects cats and dogs may cross-infect ferrets.

Giardiasis may be seen in ferrets housed in pet store settings. Cryptosporidiosis is a common finding in young ferrets and may persist in immunosuppressed individuals for months. No treatment exists in ferrets and one must keep in mind the zoonotic potential in the immunocompromised human population.

Ear mites often produce a persistent brown-red aural discharge without clinical significance. These parasites also cross-infect dogs and cats. Ear swabs are the key to diagnosis.

Heartworm disease (*Dirofilaria immitis*) occurs in ferrets, especially in endemic areas. Heartworm prevention is unapproved but recommended.

Flea infestation (*Ctenocephalides spp.*) is a common finding in ferrets housed with dogs and cats. Flea control methods for cats, particularly Advantage (Bayer, Shawnee Mission, KS) and Revolution (Pfizer, New York, NY), have been used but are not approved. These topical medications are usually applied in smaller doses (Hillyer and Quesenberry 1997).

URINALYSIS

Collection is achieved by one of three methods. Gentle expression, catheterization, and cystocentesis have all

Table 11.2. Urinalysis normals for ferrets.

Color	Clear to yellow
Specific gravity	1.015–1.055
Ph	6.0–7.5
Protein	0–1
Glucose	0–Trace
Ketones	Negative
Bilirubin	Negative
Occult blood	Negative
WBC	0–5
RBC	0–3
Casts	Occasional
Crystals	Occasional
Epithelial cells	0–Few
Bacteria	Negative
Urine volume (ml/24 hr)	8–140 ml (Mean 26–28 ml)

Source: Antech Diagnostics.

been successfully used. Catheterization is difficult in both males and females due to the small size of the urethra and the anatomically challenging os penis. There are manufacturers that produce specialized equipment for these purposes (Cook Veterinary Products, Queensland, Australia). However, size 3.5 French red rubber catheters have been successfully used to catheterize male ferrets.

Due to the activity of the animal, cystocentesis may be best performed under anesthesia using a 25-gauge needle attached to a 1-cc or 3-cc syringe. Care should be taken to avoid using a large needle because it may lacerate the bladder.

Urine dipstick, specific gravity, and sedimentation are used for standard analyses. Urinalysis normals are presented in Table 11.2. Urine culture should be performed in cases of suspected kidney or bladder infection, preferably using a sample obtained via cystocentesis or sterile catheterization.

EMERGENCY AND CRITICAL CARE

The normal life span of a ferret is five to seven years. In an emergency, as with any animal, a history and physical examination are crucial in determining the magnitude of the situation. Insulinoma, adrenal gland disease, and cardiomyopathy occur most often in older ferrets. Mediastinal lymphosarcoma, diarrhea, or foreign body ingestion are found commonly in emergencies of young animals. Infectious diseases affect ferrets of any age and are a consideration in an environmental setting in which people have respiratory illness or where new ferrets have been introduced.

Ill ferrets require minimal handling. Young and old ferrets are susceptible to green slime disease (epizootic catarrhal enteritis). Vaccine reactions were more common with previous vaccine protocols but have improved with the introduction of the new ferret distemper vaccine (Purevax Ferret Distemper, Merial, Inc., Athens, GA).

Standard methods of restraint for ferrets include wrapping the ferret in a towel or grasping the nape of the neck. TPR, physical examination, and history are important to establish a good baseline.

Hospitalization of critical ferrets requires a quiet, temperature-controlled cage with oxygen capabilities.

Anorexic ferrets are at risk due to hypoglycemia or hepatic lipidosis. The gums of the lethargic ferret may be rubbed with supplements containing high levels of sugar to provide an immediate energy boost to the ferret until other life-saving measures may be performed. Later on, force-feeding A/D Diet (Hill's Pet Nutrition, Inc., Topeka, KS), Eukanuba Recovery Diet (Proctor and Gamble, Cincinnati, OH), or Critical Care Diet for Carnivores (Oxbow, Murdock, NE) via syringe or tongue depressor provides good nutritional support. Other preparations are available or can be formulated in the hospital.

Basic diagnostic tests include a blood chemistry, hematology, and fecal examination. A blood glucose can be performed on a human glucometer or blood chemistry analyzer, or with less accuracy using a blood glucose stick. The blood chemistry analyzer offers the best accuracy providing the blood sample has been properly processed. The primary venipuncture site in ferrets is the jugular vein with the saphenous and cephalic veins serving as secondary sites.

Catheter placement is intravenously either in the lateral saphenous or cephalic veins. Jugular catheterization can be used but is not tolerated well by ferrets. They often become depressed due to the required bandaging around the neck. Cut downs of the jugular and cephalic veins in severely dehydrated ferrets may be a consideration. Sometimes the vascular system of the dehydrated patient may require re-hydration with fluids delivered via the subcutaneous route hours prior to attempted placement of IV or IO catheters.

Intraosseous catheter placement can be performed in the humerus, femur, or tibia; the femoral placement is best. This procedure is best done under anesthesia. Anesthesia may not be a safe option in animals that are severely debilitated. This procedure is painful and may require local block of the periosteum and surrounding soft tissue.

The fluid administration requirement for ferrets is 70 ml/kg/day. Dehydration and losses are the same as in other small animals. With critical animals it is important to use the IV or IO route. Use of an IV pump designed for small mammals is recommended.

Medications are administered via IV or IO catheters, IM injection in the quadriceps, and oral routes. Oral preparations are accepted best in liquid form because pill medication is difficult to administer in ferrets. Oral medications may be made more palatable with special flavorings that encourage better compliance from the patient.

Cystocentesis may require sedation due to the thin wall of the bladder and the potential for laceration. Ultrasound-guided centesis is also a consideration.

Urethral catheterization requires anesthesia in all patients regardless of condition. Locating the urethral opening is a challenge in both males and females. Male ferrets present more often in an emergency situation due to urethral obstruction from prostatic disease secondary to adrenal gland problems or cystic calculi (Orcutt 1998).

SEX DETERMINATION

Sex determination is not as difficult as in many small mammals. Adults are similar to the dog. Neonate males have a urogenital opening on the ventral abdomen. Female ferrets have a narrow anogenital distance (Fox 1998, 106) (Figure 11.3).

TECHNIQUES

Urine Collection (Sterile)

Cystocentesis: Use a small syringe attached to a 25-gauge needle. Palpate the bladder in the caudal abdomen or use an ultrasound-guided technique.

Urinary catheterization: Use a 3.5 French red rubber or other specialty catheter, nasolacrimal cannula or small gauge needle, water-based lubricant, sterile gloves, hemostats, forced-air warming blanket, and gas anesthesia.

Males: The male anatomy is complicated by the J-shaped os penis and the small diameter penile urethra.

a. Prepare supplies and anesthetize the patient.
b. Estimate the length of the catheter from the center of the urinary bladder to the urethral entrance.
c. Position the ferret into ventral recumbency and retract the prepuce.

d. Use the nasolacrimal cannula or a blunt-tipped needle as a stylet, and insert the lubricated tip of the cannula or catheter into the urethra orifice. Keep in mind that the orifice is not directly at the tip of the penis but ventral to the end of the penis. There is often a small flap of penile tissue that must be elevated to access the urethral opening.
e. Advance the catheter until urine begins to flow.

Females:

a. Prepare supplies and anesthetize the patient.
b. Place the animal in ventral recumbency with elevated hind quarters.
c. Aseptically prepare the vulva and perivulvar area.
d. Locate the urethral opening using a vaginal speculum or otoscopic cone.
e. View the urethral opening on the ventral floor of the vaginal vestibule, approximately 1 cm cranial to the clitoral fossa (Quesenberry and Carpenter 2004).
f. Insert the catheter and advance until urine flow is achieved.

Collect voided sample from examination table or empty litter box: Many ferrets will urinate and defecate after their temperature is taken.

TPR

The same procedure employed with the dog and cat is used in the ferret.

Medication Administration

Injectable medications and fluid administration require proper restraint.

IV sites: Normally given via IV catheter

a. Jugular vein
b. Cephalic vein
c. Lateral saphenous vein

IM sites:

a. Quadriceps
b. Lumbodorsals
c. Triceps
d. Semitendinosus and semimembranosus. Use caution to avoid the sciatic nerve.

Subcutaneous sites: Can be given in a fold of skin anywhere along the dorsum.

Per os: Administered by tilting the head back and placing the syringe through the side of the mouth or placing the syringe in side of the mouth while ferret is standing.

Venipuncture (Figure 11.7)
Jugular vein:

a. Sternal recumbency with one hand pulling the front legs off the table and the other pulling the head back.
b. Using a towel, wrap the ferret tightly with only the animal's head exposed. With the animal in dorsal recumbency the ferret's head is flexed dorsally toward the person responsible for drawing the blood sample. The assistant should apply light pressure to the vein on either side of the manubrium and the sample is drawn from the jugular vein.
c. The ferret may be positioned similar to a cat for a jugular venipuncture. The head is elevated dorsally, the front legs are extended downward, and blood is drawn with the needle approaching the same direction as the head.

Cephalic vein:

a. Use normal restraint using the scruff of the neck.
b. Extend the foreleg.
c. Hold off the vein.
d. Draw the sample using a 25- or 22-gauge needle.

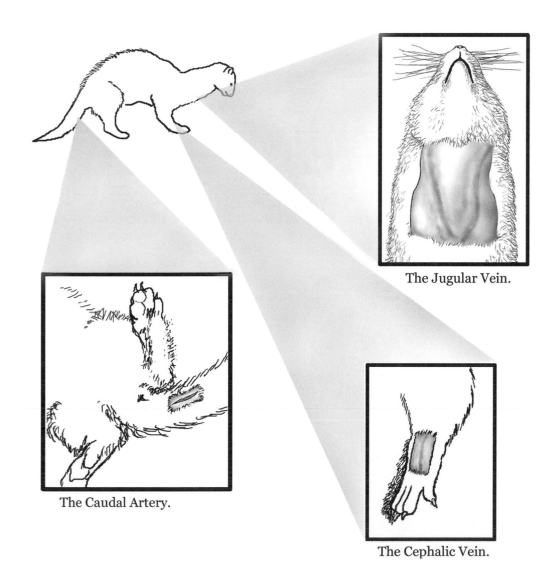

The Jugular Vein.

The Caudal Artery.

The Cephalic Vein.

Figure 11.7. Venipuncture sites. (Drawing by Scott Stark.)

Saphenous vein:

a. Used as a last resort.
b. The technique is the same as for the cephalic vein.

Cranial vena cava: This site has become more and more popular as veterinary personnel become comfortable with its use. The risk of cardiac puncture is low due to the length of the vena cava and caudal thoracic placement of the heart along with the proper use of short needles and proper placement. Sedation or anesthesia may be required unless the patient is calm and adequately restrained. Practice with an anesthetized ferret can aid in mastery of this venipuncture (Lennox 2009).

a. The ferret is restrained in dorsal recumbency with its neck extended. Alternatively, it can be wrapped in a towel.
b. Choose a one-half inch needle of 25- or 27-gauge.
c. Insert the needle in the area to the right or left of the manubrium of the sternum at a slight angle, aiming it toward the opposite hip.
d. Advance the needle while applying negative pressure. Deep penetration is not necessary because the vessel is fairly close to the surface at the cranial aspect of the sternum.
e. Look for a flash. Once one is obtained, blood should be obtained with ease. If no blood is seen, redirecting the needle may be necessary or the needle may go through the vessel.
f. Use of this technique is strongly recommended only by experienced veterinary team members.

IV Catheter Placement
Sites: Include jugular, saphenous, and cephalic veins (Figure 11.8).
Technique:

a. Materials required: 24- or 26-gauge IV catheter, clippers and surgical preparation supplies, tape, flush, tourniquet if needed.
b. Prepare the site using aseptic technique.
c. Apply a tourniquet as needed.
d. Use a 22-gauge needle to penetrate the skin lateral to the vein in the area where the catheter will enter just prior to entering the vein. In general, ferret skin is difficult to penetrate.
e. Visualize the vein, insert the needle, and advance the catheter until blood enters the hub of the needle.
f. When the catheter is properly seated in the vein and blood is flowing freely from the catheter, flush the catheter thoroughly with about 0.2 to 0.3 ml hepa-

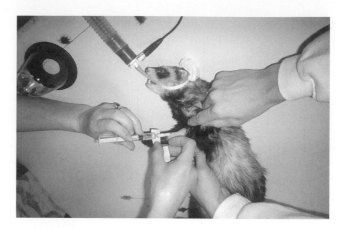

Figure 11.8. Cephalic catheter placement. (Photo courtesy of Dr. Sam Rivera.)

rinized saline and replace the cap. Remember that a smaller amount of flush will be used to accommodate the smaller patient.
g. A small drop of surgical glue may be placed at the catheter-skin junction. Tape the catheter in place, taking care not to apply too much pressure to the skin and resulting constriction of the vein.
h. Connect the IV line to the patient using a minidrip set and/or an IV pump with the potential to calibrate fluid rates for smaller patients.

Intraosseous Catheter Placement
Sites: Include humerus, tibia, and femur (Figure 11.9).
Technique:

a. The femur is the best site that causes the least restriction in movement.
b. Use 20- or 22-gauge catheters. A stylet or larger needle may be used to create a pilot hole, or entry point, for the catheter.
c. General anesthesia is recommended except in debilitated individuals. Local anesthetic blocks may be used for the surrounding soft tissue and periosteum.

Enema
Materials needed: Small rubber urinary catheter, water-based lubricant, enema solution (warm soapy water), syringe.
Technique:

a. Insert the lubricated tip of the rubber urinary catheter into the rectum of the restrained animal.
b. Attach the syringe full of enema solution to the end of the catheter and gently flush the colon using constant steady pressure.

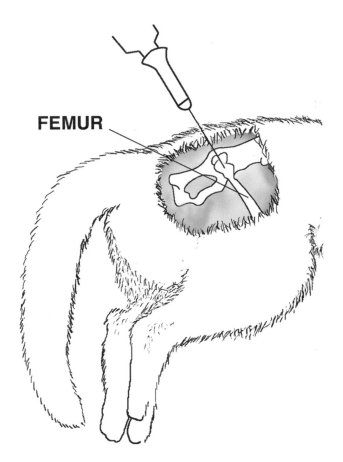

FEMUR

Figure 11.9. IO catheter location. (Drawing by Scott Stark.)

c. Remove the catheter and cleanse the surrounding skin.

Bandage and Wound Care

The same procedures used on other small animals may be used with ferrets. A separate small mammal bandage box with ready-to-go materials may be used. The materials should include small-scale items, such as small scissors and one-half inch tape or materials cut to scale from larger diameter supplies.

Blood Transfusion

Blood transfusions may be used if a local donor system is in place. Many facilities that see large numbers of ferrets may keep healthy donor ferrets on site in case a transfusion is needed. Other ferrets may be privately owned and available as needed on an emergency basis.

Donor ferrets, similar to their canine and feline counterparts, require regular screening for disease through physical examination, baseline blood work evaluation, fecal examination, assessment of adrenal hormone levels, and possibly radiographic and ultrasonographic examination. These ferrets also need preventive medical care, including heartworm prevention, regular deworming, and vaccination for rabies and canine distemper viruses.

The amount of blood available for transfusion is based upon body weight. The compatibility of donor and recipient ferrets should be determined according to previously described methods in canine and feline practice. The donor ferret should be sedated with gas anesthesia to avoid any struggling and to provide a complication-free needle stick, which will prevent contamination of the sample with disruptive clotting factors. The transfusion recipient may receive the blood sample via fluid pump. Prior to transfusion, necessary premedication with anti-histamines may be performed to minimize transfusion reactions.

The donor ferret should be kept warm, receive replacement fluids and, depending upon the amount of blood removed, will then be designated as unavailable for transfusions for a period of time as determined by the veterinary facility.

Euthanasia

Euthanasia is best performed by sedating the patient using chamber or mask induction with gas anesthesia. As an alternate method, telazol (0.2 cc/10 lb IM) may also be used. After the ferret has been sedated, the euthanasia solution can be administrated via the IV or intracardiac routes.

REFERENCES

Bell JA. 1999. Ferret nutrition. Veterinary Clinics of North America. *Exotic Animal Practice, Critical Care*, January, 169–192.

Fox JG. 1998. Biology and Diseases of the Ferret. 2nd ed. Philadelphia: Lea and Febiger. 5–106.

Garner MM, Ramsell K, Schoemaker NJ, Sidor IF, Nordhausen RW, et al. 2007. Myofasciitis in the ferret. *Vet Pathol* 44(1): 25–38.

Hillyer EV, Quesenberry KE. 1997. Ferrets, Rabbits, and Rodents, Clinical Medicine and Surgery. Philadelphia: W.B. Saunders Company. 4–70.

Lennox AM. 2009. Proceedings of the North American Veterinary Conference, 1867–1870.

Orcutt CJ. 1998. The Veterinary Clinics of North America. *Exotic Animal Practice, Critical Care*, September, 99–126.

Quesenberry KE, Carpenter JW. 2004. Ferrets, Rabbits, and Rodents, Clinical Medicine and Surgery. St. Louis: W.B. Saunders Company. 21–22.

CHAPTER TWELVE

Rabbits

Douglas K. Taylor, Vanessa Lee, Deborah Mook, and Michael J. Huerkamp

INTRODUCTION

The domestic rabbit (*Oryctolagus cuniculus*) is a lago-morph of the family Leporidae that descended from wild rabbits found originally in the area of modern day Spain. Cottontail rabbits are related, but in the genus *Sylvilagus*. The early domestication of the rabbit began in western Europe and northwestern Africa in the first century B.C. By the mid-1600s, rabbits were raised all over Europe for meat and fur and were in the course of dissemination all over the world via sailing vessels that stocked them as a source of meat supply. Female rabbits are called "does," males are "bucks," and neonates are termed "kits." Those rabbits raised for food are termed "fryers."

Rabbits are attractive as pets because they are quiet, gentle, and relatively odor-free, they rarely bite, and they can be trained to use a litter box. They generally enjoy good health if kept under sanitary conditions; receive adequate water and nutrition; and are protected from predators, environmental extremes, drafts, and trauma. Today in the United States, in addition to being kept as pets, rabbits are exhibited for showing, used in scientific research, and used for food and fur production. Depending upon the locale and nature of the veterinary practice one could be presented with rabbits from any of these general areas of use.

BEHAVIOR

Rabbits are a generally timid and often submissive prey species with a propensity for chewing and gnawing. If given the space and social opportunities, they will chase, jump, gambol, rear, bat at objects, gnaw, and explore (Bayne 2003). Episodes of cavorting and exploration tend to be intermittent and interspersed with longer periods of huddling or resting against a wall or surface. Overall, rabbits are generally quiet, not particularly playful with humans and tend to urinate and defecate in a chosen area, which facilitates litter box training. If caged, those of a timid nature retreat to the back of the enclosure when approached and may thump a hind foot–the latter is a general warning or alarm call. Aggressive rabbits may growl or grunt, charge, flail with the front feet, and attempt to bite. Biting is fairly rare, but rabbits may scratch, especially with the powerful rear limbs. They scent mark by rubbing the chin on objects and they enjoy chewing on wire, wood, cardboard, paper, hay, or other materials they encounter. Sexually intact rabbits of either gender, but particularly males, may fight, and this should be taken into account in counseling owners toward neutering or recommending individual housing. Compatible groups of does, particularly if formed in small clusters while young, can be maintained for lengthy periods of time (Bayne 2003). Sexually intact, mature rabbits of either gender may also spray urine and mark territory (Stein and Walshaw 1996).

Abnormal and stereotypic behaviors that might be elicited during the acquisition of a history include cage bar chewing, excessive fur plucking, psychogenic water consumption, head swaying or weaving, head pressing, obsession with pawing or digging at the cage floor or food hopper, rapid circling, or sitting with the head lowered (Bayne 2003). Although not backed by any scientific evidence, stereotypies and abnormal behaviors are most likely to be disproportionately high in rabbits kept singly and confined to hutches as compared to those that are more free-roaming in the home. As such, the rabbit hutch should be designed and outfitted to encourage species-typical behavior and enhance the well-being of the inhabitant.

In confined conditions, enrichment devices have been documented to decrease the incidence of undesirable behaviors and increase overall activity of rabbits (Bayne 2003, Johnson et al. 2003). The devices that have been used most successfully to encourage the species-typical nudging, playing, and investigative behaviors of rabbits are chew-resistant plastic toys and balls, Nylabone® products, sections of PVC tubing, metallic washers suspended from chains, stainless-steel rabbit rattles on spring clips, and hay and other food items specially formulated for rabbits (Bayne 2003, Johnson et al. 2003).

Mating of rabbits should be supervised because does may be aggressive toward bucks. A buck will circle a receptive doe and then quickly mount and copulate. Mating is an amusing ritual to observe as the post-coital male swoons off of the back of the doe. Kits are born in a nest that the doe makes from hair plucked from the dewlap and other materials that it may scavenge from the cage or environment. The kits are born hairless and blind, an attribute that differentiates rabbits from hares, which are born furred and with open eyes. A doe typically nurses the kits only once per day. Lactation peaks at three weeks postpartum. The kits start eating solid food at two weeks of age and cecotrophy commences about a week later. Weaning should be done at five to six weeks.

ANATOMY AND PHYSIOLOGY

Rabbits have a number of distinguishing morphophysiologic attributes that make them interesting and differentiate them from more traditional pets. For example, rabbits importantly use cecal bacterial fermentation in digestion, cannot vomit, have a narrow pylorus, and engage in cecotrophy. In some part due to the latter three characteristics, they rarely have an empty stomach. They have large, accessible veins and arteries in the ears, facilitating fluid administration, intravenous injection of therapeutic agents, blood-gas analysis, and direct blood pressure measurement. The ears, in addition to high vascularization, serve in sound gathering and heat dissipation and are highly sensitive and fragile. Consequently, rabbits should never be restrained or carried by the ears.

Rabbits have a high muscle-to-bone ratio. While 13% of the body weight is comprised of bone in the cat, only 8% is bone in the rabbit (Harkness and Wagner 1989). Because they are engulfed in large muscle masses, the long bones and lumbar spine are particularly at risk of fracture or luxation, respectively. For rabbits used as pets and in research, this is an unfortunate characteristic that can be attributed to a heritage of development for maximal meat production. Three in five rabbits will have atropinesterase in the serum, which rapidly hydrolyzes atropine, essentially rendering the agent unpredictable to worthless in effect. Like cats, rabbits are prone to laryngospasm and may be a challenge to intubate owing to the combination of a small glottis, narrow oropharynx, relatively large and fleshy tongue, and other anatomic factors. The skeletal anatomy of the rabbit is shown in Figure 12.1.

The predominant white blood cells are lymphocytes and heterophils, the rabbit equivalent of a neutrophil (Color Plate 12.1), which may be mistaken for an eosinophil because of the presence of numerous small intracytoplasmic eosinophilic granules. Unlike cats and dogs, lymphocytes are generally more common than granulocytic cells (heterophils). Basophils (2% to 7%) are more common in rabbits than other species (Harkness and Wagner 1989). Reticulated red blood cells may also be encountered more frequently in rabbits than in dogs or cats.

Clinical chemistry values observed in rabbits are not remarkable as compared to dogs and cats with the exception of serum amylase and calcium levels.

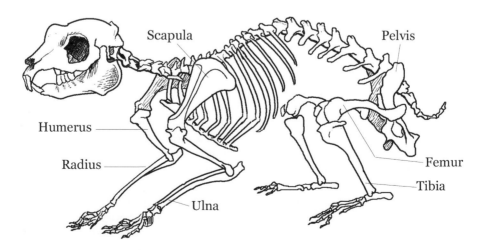

Figure 12.1. Rabbit skeletal anatomy.

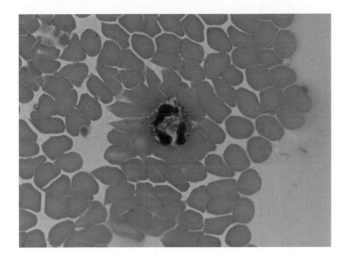

Plate 12.1. Rabbit blood smear showing heterophil. (Photo courtesy of Dondrae Coble.) (See also color plates)

Calcium is absorbed from the gut efficiently at a high rate. Consequently, blood levels relate directly to dietary levels, often resulting in a dietary nonpathogenic hypercalcemia. Rabbits on high calcium diets may have blood levels meeting or exceeding 15 mg/dL. Calcium is cleared from the blood by the kidney and excreted in the urine. Most other species excrete calcium primarily in the bile (Cheeke 1987). Rabbits are susceptible to arteriosclerosis as a consequence of dietary calcium imbalance or vitamin D excess. Serum amylase values are considerably lower than those found in dogs and cats (McLaughlin and Fish 1994). Blood gas values of normal rabbits and their interpretation are essentially identical to other species.

Reproductively, does have a duplex uterus with each uterine horn having its own cervix and eight to ten mammary glands. Does can rebreed within twenty-four hours of parturition, termed "kindling" in the parlance of rabbit users, and produce up to eleven litters per year. Kits may show growth rates of up to 35 to 40 grams per day. Like cats, ovulation in rabbits is coitus-induced. Unlike cats, the receptive does are not likely to drive owners to distraction, but intact bucks, especially those that are house pets, regularly mount seemingly everything in sight, and not uncommonly the owner's slippered foot after sitting down in the evening to relax. The inguinal canals remain open for the life of the buck and the testicles may interchangeably be found in the scrotum or retracted into the abdomen. Herniation of other intraabdominal organs is prevented by large fat depots immediately covering the canals (Swindle and Shealy 1996). Figure 12.2 shows rabbit visceral anatomy.

The rabbit is most interesting and unique from the perspective of digestion. It is a nonruminant herbivore dietarily preferring the tender, succulent parts of plants. The teeth are open-rooted and grow continuously. The normal dental formula is I2/1, C0/0, PM 3/0, and M3/3, and is unique because the upper dental arcade includes two sets of incisors with a small, secondary pair, the peg teeth, situated immediately to the lingual side of the larger labial pair. The single pair of lower incisors occludes with the upper secondary incisors. The void between the incisors and premolars that is devoid of canine teeth is called the diastema (Figure 12.3). The incisors may grow at a rate of up to 1 cm/ month.

Rabbits have a glandular stomach that functions essentially as a storage organ. The cardiac sphincter has tone to the degree that true vomiting is prevented. The stomach is never empty and even after a twenty-four-hour fast will typically be more than half full (Griffiths and Davies 1963). The stomach of the adult rabbit is noteworthy for having a gastric pH that is significantly lower than that of other species (Cheeke 1987). This renders the upper gastrointestinal tract sterile, serving partly to protect against the oral route of inoculation by pathogens. The gastric pH is higher in sucklings, permitting bacterial colonization of the hindgut by cecotroph-oral inoculation from adults in the population. Unfortunately, it also provides a window of opportunity for entry of bacterial gastrointestinal pathogens, particularly at or around the time of weaning.

The small intestine, similar to most species, is the major site of acid neutralization, protein and carbohydrate digestion, fat emulsification, and absorption of many nutrients. Rabbits are hindgut fermenters, similar to the horse, with digestion characterized by selective excretion of fiber, cecal fermentation, and reingestion of cecal contents. The spacious cecum, comprising about 40% of the total gastrointestinal capacity, is a site of constant peristalsis with mixing and remixing of its contents and where an intricate and delicate relationship exists between nutrients, the microflora, and motility. It is the primary site of bacterial fermentative digestion and water absorption. The anaerobic flora important in cecal fermentation are comprised of *Bacteroides* and other species (Cheeke 1987, Davies and Davies 2003).

Fermentation of carbohydrates results in the production of volatile fatty acids, in a process similar to that of rumination, which are absorbed through the cecal wall and used as a source of energy (Cheeke 1987). The colon, characterized anatomically by serial sacculations (termed haustrae), contracts and moves

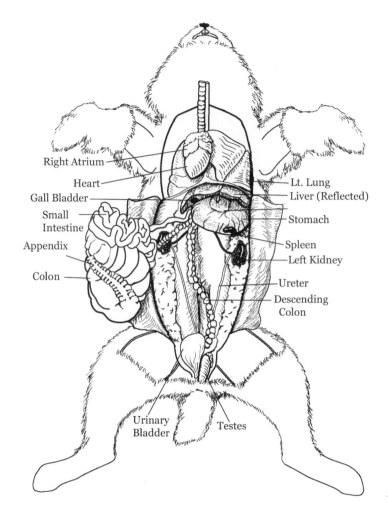

Figure 12.2. Rabbit visceral anatomy.

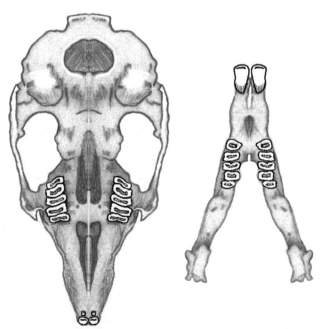

Figure 12.3. Rabbit dentition.

fluid and small digestible particles back into the cecum and propels large pieces of fiber distally where they are formed into the excreted hard pellets that are typically observed in litter boxes and fecal pans.

At intervals, the cecum contracts and the fluid, protein, and vitamin-rich cecal contents are expelled into the colon, formed into small, soft balls, covered with mucin, consumed directly from the anus, and swallowed whole by the rabbit (Davies and Davies 2003). This process is known as cecotrophy and it serves to recycle vitamins, amino acids, volatile fatty acids, and digested bacteria to the upper GI tract for absorption or further digestion as needed (Davies and Davies 2003). The unique separation of the nutritive products of cecal fermentation and fecal waste allowing for the reingestion and absorption of bacteria and their by-products in the small intestine results in more efficient use of forage proteins than rumination. It is enabled by the fusus coli, a muscular thickening at the termination of the transverse colon exclusive to lagomorphs that regulates contractions that separate

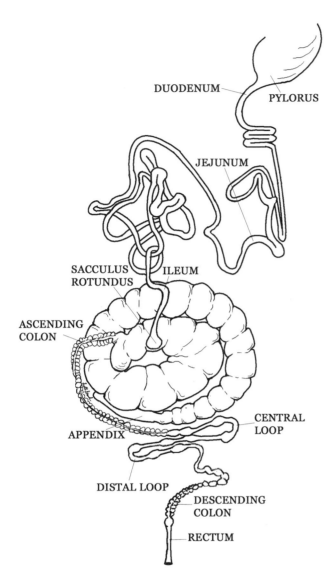

DUODENUM — PYLORUS

JEJUNUM

SACCULUS ROTUNDUS — ILEUM

ASCENDING COLON

CENTRAL LOOP

APPENDIX

DISTAL LOOP

DESCENDING COLON

RECTUM

Figure 12.4. Rabbit GI tract.

Anatomically, the rabbit gastrointestinal tract is also unique with respect to the presence of a lymphoid mass, the sacculus rotundus, at the termination of the ileum into the cecum. Lymphoid tissue is also found in the appendix at the cecal tip (Figure 12.4).

BIOLOGIC AND REPRODUCTIVE DATA

In the interpretation of laboratory tests, one should ideally rely upon a normal reference range for the species provided by the diagnostic laboratory that has conducted the test(s). When such values are not provided by the laboratory, the ranges in the tables that follow can be used as an approximation of what can be expected in the normal healthy rabbit (Tables 12.1, 12.2, 12.3). However, one should appreciate that "normal values" may be influenced by laboratory variation, sample collection technique (e.g. extent of restraint), type of anesthesia (Gonzales et al. 2005), hemolysis, post-collection sample handling (e.g. refrigeration), time to centrifugation, centrifugation characteristics, breed and age of the subject, and other factors. The numeric data provided in the tables below are normal values obtained from research populations of rabbits that were of fairly uniform genotype and age and maintained under standard conditions. They are presented as the normal distribution about the mean of a healthy population of rabbits. Presentation of values in this format merits several comments. First, some parameters may not have a Gaussian distribution and a normal distribution may not apply. Second, 5% of normal, healthy animals have values that lie outside and at the extremes of the normal range. The interpretation of laboratory data, as in any other circumstance with any other species, should take into account for interpretation the history, findings from a physical examination, and results of any other diagnostic tests.

HUSBANDRY

Rabbits can be housed either indoors or outdoors, the latter with appropriate shelter from the elements. Rabbits can be litter box trained and, for this reason, make suitable indoor pets, but their proclivity for gnawing is a drawback. Furniture, carpets, window dressings, toys, electrical cords, and shoes provide numerous indoor targets for gnawing. Wherever they are housed it is critical to protect rabbits from drafts, temperature extremes, predators, flying insects, and environmental intoxicants. Rabbits are cold-weather tolerant and are best kept at temperatures of 55°F to

digestible from indigestible material (Davies and Davies 2003).

Morphologically, the cecotrophs appear as clumps of smaller, soft, moist fecal pellets that glisten from their gelatinous coat. This mucus-like membrane serves to protect the cecotrophs, and fermentative commensals contained therein, from the gastric pH. Cecotrophs are also called "night feces" or "soft feces." As a general rule, cecotrophy generally follows about four hours after consumption of a meal (Davies and Davies 2003). While wire caging has no effect upon cecotrophy given the consumption of the cecotrophs directly from the anus, the act can be prevented through the application of an Elizabethan collar.

Table 12.1. Hematology and blood coagulation values.

Parameter	Normal distribution	Reference
Total WBC ($10^3/\mu l$)	4.6–13.2	Wolford et al. 1986
Heterophils (%)	<50%	Wolford et al. 1986
Lymphocytes (%)	>50%	Wolford et al. 1986
Monocytes (%)	0–3%	Wolford et al. 1986
Eosinophils (%)	0–2%	Wolford et al. 1986
Basophils (%)	0–7%	Wolford et al. 1986
Platelets ($10^3/\mu l$)	300–700	Wolford et al. 1986
PCV (%)	33–45	Wolford et al. 1986
RBC ($10^6/\mu l$)	5.5–7.5	Wolford et al. 1986
Hemoglobin (g/dL)	11–15	Wolford et al. 1986
MCV (fl)	56–66	Wolford et al. 1986
MCHC (%)	32–36	Wolford et al. 1986
MCH (pg)	19–22	Wolford et al. 1986
Reticulocytes (%)	<4	Wolford et al. 1986
Bleeding time (minutes)	0.8–2	Livio et al. 1988
Clotting time (minutes)	1.1–5.5	Livio et al. 1988
OSPT (seconds)	7.9–17.9	Gentry 1982
APTT (seconds)	19.5–22.5	Gentry 1982
Prothrombin time (seconds)	6.9–8.1	Lee and Clement 1990
Thrombin time (seconds)	5.7–14.1	Lee and Clement 1990

Table 12.2. Clinical chemistry values.

Parameter	Normal distribution	Reference
AST (U/L)	0–30	Yu et al. 1979
ALT (U/L)	0–60	Yu et al. 1979
GGT (U/L)	0–8	Hewitt et al. 1989
SAP (U/L)	0–139	Hewitt et al. 1989
CPK (U/L)	<700	Hewitt et al. 1989
BUN (mg/dL)	9–22	Hewitt et al. 1989
Creatinine (mg/dL)	0.6–1.5	Hewitt et al. 1989
Glucose (mg/dL)	86–137	Hewitt et al. 1989
Amylase (U/L)	270–700	Yu et al. 1979
Total bilirubin (mg/dL)	0.4–9.2	Yu et al. 1979
Sodium (mEq/L)	138–150	Gillett 1994
Chloride (mEq/L)	92–120	Gillett 1994
Calcium (mg/dL)	6–15	Yu et al. 1979 Hewitt et al. 1989 Gillett 1994
Phosphorus (mg/dL)	3–5	Yu et al. 1979
Potassium (mEq/L)	3.5–7	Gillett 1994
Total protein (g/dL)	5.3–7.6	Yu et al. 1979
Albumin (g/dL)	3.1–4.7	Yu et al. 1979

72°F or slightly below and 30% to 70% relative humidity (Patton 1994). Rabbits can be housed outdoors if protected from cold below 40°F in the winter and excessive heat in the summer.

Protection from cold, drafts, and moisture in winter can be accomplished by providing a covered nesting box containing straw, shavings, or other insulative bedding. In hot weather, generally temperatures above 85°F, rabbits require shade and plenty of cool water. Heat stress is a significant risk at this temperature and above. In extreme heat, consideration should be given to moving the hutch to a breezy garage or patio with a fan. Moving the rabbit indoors to an air conditioned area may be too much of an acute environmental stressor and such drastic actions on the part of an owner should be discouraged.

Plans for rabbit hutches and nesting boxes can be obtained from libraries, extension agents, or feed companies. Assembled cages suitable for rabbits often can be obtained from pet stores. At a minimum, rabbits confined to cages should be given sufficient floor space to stretch out to full length with sufficient head room to permit sitting on the haunches. Hardware cloth of 1.25- × 2.5 cm-grid is suitable for flooring, but the animal should have access to other surfaces as well because wire flooring can predispose the rabbit to

Table 12.3. Normative and reproductive values.

Parameter	Normal distribution	Reference
Life span (years)	5–7 (15 maximum)	Gillett 1994
Gestation (days)	31–32	Gillett 1994
Litter size (kits born)	4–10	Gillett 1994
Weaning age (weeks)	5–6	Gillett 1994
Rectal temperature (°F)	101–104	Gillett 1994
Heart rate (bpm)	200–300	Gillett 1994
Respiratory rate (bpm)	30–60	Gillett 1994
Blood pressure, systolic (torr)[1]	90–130	Gillett 1994
Blood pressure, diastolic (torr)[1]	80–90	Gillett 1994
Food intake (g/kg/day)	50	Harkness and Wagner 1989
Water intake (ml/kg/day)	100	Harkness and Wagner 1989

[1]Blood pressure values are given for instrumented conscious rabbits with central arterial catheters. Values average 10 torr less if the central auricular artery is used (Edwards et al. 1959).

pododermatitis. Wire flooring should be cleaned regularly to remove suspended hair and feces. Sexually mature rabbits, whether male or female, should be individually housed, known to be compatible, or closely monitored because they may attack one another. Attempts at environmental enrichment should focus on providing hiding places, material for chewing (cardboard, paper), or nutritional supplements such as hay.

NUTRITION

Rabbits should be fed a rationed amount of pellets supplemented with free choice hay and small amounts of fresh foods. Rabbits should be fed and will readily eat extruded pelleted diets specially formulated for their species. These can be found in feed mills and major pet stores. Pelleted diets should be stored at 72°F or lower and used within three to six months of the milling date (PMI Nutrition International 1998). Pelleted diets are nutritionally complete and typically contain 14% to 18% crude protein, 40% to 50% carbohydrate, 2% to 4% fat, 10% to 22% crude fiber, and appropriate vitamins and minerals in the proper balance. Indigestible fiber, although discriminately excreted and not an important source of nutrients, is important in digestion; normal health; and the prevention of fur pulling, gastric trichobezoars, enteritis, mucoid enteropathy, and other gastrointestinal maladies (Cheeke 1987). Fiber stimulates ceco-colonic motility promoting the peristaltic activity critical to the hindgut fermentative process. Without sufficient long particle length (>0.5 mm) fiber, hypomotility is induced, floral alterations occur, the digestive process grinds to a halt, and disease may be induced (Davies, et al. 2003). For growth, 10% to 15% dietary fiber is optimal, while less than 10% predisposes to GI disease. Adult rabbits should be kept on rations containing 15% to 22% fiber.

The pelleted diet should be supplemented with hay because this indigestible fiber helps maintain a healthy weight, gut motility, and dental health. Timothy and alfalfa hay are available in many pet stores, but alfalfa has high calcium content and so should not be given to rabbits predisposed to urinary sludge.

Fresh greens and vegetables can also be given in small quantities. Suitable greens include cabbage, cauliflower leaves, broccoli leaves, kale, turnip greens, and mustard greens. Other greens, such as sunflower leaves, carrot tops, or green bean vines, can also be offered. There is little to no information on the effect of herbs on rabbit nutrition or health and they should be used with caution. Overfeeding of fresh greens predisposes to starch overload, cecal pH extremes, and enteric diseases. In addition, to prevent gastroenteritis, it is important not to feed spoiled foods or those discarded in the trash at restaurants or groceries.

Another option is to permit grazing on clover or dandelions under supervised conditions in a fenced, covered enclosure in the yard. This should only be done in areas where fertilizers, herbicides, and pesticides have not been used. This practice also carries some risk of exposure to parasite oocysts shed by wild rabbits other forms of wildlife, dogs, cats, and other species. Grazing on forages other than clover or dandelions is not recommended. For example, crown vetch contains glycosides that may be toxic and Bermuda grasses, kudzu, and birdsfoot trefoil have low feeding value (Cheeke 1987).

Some rabbits may relish human breakfast cereal products, such as shredded wheat biscuits or grain cereals, as a treat. Fruits, whole grains, fat-based treats, and high carbohydrate supplements should be avoided (Davies et al. 2003). It is not necessary, and may actually be harmful in some cases, to supplement a proper pelleted diet with minerals.

As a rule of thumb, a rabbit generally consume 5% of its body weight in dry feed and 10% in water. Rabbits kept as pets or used in research typically are limit fed pelleted diets, while those grown for food production or that are lactating are fed *ad libitum*. Peak food consumption in *ad libitum* fed rabbits is biphasic, occurring in the interval from late afternoon to approximately midnight and again shortly after dawn (Davies and Davies 2003). Limit or controlled feeding is done by feeding 50% to 75% of the *ad libitum* consumption once per day and is important in preventing obesity and urolithiasis and otherwise optimizing health.

For a medium-sized rabbit (4- to 6-kg adult), limit feeding is done by providing 120 to 180 g pelleted diet /day. This translates to 3 to 4 oz or about 2/3 cup. Administration of the ration by limit feeding encourages daily observation of the pet and prompt detection of anorexia as a tip-off to an underlying health problem. Pregnant does should be fed 175 to 225 g/ day and at parturition they should be gradually increased over a few days to ad libitum feeding. Limit feeding is especially important at weaning during the dietary transition from milk-based diet to plant-based food when there may not be sufficient brush border enzymes in the gut to digest plant carbohydrates and protective maternal antibodies are waning. Limit feeding of weanlings protects them from osmotic overload, pH extremes, and enteric disease. Weanlings of medium-sized breeds should be given 60 g/kg/day up to a maximum of 120 to 180 g/day.

Rabbit kits are entirely dependent upon milk until ten days of age and then they progressively begin to consume solid foods and maternal-origin cecotrophs up until weaning at around four weeks of age (Davies and Davies 2003). Kits typically nurse once daily with ingested milk forming a semi-solid curd protected in the stomach by an antimicrobial fatty acid product formed by the action of the kit's digestive enzymes on the milk; this is called "stomach oil" or "milk oil" (Davies and Davies 2003). This curd gradually passes into the intestine over the time between feedings (Davies and Davies 2003). Rabbits fed on milk substitutes or milk from another species fail to develop the protective fatty acid products and are devoid of colostral antibody, making them susceptible to bacterial enteric infections (Davies and Davies 2003).

Water should be given free choice and is generally consumed at twice the feed intake quantity or about 100 120 ml/kg/day. Water consumption varies with factors such as environmental temperature, diet com-position, and health (e.g. lactation). Lactating does consume water up to 90% equivalent of their body weight daily (Harkness and Wagner 1989).

COMMON AND ZOONOTIC DISEASES

The medical management of rabbits can generally be accomplished by meeting a few basic goals. The tenets of preventive care are good nutrition and sanitation combined with protection from predators, drafts, environmental extremes, environmental intoxicants, and trauma.

Rabbits commercially reared are often raised in pole barns and, for the most part, are free of infectious agents. *Pasteurella*-free flocks are not uncommon, but most sources have some problems with coccidiosis, encephalitozoonosis, and, on occasion, internal and/or external parasites. New Zealand white and Dutch belted rabbits are often available as specific pathogen-free animals from rabbitries. Other outbred stocks or domestic breeds are generally not pathogen-free and typically are colonized by *Pasteurella multocida*. Rabbits obtained from pet stores, unless the vendor can make a specific claim otherwise, should be assumed to be *Pasteurella*-infected. Clients considering the purchase of a rabbit should be counseled to obtain it from a source with a *Pasteurella*-free colony or to obtain a kit at weaning or as close to weaning as possible. This is arguably the best advice, from a preventive medicine standpoint, that can be given to a client desiring a pet rabbit.

In private practice, a domestic or wild rabbit is most likely to be encountered in the clinic for interventional purposes rather than preventive medicine. There are no effective vaccines for specific rabbit diseases available in the U.S., for example, and, other than neutering over-sexed males or performing ovariectomies on females, there is little in the way of preventive medical procedures that a rabbit owner may seek proactively. However, clients that otherwise own dogs or cats may seek the advice of a clinic in providing proper care for their rabbits. Knowing a little bit about rabbits may not only be good for the occasional rabbit patient, but it may also be valuable in maintaining business.

The most common presentations of rabbits to a veterinary clinic are for abscesses, malocclusion, elective surgical procedures such as ovariohysterectomy and orchiectomy, and possibly nail trimming. Rabbits also may experience respiratory, gastrointestinal, or integumentary illnesses, as well as neoplasia. The rabbit diseases of greatest clinical importance are grouped into those affecting the respiratory, digestive, and integumentary systems and by infectious, inherited, or traumatic/environmental etiology.

Respiratory Infectious Diseases

Bacterial upper respiratory tract disease in rabbits is commonly referred to as "snuffles," and is characterized by sneezing, mucopurulent nasal discharge, and conjunctivitis. This syndrome is the most common infectious illness in pet rabbits, and the usual etiologic agent is the bacterium *Pasteurella multocida*. The organism is part of the normal nasal flora of cats, as well, but the serotypes that cause disease in rabbits differ from those in cats. Other bacteria have been identified in cases of rabbit snuffles, including *Bordetella bronchiseptica* and Staphylococcal species, but their importance to the pathogenesis is unknown and may be trivial (Deeb and DiGiacomo 2000). In rabbitries and/or pet stores where *Pasteurella* is enzootic, up to 90% to 100% of adult rabbits are infected. Inapparent carriers of *Pasteurella* occur frequently, and subclinical infections localized to the nasal passages or tympanic bullae are common. On the other side of the clinical spectrum, the bacterium may cause a chronic, progressive, incurable, potentially fatal, multi-systemic disease, starting with the upper respiratory tract. Most commonly, the syndrome presents with frequent sneezing or mucopurulent nasal discharge (Langan et al. 2000).

Pasteurella may be transmitted from rabbit to rabbit by direct contact, close contact aerosol, or, less frequently, venereal routes. The role of fomites in transmission is unclear. *Pasteurella multocida* is harbored in the nasal cavity and/or tympanic bullae where it may remain localized. Harborage in these areas protects the bacterium from antibodies and administered antibiotics. The organism is capable of dissemination from the nasal passages to other parts of the body, leading to a constellation of clinical manifestations including conjunctivitis, skin abscesses, inner ear infection, pyometra, orchitis, pneumonia, or septicemia.

In a rabbits with suppurative clinical signs, diagnosis of pasteurellosis can easily be confirmed by bacterial culture. When septicemic Pasteurellosis is suspected, the organism should be recoverable from the blood. Asymptomatic carriers may prove more difficult to diagnose, because even deep nasal swabs may not identify all organisms. When carriers are suspected, deep nasal swabs may be attempted under anesthesia/sedation, for both culture and polymerase chain reaction amplification, using an alginate swab. Alternatively, the serum can be assessed for antibodies against *Pasteurella multocida* that may be suggestive of exposure and infection (Sanchez et al. 2004).

There are no effective vaccines, commercially available or otherwise, to prevent pasteurellosis or control its clinical signs, although there have been many attempts at generating them. Veterinary care is primarily supportive and symptomatic, and may be dissatisfying for all parties. Antibiotics, such as marbofloxacin (Rougier et al. 2006), sulfas, chloramphenicol, tetracyclines, or enrofloxacin, may be given for a month or more and result in improvement of clinical signs, but it is difficult to eliminate the organism. Upon completion of a course of therapy, symptoms may recrudesce and worsen over time. Consequently, for the most severe cases, antibiotics may simply buy time for an owner to come to terms with the prospect of euthanasia. Less severe cases may improve and stabilize, but animals may remain carriers. Supportive care delivered by a veterinary technician is symptom-directed and may include regular cleaning of obstructed nares, flushing of the nasolacrimal duct in cases of severe conjunctivitis, nebulization or vaporizer treatments, and excision or incision/drainage of abscesses.

The proportion of rabbits with pasteurellosis increases as rabbits age. By adulthood, 90% or so of animals from a rabbitry with enzootic infection become colonized. Preweanling rabbits have a low rate of infection and early weaning can be used as a tool to obtain Pasteurella-free animals. Additionally, treatment of pregnant does prior to kindling and through lactation with antibiotics such as furazolidone, oxytetracycline, or sulfaquinoxaline in the diet or drinking water suppresses the bacterium and promotes the weaning of pathogen-free kits.

Diseases of the Digestive System

Rabbits, particularly weanlings and young kits, are commonly subject to diarrheal disease. Infectious agents that play an important part in the gastrointestinal illnesses of rabbits include coccidia; rotaviruses and coronaviruses; and the bacterial agents *E. coli*, *Lawsonia*, and *Clostridium*. Diet plays a vital role in maintaining gastrointestinal health, and the provision of a high fiber diet will in many cases be preventative or ameliorative.

Coccidiosis, caused by enteric or hepatotrophic species of the genus *Eimeria*, is a major disease problem in young rabbits. Infection can be subclinical or mild, but clinical disease is characterized by fulminant diarrhea, and occurs in juveniles, especially recent weanlings, kept under poor conditions or stressed by transportation. Unlike enteric coccidial species, *Eimeria stiedae* parasitizes the liver and bile duct. Infection is often subclinical, but in young rabbits the agent may cause fatal hepatic failure characterized by icterus, hepatomegaly, elevated hepatic enzymes, wasting, and anorexia. The transmission of coccidia in rabbits is by the fecal-oral route and the diagnosis is made by fecal examination for oocysts or at necropsy. Administration of sulfa drugs, ivermectin, and/or toltrazuril are treatment options (Cam et al. 2008). Because oocysts require a day or more to sporulate at room temperature, the ingestion of night feces is not considered to play a role in the dissemination of disease, and aggressive sanitation is an effective means of control. If housing and fomites are not cleaned effectively, oocysts remaining in the environment may be a source of reinfection for months. Vitamin E deficiency may potentiate coccidiosis.

Rotavirus is enzootic in many rabbitries where it is of mild pathogenicity. It destroys enterocytes that synthesize disaccharidases, consequently causing diarrhea due to maldigestion. Infection may be fatal in young kits that are not protected by maternal antibodies under epizootic conditions. As with enteric viral diseases of other species, treatment is directed at supportive care.

Coronaviruses have been found in association with diarrhea in young rabbits. One survey of commercial rabbitries in North America showed a prevalence of antibodies detected by serology to be as much as 40% (Deeb et al. 1993). Definitive diagnosis requires demonstration of coronaviral particles in gut contents by electron microscopy. Thus, diagnosis of pet rabbits is unlikely, and treatment remains directed at supportive care.

Clostridial enterotoxemia is caused primarily by *Clostridium spiroforme*. This Gram-positive, anaerobic bacterium is not normally a part of the gastrointestinal flora or is suppressed to a very low and nonpathogenic level in healthy adults. The normal gut microflora is protective, and its disruption appears to be required for colonization by *C. spiroforme*. Changes caused by weaning, following environmental stress, or by disruption of the normal flora through concurrent infection or the use of antibiotics with anaerobic and Gram-positive spectra can be predisposing factors. Antibiotics that have been incriminated in the disease include clindamycin, lincomycin, ampicllin, penicillin, metronidazole, and erythromycin. These antibiotics should be used clinically with caution, with the informed consent of the client, and not on a herd-wide basis.

Clinical signs include anorexia, wasting, and diarrhea, and are usually the result of enterotoxins which damage normal gut function. The disease is suspected based on a combination of signalment (the condition usually occurs in young rabbits) and a history of recent change in environment and clinical signs. Gram stains

of gut contents may show typical coiled bacteria. Anaerobic culture can positively identify the organism, and several methods exist to assay for the enterotoxin. Treatment consists of a combination of nursing care, fluid therapy, antibiotics, and increasing the fiber content of the diet, aiming toward a normalization of the gut microflora. The importance of sanitation, for removal of spores from the environment, should be stressed to the client.

Tyzzer's disease is caused by *Clostridium piliforme*, a Gram-negative obligate intracellular bacterium with vegetative and spore forms. Like coccidiosis, it causes disease most commonly in recent weanlings, especially in the face of crowding, poor sanitation, or deprivation of food or water. Natural infection is thought to be by ingestion of spore-contaminated food or bedding. The spores are hardy and can persist in the environment for years. Mortality can be acute and high. The diagnosis can be difficult to establish and is often made using special stains (silver) of specimens obtained at necropsy. Serologic assays exist for the agent, but suffer from non-specific cross-reactivity leading to false positives.

Enteropathogenic strains of *E. coli* are also important pathogens of young rabbits. The bacterium is normally found as part of the commensal flora, but proliferates in the cecum in disease-causing yellow diarrhea and leads to high mortality within forty-eight hours (Wales et al. 2005). Sucklings within two to eight days of birth and weaned kits less than three months of age are most at risk. The organism can be identified by culture, and characterization of the isolate assists in predicting its virulence. Good sanitation, fluid therapy, body temperature maintenance, and antibiotics are important in treatment.

Lawsonia intracellularis is the cause of proliferative enteropathy and typically afflicts young rabbits. Although infection is characterized by a one- to two-week course of diarrhea, depression, and dehydration, it is rarely fatal. The organism is difficult to culture; histopathology or molecular diagnostic assays are usually necessary (Horiuchi et al. 2008). Severely diarrheic rabbits require fluid therapy and body temperature management.

There are few helminth parasites of clinical importance in domestic rabbits. The rabbit pinworm, *Passalurus ambiguus*, is not contagious for humans and is largely nonpathogenic. It is found in the cecum and large intestine of wild rabbits and occasionally domestic or laboratory rabbits. The life cycle is direct and infection is acquired by ingestion. The diagnosis may be made by demonstration of oocysts by fecal floatation examination techniques or observation of expelled adult nematodes on the feces. The eggs (43 um × 103 um, flattened on one side) are laid in embryonated, infective form. Common anthelmintic agents used in dogs and cats, such as ivermectin, fenbendazole, and pyrantel pamoate, have high efficacy in rabbits (Carpenter et al. 2001, Curtis and Brooks 1990, Düwel and Brech 1981).

Mucoid enteropathy syndrome is a mucoid diarrheal disease of grave prognosis that is particularly severe in weanling rabbits. The pathogenesis remains largely conjectural, but dietary factors have been implicated. Commercial rabbit feed is high energy and low in fiber, and rabbits on low fiber diets have lower acetate levels. This fatty acid is thought to be a component of the protection offered by the normal gut environment. When levels are low, microorganisms may proliferate, further altering the fermentative microflora. The imbalance, in the presence of as yet unidentified microorganisms, progresses to profuse, mucoid diarrhea (Percy and Barthold 2007). Affected rabbits are thin with a hunched posture, anorectic, dehydrated, hypothermic, and mildly bloated. Dietary change and other stressors, such as painful injections, overheating, or inadvertent water deprivation (including excessively warm, yet plentiful, water in the summer months), may also predispose to disease. Treatment is generally unsuccessful with the case fatality rate approaching 100%. This is clearly a disease in which an ounce of prevention is worth a pound of cure. Mucoid enteropathy can be prevented by feeding high fiber rations and restricting the pelleted diet to 60 g/kg body weight.

Gastric stasis syndrome may occur in rabbits of all ages, and generally presents as an anorectic rabbit with decreased or no fecal production, but otherwise appears normal. It may be possible to palpate a doughy mass (the stomach) in the cranial abdomen, but abdominal palpation may also be normal. Gut stasis can be caused by environmental changes, stress (including postoperative stress), or excessive amounts of a high energy, low fiber diet. The gut contents may or may not be predominantly composed of hair, and the presumptive diagnosis of trichobezoar may occasionally be made more rapidly than is warranted. Due to gastric hypomotility, the stomach contents, whether hair or ingesta, become dehydrated and difficult to pass. Treatment consists of rehydrating the contents of the stomach, maintaining hydration of the animal, and stimulating motility. The rabbits should be force-fed liquids and/or fruit and vegetable purees (e.g. baby food). The use of pineapple juice for the bromelin has been advocated as a method for breaking down the mass. The juice may well work, but the mechanism of action is more likely to be based on the hydration of the mass than a chemical decomposition. If necessary, the rabbit should be administered subcutaneous or intravenous fluids. Provided there are no signs of impaction, metoclopramide for three to five days should assist in restoring normal gastrointestinal motility.

Additionally, it is important to appreciate that healthy rabbits commonly harbor gastric trichobezoars without pathologic effect. Slaughter checks of 208 healthy rabbits in one study, for example, showed that 23% had trichobezoars (Leary et al. 1984). In the same study, infusion of rabbit stomachs with latex causing a large space-occupying mass had no effect on the immediate or long-term health of the rabbits. Consequently, trichobezoars can be incidental findings in rabbits and should not be considered to be pathologic until proven otherwise.

Integumentary Infectious Diseases

The most important integumentary disease of rabbits is ear mite infestation by the ectoparasite *Psoroptes cuniculi* (Figure 12.5). The condition, most properly called otoacariasis, may be referred to as ear mange or ear canker by rabbit keepers. Exudate and inflammation in the ear canal can be extensive and the mites may also parasitize periauricular areas, including the face and neck. Transmission of the parasite is direct from rabbit to rabbit and the life cycle requires twenty-one days for completion. Tens of thousands of mites may be found on a single animal (Bowman et al. 1992). Mites can survive off of the host for weeks at a time (Hess 2004). Infestation causes pruritus, head shaking, stress, and competition for nutrients. The ears may be painful to touch and, in advanced cases, are heavily encrusted with exudate. The mites are large enough to

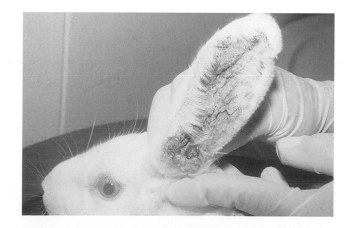

Figure 12.5. Ear mite infestation.

be seen with the unaided eye, but the diagnosis usually is made by otoscope examination of the large adults (males, 431 to 547 um × 322 to 462 um; females, 403 to 749 um × 351 × 499 um) in the aural canal or microscopic observation of mites from exudate swabbed from the ear.

Treatment is with ivermectin by SC injection every two weeks for a total of three treatments, and aggressive environmental sanitation (Curtis and Brooks 1990, Wright and Riner 1984). Although the antiparasitic agents selamectin and moxidectin are not labeled for rabbits, both have been used to eradicate *Psoroptes cuniculi* without ill effects (McTier et al. 2003, Wagner and Wendlberger, 2000). Alternative methods for treatment, including topically applied ivermectin and oils, have been advocated (Fichi et al. 2007) and may be effective, but thorough environmental sanitation is still required and cases treated thusly should be closely monitored.

Venereal spirochetosis is caused by a spirochete bacterium, *Treponema paraluis cuniculi*. The disease is known by a number of synonyms including treponemiasis, cuniculosis, vent disease, and rabbit syphilis. Transmission may be horizontal by the venereal (coitus) or extragenital (facial-genital contact) routes. Fomite inoculation is also a possibility. In contrast to many other infectious diseases of rabbits, young rabbits are relatively resistant to infection, but incidence increases with time in a breeding program. Following infectious contact, organisms localize and proliferate at mucocutaneous junctions, causing erythema and edema of prepuce, vulva, scrotum, perineum, or anus. The nose, eyelids, lips, and extremities can also be affected. The lesions become vesicular; exude serum; and then become dry, scaly, and crusty. In the natural course of the disease, lesions persist for *at least* one to three months and often for five months or so (Delong and Manning 1994). During the course of infection, the bacterium then colonizes regional lymph nodes where it remains even after lesions fade. Overt clinical disease is then precipitated by stress. Venereal spirochetosis may be confused with and should be differentiated from traumatic or chemical dermatitis, localized nontreponemal bacterial pyoderma (e.g. "hutchburn"), dermatophytes, and ectoparasites. The diagnosis of treponemiasis is by history, physical examination, and *in vitro* tests such as darkfield microscopy and various serologic assays.

Penicillins, given for periods ranging from five to twenty-eight days, are the treatment of choice. A less intensive penicillin regimen involving weekly injections for a total of three treatments has also been advocated (Delong and Manning 1994). Lesions generally resolve and the organism will be eliminated within three weeks of the start of treatment.

Ulcerative pododermatitis presents as decubital ulcers, typically on the plantar surfaces of the hind feet (Figure 12.6). Superficial ulcers and scabs may progress, without intervention, to abscesses or granulomas, and further progression could lead to osteomyelitis or sepsis. The lesions are pressure-induced and predisposed commonly by a genetically-related decrease in hair density on the feet. Poor sanitation, excessive environmental moisture, foot stomping, large adult size, and wire-bottomed caging all may be contributory factors. Treatment consists of debriding and cleaning the site, and topical application of antibiotic creams with bandaging and rebandaging for weeks at a time.

Other interventions should include improving sanitation and changing the flooring from wire to flat metal slatted flooring or solid flooring with use of a litter box. The latter, however, may become soiled and aggravate problems. When rabbits must be kept on wire the strategic placement of a flat, solid resting board in an area of the cage preferred for rest and away from areas used for urination/defecation may be helpful. Successful treatment is lengthy and the condition often recrudesces, particularly if housing conditions are not changed. *Staphylococcus aureus* is the most frequently identified associated organism (Percy and Barthold 2007).

Moist dermatitis (blue fur disease) may be seen in the perineal area subsequent to urine or diarrhea scald, known colloquially as "hutch burn," or around the face, neck, or dewlap as a consequence of malocclusion or continual moistening of the fur by drinking from a water bowl. The latter presentation may be called "slobbers" by fanciers and breeders. The initial

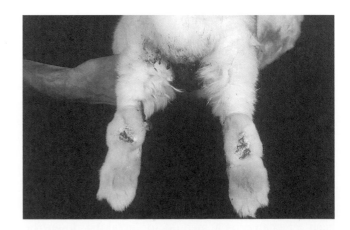

Figure 12.6. Pododermatitis.

physical insult may lead to secondary bacterial dermatitis caused by the bacterium *Pseudomonas aeruginosa*, which originates from feces or fecal-contaminated drinking water. *Pseudomonas* species elaborate a blue-green pigment that discolors the affected area. Rabbits so afflicted are often described as having blue fur. The treatment is by correcting the initiating cause, drying the environment, clipping fur in the area of any lesions, and treating the lesions with astringents and topical or systemic gentamicin. The condition is prevented by good sanitation, controlling obesity, and not offering water from bowls or crocks.

Necrobacillosis (Schmorl's disease) is a syndrome that most commonly refers to dermatitis of the face and neck area caused by excessive salivation, usually due to malocclusion or other dental disease. Skin lesions may be found elsewhere on the body, however, and infection is typically associated with filthy conditions or skin trauma. The microorganism generally associated with this condition is the Gram-negative anaerobic bacterium, *Fusobacterium necrophorum*. This bacterium is a normal inhabitant of the gastrointestinal tract and causes ulceration and necrosis of the skin when inoculated into it. Fecal contamination from cecotrophy may be a source of oral inoculation. The diagnosis is made by a combination of clinical signs and anaerobic bacterial culture. Treatment consists of debriding wounds and applying topical antibiotics. Systemic drugs with an anaerobic spectrum such as penicillins, cephalosporins, or chloramphenicol may be used in severe cases. Prevention is achieved by maintaining a high level of sanitation, providing dental care where indicated, and eliminating sources of trauma such as coarse feed or sharp edges in cages.

Fly strike is not uncommon in rabbits housed outdoors. Larvae of *Cuterebra* species can be found in the subcutis, causing 1- to 3-cm swellings, each housing a single larva and each having a breathing hole. Larvae should be surgically removed carefully, so as not to damage them, because crushed larvae can cause an anaphylactic reaction. Maggots of non-*Cuterebral* species may be found anywhere on the body, but have a predilection for the perineal skin folds of aged or obese rabbits. For all fly species, the treatment is to remove the larvae and clean the wound site under sedation, provide antibiotics and fluid therapy, and administer ivermectin for two doses at two-week intervals. Preventive strategies consist of fly control measures including screening outdoor pens.

Mastitis can occur in lactating does, and also is possible independent of lactation. The offending bacteria are typically *Staphylococcus aureus*, streptococci, or *Pasteurella* (Pare et al. 2004). Treatment consists of antibiotics, warm compresses, fluid therapy, and, where indicated, incision and drainage.

Other Infectious Diseases

Cerebral larval migrans and fatal central nervous system disease may be seen in rabbits that acquire aberrant infections with *Baylisascaris* species. Disease may occur where raccoons or skunks contaminate stored feed or hay, gain access to barns or cages housing rabbits and defecate from the cage top into the interior of the cage, or where pet rabbits have grazed contaminated forage or been housed on contaminated hay (Deeb and Digiacomo 1994, Jensen et al. 1983, Kazacos and Kazacos, 1983). Signs of infection include progressive torticollis, ataxia, tremors, and falling (Deeb and Digiacomo 1994). The diagnosis is based on clinical signs and histopathology, but fresh minced brain can be placed in a Baermann apparatus to separate the larvae for specific identification. The condition is untreatable. Rabbits are a dead-end host for this disease and cannot pass it on to humans.

There are a number of other infectious diseases of rabbits that are not likely to be encountered in pet rabbits, but are worth mentioning. *Obeliscoides cuniculi*, the rabbit stomach worm, is common in wild rabbits and may be found in laboratory rabbits that are fed contaminated feed or grazed on contaminated forages. It is a trichostrongyle, embedding in the gastric mucosa with a direct life cycle with shedding for sixty-one to 118 days (Jenkins 2004). Staphylococci may cause septicemia, suppurative disease (including cutaneous abscesses or mastitis), and conjunctivitis. It is most severe and common in young or distressed animals. Rabbit hemorrhagic disease (RHD) is caused by a calicivirus and targets rabbits after weaning. The disease is acute and highly fatal, showing few clinical signs. The virus usually presents as an explosive outbreak with high mortality in rabbitries, with rabbits succumbing to a severe and widespread intravascular coagulopathy (Xu and Chen 1989, Percy and Barthold 2007). Slaughter and disinfection are standard procedures in rabbitries where outbreaks have occurred. Rabbits are also susceptible to toxoplasmosis (Leland et al. 1992) and may be an accidental host for the canine heartworm (Narama et al. 1982) and other dirofilarial species if housed outdoors.

Inherited Diseases

Buphthalmia (glaucoma, ox eye) is not uncommon in New Zealand white rabbits and is due to inadequate drainage of aqueous humor from the anterior chamber (Tesluk et al. 1982). It occurs unilaterally or bilaterally and is usually detectable by the time the rabbit is three to five months old. Buphthalmia in rabbits is characterized by megaloglobus, increased intraocular pressure, and increased corneal diameter. The condition is generally not painful, at least in the early stages, but may cause blindness. Medical treatment with antiglaucomatous agents generally is not successful. Consequently, affected rabbits should be monitored regularly for pain or distress. Clients should be cautioned not to breed affected rabbits.

Splay leg, a developmental musculoskeletal disorder, is seen in young rabbits; the rear limbs splay and will not bear weight (Cohen 1969, Deeb and Carpenter 2004). The condition varies in severity, with relatively mild cases showing only clumsiness when ambulating, to severe cases, which are completely paralyzed. In the latter cases, euthanasia is warranted. As is the case with most inherited disorders, clients should be cautioned not to breed affected rabbits.

Depending upon the breed and genotype, rabbits may be afflicted by any number of other genetic and metabolic diseases including epilepsy, hydrocephalus, arteriosclerosis, cataracts, Pelger-Huet anomaly, cleft palate, lymphosarcoma, and hypertension (Lindsey and Fox 1994). Arteriosclerosis is a polygenic or familial trait that can be seen in all breeds, with calcified vessels visible on radiographs. Clinical signs are vague and may include general malaise, lethargy, and weight loss. Hydrocephalus is often associated with dwarfism and brachygnathia, although vitamin A deficiency in pregnant does will produce identical clinical signs in offspring (Cohen 1969, Lindsey and Fox 1994).

Skeletal, Traumatic, and Environmental Diseases

Malocclusion of the incisors (mandibular prognathism, walrus teeth, and buck teeth) may be inherited due to the shortening of the maxillary skull relative to the mandible of normal length with the lower incisors extending cranial to the upper incisors and growing into the mouth. Malocclusion may also be caused from tooth loss due to trauma. More commonly, malocclusion results from high-energy diets causing excessive tooth growth and resulting in teeth that are not worn down adequately (Crossley and Aiken 2004). Uncontrolled growth of the incisors or "spikes" which develop as a result of incomplete or inadequate wearing of teeth leads to functional anorexia and wasting with variable drooling and oral lesions. The treatment for malocclusion is periodic tooth trimming with an appropriate power dental bur or extraction. The owner should be counseled against breeding the animal when the cause is suspected to be genetic.

Traumatic vertebral subluxation or fractures may occur secondary to struggling against restraint, improper handling or sudden jumping, or startling a caged rabbit. Injury is predisposed by the high muscle-to-bone ratio in rabbits. The lumbosacral joint acts as a fulcrum for the hind limbs with subluxation or fracture generally occurring at L7 or the caudal vertebrae. Diagnosis is made by clinical signs (i.e. posterior paresis or paralysis, loss of pain sensation, urinary retention, and fecal incontinence), palpation, and/or radiography. Sequellae include decubital sores and perineal dermatitis from urine scald, along with uremia from urine retention. To treat, provide shock doses of methylprednisolone sodium succinate if the injury is acute. Long-term prognosis depends on the degree of injury, with mildly injured rabbits responding to a course of treatment including bladder expression and anti-inflammatory drugs. Severely injured rabbits are likely incurable and may require euthanasia.

Pregnancy toxemia is uncommon, but may be seen especially in Dutch or Polish breeds. It is most common in pregnant does in the last week of pregnancy, but a similar metabolic toxemia may also be seen in pseudo-pregnant, postparturient, or obese does. Obesity and fasting are considered to be predisposing factors, and there is some evidence that hereditary factors play a role. There is often hepatic fatty infiltration and necrosis. Clinically-affected animals are depressed and have acetone breath, dyspnea, and decreased urine production. Abortion, incoordination, convulsions, and coma may precede death. Death without premonitory signs can be a presentation. Treatment with lactated Ringers or 5% dextrose, steroids, and empiric use of calcium gluconate is recommended, but is rarely successful. Prevention is accomplished by providing an adequate nutritional plane, including a high-energy diet late in gestation balanced with obesity prevention.

Neoplasia

Retrospective assessments of tumor incidence in rabbits are confounded by the fact that case reports and historical surveys have been largely derived from colonies of research animals in which rabbits, for the most part, rarely live longer than one to two years (Weisbroth 1994). While tumor incidence increases with age, there is no comprehensive tumor incidence information for aging rabbits.

Uterine adenocarcinoma is the most common neoplasm of female rabbits with a high incidence in the Dutch, Californian, and New Zealand white breeds. The incidence is less than 5% in does under two years of age, but in certain populations it may affect 80% of does over five years of age (Percy and Barthold

2007). Clinical signs include vulvar bleeding, anemia, and a palpable abdominal mass. The prevention and attempted treatment of the disease is by ovariohysterectomy (OHE). Unless does are to be bred, OHE is recommended universally. In young rabbits, the most common neoplasm is lymphosarcoma. Unlike other species, in which lymphoid organs are the most common sites of involvement, in rabbits it is the kidney and gastric mucosa (Percy and Barthold 2007). Interstitial cell tumors and seminomas have been reported in male rabbits (Weisbroth 1994). Other neoplasms that have been reported with some frequency in rabbits include embryonal nephroma, leiomyoma/leiosarcoma, lymphosarcoma, cutaneous papilloma, and mammary adenocarcinoma (Weisbroth 1994).

Zoonotic Diseases

Domestic rabbits harbor few zoonoses of any significance, with dermatophytosis ("ringworm") arguably the most important. *Trichophyton mentagrophytes* is most common, but *Microsporum canis* and other species may cause infection (Bergdall and Dysko 1994, Vogtsberger et al. 1986). Typical red, raised lesions are usually found around the head and ears, and diagnosis can be made from a skin scraping placed in dermatophyte test medium or cleared with 10% KOH. There is a demonstrated association with marginal husbandry practices, poor nutrition, environmental or internal stress factors, overcrowding, excessive heat and/or humidity, genetics, ectoparasites, extremes of youth or old age, and pregnancy. Direct contact or fomite transmissions are not uncommon and rabbits may be asymptomatic carriers (Lopez-Martinez et al. 1984). The disease is readily transmissible to humans. Individual animals can be isolated and treated with griseofulvin (orally or topically in DMSO) or topical povidone iodine (Bergdall and Dysko 1994).

Salmonellosis, often presenting as a peracute fatal disease subsequent to a stressor (e.g., anesthesia, environmental extremes), has been reported in rabbits. The diagnosis is based on culture and identification of the organism from blood, bile, feces, lymph nodes, or affected organs. Treatment is ineffective in eliminating the carrier state and, due to the public health risks, infected animals should be euthanized.

Rabies virus has been identified in pet rabbits in New York state, serving as a reminder that any pet animal with access to the outdoors requires adequate protection. There are currently no rabies vaccines available for pet rabbits.

Yersinia pseudotuberculosis is acquired by ingestion and causes emaciation and swollen lymph nodes with variable incidence of septicemia or diarrhea. *Listeria monocytogenes* causes acute, sporadic disease in many species. In rabbits, it most commonly causes septicemia, abortion, and fatality of pregnant does.

Encephalitozoonosis, caused by the protozoan *Encephalitozoon cuniculi*, has a tropism for the brain, kidney, and eyes, and may cause neurologic signs, primarily head tilt, in rabbits. It may also infect immunocompromised humans, with diarrhea, renal disease, and keratoconjunctivitis associated with encephalitozoonosis in AIDS patients. Encephalitozoonosis may be found in up to 30% of asymptomatic rabbits in certain colonies, and a survey of neurologic pet rabbits revealed 69% to be seropositive (Harcourt-Brown and Holloway 2003). In cases in which encephalitozoonosis is suspected, definitive diagnosis is difficult because it has historically relied on visualization of lesions in brain tissue or PCR of the same. Thus, antemortem diagnosis is based on clinical signs and serology, although a recent report cites positive PCRs obtained from liquefied lens material in cases of uveitis and lens rupture (Kunzel et al. 2008). Infection is acquired by ingestion, usually of food contaminated with infected urine, or nasal inoculation. Little scientific evidence is available regarding treatment of rabbits for encephalitozoonosis, although albendazole and corticosteroids have anecdotally resulted in improvement in some cases (Harcourt-Brown and Holloway 2003), and fenbendazole has been shown to resolve others (Suter et al. 2001).

Certain ectoparasites, such as the fur mite *Cheyletiella parasitovorax*, and burrowing sarcoptid mites may be transmissible from rabbits to humans. Of lesser importance are diseases such as leptospirosis, tularemia, and endoparasitism. *Francisella tularensis*, the etiologic agent of tularemia, rarely infects domestic lagomorphs, but may cause acute, febrile disease. It is noteworthy that exposure to wild rabbits is associated with the vast majority of human cases. Zoonoses generally can be prevented by wearing gloves and long-sleeved clinical garments when handling rabbits and hand-washing upon the removal of gloves.

TAKING A HISTORY

The basic fundamentals of the history for rabbits are similar to those for other animals, and are summarized in Table 12.4. As with other species, the first information to document should be the signalment. Certain rabbit breeds may be predisposed to particular diseases, so breed is an important component of the signalment, as it would be for dogs. There are currently forty-seven breeds in the United States recognized by the American Rabbit Breeders Association (ARBA),

Table 12.4 History questions for rabbit owners.

Topic	Questions	Comments
Signalment	Age Sex Neutered status Breed	Owners may not be correct about the sex of the rabbit and education might be necessary. The age when the animal was neutered may also be relevant.
Acquisition	Location (pet store, breeder, etc.) When the animal was acquired	How many owners the animal has had may be important for behavioral problems.
Housing	Cage type Flooring substrate Exercise amount/frequency Frequency of cage cleaning	If the animals have wire bottom cages, ask about access to areas away from the wire. Amount of time per day or week available out of the cage for exercise is important.
Environment	Other animals in the house Indoors/outdoors Potential environmental hazards	Newly acquired rabbits or wild animals may be a source of infectious disease. Rabbits may like to chew objects when roaming the house.
Diet	Types of food: hay, pellets, fresh foods Amount offered and eaten	Make sure to ask about treats and if the pellets are just pellets or have other items (corn, seed, etc.).
Animal	Changes in feces or urine Changes in appetite or diet preferences Changes in behavior Coughing, sneezing, or nasal discharge Any medications, including herbal and nutritional supplements	If there are changes in appetite/drinking, ask about any environmental changes such as a new diet, stressful situation, or new water or food dispensers.

ranging in size from 1 kg dwarf/small breeds to 5 to 8 kg or greater giant breeds. Many of these breeds can have multiple colors called "varieties." Rabbit breeds are made distinctive by a combination of body size and shape, ear carriage, and pelt coloration. If the ears "flop" down alongside the head, rather than stand erect, the breed is of the lop-eared variety. Some non-show grade lops may have one or both ears "helicopter" by projecting horizontally. Many rabbits presenting to a veterinary practice, particularly if acquired from a pet store, are not purebreds or do not meet the breed standards. However, some breeds are commonly seen, such as the Dutch, Holland lop, Mini-lop and Rex (Table 12.5). The best method to become familiarized with rabbit breed is to visit the ARBA web site at: http://www.arba.net.

The realities of rabbit medicine are such that most are presented to a clinic for intervention for a clinical problem and there are few presentations for wellness exams, which requires a detailed history about both the routine care of the animal and the presenting complaint. To obtain accurate information, it is important to be non-judgmental and carefully ask questions because owners may be reluctant to admit what they do not perceive as the "correct" answer. The diet is

perhaps the most significant question for many rabbit owners. This requires specifically asking not only what is offered, but what the animal actually eats. Unfortunately, many commercial rabbit pellets are mixed with unhealthy items such as corn and seeds, and rabbits may selectively eat high carbohydrate and high fat items, leading to obesity or gut stasis (Harcourt-Brown 2002). Pellets can also be composed of different types of hay that may have different nutrient values.

After questions about husbandry, the general questions about the rabbit are similar to those for other animals. Decreased appetite/anorexia is one of the most common presenting complaints for rabbits, but this can indicate a wide variety of diseases. Respiratory, dental, dermatological, and gastrointestinal problems are common issues for rabbits presenting to the veterinarian. Sometimes rabbits, especially unspayed adult females, may present because of increased aggression. The etiology for aggression can vary from hormonal, normal exploratory behavior, overzealous grooming, pain, deafness, and even infectious diseases, so these are all important aspects of the history to address in addition to the standard questions (Harcourt-Brown 2002).

Table 12.5. Common purebred rabbit breeds.

Breed	Size range (lbs)	Color and markings	Other characteristics
Californian	8–10.5	White with colored nose, ears, tail, and feet	Compact body type and pink eyes
Checkered giant	>11	White with colored nose, ears, eye-rings, cheek spots, a stripe down length of spine, and a pair of spots on each side of body	Hare-like posture
Dutch	3.5–5.5	White forequarters and thorax with ears, cheeks, and back half of body colored	Short, blocky, compact body type
Himalayan	4–5	White with colored nose, ears, feet, and tail	Small and slender body type with a long, pointed head, erect ears, and pink eyes
Holland lop	<4	Variable	Short, blocky, compact body type
Rex	7.5–10.5	Variable	Short and upright fur
Mini-lop	4.5–6.5	Variable	Short, blocky, compact body type
New Zealand white	9–12	Albino	Compact body type

PHYSICAL EXAMINATION AND PREVENTIVE MEDICINE

As with cats, clients should be advised to bring the rabbit to the clinic concealed in a secure carrier in which the rabbit should remain until in the exam room. A normal rabbit typically rests compactly on all four limbs with its mouth closed and regular twitching of the nostrils. A rabbit presenting with severe pain will show a hunched posture and immobility and may grind its teeth. Those in acute pain or distress, especially upon handling, may emit a haunting, high pitched cry. Many an amiable rabbit will become aggressive if in chronic pain or distress.

An appreciation of the normal protrusion of the eyes is necessary to recognize buphthalmia or exophthalmia. The eyes may protrude more in some breeds, males during breeding season, and when fearful (Harcourt-Brown 2002). Rabbits may not menace because of their natural tendency to freeze, so this response is not an adequate test for vision (Vernau et al. 2007). Ocular examinations can be done as for other species, but keep in mind the caveat that atropine may be unreliable or ineffective as a mydriatic owing to the presence of serum atropinesterase in many rabbits. There should be no ocular or nasal discharge. Periocular depilation or discharge may suggest conjunctivitis or dacryocystitis/nasolacrimal duct obstruction that can occur with bacterial infections or malocclusion. Dacryocystitis is usually secondary to dental disease, particularly of the incisors. Conjunctivitis can be associated with primary bacterial infections, environmental irritants, or eyelid abnormalities, or it can be secondary to dacryocystitis or an upper respiratory infection (Harcourt-Brown 2002). Conjunctivitis in combination with nasal discharge is commonly caused by *Pasteurella multocida*. Throughout the examination be mindful of sneezing or evidence of obstructed breathing that may suggest pasteurellosis. Rabbits are fastidious groomers; therefore, the eyes and nose may be dry while the inside of the front paws has evidence of discharge that has been groomed away.

The ears should be examined for crusts or discharge that may indicate bacterial or mite infections. Lop-eared rabbits in particular are prone to accumulations of exudate in the ear canals. The scrotum of mature males and the internal pinnae of the ears are the only hairless areas on a normal rabbit. Alopecia should be noted, but small areas of alopecia can occur normally as part of the molting process in some breeds. Mature females can have a large fold of skin over the throat called a dewlap, which is particularly prone to dermatitis in animals that drink from water bowls or have excessive saliva secondary to dental disease. Older castrated males can develop skin folds as well, so do not confuse these with a female's dewlap.

The hair should be examined for evidence of parasites, especially on the dorsum, such as fleas or

Cheyletiella. If the rabbit spends time outside, look carefully through the hair for signs of maggot infestations or *Cuterebra* larvae. *Cuterebra* larvae cause cystic structure or fistulas, and usually the small breathing hole is the only superficial indication of their presence. Skin turgor is the best assessment for hydration, and rabbits do not tend to develop appreciably sunken eyes. When dehydrated, the skin can become wrinkled and the hairless skin on the scrotum of the males or the inguinal skin in females/neutered males is the best place to assess skin tenting.

Gentle palpation of the trunk should show the vertebrae and ribs to be detectable, but not pronounced. The abdominal organs, such as the stomach, kidneys, and spleen, can be easily palpated. With respect to vital signs, the heart rate (130 to 325 beats per minute) and respiratory rate (thirty to sixty breaths per minute) are more rapid than other more commonly encountered species. Temperature is not usually taken during the exam unless the animal is critical, but the body temperature of the domestic rabbit is significantly higher than that found in other species. The normal range is 101°F to 104°F (Harkness and Wagner 1989). Animal and human tympanic thermometers are sometimes used, but these produce more variable readings and may read lower than rectal temperatures, although implantable microchip transponders correlate well with rectal temperature (Chen and White 2006). Ausculted airway sounds should be short, regular, and rapid in progression with obviously dry bronchovesicular sounds. Auscultation of gut sounds may be helpful if the rabbit has a decreased appetite, but keep in mind that gut sounds are not always present, even in healthy animals.

As described in the restraint section, cradle or lift the animal to look at the ventrum. The chain of mammary glands of intact does should be palpated for evidence of mastitis. Not only lactating or pseudopregnant does are susceptible to this condition, but also non-gravid females with uterine hyperplasia or adenocarcinoma (Mullen, 2000). The urinary and genital openings are located immediately below the anus (Figures 12.7, 12.8). The testes descend at about twelve weeks of age in the buck, but, due to the open inguinal canals, may be present in the scrotum or retracted partly into the abdomen. The testicles can be gently manipulated from the inguinal canals into the scrotum for palpation by applying mild pressure in the cranial inguinal area. Look for any signs of crusts in the genital region suggestive of ectopic ear mites or syphilis. Rabbits have inguinal glands, which are folds of skin by the anal orifice that normally have a brown, foul smelling deposit. At this time, also look at feet for

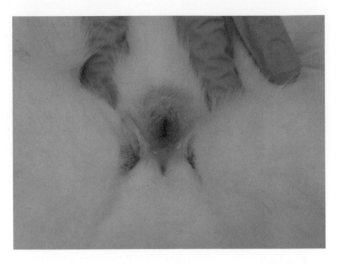

Figure 12.7. Sex determination of a female rabbit. (Courtesy of Dondrae Coble.)

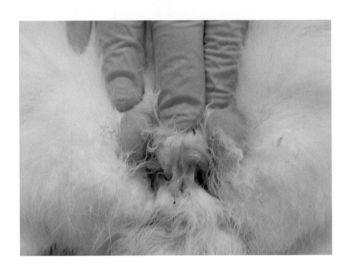

Figure 12.8. Sex determination of a male rabbit. (Courtesy of Dondrae Coble.)

length of nails and evidence of pododermatitis. Obese or mature, potentially arthritic animals may have urine scald or the presence of a fecal impaction in the fur and perineal skin folds because of their inability to groom themselves.

The oral exam is usually the least appreciated part of the physical, so it is often saved for last. A non-invasive indicator of dental disease may be saliva staining around the mouth. The incisors can be easily viewed for length and symmetry by retracting the lips. Dwarf rabbits in particular are prone to congenital incisor malocclusion (Figure 12.9). The molars are difficult to examine without sedation, except in the hands of experienced and skillful individuals. An otoscopic cone, commonly used for examining dog ears,

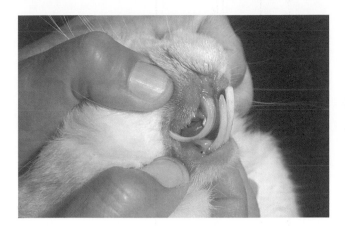

Figure 12.9. Malocclusion.

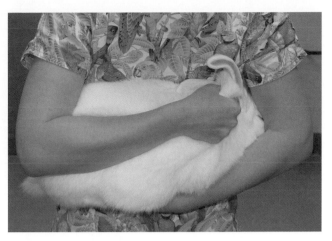

Figure 12.10. Restraint for transport. (Courtesy of Vanessa Lee.)

or stainless steel nasal speculum with an attached light source can be used to aid visualization in an awake and appropriately restrained patient. Although personnel can become quite adept at this technique, it is not a substitute for an anesthetized exam if intraoral disease is suspected.

There are no vaccines or monthly prophylactic dewormers standardly recommended for pet rabbits in the United States. Owners should bring their rabbits for a wellness check when they are first obtained and for annual exams thereafter with blood work and screening tests as recommended by the veterinarian. Fecal exams may also be recommended, especially in new rabbits or those housed outdoors. The best preventive health measure is to spay female rabbits at about five months of age, depending on the breed, to eliminate the potential for uterine adenocarcinoma. Neutering both males and females decreases the chance of aggressive behaviors. Remember that males should be separated from intact females for about four weeks after neutering, because they can maintain fertile sperm during this time period.

RESTRAINT

Rabbits are at significant risk of injury from improper handling due to their general timidity and musculoskeletal conformation. Something seemingly as innocuous as permitting a rabbit to leap from one's arms into a cage may result in a vertebral luxation or fracture, especially of the caudal lumbar vertebrae. Additionally, if rabbits are improperly restrained, they may inflict painful scratches to a handler from the claws on their powerful rear limbs.

The safest way to transport a rabbit is in a small carrier suitable for a cat, but this is not always practi-

cal. One appropriate method of restraint is to grasp the scruff of the neck with one hand and support the body and hindquarters with the other arm. While in this position, use the scruff to tuck the head of the rabbit into the crook of the elbow of the arm, which is used to support the body weight (Figure 12.10). This will conceal the rabbit's eyes and make it less likely to become startled. Never handle a rabbit by the ears or allow its back feet to dangle. When returning a rabbit to its cage, carrier, or setting it on a surface, such as an examination table, do not allow it to leap or hop from the arms because this a common time for back injuries. If possible, place the rabbit down rear end first, especially when placing it back in the cage. This way, the rabbit is less likely to kick from your arms, which predisposes it to back injury. Alternatively, continue to grasp the scruff of the neck with one hand and support the hindquarters with the other and place it on the surface with the rabbit's head concealed in the elbow throughout the process. It will be disinclined to jump and instead often will simply turn away from the handler. Remember that even a seemingly immobilized rabbit can kick its back legs and obtain a back injury.

For examination, rabbits should be placed on an examination table and never left unattended due to the risk that they may jump off of the table. A bathmat or large towel can help the animal have traction and feel secure so that it is less likely to kick while trying to gain its footing. When restraining a rabbit, stand facing the flank of the patient while placing one hand gently over the thorax and the other upon the hindquarters, with the purpose of maintaining the position of the rabbit should it attempt to make a sudden and dangerous jump forward. If alone, the hindquarters can be braced against the restrainer's abdomen. With one hand on the thorax, the other can be used for the physical exam. Most rabbits, providing they are not agitated, will sit quietly in a compact posture, occasionally raising the head to look about or sniff. Examining the ventrum and genital region is very important but can be difficult to do safely, and is easiest done with an assistant. Some animals will become immobile when placed in dorsal recumbency, which can be advantageous for the exam, but realize that some argue that the animal is "freezing" because of undue stress (Harcourt-Brown 2002, Mader 2004). One technique is to cradle the rabbit in one arm with each foot securely held with each hand. Some rabbits may be too large or unruly to safely do this, so they can be lifted, allowing them to rest the rear legs on the table for observation.

An oral exam requires two people if the animal is not sedated. It is easiest to wrap the animal in a towel and tuck the back end into the restrainer's abdomen (Figure 12.11). Place each arm along the flanks to restrain the body, leaving the hands free to restrain the head and neck area. The restrainer should be careful not to occlude nasal passages because rabbits are obligate nasal breathers and will not breathe through their mouth, even though is it open during the exam. Chemical restraint with inhalants (often isoflurane or sevoflurane) or injectable anesthetics are useful for radiography, thorough oral exam, or collection of laboratory samples. For administration of oral medications or assisted feeding, the rabbit can be similarly wrapped in a towel and either restrained on a table or in the restrainer's lap. While holding the head with one hand, use the other to insert the syringe or pill giver into the commissure of the mouth at the proximity of

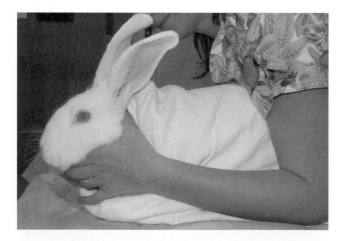

Figure 12.11. *Restraint using a towel. (Courtesy of Vanessa Lee.)*

the diastema and administer the agent. Restraint for specific procedures is further described in "Clinical Techniques."

RADIOLOGY

The common indications for radiography include confirmation or evaluation of dental disease, vertebral luxation, limb fracture, respiratory disease, and gastrointestinal diseases or other intraabdominal disease such as uterine adenocarcinoma. Positioning for radiography is often facilitated by the use of sedation or general anesthesia. Otherwise, it is not possible to stretch the rabbit and properly position it for lateral or ventrodorsal views without risking serious injury to the animal or movement during the exposure, which may degrade the quality of the image. The DV view, rather than the VD, is preferred in rabbits because it minimizes the risk of torso rotation along its sagittal axis, enhances spinosternal alignment, and does not impair respiration. In general, and because of the relatively rapid respiratory rate, short exposure times (0.017 second) are most desirable (Morgan and Silverman 1984).

If the practice encounters a significant number of lapine patients, it is most advantageous to develop a technique chart for the various anatomic structures given the capacity of the X-ray generator, the film speed commonly available, and the qualities of the intensifying screen. An alternative is to use a feline technique chart, but to shorten the exposure time, compensate with increase mA, and, given the less dense bones, reduce the KVp to preserve resolution. Without a custom technique chart, a good starting point for rabbits is to use a focal film distance of 40 inches and an intensifying screen. For a thoracic exposure, use 60 kilovolts, 300 milliamperes, and an exposure time of 0.008 second for an 8-cm thick chest (Morgan and Silverman 1984). For a similarly thick abdomen, increase the exposure time to 0.034 second, reduce the mA to 100, and reduce kVp to 58 (Morgan and Silverman 1984).

Dental radiographs should include lateral, DV/VD, and two lateral oblique skull films; rostral and intraoral views may also be helpful (Capello and Gracis 2005). Obliques are used to thoroughly evaluate the tooth roots, and are obtained by placing the animal laterally and rotating the side of the mouth that is facing upward dorsally approximately 10 to 20 degrees.

Mammography films and high quality dental radiographic units obtain the best images, but standard radiographic machines are adequate for most diagnostic purposes. Be very careful when positioning a

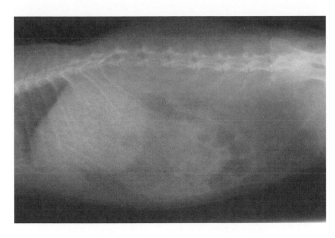

Figure 12.12. Lateral radiograph. (Courtesy of Ryan Cheek.)

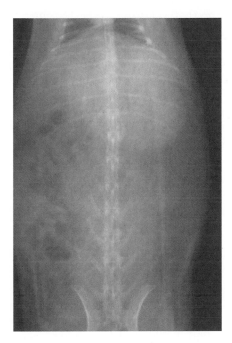

Figure 12.13. VD radiograph. (Courtesy of Ryan Cheek.)

sedated animal for radiographs, especially a rostral view, because flexing the neck can obstruct the airway. The neck should always be extended whenever possible (Figures 12.12, 12.13).

ANESTHESIA

Rabbits may present an anesthetic challenge to veterinarians or veterinary technicians unfamiliar or inexperienced with them. However, because virtually all drugs, equipment, and resources necessary for safe and humane anesthesia of rabbits are available in most

veterinary clinics, this does not need to be the case. The rumors regarding rabbit anesthesia, for example, that rabbits are difficult to intubate, can be overcome by a veterinary technician who is knowledgeable and balances caution with confidence. In any event, it is important to keep the rabbit calm and isolated from perceived threats such as noisy dogs. A frightened rabbit can be so permeated with catecholamines that anesthesia can be adversely affected (Jenkins 2000).

Preanesthesia

As with other companion animals, obtaining a thorough history and a preanesthetic physical examination are important in detecting underlying medical conditions, such as rabbit pasteurellosis, that may complicate anesthesia. For rabbits, the nares should be examined for rhinorrhea suggestive of bacterial respiratory disease, the thorax should be carefully auscultated for evidence of cardiac or pulmonary disease, and the rectal temperature should be determined. Once admitted to the clinic, rabbits should be kept in escape-proof cages in a quiet area.

Rabbits have high metabolic energy requirements and are unable to vomit; therefore, the need for preoperative fasting is a topic of debate. Mature, non-obese rabbits may be fasted for twelve hours to decrease the amount of ingesta in the cecum and stomach that may result in anesthetic overdosages due to overestimating the real body weight. In addition, rabbits breathe primarily by diaphragmatic movement, so fasting to decrease stomach volume will enhance respiration during anesthesia. However, this may have variable effect due to cecotrophy and given that rabbits will drink water to excess when fasted (Chew 1965). Fasting may also cause mild metabolic acidosis or postoperative gastrointestinal disturbances (Flecknell et al. 2007). Short preoperative fasting periods between two hours (Jenkins 2000) and up to four hours (Heard 2004) are recommended. Fasting in excess of twelve hours is contraindicated because it may promote hypoglycemia and more severe metabolic acidosis and, in young rabbits or adults of small breeds, fasting for more than a few hours may induce the same conditions. Fasting of obese, pregnant, or postparturient rabbits is contraindicated because it may predispose to ketosis and liver necrosis.

Preanesthetic medications are not typically used, with the exception of anticholinergic drugs, because single injection anesthesia techniques have been developed that minimize the handling stress and eliminate the discomfort associated with multiple injections. A sedative or tranquilizing preanesthetic agent should be used if, in the opinion of the anesthetist, the animal would benefit from such agents. Serum and tissue atropinesterases found in many rabbits render the anticholinergic agent atropine sulfate of unpredictable efficacy. In the presence of atropinesterase, atropine must be given in high doses (1 to 2 mg/kg) with redosing every ten to fifteen minutes (Lipman et al. 1997). Therefore, 0.01 to 0.02 mg/kg subcutaneous (SC) administration of glycopyrrolate, a quaternary ammonium parasympatholytic, should be administered to reduce salivary and bronchial secretions and prevent vagal bradycardia.

Types of Anesthetic Agents Used in Rabbits

For practical purposes, anesthetics used in rabbits can be divided into injectable and inhalation agents. Historically, injectable drugs have been popularly used for anesthesia of rabbits because they are inexpensive, require no specialized equipment as do inhalant agents, and are typically safe and effective. However, disadvantages attendant to anesthesia by injection include the lack of precision in anesthetic depth control, prolonged recovery time, and physiologic changes such as hypotension, hypoxemia, and acid-base disorders associated with some agents. For uncomplicated procedures involving healthy animals, these drawbacks may not be of consequence, but when used in ill animals, some injectable agents carry unacceptable risk of untoward events.

Ketamine HCl is the anesthetic agent most commonly used in rabbits, but as a sole agent, it does not provide sufficient analgesia or muscle relaxation for surgical purposes at any dose. For minimally invasive diagnostic procedures requiring immobilization (i.e. radiography); surgical procedures of moderate intensity (i.e. wound suturing, tissue biopsies) lasting less than thirty to forty-five minutes; or anesthesia permitting preparation of a surgical field, placement of intravascular catheters, and intubation for subsequent administration of gas anesthetics, ketamine is most commonly combined with xylazine HCl or medetomidine and given intramuscularly as a single injection into the cranial muscles of the thigh or the lumbar epaxial musculature. The ketamine dose is 35 to 45 mg/kg with xylazine (5 mg/kg) given IM or IV, and 15 to 25 mg/kg with medetomidine (0.5 mg/kg) (Flecknell 1996, Flecknell et al. 2007, Orr et al. 2005)) given SQ. It is worth noting that some question the effectiveness of SQ administration, but it continues to be administered commonly in this way. The combination of xylazine and ketamine alone may be unreliable in inducing and/or maintaining an adequate anesthetic plane for an appreciable period of time and will not provide adequate analgesia for procedures with intense sympathetic stimulation such as laparotomy and thoracot-

omy; therefore, the use of ketamine combined with medetomidine is gaining favor. Additionally, ketamine/medetomidine has been shown to maintain cardiovascular parameters more effectively than ketamine/xylazine when administered IM (Difilippo et al. 2004). While there are choices for the route of administration for ketamine/medetomidine, it has been shown that SQ administration causes less discomfort for the patient (Williams and Wyatt 2007).

Anesthesia with either combination is fully induced within ten to fifteen minutes and typically lasts twenty-five to forty-five minutes, but total time unconscious may be up to two hours (Flecknell 1996). When ketamine/xylazine must be used, 0.1 mg/kg butorphanol tartrate or, less ideally, 0.75 mg/kg acepromazine maleate, can be given to augment muscle relaxation and analgesia. These triple combination regimens provide anesthesia lasting sixty to ninety minutes. Acepromazine should be used with caution in ill animals, however, because it may further contribute to hypotension, bradycardia, and respiratory depression. If it is necessary to further extend anesthesia, incremental doses of one half the original ketamine dose can be given.

Telazol (Aveco Co. Inc., Fort Dodge, IA), tiletamine combined with zolazepam, has been shown to be nephrotoxic for rabbits at doses of 7.5 mg/kg and its use is contraindicated (Brammer et al. 1991, Doerning et al. 1992). It is possible that the reported toxic effects of telazol are breed-specific and there are those who advocate its use. This being the case, the authors recommend judicious use of this anesthetic agent, should it be chosen.

If for some reason, such as debilitation or disposition, injection is not feasible, the intranasal route is an option for administration of induction agents (Robertson and Eberhart 1994). The onset of effect is generally rapid (less than three minutes) and the duration of effect may be thirty minutes or more. Midazolam alone for sedation and xylazine-ketamine for low grade anesthesia can be given effectively by this route (Robertson and Eberhart, 1994).

For procedures anticipated to last one to four hours, when inhalation anesthesia is unavailable, and the patient is healthy, administration of a constant infusion of xylazine and ketamine can be done. Over comparable periods of time, anesthesia by controlled infusion provides stable anesthesia with a decreased total anesthetic drug requirement and reduced recovery time as compared to anesthetics given periodically by multiple bolus (Wyatt et al. 1989). Rabbits to be anesthetized by intravenous infusion are first given xylazine (5 mg/kg) and ketamine (35 mg/kg) by intramuscular injection to induce anesthesia. Following placement of an indwelling catheter in a lateral ear vein, as described elsewhere, a constant infusion of xylazine (0.04 mg/kg/minute) and ketamine (0.4 mg/kg/minute) can be given in 0.9% saline. A working infusion solution is made by adding 4 ml of ketamine HCl (100 mg/ml) and 2 ml of xylazine (20 mg/ml) to 94 ml 0.9% saline. The infusion solution is given at a rate of 6 ml/kg/hour to maintain anesthesia. This method of anesthesia should be done with an infusion pump or precisely controlled use of a mini-drip (60 drops/ml) and vital signs should be monitored closely.

The use of inhalation anesthesia is feasible in rabbits and often preferred for procedures lasting two or more hours because it is precise, rapidly adjustable, and safe and effective. In addition, postoperative recovery is more rapid and less complicated than with injectable anesthetics. An Ayre's T-piece or other non-rebreathing circuit is most appropriate for rabbit inhalational anesthesia (Flecknell 1996). For anesthetic induction, an intravenous injection of propofol (1.5 mg/kg slowly to effect) or an SC or IM injection of xylazine and ketamine are preferred.

The use of ultra-short-acting thiobarbiturates is not recommended due to their narrow margin of safety, slow elimination in obese animals, and resultant respiratory depression or fatal apnea that can occur if intubation is not performed in a timely manner. Induction using a mask or induction chamber is not recommended because of the high incidence of struggling, distress vocalization, and breath-holding (Flecknell 1996, Hedenqvist et al. 2001). This technique is commonly used in practice, however, and can be done without harm to the patient with proper restraint (Figure 12.14).

The anatomy of the rabbit oropharynx makes endotracheal intubation challenging (Tran et al. 2001). The oral cavity is long and narrow, the mandible has a limited range of abduction, and entry into the oral cavity is partially occluded by the large incisors and cheek teeth. The tongue protrudes dorsally; the epiglottis is relatively large, U-shaped, soft, and flexible; and the larynx slopes ventrally. Just beyond the epiglottis is a deep sagittal niche, bordered on both sagittal recesses by the friable hamuli epiglotti which are easily damaged. Additionally, laryngeal tone and the propensity to laryngospasm are high. All of these factors combine to obscure visualization and access to the glottis and make endotracheal intubation of the rabbit challenging.

These challenging anatomic features aside, rabbits can be reliably and easily intubated by an experienced

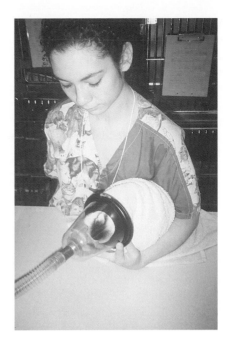

Figure 12.14. Inhalation anesthesia using a face mask.

technician. Prior to intubation, diazepam or midazolam can be given IV to effect if additional relaxation is necessary. Intubation should be done with a transparent, cuffed (e.g. Murphy), 14-cm long, 3- to 4-mm internal diameter endotracheal (ET) tube for rabbits weighing 3 to 6 kg or an uncuffed 1- to 2.5-mm endotracheal tube for rabbits weighing less than 3 kg. The key to intubation by direct visualization is to bring the mouth, larynx, and trachea into linear alignment by positioning the rabbit in dorsal recumbency and hyperextending the head. One way this can be achieved is by placing a rolled towel under the cervical spine or permitting the head to overhang a table edge. The tongue should be retracted laterally through one of the diastema, the bilateral spaces between the incisors and premolars, to prevent laceration on the incisors and an inverted laryngoscope with a #1 Miller blade should be inserted into the contralateral diastema and maintained either between the incisors in alignment with the midline or lateral to the incisors at a slight angle to the sagittal plane of the body. Gentle pressure should be directed ventrally with the blade tip while slight rostrodorsal traction is placed on the head until the epiglottis and arytenoid cartilages are seen.

To assist in intubation a metal dowel or cotton-tipped applicator used as a stylet to prevent bending of the tube can be employed. If a 3-mm or larger internal diameter ET tube is used, intubation can be done using the polypropylene guide technique (Gilroy

1981). A 56-cm, 8 French polypropylene catheter should be passed through the endotracheal tube lumen from the connector to the distal end until the blunt catheter tip extends 15 to 20 cm past the bevel. Under direct visualization using a laryngoscope, the tip of the catheter should be cautiously advanced through the diastema, past the vocal folds, and into the trachea. Once the guide is in the trachea, the laryngoscope can be removed and the ET tube advanced as a sheath over the stationary catheter into the trachea. Following intubation, the stylet or guide should be immediately removed and the ET tube secured. Alternative intubation aids are described in the literature, including otoscopes (Heard 2004) as well as endoscopes (Tran et al. 2001).

If preferred, intubation can be performed blindly. After induction, the rabbit should be placed in sternal recumbency with the head extended dorsally such that the alignment of mouth, larynx, and trachea is perpendicular to the table surface. An endotracheal tube should then be advanced to the proximal aspect of the larynx. This can be confirmed by visualizing the fogging of the tube interior with every exhalation and listening for respiratory sounds through the endotracheal tube. The position of the tube should be adjusted until the sounds are at maximal intensity. At this point, the endotracheal tube should be gently advanced into the trachea. If breaths are shallow, it is sometimes helpful to have an assistant administer gentle chest compressions and to advance the tube timed with the release of a compression (inhalation). A cough reflex often confirms correct insertion. A capnograph can also help to confirm proximity of the tube tip at the oropharynx. This blind technique carries a risk of trauma and should be abandoned in favor of direct observation if intubation is not successful after several gentle attempts.

Regardless of the intubation technique, intubation should never be forced, because the trachea, tracheal bifurcation, and tissues of the oropharynx are easily damaged and the vagus nerve may be stimulated. Correct placement in the trachea should be further confirmed by visualizing the respiration-associated condensation of water vapor on the internal surface of the endotracheal tube, by auscultation in conjunction with manual respiration using an Ambu bag, or capnography. Mechanical ventilation should not be done until intubation is confirmed, because overzealous ventilation into the stomach can lead to acute dilatation and rupture.

There is no consensus on the use of topical anesthetics to enhance intubation. While spraying of the pharynx, larynx, and trachea will reduce the risk of laryngospasm and enhance passage of the tube, it also suppresses the convenient forward motion of the glottis during swallowing that may enhance intubation. If a topical anesthetic is desired, lidocaine 10% oral spray should be judiciously misted on the glottis to prevent laryngospasm and facilitate intubation. Topical benzocaine should not be used, because it may cause methemoglobinemia.

An alternative to endotracheal intubation to maintain a patent airway during inhalation anesthesia is the use of a laryngeal mask airway (LMA). The principle advantage that the LMA can offer over an ET tube is that it requires less technical skill to place, which is highly beneficial for those with little experience or in cases of emergency. LMAs have been used in human pediatric patients for many years and their use in rabbits has been recently described (Kazakos et al. 2007, Smith et al. 2004). These reports indicate that LMAs size 1 to 1.5 perform the best. One problem with the use of LMAs is the possible inability to completely protect the airway from gastric contents; however, in a species with the inability to vomit such as the rabbit, this should not be a concern.

Once intubated, the rabbit should be connected to a gas anesthesia machine with a closed breathing circuit for ventilation with a mechanical respirator at a rate of thirty to forty breaths per minute and a tidal volume of 11 to 15 ml/kg. The inspiration-to-expiration ratio should be 1:2 or 1:3 and airway pressures should not be permitted to exceed 20 cm H$_2$O because barotrauma will occur at higher pressure (Reuter et al. 2005). Gas flow rate of 200 ml/kg is sufficient (Heard 2004). If mechanical ventilation is not available, spontaneous ventilation should be accommodated with a semi-closed pediatric breathing circuit. Spontaneous respirations should be regular and deep and occur at a rate of fifteen or more breaths per minute. The anesthetist should be cognizant of the risk of apnea in this circumstance and be prepared to evaluate the depth of anesthesia and assist ventilations.

Anesthesia should be maintained with 2% to 3% isoflurane in 100% oxygen. This requirement for relatively high isoflurane concentration in rabbits is due partly to their tendency to take shallow breaths compared to other species, although intubation and mechanical ventilation can reduce the requirement. Although not routinely done because combination anesthetic regimens can allow for the reduction of gas concentration needed to maintain anesthesia, yohimbine or atipamezole can be given shortly after gas anesthesia is commenced to reverse the hypotensive effects of xylazine or medetomidine if those agents were used at induction.

Perioperative Considerations

While anesthetized, rabbits should have bland oph-thalmic ointment placed in the eyes to prevent exposure keratitis. The maintenance of normothermia from induction through recovery is very important and can be accomplished through the use of circulating water blankets such as the Gaymar-T (Gaymar, Orchard Park, NY) or hot air blankets such as the Bair Hugger (Arizant Healthcare, Eden Prairie, MN)(Sikoski, Young, and Lockard 2007). An intravenous catheter should be placed for administration of parenteral fluids. Because fasting generally induces mild metabolic acidosis, warmed lactated Ringer's solution, providing the kidneys are functioning normally, or half-strength saline-dextrose solutions with sodium bicarbonate supplementation are most ideal for fluid administration in surgery. These should be given at a rate of 10 to 20 ml/kg/hour via a 60-drop/ml intravenous fluid administration set. If it is desirable to gain arterial access for blood-gas analysis or blood pressure monitoring, a 22-gauge catheter can be placed in the central auricular artery and secured with a heparin-lock (for blood gases) or connected to a transducer (for continuous arterial pressure monitoring).

Anesthesia Monitoring

Because controlled ventilation may increase mean intra-thoracic pressure, decrease venous return, compromise cardiac output, and cause hypotension, blood and airway pressure should be monitored. The systolic/diastolic arterial pressure of an anesthetized rabbit is approximately 95/75 (Huerkamp 1995). As a rule, arterial pressures should not be permitted to decrease below 80/60. Intubated animals undergoing lengthy procedures should have cuffed tubes deflated, rotated, and reinflated hourly because there is evidence suggesting injury can occur during prolonged procedures (Phaneuf et al. 2006), while those that are not intubated should be positioned to maintain an open airway. Alterations in heart rate and blood pressure are the most reliable indicators of anesthetic depth with changes of 20% or more from baseline usually mandating modifications in management to ensure an adequate plane of anesthesia. The monitoring of heart rate and rhythm can be done with an esophageal stethoscope or electrocardiography. In addition to direct blood pressure monitoring via the central auricular artery, indirect monitoring can be attempted with cuffs placed on a limb. Capnography (end tidal CO_2 determination), blood-gas analysis, and pulse oximetry are useful in evaluating the adequacy of ventilation. Ventilation-perfusion efficiency can also be assessed through observation of mucous membrane color and capillary refill time.

Where sophisticated cardiovascular monitoring is not practical, reflex assessment is the most accurate determinant of adequate anesthesia depth. Traditional reflexes used in the monitoring of rabbit anesthesia include righting, palpebral, corneal, pedal withdrawal, and pinna reflex. The pinna reflex is the most accurate measure of depth of anesthesia followed by pedal withdrawal, corneal, and palpebral reflexes, in that order. Corneal reflex may be preserved until very deep levels of anesthesia are reached. Muscle tone, jaw tone, and purposeful movements in response to surgical stimuli may also be used as indicators of anesthesia depth. When reflex assessment is used as the sole determinant of anesthetic depth, more than one reflex should be monitored to ensure adequate anesthesia. At a minimum, anesthetic depth should be monitored temporally by constantly assessing reflexes, cardiac rate and rhythm, and respiratory rate.

Analgesia

Rabbits experiencing pain often exhibit changes in appetite, reduced grooming, reduced activity, and teeth grinding (bruxism), and monitoring for such behavior can help the technician effectively manage pain (Kohn et al. 2007). As a general rule, analgesics should be first administered before the animal is fully recovered from anesthesia, but stable, and should be continued for the next forty-eight to seventy-two hours. Rabbits may self-mutilate areas that are painful or irritating and if self-mutilation is a concern, a 12-inch Elizabethan collar can be used in conjunction with administration of analgesics. Be aware that rabbits typically tolerate these collars very poorly and long-term maintenance will prevent cecotrophy, which could lead to B vitamin and other nutritional deficiencies.

There are essentially two classes of drugs available for pain management, nonsteroidal anti-inflammatory drugs (NSAID) and opioids. Often, analgesia is most effectively provided by using these agents in combination. NSAIDs inhibit the production of chemical mediators such as prostaglandins that activate peripheral nociceptors and are sufficiently potent to treat musculoskeletal, incisional, and acute, mild visceral pain. There are several effective NSAIDs from which to choose, but the authors prefer newer, more specific inhibitors of cyclooxygenase 2 activity such as meloxicam, a drug which can be given orally or injected subcutaneously once per day at 0.3 or 0.2 mg/kg respectively. These newer NSAIDs are often as effective as some opioids for the control of pain.

Opioid agents act by binding to specific receptors in different parts of the nervous system. Those most commonly used are buprenorphine, butorphanol, fentanyl, morphine, meperidine, and oxymorphone; all are controlled substances. Opioids are typically used in their injectable form, but fentanyl is also available as a dermal patch, which is advantageous because it abrogates the need to handle the patient for drug administration. A 25 ug/hour fentanyl patch can be used and should be applied before or at the time of the painful procedure (Foley et al. 2001). Because twenty-four hours is required for dermal fentanyl to reach therapeutic levels, administration of an additional agent such as an NSAID during that time period and beyond if necessary should be considered.

Opioid agonist-antagonists, such as butorphanol, or buprenorphine, have relatively long half-lives and offer the advantage of attenuating or ablating visceral pain while minimizing the undesirable respiratory and cardiovascular side effects compared to morphine and meperidine. Buprenorphine can be given by injection every six to twelve hours to rabbits (0.01 to 0.05 mg/kg IM, SC). Anecdotally, the authors have observed frequent cases of postoperative anorexia and ileus in rabbits given intensive treatment with buprenorphine injections. In these cases, appetite return was associated with discontinuance of analgesic treatment. Buprenorphine given at the high range of recommended levels in rats has been shown to cause anorexia and weight loss (Jablonski et al. 2001). Others have also questioned the efficacy of buprenorphine in rabbits (Wixson 1994).

Immediate Post-anesthetic Care

Following completion of surgery under inhalation anesthesia, recovery is rapid and rabbits typically are conscious and regain the righting reflex within twenty to thirty minutes. The most likely causes of delayed or complicated recovery from general anesthesia are hypothermia and anesthetic overdosage followed by complications related to lengthy procedures or a presenting medical condition such as hypoglycemia and dehydration. Anesthetic agents impair central and peripheral thermoregulatory mechanisms and rabbits are prone to radiative and conductive heat losses because of their relatively high body surface area to body weight ratio. Because the pharmacokinetics of anesthetic metabolism are partially temperature dependent, maintaining body temperature is critical to recovery from anesthesia. Ideally, recovering animals should be kept in an escape-proof incubator on a clean, dry towel or blanket. The use of an incubator permits careful control of the ambient temperature and enables supplemental oxygen administration. Recovery should not be done on metal flooring or in suspended wire cages because heat loss will be accelerated.

If an incubator is not available, supplemental heating can be provided with a water-circulated heating pad or a heat lamp judiciously placed outside of the cage. It is important to remember that rabbits are gnawing species that, left unattended following recovery, may mutilate heating pads or wiring. The ambient temperature in the recovery area should be 29°C to 32°C. The temperature of the animal and the recovery area should be monitored as regularly as for dogs and cats.

Animals slow to recover from anesthesia should be turned every thirty to sixty minutes to prevent hypostatic lung congestion and should be given warmed, parenteral fluids to compensate for metabolic needs and for losses during surgery. Extubation should be done only when chewing begins or coughing is elicited. If not done beforehand, yohimbine or atipamezole can be given to reverse the effects of xylazine and medetomidine. Where reversal is not possible, respiratory depression can be treated with 2 to 5 mg/kg doxapram given SC or IV every fifteen minutes.

COMMON SURGICAL PROCEDURES

The duties of a veterinary technician supporting a surgical procedure for a rabbit are identical to those duties for other species, with the focus on preoperative preparation of the surgical patient and intraoperative support of the procedure, including anesthesia management. The surgeon and operating room attendants should prepare and dress as for procedures done on other pet species. Sterile instruments and draping should be used. When post-op care is expected to be extensive, a nasogastric tube can be placed to permit feeding of liquid diets and evacuation of any gastric gas (Mullen 2000). Rabbits with a history of pasteurellosis should be started on a preoperative course of antibiotics for a duration (days) sufficient to suppress any clinical manifestations or prevent septicemia (one to two hours pre-operatively IV).

As would be customary in any species, the fur at the surgical site should be clipped and the skin should be decontaminated with alcohol and disinfectants. Rabbits have thick hair coats and thin skin, which renders clipping of the hair from a surgical site more time-consuming and puts a premium on clipper blade sharpness. It is critical that sharp, spare blades be available and that all clipper blades be properly cleaned and restored after use. The rabbit skin easily lacerates or tears in cases in which clipping is done hurriedly or carelessly or where dull clipper blades are used. The technician should concentrate on keeping the skin taut in front of the clipper blade and the head of the blade flat against the skin. The best skin preparation comes from using a combination of no. 10 and no. 40 blades to prepare the skin. This is an area where patience and careful attention to detail are most important. In fact, gentle handling of the skin perioperatively and all tissues intraoperatively is critical in reducing the incidence of postoperative automutilation of incisions for which rabbits are notorious. Some people choose to wear a mask while shaving a rabbit to preclude floating hair from entering their mouth or nose.

The surgical procedures most commonly performed in rabbits include spay, castration, drainage of abscesses, cutaneous mass excision, and exploratory laparotomy. Enucleation, perineal dermatoplasty in cases of relentless urine scald, cystotomy, large bowel, and renal surgical procedures have also been described in rabbits (Mullen 2000, Jenkins 2004). Castration and ovariohysterectomy (OVH) are often done for the same reasons that these procedures are done in dogs and cats. Castration should be recommended to clients as a measure for bucks housed indoors to prevent urine spraying and mounting, reduce aggression toward other rabbits and owners, and eliminate the risk of testicular cancer. OVH is recommended as a preventive measure for group-housing and uterine diseases such as uterine adenocarcinoma. Both procedures are performed with the patient in dorsal recumbency. The surgical approaches for these two procedures are similar to those used for dogs and cats, with castration commonly done by the scrotal approach (Jenkins 2000), prescrotal approach, or abdominal midline incisions for crytorchidism (Swindle and Shealy 1996). The OVH requires a standard, mid-line abdominal approach, and surgical site preparation should reflect this. It is important to express the urinary bladder during preparation for an OVH to avoid complications during surgery.

A variety of other surgical procedures can be safely performed in rabbits, and the preparation of the surgical site varies by location and surgeon preferences. Cystotomy is indicated for urolithiasis. Although the bladder wall is thin, which may be discouraging to some surgeons, it holds suture well (Mullen 2000) and can be closed in a single layer (Swindle and Shealy 1996). Most rabbits with urolithiasis are overweight and probably overconsuming calcium (Mullen 2000); therefore, the post-operative instructions given to the owner should include an exhortation to limit feed and not provide mineral supplementation. Exploratory laparotomy is required in cases of gastrointestinal obstruction from trichobezoars, other foreign bodies, or space-occupying lesions. Enucleation may be necessary for ocular trauma, severe buphthalmia, or retrobulbar abscess. The retrobulbar venous sinus is extensive and there is a risk of severe and difficult-to-control hemorrhage (Mullen 2000). It is important to have considerable sterile methylcellulose on hand to pack the ocular defect. Likewise, bulla osteotomy for drainage of middle ear infections, such as for pasteurellosis, is fraught with risks of post-operative pain and drainage complications (Swindle and Shealy 1996) and is a procedure probably best referred to a specialty surgical practice.

Absorbable polymer suture materials, such as monofilament polyglyconate, are preferred by many for internal use, due to their minimally reactive nature. Because they are not exposed and are less likely to be chewed, subcuticular sutures are preferred for skin closure. Generally, sutures in sizes appropriate for cats (3-0, 4-0, and 5-0) are most appropriate for rabbits. Cyanoacrylate tissue adhesives also provide satisfactory closure, as long as they are used in clean, dry, incisions. Wound clips are a viable alternative and are advocated by some for skin closure. Regardless of which material is used for skin closure, it is important to keep in mind the proclivity of rabbits for chewing at their wound closure materials and monitor animals closely during the wound healing period.

Following acute recovery from anesthesia, the most reliable indicator of post-operative well-being, including the effectiveness of analgesia, is the daily assessment of body weight and food and water consumption. Because rabbits are prone to hypoglycemia because of high metabolic rates and, in juvenile animals, limited fat reserves, a nutritious pelleted diet should be provided as soon after surgery as feasible. Inappetant animals can be offered supplements such as hay, other supplements, or treats as described under "Nutrition," or herbivore liquid dietary products. In some cases, the stress associated with surgery will cause pH changes in the cecum that result in alterations of commensal and fermentative bacteria. When chronic anorexia and ileus that is nonresponsive to treatments described above is the result, specific bacteriotherapy, as described in the "Critical Care" section, may be useful in recolonizing the gastrointestinal tract.

PARASITOLOGY

The most important diagnostic tools used in the diagnosis of parasitism in rabbits are essentially the same as for dogs and cats. These comprise the fecal floatation examination, fur exam, skin scraping, and examination of the ear canals. With respect to skin scrapings, bear in mind that the skin of rabbits is thin relative to dogs and cats and may lacerate easily. The examination of the ear canals should be done using an otoscope. This is sufficient in many cases to diagnose aural acariasis caused by *Psoroptes cuniculi*. The mites are easily seen with low magnification crawling in the beam of light emitted from the otoscope. The diagnosis can be confirmed, and mites demonstrated for the owner, by swabbing exudate from the canal with a cotton-tipped applicator and mineral oil and examining it under a microscope. For rabbits housed outdoors, one important consideration is that flies are attracted to rabbit droppings and owners may confuse the recently hatched fly larvae with parasites.

URINALYSIS

The urine pH ranges from 6 to 8.2 with alkaline urine (pH > 8) generally associated with good health and acidic pH with anorexia or fasting. The normal range of urine specific gravity is 1.003 to 1.036 with 1.015 representing the normal mean in a healthy population of rabbits (McLaughlin and Fish 1994). The urine typically is turbid due to calcium carbonate excretion and is also pigmented ranging from light yellow to orange to various combinations of red with brown. Certain porphyrin pigments in the urine may cause a reddish appearance and elicit concerns of hematuria (Garibaldi et al. 1987). Consequently, any suspected cases of hematuria in the rabbit should be confirmed by complete urinalysis. The most likely causes of hematuria are from uterine adenocarcinoma, uterine polyps, uterine hyperplasia, abortion, urolithiasisis, cystitis, septicemia, DIC, and certain renal diseases.

The urine should be free of protein, casts, blood, glucose, ketones, and bilirubin. An occasional white blood cell per high-powered field in an examination of the sediment is within the realm of normal. The urine output ranges from 20 to 350 ml/kg/day and is influenced by many factors related to the diet, animal, and environment (McLaughlin and Fish 1994). Ammonium magnesium phosphate (struvite) and calcium carbonate are the two most common uroliths of rabbits (Bergdall and Dysko 1994). Struvite uroliths are usually the consequence of urinary tract infection. Calcium carbonate uroliths may precipitate and form uroliths when the urinary pH exceeds 8.5 (Leck 1988). Infection, inadequate water intake, genetic predisposition, metabolic disturbances, and nutritional imbalances enhance the development of urolithiasis.

CLINICAL TECHNIQUES

Blood Collection

Blood is most often obtained from the ear arteries or veins or jugular or saphenous vein, and may also be collected from the cephalic (Figures 12.15, 12.16). Blood collection from the ear vessels carries a risk of hematoma or bruising that may be unacceptable to an owner. It also has a small risk of thrombosis and subsequent sloughing of the skin, which is more likely in breeds with small ears or if the artery is used (Mader 2004, Harcourt-Brown 2002). The preferred location depends on the techniques developed by the phlebotomist. Rabbit blood can clot quickly, so heparinizing the syringe and needle may be helpful.

The auricular artery is central, while the veins are found along the margins of the ear (Color Plate 12.2). The hair may be shaved and a warm towel may be applied to help dilate the vessel. A topical anesthetic, such as EMLA cream or lidocaine cream, can be used in an awake animal to reduce head shaking. These agents may reduce the restraint that is required, but keep in mind the time it takes for the creams to have an effect (Flecknell et al. 1990). The size of the needle depends on the size of the vessel, and generally a 22- to 27-gauge needle is used. The needle is inserted into the vessel and if the vessel is large enough may be aspirated with a syringe. For small breeds, suction from a syringe may collapse the vessel and so blood can be collected as it drips from the needle hub. Upon removal of the needle, it is necessary to apply pressure for three to five minutes if using the artery and monitor thereafter for ten to fifteen minutes recrudescence of bleeding; less time may be needed if using a vein.

The lateral saphenous is easily accessible in an appropriately restrained rabbit. The restrainer should hold the animal wrapped in a towel in his lap and hold off the back leg just below the stifle. The vein is seen where it crosses from medial to lateral, usually in the area of the middle third of the lateral tibia. Sometimes the vessel can be visualized with just alcohol, but often shaving is required. A butterfly catheter attached to a syringe is often the easiest way to obtain blood.

The jugular can be used in some cooperative awake patients, but this technique may require sedation. If the animal is sedated, place it in dorsal recumbency and shave the neck area. If the animal is awake, it can be restrained in the same way as a cat for jugular venipuncture. The rabbit is wrapped in a towel and held at the edge of the table. One hand is used to hold the head up and the other restrains the front legs. Venipuncture from the cephalic is difficult, particularly in small breeds.

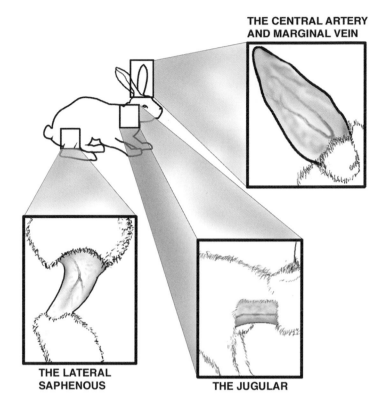

THE CENTRAL ARTERY
AND MARGINAL VEIN

THE LATERAL
SAPHENOUS

THE JUGULAR

Figure 12.15. Venipuncture sites.

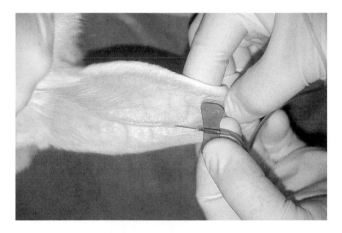

Figure 12.16. Blood sampling using the central auricular artery with a butterfly catheter. (Courtesy of Ryan Cheek.)

Placing a Catheter

The marginal ear veins and cephalic are the easiest and most frequently used to place an intravenous catheter. As with venipuncture, catheterization of the ear vessels carries a small risk of necrosis, so the cephalic is often used (Mader 2004, Harcourt-Brown 2002). The saphenous can also be used for venous access, and the central ear artery can be used if arterial access is needed

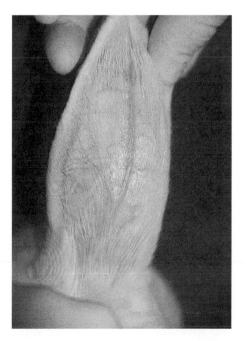

Plate 12.2. Marginal lateral ear vein on the left and the prominent central auricular artery. (Photo courtesy of Ryan Cheek.) (See also color plates)

for direct blood pressure measurement or periodic blood-gas analysis in surgery. For any catheter, an E-collar may be used to prevent the animal removing it, but should be avoided in cooperative animals. E-collars can be stressful and prevent the animal from engaging in cecotrophy, so they are not ideal for long-term use.

The principles of preparation are the same as for other species, but the animal may require sedation for vasodilation and to enhance cooperation. As with venipuncture, EMLA cream may facilitate placement of the catheter in an awake patient. A 24-gauge catheter is appropriate for most rabbits, but a 22-gauge may be used in large vessels of some large rabbits. Occlude the vessel by compressing proximal to the location of the catheter. After puncture of the vessel wall, the catheter should be advanced over the stylet and into the vessel lumen. The thin walls of the vessel make it easy to visualize the threading of the catheter into the lumen of the vein to the hub. Due to the relative small volume of blood in the vein and the low venous blood pressure, it is unlikely to obtain a backflow of blood into the catheter flange or hub. If in doubt, a small quantity of saline can be injected via the catheter for observation of the telltale blanching of the vessel with infused fluid. For the ear, a roll of four to five gauze 4 × 4 sponges should be placed in the concave pinna and then the catheter secured using tape in a butterfly application and a circumferential wrap of tape over the roll of gauze in the ear. The IV line should also be secured with a circumferential wrap of tape. The principles of fluid therapy are identical to those for other species. See Figure 12.17 for illustrations relating to placing an IV catheter.

Intraosseous infusion is indicated when intravenous access is not possible or difficult and a delay in access may affect survival. The common locations for catheterization are the humerus, tibial crest, and femur. A 20- to 22-gauge spinal needle that is about half the length of the bone is appropriate for most situations. If a spinal needle is not available, use an appropriately sized hypodermic needle. If the hypodermic needle plugs, a thinner, sterile Kirschner wire can be used as a plunger to push bone cortex from the needle lumen (Anderson 1995). The procedure is done using a similar approach and equipment as for cats and can be done in kits as small as 200 grams, although potential risk to active growth plates must be considered in juvenile animals (Bielski et al. 1993, Harcourt-Brown 2002).

Preparation of the area should follow strict aseptic technique because of the risk of osteomyelitis, and if it is necessary in an emergency situation in a conscious

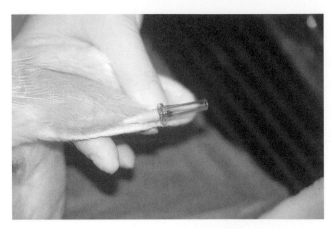

A

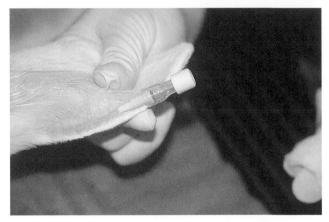

B

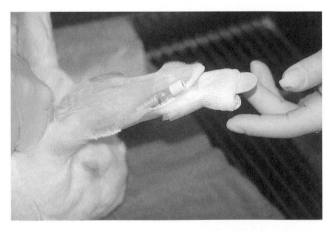

C

Figure 12.17. (A) Initial insertion of the catheter in the vein; note the "flash." (B) The catheter is seated into the vein and the cap has been applied. (C) A tongue depressor was added for additional support.

animal, a local anesthetic such as lidocaine can be used. The humerus may be the easiest location for placement, where the needle is inserted through the greater trochanter (Harcourt-Brown 2002). For the tibial crest, the needle should be inserted at the medial aspect of the proximal tibia of the flexed stifle at an angle of about 30 degrees (Anderson 1995, Bielski et al. 1993, Otto and Crowe 1992). Because of the curved cortex of the tibia, it may be difficult to keep the needle in the medullary cavity and instead go into the cortex. The femur can be difficult because of the well developed trochanteric fossa, and the catheter often needs to pass through three layers of cortical bone. Although placement of the catheter may be more difficult in the rear leg, some rabbits may be less inclined to disturb a catheter that is not by the face (Jenkins 2004).

For any location, the needle should be advanced in a distal direction away from the physis until there is a dramatic reduction of resistance, indicating penetration of the marrow cavity, and one aspirates slightly to obtain marrow to confirm that the needle is in the desired location. Once in the marrow cavity at the desired depth, the needle should be sutured to the skin and protected and further immobilized with a sterile wrap and bulky bandage. Any drug, agent, or fluid that can be safely given intravenously can be given by the intraosseous route. The maximal rate of infusion is about 10 ml/minute by this route (Anderson 1995).

Bandaging and Wound Care
The principles of bandaging and wound care are essentially the same for rabbits as they are for other species. Ulcerative pododermatitis is one of the most frequent indications for bandages, and these bandages are generally well-tolerated by the rabbits being treated. Bandages of the feet should relieve pressure on the affected area, such as with a doughnut bandage. The bandages should extend above the hock and be secured at the proximal aspect with loosely wrapped adhesive tape extending from the bandage to the fur, so that the bandage is not kicked off.

Rabbit skin is very thin, so bandages must be changed frequently and carefully observed for signs of urine contamination, irritation, constriction, or slippage. Tight or contaminated bandages can themselves cause dermatitis and even tear the skin. As opposed to dogs, dermatitis should not be treated with ointments containing steroids because rabbits are particularly sensitive to their side effects, including adrenocortical suppression, delayed wound healing, and immunosuppression (Graham 2004). If topical antibiotics are used, make sure the animals cannot ingest the ointment because of their sensitivity to some antibiotics.

Urine Collection
Urine may be collected from rabbits into a clean cage pan, by catheterization as for cats, by cystocentesis, or from anesthetized rabbits by expression. The bladder wall is thin and susceptible to trauma or puncture; therefore, cystocentesis, manual expression, or catheterization should be done with care. If doing cystocentesis, use a small needle appropriate for the patient (23 to 25 gauge).

Administration of Medication

Intravenous Injection
The marginal ear veins are the easiest to access for IV injection, but the cephalic and saphenous can also be used. The technique is the same as described for venipuncture. Typically volumes of up to 5 ml can be given by bolus by this route (Flecknell 1987). Be careful not to inject into the central auricular artery, which may be fatal (O'Malley 2005).

Per Os
Rabbits may accept oral medications when mixed with small amounts of preferred food items, such as bananas or bread. Rabbits can be difficult to pill, but may accept palatable medications when placed through the diastema as far back in the mouth as possible. A pill "gun," as used in cats, may be useful for this procedure. Alternatively, the pill should be crushed and given in suspension. Suspensions or liquid medications may be eaten from the syringe if palatable, and rabbits usually like sweet formulations such as juice or fruit baby foods. Otherwise, the rabbit can be restrained as previously described and volumes should be limited to less than about 5 ml of liquid. In some cases it may be tempting to give drugs via the drinking water; however, this is imprecise. Depending on their level of consumption, the palatability of the liquid, and stability of the drug, animals may be overdosed or underdosed.

Subcutaneous Injection
The methodology for a subcutaneous injection is the same as for other species with the interscapular region preferred. A 21- to 25-gauge needle should be inserted under the lifted loose skin over the scapulae and parallel with the underlying muscle. Volumes of 10 to 20 ml/kg can be given by this route (Harcourt-Brown 2002).

Intraperitoneal Injection
This route is rarely used in rabbits, but should be considered in neonates or moribund, hypothermic animals in which vasoconstriction may be pronounced and there is a need to rapidly attempt fluid therapy or

administer medications. For intraperitoneal injection, the rabbit ideally should be held on its back with the head slightly lower than the hindquarters to allow the stomach and intestines to fall cranially. However, if dorsal recumbency is at all resisted, the animal can be positioned on its side or in ventral recumbency. A second individual should insert a 21- to 25-gauge needle at a 45 degree angle through the skin and abdominal wall slightly to the right and just caudal to the umbilicus. Aspirate before injecting to reduce the chance of injecting into an organ. For fluid therapy or injection of a volume of material in excess of a few milliliters and to prevent accidental laceration of the internal organs, a catheter can be inserted and the stylet immediately removed after puncture of the abdominal wall. Volumes of up to 100 ml of warmed fluids can be given to a 4- to 5-kg rabbit by the IP route (Flecknell 1987).

Intramuscular Injection

The restraint for injection is similar to that for examination, remembering to always hold the hindquarters and keep the rabbit from jumping forward with the other hand. If alone, the animal should be held with the flank against the restrainer's side/abdomen and the head tucked into the elbow of the dominant arm, with the dominant arm wrapped around the exposed flank of the animal and the hand curled around and restraining the hindquarters. The free hand is then used for the injection. Fractious rabbits may need two people for injection or to be wrapped in a towel. Lumbar muscles (cranial to the pelvis) or the cranial aspects of the rear leg (quadriceps) are the sites of choice to avoid damage to the sciatic nerve (Mader 2004). Aspirate to confirm that blood is not obtained before injecting. Any volume greater than 0.5 ml/kg should be divided and given in two sites.

Teeth Trimming

Conventional dog nail trimmers should not be used for trimming the incisors because of the risk of complications, including longitudinal fissures, periodontal abscesses, and damage to the germinal tissue (Gorrel 1996, Malley 1996). Nail trimmers can also leave sharp edges that may lacerate the tongue, cheek, or lips. Ideally, the teeth should be reduced using high speed dental equipment with a water-cooling system (Capello and Gracis 2005). Alternatively, a Dremel® tool (Dremel, Racine, WI) can be used, but these have a lower speed and increased torque that increases the chance of thermal damage to tissues. These procedures generally require sedation, although rarely veterinary personnel may be able trim the incisors in a conscious

animal. This should be done, however, with great caution and the obvious consent of the owner. Specialized equipment is available that significantly aids rodent and rabbit dentistry (Cappello and Gracis 2005), but readily available items can also be useful, such as a tongue depressor or the barrel of a syringe through the diastema to serve as a gag to open the mouth slightly and as a backstop when trimming the incisors. Extraction is also an option for severely affected teeth, but is much more difficult for cheek teeth than incisors. Rabbits can actually do very well with all of their incisors extracted by using their lips for prehension. In cases of malocclusion, teeth trimming may need to be repeated every six to eight weeks for the lifetime of the animal (Swindle and Shealy 1996).

Nail Trimming

Nail trimming can be done with any conventional nail trimmer used for dogs or cats. The quick is generally easy to visualize, and overly aggressive trimming causing bleeding should be managed as for dogs and cats. Owners can be taught to trim the nails of their pets because nails may grow long with rapidity in sedentary animals. Similar to dogs, declawing should not be done in rabbits unless medically necessary for a particular digit. Unlike cats, rabbits use the last phalanx for weight bearing and traction, and removal can lead to abnormal weight distribution and foot injuries. Excessive scratching should be dealt with by behavior management and frequent nail trims.

Assisted Feeding

Nutritional support is important for rabbits that are anorexic because, like cats, they are predisposed to hepatic lipidosis. Critical care diets specifically for herbivores are available (Critical Care, Oxbow Animal Health, Murdock, NE), but ground-up pellets can be used as well. Many rabbits can be syringe fed by restraining the animal with a towel and gently placing a catheter tip syringe in the diastema as previously described. Rabbits that do not readily accept food from a syringe may be tube fed.

Restraint for tube feeding is similar to that used for oral examination. A second person should place an oral speculum behind the incisors, in the diastema. Select a tube that should be larger than the trachea and premeasure to the last rib on the left side and mark the tube. Once the tube is passed, proper placement can be confirmed by aspirating stomach contents or injecting 5 to 10 ml of air through the tube while auscultating the stomach for the telltale sounds of bubbling fluid or turbulent airflow. The tube should be easy to pass, and if the rabbits struggles excessively the procedure should be stopped. The animal may need to be sedated for this procedure.

If a suitable mouth gag is not present on the premises, a gag can be made by taping two tongue depressors (0.75 inch width) in flat alignment with medical adhesive tape. A hole should be bored through the center of the taped tongue depressors, using a scissors tip or other sufficiently sharp instrument, of such size to permit passage of the stomach tube. An alternative is to remove the plunger from a syringe, bore a hole through the cylinder walls, and use the empty barrel as a gag. Mouth gags for rabbits should be of sufficient height or diameter to prohibit occlusion of the incisors and sectioning or damage to the tube. Tongue depressors that are 0.75 inches wide or the barrel of a 10-ml syringe are generally sufficient as gags for rabbits 4 to 6 kg in weight.

Although of arguable value given the confounding effects of the bactericidal low gastric pH, force-feeding may be attempted for transfaunation in cases of cecal dysbiosis. This procedure is accomplished by outfitting a healthy donor rabbit with an Elizabethan collar overnight to prevent cecotrophy. The collected cecotrophs should be mixed and suspended in warmed (37°C), nonbacteriostatic saline and strained through gauze prior to administration with a stomach tube. A volume of 40 to 60 ml of this suspension can be safely given to a 4- to 5-kg rabbit using a 12 French, 16-inch Sovereign Feeding Tube (Kendall Co., Mansfield, MA).

If a permanent tube is needed, nasogastric tubes can be placed using a technique similar to that used in cats. The disadvantage of nasogastric tubes is that solutions designed for nutritional support of rabbits will clog a tube this small. Although it is common to use human nutrition products such as Ensure for rabbits, these are not ideal for herbivores. Solutions available for herbivorous reptiles will pass through these tubes, although no solution will be able to provide appropriate insoluble fiber because it would clog the tube (Paul-Murphy 2007). Surgical placement of pharyngostomy and gastrotomy tubes have also been described (Smith et al. 1997, Rogers et al. 1988).

SEX DETERMINATION

Gender determination in rabbits is similar to that in cats with the exception that does also show sexual dimorphism by virtue of a pendulous fold of skin at the caudal mandibulocervical region. This redundant skin is termed the "dewlap." The vulva in does is located directly below the anus (Figure 12.7). The ensheathed penis of the buck is also located directly below the anus, similar to cats, and it has an obvious scrotum with palpable testes (Figure 12.8). However, due to open inguinal canals the testes may migrate back and forth from the scrotum to the abdomen.

EMERGENCY AND CRITICAL CARE

Emergency and critical care are action-oriented and immediate with the goals of interventions being to stabilize the rabbit and afford the opportunity to then pursue the diagnosis of the primary problem. There may be any number of presentations requiring critical care, including gastrointestinal disorders, trauma, environmental exposure (hypothermia, hyperthermia), intoxications, respiratory distress, neurologic symptoms, and urinary obstruction. Identical presentation directed interventions constitute the tenets of care including fluid therapy, body temperature maintenance, oxygen administration, and control of hemorrhage. If in shock, rabbits rarely present in a compensatory stage as may be seen in dogs and birds, and instead usually have signs of decompensation such as hypothermia, bradycardia, hypotension, pale mucous membranes, and prolonged capillary refill time (Lichtenberger 2007). Rabbits are obligate nasal breathers, so a rabbit that is open mouth breathing is in severe respiratory distress. Acute respiratory distress can occur with bacterial infections of nasal passages, bacterial pneumonia, trauma, or cardiac disease (Paul-Murphy 2007).

If CPR is required, immediate action is directed at the "ABCs" of emergency care as in other species: Airway, Breathing, and Circulation. An airway should be established with either intubation or a tracheostomy tube and the animal placed on oxygen. If an airway cannot be established, high flow oxygen with tight-fitting mask can be used at a rate of twenty to thirty breaths/minute, but monitor the animal for signs of bloat (Lichtenberger 2007). Chest compressions at a rate of at least eighty times/minute and medications are used to address circulatory issues, but remember that some rabbits have serum atropinesterases so atropine is not the preferred anticholinergic if one is indicated.

More advanced care and monitoring includes intravenous fluids, ECG, blood-gas analysis, end tidal CO_2 measurements, and temperature. The use of corticosteroids in shock therapy is controversial in dogs and cats and not recommended for rabbits (Lichtenberger 2007). The treatment may also need to include addressing metabolic disturbances that may be the cause or consequence of the shock.

In addition to shock, hypothermia is a risk in sucklings, rabbits housed outdoors in winter, and those recovering from anesthesia, especially if room-temperature fluids were administered. Therapy centers on slowly warming the animal and restoring circulation with warm, isotonic fluids in conjunction with an external heat source such as warm water bottles, water-circulated heating pads, or a Bair-Hugger. The goal in treating hypothermia, as it is with other species, is to raise the body temperature slowly. Otherwise, in theory, the cure may be worse than the disease. A rapid rise in body temperature without control may increase brain metabolic demands above that which can be provided and expose the heart, liver, and lungs to cold, acidotic blood from the periphery. Overzealous body warming also could result in hyperthermia. Failure to restore fluids in any hypothermic animal can result in acute tubular necrosis. Hypoxemia should be considered as a possible complication in downer and hypothermic animals, and animals may require oxygen delivered via a face mask.

Hypoglycemia is generally a risk in neonatal or small breed animals either on an inadequate nutritional plane or recovering from surgery. High metabolic energy demands and low depot fat reservoirs coupled with postoperative anorexia make these animals particularly at risk. It could be a companion to hypothermia. In a pinch, however, response to glucose therapy can be used as a diagnostic tool. Acute hypoglycemia should be treated as for other species by intravenous or oral bolus of 50% dextrose (e.g. 2 ml/kg). Parenteral administration of glucose is preferred because excessive administration of oral carbohydrates may create conditions that upset the enteric microflora and predispose to cecal dysbiosis. For those animals that are both hypoglycemic and hypothermic, intravenous glucose provides fuel to the brain during rewarming.

Hyperthermia is associated with rectal temperatures higher than 104°F. Rabbits are prone to hyperthermia if housed outdoors because they cannot sweat or effectively pant. It may also be caused iatrogenically by overzealous rewarming during anesthetic recovery or can be associated with certain toxicoses. The treatment, as for other species, is to cool the rabbit slowly. Hyperthermia can be treated with room-temperature intravenous fluids and tepid water, especially on the ears. Animals need to be monitored for kidney failure and other metabolic abnormalities.

Rabbits may present with a variety of gastrointestinal emergencies, such as ileus, diarrhea, gastric dila-

tion, and obstruction. Ileus and diarrhea can both lead to life-threatening enterotoxemia and dehydration. Ileus is more common than diarrhea, and is a common problem given the intricate, complex and delicate interrelationship between diet, other environmental factors, the commensal, fermentative microflora, and gut motility in rabbits of all ages. Diarrhea can also occur due to these factors or associated with other conditions, such as infection or antibiotic administration.

Fluids and nutritional support are the most important aspect of treatment for these animals. Even if there is no appreciable fluid loss because rabbits cannot vomit and diarrhea is not observed, colonic hypomotility leads to decreased water absorption and dehydration (O'Malley 2005). Cecotrophs contain high levels of vitamins B and K, so supplementation of B vitamins in particular should be considered for animals that are unable or unwilling to eat their night feces. Additional treatment may include analgesics, motility agents, antibiotics, anthelmintics, anti-ulcer medications, or other agents as indicated. For diarrhea, transfaunation with cecotrophs collected from a healthy donor rabbit to re-establish the enteric flora may be considered. It should be noted that yogurt and many commercial probiotics have not been shown to be effective in floral reconstitution for rabbits (Myers 2007).

Gastric dilation is rare, but must be excluded in an anorexic rabbit, because the animal may need to be decompressed and prokinetic agents may be contraindicated. Gastric dilation can occur secondary to small intestinal obstruction because of the inability to vomit, leading to fluid and gas accumulation in the stomach. This must be differentiated from gut stasis based on radiographs. Initial treatment includes passage of a stomach tube to decompress and fluid therapy, with subsequent decisions regarding whether surgery is necessary (Harcourt-Brown 2007).

Traumatic presentations may include fractured limbs, traumatic vertebral luxation or fractures, and fight-related lacerations, including those of the scrotum. Limb fractures should be stabilized by splinting if possible, but often this is difficult and surgery may be indicated. Radiography should be done to characterize the fracture and permit the development of a plan for reduction and stabilization. Unfortunately, vertebral injuries are rarely curable and often euthanasia is the most humane option. Rabbits presenting acutely for vertebral injury should be radiographed to confirm the diagnosis and should be kept clean, padded to retard the development of decubital ulcers, and provided fluid and dietary therapy as needed. Spinal surgery is not commonly done in rabbits, but a referral center can be contacted to determine if someone is capable of performing this procedure. For especially dedicated and competent owners, the use of carts has been described for paraplegic rabbits (Boydell 2000).

Trauma to the scrotum or testes may require surgical castration. Steroids for trauma should be used with caution in rabbits because they are sensitive to their side effects (Paul-Murphy 2007).

The principles of treatment for toxin exposure are also similar to those for cats and dogs, with some notable exceptions. Emetics such as apomorphine are ineffective for the physiologic reasons mentioned. It may also be necessary to apply an E-collar for seventy-two hours to keep rabbits from eating cecotrophs that may still contain the toxic substance. Therapy should involve fluid administration, gastric lavage, bathing, and activated charcoal as indicated, depending on the substance and route of intoxication. Toxicoses have been associated with a variety of chemicals, pesticides/rodenticides, antibiotics, tiletamine, and various household plants (Johnston 2008). Although rabbits are resistant to many plant toxins such as ragwort, nightshade, comfrey, and laburnum, they are sensitive to aflatoxins that may be present in the feed (Harcourt-Brown 2002). Lead toxicosis can occur in rabbits in older houses that like to chew the baseboards, which can cause anorexia or neurologic signs. Fipronil (Frontline®) or high doses of permethrins or pyrethrins can be toxic, especially in small rabbits.

Hemorrhage should be controlled by stopping the bleeding, including surgical interventions, if needed. Intravenous fluids should be given for significant blood loss. Transfusion should be considered for rabbits based on the same principles as in small animals, and although it is used clinically, blood groups have not been studied in rabbits and a cross-match is recommended (Lichtenberger 2004). Rest, oxygen therapy, iron supplementation, and nutritional support may also be important in the treatment of anemia. The most likely causes of hemorrhage are trauma and internal hemorrhage or hematuria in intact does from uterine adenocarcinoma.

EUTHANASIA

Methods should conform to those listed as acceptable by the 2007 *AVMA Guidelines on Euthanasia*. In a practice setting, the most preferable method is by injection of a barbiturate overdose (50 to 100 mg/kg) into the lateral marginal ear vein. This can be facilitated by first sedating or anesthetizing the rabbit as described in the preceding section on surgical anesthesia.

REFERENCES

Anderson NL. 1995. Intraosseous fluid delivery in small exotic animals. In: Kirk's Current Veterinary Therapy XII: Small Animal Practice, Philadelphia: W.B. Saunders Co. 1331–1335.

Bayne K. 2003. Environmental enrichment of nonhuman primates, dogs and rabbits used in toxicologic studies. *Toxicologic Pathology* 31*(Suppl)*: 132–7.

Bergdall VK, Dysko RC. 1994. Metabolic, traumatic, mycotic and inherited diseases and variations. In: The Biology of the Laboratory Rabbit, 2nd ed., edited by Manning PJ, Ringler DH, Newcomer CE, Orlando: Academic Press. 293–319.

Bielski RJ, Bassett GS, Fideler B, et al. 1993. Intraosseous infusions: Effects on the immature physis—an experimental model in rabbits. *J Ped Orthopedics* 13(4): 511–515.

Boydell P. 2000. Nervous system and disorders. In: Manual of Rabbit Medicine and Surgery, edited by Flecknell PA, 57–62. British Small Animal Veterinary Association.

Bowman DD, Fogelson ML, Carbone LG. 1992. Effect of ivermectin on the control of ear mites (*Psoroptes cuniculi*) in naturally infested rabbits. *Amer J Vet Res* 53: 105–109.

Brammer DW, Doerning BJ, Chrisp CE, et al. 1991. Anesthetic and nephrotoxic effects of Telazol in New Zealand white rabbits. *Lab Anim Sci* 41(5): 432–435.

Cam Y, Atasever A, Eraslan G, Kibar M, Atalay O, Beyaz L, et al. 2008. *Eimeria stiedae*: experimental infection in rabbits and the effect of treatment with toltrazuril and ivermectin. *Exp Parasitol.* 119(1):164–172.

Capello V, Gracis M. 2005. Rabbit and Rodent Dentistry Handbook, edited by Lennox AM. Lake Worth: Zoologic Education Network Inc.

Carpenter JW, Mashima TY, Rupiper DJ. 2001. Exotic Animal Formulary, 2nd ed., 301–326. Philadelphia: W.B. Saunders Company.

Cheeke PR, Cunha TJ. 1987. Rabbit Feeding and Nutrition. Orlando: Academic Press.

Chen PH, White CE. 2006. Comparison of Rectal, Microchip Transponder, and Infrared Thermometry Techniques for Obtaining Body Temperature in the Laboratory Rabbit (*Oryctolagus cuniculus*). *J Am Assoc Lab Anim Sci* 45: 57–63.

Chew RM. 1965. Water metabolism of mammals. *Physiol Mammal* 2: 43–178.

Cohen C. 1969. Genetics of the Rabbit. In: Laboratory Animal Medicine, NAS Publication 1724, Washington DC.

Crossley DA, Aiken S. 2004. Small Mammal Dentistry. In: Ferrets, rabbits and rodents: clinical medicine and surgery, edited by Quesenberry KE and Carpenter JW, St. Louis: W.B. Saunders Co. 370–382.

Curtis SK, Brooks DL. 1990. Eradication of ear mites from naturally infested conventional research rabbits using ivermectin. *Lab Anim Sci* 40: 406–408.

Davies RR, Davies JA. 2003. Rabbit gastrointestinal physiology. Veterinary Clinics of North America. *Exotic Animal Practice.* 6(1):139–153.

Deeb BJ, Carpenter JW. 2004. Neurologic and Musculoskeletal Diseases. In: Ferrets, rabbits and rodents: clinical medicine and surgery, 2nd ed., edited by Quesenberry KE and Carpenter JW, St. Louis: W.B. Saunders Co. 203–210.

Deeb BJ, DiGiacomo RF. 2000. Respiratory diseases of rabbits. *Vet Clin North Am Exot Anim Pract* 3(2): 465–480, vi–vii.

Deeb BJ, DiGiacomo RF, Evermann JF, Thouless ME. 1993. Prevalence of coronavirus antibodies in rabbits. *Lab Anim Sci* 43:431–433.

Deeb BJ, Digiacomo RF. 1994. Cerebral larval migrans caused by *Baylisascaris* species in pet rabbits. *JAVMA* 205:1744–1747.

Delong D, Manning PJ. 1994. Bacterial Diseases. In: The Biology of the Laboratory Rabbit, 2nd ed., edited by Manning PJ, Ringler DH, Newcomer CE, Orlando: Academic Press. 131–170.

Difilippo SM, Norberg PJ, Suson UD, Savino AM, Reim DA. 2004. A comparison of xylazine and medetomidine in an anesthetic combination in New Zealand White Rabbits. *Contemp Top Lab Anim Sci* 43: 32–34.

Doerning BJ, Brammer BW, Chrisp CE, et al. 1992. Nephrotoxicity of tiletamine in New Zealand white rabbits. *Lab Anim Sci* 42(3): 267–269.

Düwel D, Brech K. 1981. Control of oxyuriasis in rabbits by fenbendazole. *Lab Anim* 15: 101–105.

Edwards AW, Korner PI, Thornburn GD. 1959. The cardiac output of the unanesthetized rabbit, and the effects of preliminary anesthesia, environmental temperature, and carotid occlusion. *Q J Exp Physiol* 44: 309–321.

Fichi G, Flamini G, Giovanelli F, Otrant D, Perrucci S. 2007. Efficacy of an essential oil of *Eugenia caryophyllata* against *Psoroptes cuniculi*. *Exp Parasitol*. Feb;115(2): 168–172.

Flecknell PA. 1987. Laboratory Animal Anaesthesia: An Introduction for Research Workers and Technicians. London: Academic Press.

Flecknell PA, Liles JH, Williamson HA. 1990. The use of lignocaine-prilocaine local anesthetic cream for pain-free venipuncture in laboratory animals. *Lab Anim.* 24: 142–146.

Flecknell PA. 1996. Laboratory Animal Anaesthesia, 2nd ed., London: Academic Press. 182–193.

Flecknell PA, Richardson CA, Popovic A. 2007. Laboratory Animals. In: Veterinary anesthesia and analgesia, edited by Tranquilli WJ, Thurman JC, Grimm KA. Ames: Blackwell Publishing, 766.

Foley PL, Henderson AL, Bissonette EA, Wimer GR, Feldman SH. 2001. Evaluation of fentanyl transdermal patches in rabbits: blood concentrations and physiologic response. *Comp Med* 51: 239–244.

Garibaldi BA, Fox JG, Otto G, et al. 1987. Hematuria in rabbits. *Lab Anim Sci* 37: 769–772.

Gentry PA. 1982. The effect of administration of a single dose of T-2 toxin on blood coagulation in the rabbit. *Can J Comp Med* 46: 414–419.

Gillett CS. 1994. Selected drug dosages and clinical reference data. In: The Biology of the Laboratory Rabbit, 2nd ed., edited by Manning PJ, Ringler DH, and Newcomer CE, Orlando: Academic Press. 467–472.

Gilroy BA. 1981. Endotracheal intubation of rabbits and rodents. *JAVMA* 179: 1295.

Gonzales GA, Silvan G, Illera JC. 2005. Effects of Barbiturate administration on hepatic and renal biochemical parameters in New Zealand white rabbits. *Contemp Top Lab Anim Sci* 44: 43–45.

Gorrel C. 1996. Teeth trimming in rabbits and rodents. *Vet Rec* 139(21): 528.

Graham JE. 2004. Rabbit Wound Management. *Vet Clin Exot Anim* 7: 37–55.

Griffiths M, Davies D. 1963. The role of soft pellets in the production of lactic acid in the rabbit stomach. *J Nutr* 80: 171–180.

Harcourt-Brown F. 2002. Textbook of Rabbit Medicine. Oxford: Alden Press.

Harcourt-Brown FM, Holloway HK. 2003. *Encephalitozoon cuniculi* in pet rabbits. *Vet Rec.* Apr 5;152(14): 427–431.

Harcourt-Brown TR. 2007. Management of Acute Gastric Dilation in Rabbits. *Journal of Exotic Pet Medicine* 16: 168–174.

Harkness JE, Wagner JE. 1989. In: The Biology and Medicine of Rabbits and Rodents, 3rd ed., Philadelphia: Lea and Febiger. 9–65.

Heard D. 2004. Anesthesia, analgesia, and sedation of small mammals. In: Ferrets, rabbits and rodents: clinical medicine and surgery, 2nd ed., edited by Quesenberry KE and Carpenter JW. St. Louis: W.B. Saunders Co. 356–369.

Hedenqvist P, Roughan JV, Antunes L, Orr H, Flecknell PA. 2001. Induction of anaesthesia with desflurane and isoflurane in the rabbit. *Lab Anim* 35: 172–179.

Hess L. 2004. Dermatologic Diseases. In: Ferrets, rabbits and rodents: clinical medicine and surgery, edited by Quesenberry KE and Carpenter JW, 194–202.

Hewitt CD, et al. 1989. Normal biochemical and hematological values in New Zealand White rabbits. *Clin Chem* 35: 1777–1779.

Horiuchi N, Watarai M, Kobayashi Y, Omata Y, Furuoka H. 2008. Proliferative enteropathy involving *Lawsonia intracellularis* infection in rabbits (*Oryctolagus cuniculus*). *J Vet Med Sci.* Apr;70(4): 389–392.

Huerkamp MJ. 1995. Anesthesia and postoperative management of rabbits and pocket pets. In: Kirk's Current Veterinary Therapy XII: Small Animal Practice, Philadelphia: W.B. Saunders Co. 1322–1327.

Jablonski P, Howden BO, Baxter K. 2001. Influence of buprenorphine analgesia on post-operative recovery in two strains of rats. *Lab Anim* 35: 213–222.

Jenkins JR. 2004a. Gastrointestinal Diseases. In: Ferrets, rabbits and rodents: clinical medicine and surgery, 2nd ed., edited by Quesenberry KE and Carpenter JW, St. Louis: W.B. Saunder Co. 161–171.

Jenkins JR. 2004b. Soft Tissue Surgery. In: Ferrets, rabbits and rodents: clinical medicine and surgery, 2nd ed., edited by Quesenberry KE and Carpenter JW, St. Louis: W.B. Saunders Co. 221–230.

Jenkins JR. 2000. Surgical sterilization in small mammals. Spay and neuter. *Vet Clin N A Exot Anim Pract* 3(3): 617–627.

Jensen LJ, et al. 1983. Natural infection of *Obeliscoides cuniculi* in a domestic rabbit. *Lab Anim Sci* 30: 231–233.

Johnson CA, Pallozzi WA, Geiger L, Szumiloski JL, Castiglia L, Dahl NP, Destefano JA, Pratt SJ, Hall SJ, Beare CM, Gallagher M, Klein HJ. 2003. The effect of an environmental enrichment device on individually caged rabbits in a safety assessment facility. *Contemporary Topics in Laboratory Animal Science*. 42(5): 27–30.

Johnston MS. 2008. Clinical Toxicoses of the Domestic Rabbit. *Vet Clin Exot Anim* 11: 315–326.

Kazacos KR, Kazacos EA. 1983. Fatal cerebrospinal disease caused by *Baylisascaris procynosis* in domestic rabbits. *JAVMA* 183: 967–971.

Kazakos GM, Anagnostou T, Savvas I, Raptopoulos D, Psalla D, Kazakou IM. 2007. Use of the laryngeal mask airway in rabbits: placement and efficacy. *Lab Anim (NY)* 36: 29–34.

Kohn DF, Martin TE, Foley PL, Morris TH, Swindle MM, Vogler GA, Wixson SK. 2007. Public statement: guidelines for the assessment and management of pain in rodents and rabbits. *J Am Assoc Lab Anim Sci* 46: 97–108.

Kunzel F, Gruber A, Tichy A, Edelhofer R, Nell B, Hassan J, et al. 2008. Clinical symptoms and diagnosis of encephalitozoonosis in pet rabbits. *Vet Parasitol.* Feb 14;151(2–4): 115–124.

Leary, SL, Manning PJ, Anderson LC. 1984. Experimental and naturally-occurring gastric foreign bodies in laboratory rabbits. *Lab Anim Sci* 34: 58–61.

Leck G. 1988. Removing a calculus from the urinary bladder of A rabbit. *Vet Rec* 83: 64–65.

Langan GP, Lohmiller JJ, Swing SP, Wardrip CL. 2000. Respiratory diseases of rodents and rabbits. *Vet Clin North Am Small Anim Pract.* Nov;30(6): 1309–1335, vii.

Lee MJ, Clement JG. 1990. Effects of soman poisoning on hematology and coagulation parameters and serum biochemistry in rabbits. *Mil Med* 155: 244–249.

Leland MM, Hubbard GB, Dubey JP. 1992. Clinical toxoplasmosis in domestic rabbits. *Lab Anim Sci* 42: 318–319.

Lichtenberger M. 2004. Transfusion Medicine in Exotic Pets. *Clinical Techniques in Small Animal Practice* 19: 88–95.

Lichtenberger M. 2007. Shock and Cardiopulmonary-Cerebral Resuscitation in Small Mammals and Birds. *Vet Clin Exot Anim* 10: 275–291.

Lindsey JR, Fox RR. 1994. Inherited diseases and variations. In: The Biology of the Laboratory Rabbit, 2nd ed., edited by Manning PJ, Ringler DH, and Newcomer CE. Orlando: Academic Press. 293–319.

Lipman NS, Marini RP, Flecknell PA. 1997. Anesthesia and analgesia in rabbits. In: Anesthesia and Analgesia in Laboratory Animals, edited by Kohn DF, Wixson SK, White WJ, and Benson GJ, Boston: Academic Press. 205–232.

Livio M, et al. 1988. Role of platelet-activating factor in primary hemostasis. *Am J Physiol* 254: 218–223.

Lopez-Martinez R, Mier T, Quirarte M. 1984. Dermatophytes isolated from laboratory animals. *Mycopathologica* 88: 111–113.

Mader DR. 2004. Rabbits: Basic Approach to Veterinary Care. In: Ferrets, rabbits, and rodents: clinical medicine and surgery, 2nd ed., edited by Mader KE and Carpenter JW, St. Louis: W.B. Saunders Co. 147–154.

Malley D. 1996. Teeth trimming in rabbits and rodents. *Vet Rec* 139(24): 603.

McLaughlin RM, Fish RE. 1994. Clinical chemistry and hematology. In: The Biology of the Laboratory Rabbit, 2nd ed., edited by Manning PJ, Ringler DH, Newcomer CE, 111–127. Orlando: Academic Press.

McTier TL, Hair JA, Walstrom DJ, Thompson L. 2003. Efficacy and safety of topical administration of selamectin for treatment of ear mite infestation in rabbits. *JAVMA* 223(3): 322–324.

Morgan JR, Silverman S. 1984. Techniques of Veterinary Radiography. 4th ed. Davis: Veterinary Radiology Associates.

Mullen HS. 2000. Nonreproductive surgery in small mammals. *Vet Clin NA Exot Anim Pract* 3(3): 629–645.

Myers D. 2007. Probiotics. *J. of Exotic Pet Medicine* 16: 195–197.

Narama I, et al. 1982. Pulmonary nodule causes by *Dirofilaria immitis* in a laboratory rabbit. *J. Parasitol.* 68: 351–352.

Orr HE, Roughan JV, Flecknell PA. 2005. Assessment of ketamine and medetomidine anaesthesia in the domestic rabbit. *Vet Anaesth Analg* 32: 271–279.

Otto CM, Crowe DT. 1992. Intraosseous resuscitation techniques and applications. In: Kirk's Current Veterinary Therapy XI: Small Animal Practice. Philadelphia: W.B. Saunders Company Co.

O'Malley B. 2005. Rabbits. In: Clinical Anatomy and Physiology of Exotic Species: Structure and function of mammals, birds, reptiles, and amphibians, Philadelphia: Elsevier Saunders. 173–196.

Pare JA, Paul-Murphy J. 2004. Disorders of the Reproductive and Urinary Systems. In: Ferrets, rabbits and rodents: clinical medicine and surgery, 2nd ed., edited by Quesenberry KE and Carpenter JW, St. Louis: W.B. Saunders Co. 183–193.

Patton NM. 1994. Colony husbandry. In: The Biology of the Laboratory Rabbit, 2nd ed., edited by Manning PJ, Ringler DH, Newcomer CE, 27–45. Orlando: Academic Press.

Paul-Murphy J. 2007. Critical Care of the Rabbit. *Vet Clin Exot Anim* 10: 437–461.

Phaneuf LR, Barker S, Groleau MA, Turner PV. 2006. Tracheal injury after endotracheal intubation and anesthesia in rabbits. *J Am Assoc Lab Anim Sci* 45: 67–72.

Percy DH, Barthold SW. 2007. Rabbit. In: Pathology of Laboratory Rodents and Rabbits, 3rd ed., edited by Percy DH and Barthold SW, Ames: Blackwell Publishing. 253–308.

PMI Nutrition International. 1998. LabDiet: Product Reference Manual. SL1-5.

Reuter JD, Fowles KJ, Terwilliger GA, Booth CJ. 2005. Iatrogenic tension pneumothorax in a rabbit. *Cont Top Lab An Sci* 44(4):22–25.

Robertson SA, Eberhart S. 1994. Efficacy of intranasal route for administration of anesthetic agents to adult rabbits. *Lab Anim Sci* 44(2): 159–165.

Rougier S, Galland D, Boucher S, Boussarie D, Valle M. 2006 Epidemiology and susceptibility of pathogenic bacteria responsible for upper respiratory tract infections in pet rabbits. *Vet Microbiol.* 115(1–3): 192–198.

Rogers G, Taylor C, Austin JC, et al. 1988. A pharyngostomy technique for chronic oral dosing of rabbits. *Lab Anim Sci* 38: 619–620.

Sikoski P, Young RW, Lockard M. 2007. Comparison of heating devices for maintaining body temperature in anesthetized laboratory rabbits (*Oryctolagus cuniculus*). *J Am Assoc Lab Anim Sci* 46: 61–63.

Smith DA, Olson PO, Mathews KA. 1997. Nutritional support for rabbits using the percutaneously placed gastrostomy tube: a preliminary study. *J Am Anim Hosp Assoc* 33: 48–54.

Smith JC, Robertson LD, Auhll A, March TJ, Derring C, Bolon B. 2004. Endotracheal tubes versus laryngeal mask airways in rabbit inhalation anesthesia: ease of use and waste gas emissions. *Contemp Top Lab Anim Sci* 43: 22–25.

Sanchez S, Mizan S, Quist C, Schroder P, Juneau M, Dawe D, et al. 2004. Serological response to *Pasteurella multocida* NanH sialidase in persistently colonized rabbits. *Clin Diagn Lab Immunol.* 11(5): 825–834.

Stein S, Walshaw S. 1996. Rabbits. In: Handbook of Rodent and Rabbit Medicine, edited by Laber-Laird K, Swindle MM, and Flecknell P, Tarrytown: Elsevier Science Inc. 183–217.

Suter C, Muller-Doblies UU, Hatt JM, Deplazes P. 2001. Prevention and treatment of *Encephalitozoon cuniculi* infection in rabbits with fenbendazole. *Vet Rec.* 148(15): 478–480.

Swindle MM, Shealy PM. 1996. In: Handbook of Rodent and Rabbit Medicine, edited by Laber-Laird K, Swindle MM, and Flecknell P, Tarrytown: Elsevier Science Inc. 239–254.

Tesluk GC, Peiffer RL, Brown D. 1982. A clinical and pathological study of inherited glaucoma in New Zealand white rabbits. *Lab Anim.* 16: 234–239.

Tran HS, Puc MM, Tran JL, Del Rossi AJ, Hewitt CW. 2001. A method of endoscopic endotracheal intubation in rabbits. *Lab Anim* 35: 249–252.

Vernau KM, Osofsky A, LeCouteur RA. 2007. The neurological examination and lesion localization in the companion rabbit (*Orytolagus cuniculus*). *Vet Clin Exot Anim* 10: 731–758.

Vogtsberger LM, et al. 1986. Spontaneous dermatophytosis due to *Microsporum canis* in rabbits. *Lab Anim Sci* 36: 294–297.

Wagner R, Wendlberger U. 2000. Field efficacy of moxidectin in dogs and rabbits naturally infested with *Sarcoptes* spp., *Demodex* spp. and *Psoroptes* spp. mites. *Vet Parasitol* 93: 149–158.

Wales AD, Woodward MJ, Pearson GR. 2005. Attaching-effacing bacteria in animals. *J Comp Pathol.* 132(1): 1–26.

Weisbroth SH. 1994. Neoplastic diseases. In: The Biology of the Laboratory Rabbit, 2nd ed., edited by Manning PJ, Ringler DH, Newcomer CE, 259–292. Orlando: Academic Press.

Wixson SK. 1994. Anesthesia and analgesia for rabbits. In: The Biology of the Laboratory Rabbit, 2nd ed., edited by Manning PJ, Ringler DH, Newcomer CE, 87–109. Orlando: Academic Press.

Wolford ST, et al. 1986. Reference range data base for serum chemistry and hematology values in laboratory animals. *J Toxicol Environ Health* 18: 161–188.

Wright F, Riner J. 1984. Comparative efficacy of injection routes and doses of ivermectin against Psoroptes in rabbits. *Amer J Vet Res* 46: 752–754.

Wyatt JD, Scott RW, Richardson ME. 1989. The effects of prolonged ketamine-xylazine intravenous infusion on arterial blood pH, blood gases, mean arterial blood pressure, heart and respiratory rates, rectal temperature, and reflexes in the rabbit. *Lab Anim Sci* 39: 411–416.

Williams AM, Wyatt JD. 2007. Comparison of Subcutaneous and intramuscular ketamine-medetomidine with and without reversal by atipamezole in Dutch belted rabbits (Oryctolagus cuniculus). *J Am Assoc Lab Anim Sci* 46: 16–20.

Xu ZJ, Chen WX. 1989. Viral hemorrhagic disease in rabbits: A review. *Vet Res Commun* 13: 205–212.

Yu L, et al. 1979. Biochemical parameters of normal rabbit serum. *Clin Biochem* 12: 83–87.

CHAPTER THIRTEEN

Mice, Rats, Gerbils, and Hamsters

Anne Hudson and April Romagnano

INTRODUCTION

This chapter focuses on the mouse (*Mus musculus*), rat (*Rattus norvegicus*), gerbil (*Meriones unguiculatus*), and hamsters: golden or Syrian hamster (*Mesocricetus auratus*), European hamster (*Cricetus cricetus*), and Russian dwarf hamster (*Phodopus* spp.). They are described as follows:

Mice: Small, busy rodents; long, hairless tail; 20 to 63 g.

Rats: Large, intelligent rodents; long, hairless tail; 225 to 500 g.

Gerbils: Desert-adapted rodents but need fresh water access; produce concentrated urine; long, hairy tail; 46 to 131 g.

Hamsters: Stocky, loose-skinned rodents; cheek pouches and short tail; 87 to 130 g.

ANATOMY AND PHYSIOLOGY

Basic anatomy and physiology of mice, rats, gerbils, and hamsters is like that of other mammals, so only the significant differences are addressed in this section (Figure 13.1). Please note the following: Male mice have 50% bigger spleens then females. Rats have no gallbladder and their Harderian glands are known to produce red porphyrin staining around the eyes; this is related to stress. Some gerbils have seizures, a thymus through adulthood, and a large adrenal-weight-to-body ratio. Male hamsters have larger adrenals than females (Harkness and Wagner 1995, Quesenberry and Carpenter 2003).

The teeth of mice, rats, gerbils, and hamsters are divided into two separate functional units, the incisors and the cheek teeth. These two units are separated by a long gap called the diastema (Quesenberry and Carpenter 2003). The diastema is shorter in the mandible than in the maxilla, giving rodents their normal brachygnathic appearance (Quesenberry and Carpenter 2003).

Mice, rats, gerbils, and hamsters all share a dental formula of 2 (I 1/1, C 0/0, P 0/0, M 3/3), with hamsters having incisors at birth (Harkness and Wagner 1995). The incisors are open rooted and grow continuously; the molars do not. Incisors develop a yellow-orange color as the animal ages. Classically the incisors are used for rostrocaudal gnawing during eating. A near vertical biting motion also exists, but is more common in defensive or offensive behaviors (Quesenberry and Carpenter 2003). Gnawing naturally wears down the surface of the incisors, but a malocclusion of the incisors precludes normal wear and makes trimming of the teeth necessary. Malocclusion is especially problematic in weanlings and if not caught early can lead to starvation and death. Malocclusion can be genetic, or it can occur secondary to a fractured tooth which grows back crooked, causing misalignment of teeth and preventing proper wear.

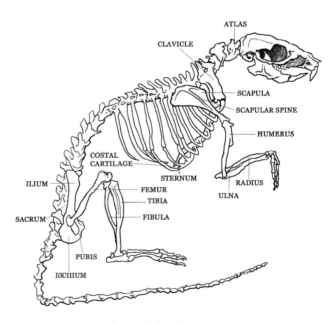

Figure 13.1. Rodent skeletal anatomy.

Rats, mice, and gerbils possess long tails; hamsters have very short tails. It is very important to exercise caution when handling the tail because improper restraint can cause trauma. In gerbils the skin can actually slip "tail-slip" or deglove with improper handling (Harkness and Wagner 1995). When held distal to the base, the animal can go into a spin and twist the distal part of the tail off in all three, which is an escape mechanism. Further, rodents, mainly rats and gerbils, can regulate their temperature via thermoregulatory activities, such as tail extension. Hence, damage to the tail can indeed affect temperature regulation in these species.

Mammary tissue is extensive, reaching cranially between the front legs and up over the shoulders, and caudally toward the inguinal area. Therefore, mammary masses can be located well away from the teats. The mammary glands are paired, with rats having four to six pairs; mice, five pairs; gerbils, four pairs; and hamsters, six to seven pairs.

Harderian glands are specialized glands located behind each eye. They secrete a substance containing porphyrin, giving the secretion a red tinge. An animal experiencing stress or illness may have a buildup of the secretions around the eyes and may appear to the client to be bleeding from the eyes and nasolacrimal duct, and hence the nares. This collection of secreted material is also referred to as "red tears" and is most common in stressed rats.

Additional glandular structures include bilateral flank glands in the hamster and a ventral gland in the gerbil (Harkness and Wagner 1995). These sebaceous glands are brown in color and play a part in mating behavior, territorial marking, and marking of pups. The animals spend time grooming these areas and are often observed rubbing the glands over surfaces.

Small rodents are seasonally polyestrus and are spontaneous ovulators. Mating behavior results in the production of a whitish-tan collection of secretions, called a copulatory plug, that is often found lying in the bedding of the cage. Most male rodent species have an os penis and open inguinal canals, allowing them to retract the testicles into the abdominal cavity (Harkness and Wagner 1995). Gentle pressure to the caudal abdomen will force the testicles into the scrotal sac.

Hamsters have large cheek pouches that extend back to their scapulae (Figure 13.2). These pouches can distend to quite a large size, allowing the hamster to transfer food and bedding from one point to another. A startled mother may move her offspring from one area to another via her cheek pouches; however, the pups can suffocate inside a pouch. Hence, great care should be taken not to disturb females with litters.

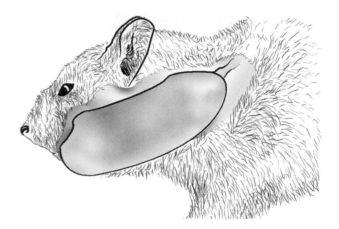

Figure 13.2. Cheek pouch.

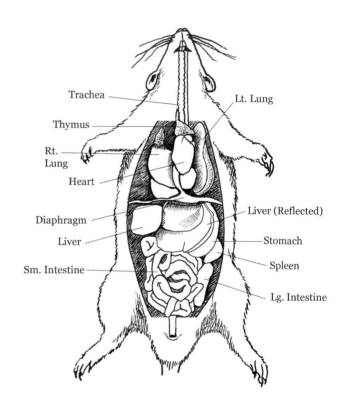

Figure 13.3. Rodent visceral anatomy.

The digestive systems of mice, rats, gerbils, and hamsters have some differences from other mammals, including an inability to regurgitate. Hamsters have an esophageal pouch that allows for pre-gastric fermentation of food prior to reaching the stomach. Rodents are monogastric, with their stomachs divided into two areas: a glandular portion and a non-glandular portion. The practice of coprophagy is believed to assimilate certain nutrients, such a B vitamins, that are produced by bacterial action in the colon (Quesenberry and

Carpenter 2003, Hillyer and Quesenberry 1997). Rats do not have a gallbladder; therefore, bile continuously flows into the duodenum. The pancreas of rodents is arranged in diffuse lobes, making palpation difficult. Brown fat in rodents seems to provide a source of energy, and is found deposited around the kidneys and thymus and between the shoulders. The rodent's visceral anatomy is shown in Figure 13.3.

BIOLOGIC AND REPRODUCTIVE DATA

It is important for a technician to know physiologic data for small rodents (Table 13.1). This aids in determining an animal's state of health and also helps answer questions that owners commonly ask. It should be noted that gerbils form monogamous pairs, which should be set up before the animals reach maturity. Attempts to separate and re-pair a mated pair will result in fighting and may result in death.

HUSBANDRY

Rodent housing should be escape proof, chew proof, and easily cleaned. A variety of metal and plastic caging is available. Solid flooring is easy to clean and may help prevent trauma to the toes, feet, and legs. Breeding animals should be housed on solid flooring. Adequate ventilation is important because the buildup of ammonia from urea breakdown contributes to upper respiratory disease (Harkness and Wagner 1989). Wire caging promotes better ventilation than plastic-shoebox-type or tunnel-type caging, but wire bottom cages are dangerous for toes, feet, and limbs and are thus not recommended. Lameness is a common sequeale to wire bottom caging. Cleaning tunnel-type cages frequently solves some of their ventilation problems. Further, plastic caging with tunnels and toys provides more environmental enrichment and exercise for the animals than simple wire caging. If kept clean, these tunnel-type caging environments are indeed best.

A variety of bedding materials have been available for sometime, including ash and pine wood shavings and corncob. More recently, various absorbent paper products, developed for rodents and birds, have become available. The paper products are safer. They are not irritating to the feet and toes, and they are designed to break down if ingested and therefore usually do not cause impactions. Wood shavings can be too rough, or pointed, and cause lesions and abrasions, especially on the feet and toes, leading to pododermatitis. Due to the sensitive respiratory system of rats, wood shavings in general are not recommended because they produce so much dust. The use of cedar wood shavings is completely contraindicated; the aromatic oils are irritating and alone can cause pododermatitis. If cleaning is performed adequately (two or more times a week), scented bedding, such as dangerous cedar shavings, is unnecessary. Further, many wood shavings have chemical products in them that can adversely affect the liver and can also cause eye damage, among other problems. Corncob is the most absorbent, but is prone to fungal growth and if fine can be ingested by some species, leading to fatal GI impactions. In summary, the most important consideration is that the bedding be clean, dry, nonabrasive, non-nutritional, and supplied in ample quantities, so that the animal can dig or burrow.

In addition to the bedding substrate, breeding animals should be provided with some form of nesting

Table 13.1. Physiological data of selected rodents.

Physiological data	Mouse	Rat	Gerbil	Hamster
Lifespan	1–3 years	2–4 years	3–4 years	18–24 months
Adult weight M/F	20–40 g/25–40 g	300–520 g/250–300 g	65–120 g/55–95 g	85–130 g/95–150 g
Body temperature °F	98–101	96.6–99.5	98.6–101.3	98.6–101.4
Heart rate (bpm)	300–750	250–450	360	300–500
Respiratory rate (bpm) 60–220	70–120	90	35–135	
Puberty	35 days	37–67 days	70–84 days	45–75 days
Estrous cycle	4–5 days	4–5 days	4–7 days	3–4 days
Gestation	19–21 days	21–23 days	24–26 days	15 days
Weaning age	21–28 days	21 days	21–30 days	20–25 days

material. Lack of appropriate nesting material can result in the death of offspring (Harkness and Wagner 1995), either through abandonment or cannibalism, as can disturbing the nest in an effort to clean the cage. Commercial nesting products such as "nestlets" are available, or white tissue paper or paper towels can be used. Do not use old cotton towels because the animals can get entangled in the cotton fibers. This entanglement can cause constrictions leading to loss of toes, feet, or limbs. Further, be sure that the cages are cleaned just prior to parturition and stocked with all that the dam will need. Ensure that the soon-to-be-lactating dam will have enough food to last about a week, and do not disturb the nest in any way. Do not handle the young at all during this time unless absolutely necessary, because cannibalism of offspring is most common within the first five days of parturition.

Exercise wheels and balls are popular with pet owners and provide the animal with a healthy activity. Routinely check the wheels for any rough or sharp areas, and caution owners using plastic balls to keep them away from stairs and other pets. Most rodent species are more active at night, so placing the animal in an area other than the bedrooms might be a good idea. A small amount of vegetable-based oil applied on the axle of a metal wheel temporarily helps eliminate any squeaking.

NUTRITION

Monogastric mice, rats, gerbils, and hamsters are omnivores and will eat anything—plant, animal, plastic, rubber, etc. if they get hungry enough or curious enough. Therefore, offer a fresh pelleted diet, such as those used for laboratory rodents, daily in ample amounts. Be sure to buy the standard rodent chow pelleted diet from a reliable dealer who sells a lot and maintains fresh stock. In addition to the pelleted diets, all rodents are coprophagic and eat a fair amount of fecal pellets, providing them with B vitamins produced by their colonic bacteria.

Pelleted diets are preferred over seed mixtures, which contribute to nutritionally related diseases. Seeds can be given, but are best saved for an occasional treat or a flushing food given during pre-breeding and breeding periods, and as a supplement during lactation. A small amount of fresh foods can be given as snacks (carrots, sliced apple, or greens) but should be removed if not eaten within four to six hours. If fresh foods are not removed, spoilage can occur, fostering both fungal and bacterial growth.

Crocks are recommended over plastic bowls that the animal may chew on and wire hoppers, which may cause facial abrasions (Harkness and Wagner 1989. Mothers with litters should have their food placed in a crock and directly in the cage on top of dry bedding for easier access.

Fresh water should be provided daily, and water bottle mechanisms need to be checked each day to ensure that they are functioning properly. Sipper tubes or drinking valves may become clogged with bedding or other foreign material, preventing the animal from having access to water. Intelligent, bored rodents are notorious for placing food or bedding directly into their water bottles through the valve. Alternately, a malfunctioning water bottle may leak into the cage or not function at all, leading to dehydration. The bottle should be mounted on the outside of the cage with only the metal tube extending into the cage. This prevents the animal from chewing any plastic or rubber parts. The water bottle should never be filled completely. An air bubble is needed to ensure the water will come out of the sipper tube when licked.

COMMON PARASITES, DISEASES, AND ZOONOSES

Many of the medical problems seen in rodents, and especially pet mice, are associated with the skin.

Acariasis is the skin condition that results from mite infestation. Most species of mites are host specific. Rodents can be affected by several species of skin mites; however, the most commonly encountered mites are the *Myobia* sp., *Myocoptes* sp., and *Radfordia* sp., which are spread through exposure to infected animals and bedding.

Signs include alopecia, dermatitis, rough hair coat, and skin lesions from excessive scratching. The rump area is typically involved and the lesions present as scaly, scabby dermatitis. These signs are most commonly seen in mice and hamsters. Further, geriatric male hamsters over 1.5 years of age typically develop dermatitis secondary to chronic kidney disease, lowered immune system, systemic disease, or malnutrition.

Some mite species can be visualized with a hand lens, or microscopically with a skin scraping. Ectoparasites can be treated with a variety of antiparasitic agents including ivermectin and amitraz (Mitaban) (Quesenberry and Carpenter 2003). Caging must be concurrently cleaned. Alopecia in mice housed in

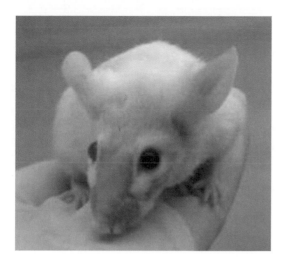

Figure 13.4. Barbering on a mouse. (Courtesy of Animal Care Services, University of Florida.)

groups may be a result of barbering rather than an infestation with an ectoparasite.

Barbering behavior occurs when dominant mice chew on the whiskers and hair around the muzzle and eyes of subordinate mice. Usually, barbering occurs in a symmetrical pattern that is consistent with all animals in the cage. Barbering is not normally associated with dermatitis but can lead to it (Figure 13.4) . Typically a cage of mice will be suspected if one mouse in an affected group is not suffering from hair loss. Usually the unaffected mouse is the dominant mouse, and it should be removed from the group to stop the cycle. Barbering is most common in female mice and can also be seen in breeding pairs (including pups). Groups of male mice are usually fine, if litters are raised together from birth. However, unknown males put together in the same cage will fight ferociously. The most commonly affected areas during fighting are the rump, back, shoulders, tail, feet, and genitals (Figure 13.5). It is not uncommon for the entire penis (including os penis) to be bitten off in severe cases of fighting. Any genital wounds should be monitored closely to ensure the animal can urinate with no problems.

Mechanical abrasions result from self trauma on cage bars, equipment, etc. This type of alopecia is husbandry related, and most commonly occurs around the lateral muzzle. Alopecia in this area is secondary to chafing on drinking valves, metal feeders, or metal cage tops, and may be followed by dermatitis.

Mange in a rat is shown in Figure 13.6. Mange is typically caused by *Demodex nanus* in rats, but is a rare condition. This condition is also rare in gerbils. *Staphylococcus aureus* ulcerative dermatitis occurs in rats secondary to self-inflicted scratching wounds or fur mite infestation, or over inflamed salivary glands.

Avascular necrosis of the tail, or ring tail, occurs in both mice and rats. Ringtail can be caused by several factors, but is most commonly associated with low humidity (less than 20%) and is more commonly seen during winter months when heating devices may be used. It is more common in laboratory rodents, but can be seen in pet mice and rats. Treatment involves tail amputation below the necrotic annular constriction.

Common endoparasites include pinworms and tapeworms. Clinical signs may not be present, but may include weight loss, diarrhea, and rectal prolapse in young animals. Detection of parasites is performed either through examination of fecal matter, through fecal floatation, or, for pinworms, by the cellophane tape test. The cellophane tape test is only about 30% accurate. A more accurate diagnosis is a cecal smear.

To perform the cellophane tape test:

1. Assemble the following supplies: cellophane tape, microscope slide, microscope.
2. Press a small piece of the cellophane tape against the perianal area. For pinworms, testing is best done in the early afternoon, around 2 pm, when the pinworm ova are exiting the animal's rectum.
3. Place the tape on a microscope slide, sticky side down, for examination (Quesenberry and Carpenter 2003, Hillyer and Quesenberry 1997).
4. Examine the slide for the slightly banana-shaped pinworm ova.

Note: Pinworm eggs are known to be sticky and very difficult to eradicate in the environment. Treatment is long and arduous.

Neoplasia occurs in rodents, with mammary tumors a common finding in females (Figure 13.7). Rats get predominately benign mammary fibroadenomas and mice get predominately malignant mammary adenocarcinomas. Extensive mammary tissue may result in the tumor being located on the abdomen or shoulders. The tumors often interfere with the animal's ability to walk normally, and chronic mechanical irritation can cause them to become ulcerated (Harkness and Wagner 1989). Systemic and cutaneous lymphoma is common in hamsters both old and young. Young hamsters develop lymphoma secondary to hamster polyoma virus (HaPV). Male gerbils get squamous cell carci-

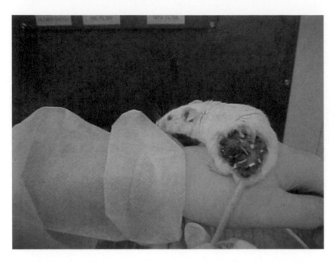

Figure 13.5. *Male rat with fight wounds on its back. (Courtesy of Animal Care Services, University of Florida.)*

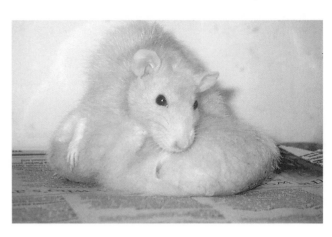

Figure 13.7. *Neoplasia in a rat.*

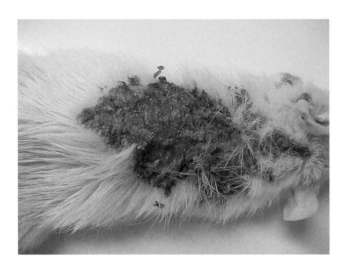

Figure 13.6. *Mange with a bacterial infection in a rat.*

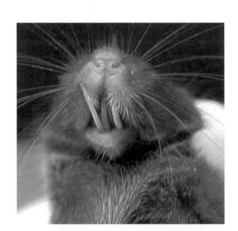

A

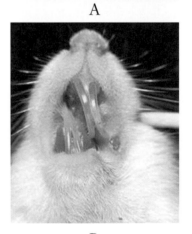

B

Figure 13.8. *(A) Malocclusion in a mouse. (B) Malocclusion in a rat. (Courtesy of Animal Care Services, University of Florida.)*

noma (SCC) of the ventral marking gland and female gerbils get ovarian granulosa cell tumors.

Malocclusion results when the continuously erupting incisors are misaligned (Figure 13.8). This misalignment prevents the teeth from being worn down during normal daily activities. Common signs of malocclusion include weight loss, drooling, and oral trauma. Malocclusion is genetic. Breeding animals with malocclusion should be avoided at all costs. Other causes include malnutrition, disease, and injury (Harkness and Wagner 1989). Periodic trimming with a dental burr, clippers, or a sharp pair of scissors must be done carefully to avoid splitting the tooth; rough edges should be filed smooth. Splitting teeth can result in the formation of abscesses.

Moist dermatitis commonly occurs in rodents that are chronically exposed to wet conditions, or in those with trauma to the skin from urine scald, diarrhea, abrasions, cuts, or other breaks in skin integrity. The most common condition affecting gerbils, facial eczema "sore nose," causes a moist dermatitis lesion on the face and nose caused by an accumulation of Harderian gland secretions. (Quesenberry and Carpenter 2003, Hillyer and Quesenberry 1997). Other causes should be ruled out, such as malocclusion, damaged crockery or caging, and abrasive bedding. Treatment involves clipping the hair from the lesion, cleaning the area, and removing any known causative agents. The veterinarian may prescribe systemic and or topical antibiotics.

Hamsters with diarrhea are often referred to as having "wet-tail" (Figure 13.9). Young animals are particularly sensitive to proliferative ileitis, especially if recently weaned. Multiple bacteria are implicated in the cause, as well as improper diet and stress. Signs are hunched posture, matted hair, watery diarrhea, lethargy, rectal prolapse, and death. Careful husbandry may help prevent the disease, and the veterinarian may prescribe antibiotic therapy (Harkness and Wagner 1989).

Gerbils are susceptible to epileptiform seizures that can result from excitement related to handling. The seizures can be mild, resulting in a dazed or hypnotic appearance, or severe, and the activity may last only a few seconds to a minute or more. There is no treatment and anticonvulsant drugs are not indicated. Exposure to frequent handling at a young age may help prevent the seizures from occurring (Harkness and Wagner 1989).

From a zoonotic perspective, the following infectious diseases are of concern because they are common and transmissible to humans: lymphocytic choriomeningitis (LCM), a virus; and *Staphacoccus* sp., *Streptacoccus* sp., *Pasturella* sp., *Klebsiella* sp., and Salmonella, bacterial diseases.

Other relatively common diseases of rodents include mouse hepatitis virus (MHV), mouse parvovirus (MPV), mouse norovirus (MNV), mycoplasmosis, sialodacryoadenitis virus, and lymphocytic choriomeningitis.

LCM is found naturally in wild mouse populations and can be passed via arthropod vectors and through bodily secretions and bite wounds. Clinical signs, if present, include a hunched posture, unthrifty appearance, photophobia, and convulsions. LCM is zoonotic; humans can become infected through contact with infected tissue, urine, or a bite wound. Clinical signs are similar to those associated with influenza and include headache, fever, muscle aches, malaise, and meningitis.

MHV is a highly contagious disease that can cause severe diarrhea and death in very young (one- to two-week-old) mice. MNV is fairly new a subclinical virus. MPV also results in enteritis, but can be both subclinical and devastating.

Chronic respiratory disease (CRD) in rodents may be caused by *Mycoplasma pulmonis*. Animals can be carriers of *Mycoplasma pulmonis* but never show any signs. CRD is very common in rats and clinical signs will be amplified if unsanitary living conditions, improper husbandry materials, and increased ammonia content are present. Respiratory disease, caused by infectious agents, is the most common health concern in rats. CRD is also referred to as murine respiratory mycoplasmosis in mice. Clinical signs include general upper respiratory signs; severe porphyrin staining around the eyes, nose, and mouth; as well as rhinitis and a possible head tilt associated with otitis. Antibiotics can be employed to help control the signs, but will never completely eradicate the disease.

Sialodacryoadenitis virus is a coronavirus related to MHV and is spread through respiratory secretions. Infection causes the cervical lymph nodes to swell and the salivary glands to become inflamed. Affected animals may continue to eat despite swelling in the neck. A very noticeable sign is chromodacryorrhea, or porphyrin staining or "red tears." The animal may be sensitive to light and develop ophthalmic lesions.

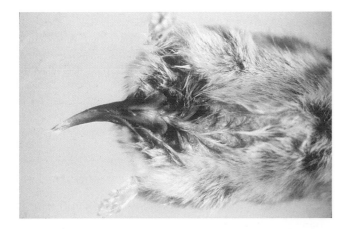

Figure 13.9. Wet tail.

Tyzzer's disease is a fatal hepatoenteric infectious disease that hamsters and gerbils may also contract. Tyzzer's is caused by *Clostridium piliforme*. Mice and rats that contract this disease can overcome it. Clinical signs in hamsters and gerbils include sudden death, listlessness, rough hair coat, and weight loss. Stress is a major contributing factor in addition to exposure to infected bedding. In general, gerbils do not contract many diseases, when compared to other rodents,

There are diseases with zoonotic potential aside from LCM, *Staphylococcus* sp., *Streptacoccus* sp., *Pasturella* sp., *Klebsiella* sp., and *Salmonella*, many of which are more common in wild rodent populations than in domestic rodents. According to the Centers for Disease Control, the risk of a human contracting Korean hemorrhagic fever or the organism responsible for bubonic plague from a pet rodent is extremely remote in the United States (CDC, personal communication). People with immunosuppression are at higher risk, and practicing good hygiene is essential. Rat bite fever is a bacterial infection causing chills, fever, myalgia, localized swelling at the wound site, and headache. It is also possible to contract hymenolepid tapeworm infection, which causes enteric disease in humans (Quesenberry and Carpenter 2003, Hillyer and Quesenberry 1997, Harkness and Wagner 1989). Other zoonotic concerns include rabies, which is extremely rare in rodents, and rodent allergies from urine and dander, which are very common and of great concern to the CDC.

BEHAVIOR

Most rodents are nocturnal but are easily awakened during the day. Gentle handling will prevent a startled animal from biting out of defense. Male mice, gerbils, and hamsters fight with each other, and should be housed alone unless raised together since birth. Hamsters of either sex are better housed singly than in groups, and should only be brought together for mating (Figure 13.10).Gerbils are known to establish monogamous pairs, but fighting in older gerbils that previously seemed to peacefully coexist may develop, and can result in serious wounds. Because many rodents are kept as pets for small children, separate housing is recommended because witnessing such activity could be traumatic.

The exception to the housing recommendation is the rat. Rats are very social animals and tend to do better if housed with a cage mate (Figure 13.11). Rats

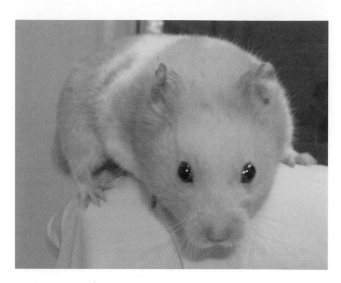

Figure 13.10. Hamsters are best kept as solitary pets.

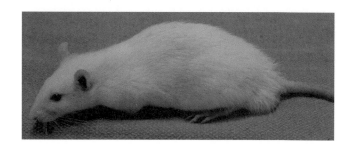

Figure 13.11. Rats are very social and non-aggressive and should always be housed with a cage mate.

of both sexes can be grouped together and females with litters can be left in communal housing with relative safety, provided conditions are not overcrowded. Females will share in caring for and nursing young animals.

Cannibalism of young may occur if nests are disturbed or the mother is overly nervous. This behavior is most often associated with hamsters and mice; gerbils seem less sensitive to disturbance and rats rarely cannibalize their offspring. It is imperative to ensure the cage is supplied with clean bedding and adequate food and water prior to parturition to prevent having to disturb the nest once the offspring have been born.

HISTORY AND
PHYSICAL EXAMINATION

Rodents should be brought to the hospital in the cage in which they are normally housed. The cage should be covered to protect the rodent from temperature changes, noise, and disease exposure. The person scheduling the appointment should advise the client not to clean the cage prior to coming into the hospital. This allows the staff to observe the condition of the cage, the presence of fecal material, type of bedding, and so on. Ideally, the client should sit away from cats and dogs once at the hospital to prevent further stress. The exam room should be stocked with urine dipsticks for immediate sampling because most rodents urinate as soon as they are handled or touched in the genital area (Quesenberry and Carpenter 2003, Hillyer and Quesenberry 1997).

As with any patient, clients should be asked where they obtained the pet, how long they have had it, what they feed it, and if this is the first time they have owned this particular species. Discuss with clients when they first noticed any signs of illness, how long the problem has existed, and what, if anything, they have done in response to the signs. Rodents must be weighed using a gram scale, and in a small container to prevent escape. Unless the practice has a thermometer specifically designed for use in rodents, forgo obtaining a rectal temperature. Standard thermometers are too large to use safely.

RESTRAINT AND HANDLING

Firm but gentle handling is important when working with rodents. They may bite out of fear, and also jump or run quickly in an effort to escape. Falls to the floor are survivable, but could easily result in fracture of the liver, feet or limbs, ribs, or spine.

Most rodents are amenable to being gently scooped up into the hands to lift them from their cages. This is indeed the best way to pick them up. Rats and mice can be briefly lifted by the base of the tail onto a table or other surface if scooping does not work with the animal in question. Gerbils should never be restrained or held by their tail. Prolonged handling of the tail can cause trauma, such as sloughing of the skin and exposing the vertebrae, especially in gerbils. Sloughing can also occur in rats and mice. Grasping the tail at its base prevents tail trauma. Use of a towel, screen or barred lid of the animal's cage gives it something to hold onto when being restrained on a table. Rodents showing signs of aggression or agitation (chattering, vocalizing, rolling onto their backs, and in gerbils, thumping of the hind feet) can be picked up with an empty plastic container or lifted with a small towel folded for thickness. Gloves may be needed to handle some rats, but they are often unwieldy and can make it difficult to feel what the animal is doing. Therefore, care must be taken to observe the animal for any respiratory difficulty. Laboratory animal supply companies (i.e., Kent Scientific, Torrington, CT) have plastic restraint devices.

To handle gerbils, mice, and rats:

1. The animal should be scooped up. The base of the tail should be gently grasped only if need be, prior to scooping.
2. The animal should then be lifted out of its enclosure, and the animal's body allowed to rest on a hand, arm, or table. A hold should be maintained on the tail while supporting the animal's body to prevent escape (gerbils are excellent jumpers) (Figure 13.12).
3. Rats can be lifted by placing a hand over the dorsum and gently pressing the forelimbs together under the rat's chin with the thumb and index finger.

To handle a hamster:

1. If the animal is awake, it can usually be scooped up gently using both hands; use caution if the hamster is sleeping because startled hamsters may bite.
2. If there is concern that the hamster may react aggressively, a piece of toweling or an empty plastic container may be used to lift the animal up.

For injections or other procedures that the rodent may object to, the animal may be scruffed:

1. It is helpful to place the rodent on a towel or the top of a wire cage while maintaining a gentle hold on the tail.
2. Slight traction should be applied to the base of the tail, which will encourage the animal to grip onto the surface with its front feet.
3. Grasp the loose skin over the neck, using the little finger of the restraining hand to hold the tail.
4. Scruffing a hamster can be more difficult; the abundance of loose skin can still permit the animal to turn and bite if the restrainer has not grasped a sufficient amount. An indication of a sufficient amount of skin grasped is when the hamster "smiles" (Figure 13.13).

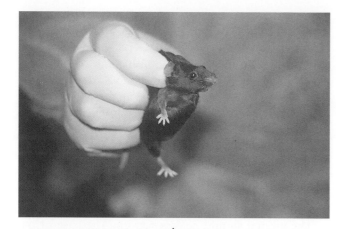

A

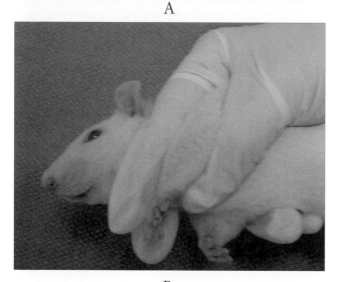

B

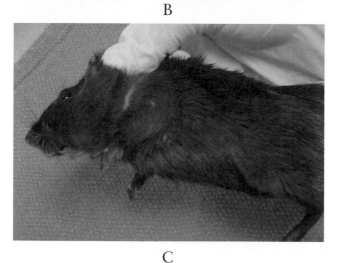

C

Figure 13.12. (A) Mouse restraint. (B) Rat restraint. (C) Gerbil restraint.

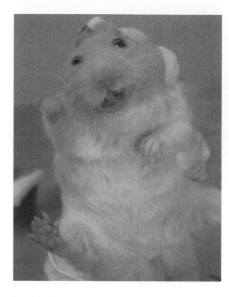

Figure 13.13. Hamster restraint.

RADIOLOGY

Sedation is usually needed for most radiography to have proper positioning. Whole-body studies are often employed due to the size of the patient. Animals may be placed in radiolucent tubing or briefly positioned with paint/masking tape. Exposure times of 1/60 of a second are best due to the rapid respiratory and heart rates of rodents.

SURGERY AND ANESTHESIA

Common surgical procedures include ovariohysterectomy, castration, tumor excision, and abscess draining. Surgical preparation is similar to that of any small animal, except pro-longed fasting of the animal prior to anesthesia is not necessary and could result in hypoglycemia, because it reduces glycogen stores in the liver. Surgical scrub solutions should be warmed, as should the surgical tables (using a warm water circulating pad), the peri-operative fluids, and the recovery incubator. This prevents unnecessary heat loss to the patient. Hypothermia is the number one killer of rodents, especially mice, that undergo surgery. All rules of aseptic technique apply, and the surgical suite and equipment should be prepared accordingly. Sterile surgical tape can be used to restrain the animal on the table post induction.

Rodents can be chamber or face-mask induced using isoflurane gas. Intubation is difficult in rodents, but they can be maintained using a face mask or a plastic syringe case modified to use as a nose cone. A non-rebreathing system should always be used (Quesenberry and Carpenter 2003, Hillyer and Quesenberry 1997).

The technician should monitor the depth and quality of respiration. The deeper the animal's anesthetic plane becomes, the more the abdominal muscles will move with each breath. The animals normally breathe with their abdomen/diaphragm. When they start to use their chest and move their forelimbs, they are having problems. Lightly anesthetized rodents will still blink when the eyelashes are touched. The palpebral reflex will be diminished as the animal enters a surgical plane. The ears or toes can be pinched to evaluate the animal's ability to react; if the animal reacts, the plane of anesthesia is still light (Quesenberry and Carpenter 2003, Hillyer and Quesenberry 1997). Ears are best on mice, and toes are best on rats.

Mucous membranes should be pink, and the color can be evaluated using the pads of the feet, ears, eyes if albino, and gingiva. Pulse oximeters are commonly found in most small animal hospitals and can be placed on the tail, tongue, or foot pad.

Recovery from surgery should be in a pre-warmed incubator as described above; the incubator should be situated in a quiet area. The technician should gently turn the animal from side to side every few minutes to prevent pooling of blood on the dependent side. Rodents will attempt to chew sutures and bandages; surgical glue, staples, or subcuticular sutures are best. Elizabethan collars are available commercially. Those with Velcro closures are tolerated the best. The sedative effects of opioid analgesics, such as buprenorphine, often are enough to prevent self-trauma to the surgical site. Nonsteroidal anti-inflammatory drugs, such as meloxicam, may also be used in rodents for minor surgery.

BANDAGING AND WOUND CARE

Rodents easily become stressed and daily wound care may do more harm than good. Wounds should be cleaned as thoroughly as possible during the initial treatment phase. The use of intact white paper towels for the first forty-eight hours post-surgery allows for easier observation, keeps the wound cleaner, and enables better drainage. After this initial time period, advise the owner to increase the frequency of bedding changes to keep the healing wounds as clean as possible.

EMERGENCY AND CRITICAL CARE

Unfortunately, many of infectious diseases of rodents are challenging to treat and historically, harsher antibiotics were known to cause fatal reactions. Today, enrofloxcin is an example of a safe and effective rodent antibiotic. It can easily be delivered through the drinking water, thus decreasing the stress of handling. Supportive care in the form of subcutaneous fluids, dextrose, calcium, adequate dietary support such as diet gel (a fluid and food combination choice), and heat and oxygen must be administered immediately.

Wet tail or proliferative ileitis in hamsters may respond to improved diet, sanitation, and aggressive supportive care, including enrofloxcin parentally initially and later in the drinking water, but the animal's prognosis is guarded (Plunkett 1993).

Animals suffering from bite wounds or lacerations may be extremely stressed and vocal. Be cautious when attempting to pick up an animal in this condition, because it may respond aggressively. The patient should be kept warm and quiet until it can be anesthetized with isoflurane, if necessary, for wound care.

SEX DETERMINATION

Males and females can be distinguished by comparing anogenital distance. The distance from the anus to the genital papilla is greater in the male than in the female. This can be difficult to assess if there are no other animals present for comparison purposes. In hamsters, the male has a rounded posterior when viewed from above due to the scrotum, whereas the female's posterior appears more square (Figures 13.14, 13.15). Male gerbils have a larger mid-ventral scent gland (Figure 13.16).

TECHNIQUES

Administration of Medications
Parenteral administration sites include IV (difficult), IM (may cause necrosis and is usually not recommended due to the small muscle mass), IP (common in lab animals), and SQ (preferred site, safest and easiest).

IV
Intravenous injection of drugs is difficult to accomplish in rodents. The most commonly used site is the lateral tail vein in mice, rats, and gerbils. Four vessels are present on the tail, two veins and two arteries. Veins

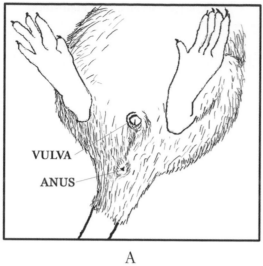

A

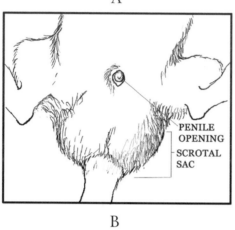

B

Figure 13.14. *Sex determination. (A) Female. (B) Male.*

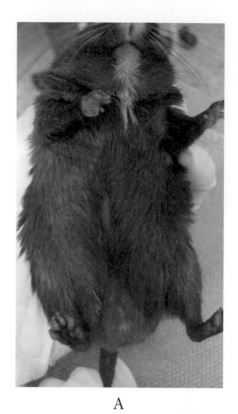

A

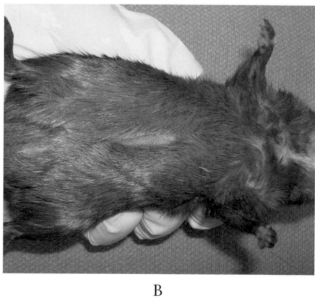

B

Figure 13.16. *(A and B) Gerbil scent glands.*

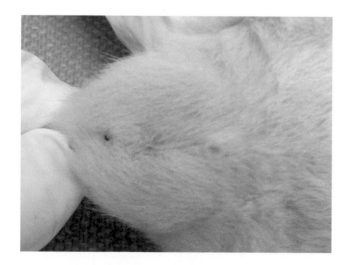

Figure 13.15. *Hamster testicles.*

are located laterally on the tail and arteries are dorsal/ventral (Figure 13.17).

For IV injection:

1. Assemble supplies: 27- to 30-gauge (mice) 22- to 25-gauge (rats and gerbils) needles, tuberculin syringes, chlorohexidine, and alcohol swabs.
2. Unless a restraint device is used, a second individual will need to restrain the animal.
3. Clean the venipuncture site with chlorohexidine and alcohol. Warming the tail with a focal heat light (penlight) may be useful to help visualize the vein and cause vasodilation.
4. Always slowly aspirate to ensure proper placement. Note that due to the low blood pressure of the mouse, there will not always be a flash of blood when in the vein.
5. Once the injection is completed, apply gentle pressure as the needle is removed to allow for clot formation.
6. Dispose of the needle into a puncture-proof biohazard container.

IM

The quadriceps muscle can be used to administer injections in all four rodents discussed. Only very small amounts of drug can safely be injected into this site due to the small size of the patient (0.05 ml in mice, up to 0.3 ml in rats) or necrosis will result. Care must be taken not to inject into the posterior thigh because irritation of the sciatic nerve may result. It may help to "pinch up" the muscle mass between the fingers of one hand while injecting with the other.

For IM injection:

1. Assemble supplies: 25-gauge needles for mice, up to 22-gauge needles for larger rats, tuberculin syringes, chlorohexidine, and alcohol swabs.

2. Have an assistant restrain the animal if a commercial restraint device is not available.
3. Always aspirate prior to administering any medication to ensure correct placement.
4. Inject drug and withdraw the needle.
5. Dispose of needle into a puncture-proof biohazard container.

IP

IP injections allow for larger volumes of drug to be injected than can be safely given IM or IV. However, SQ injections are safer than all of the above-mentioned injections, and allow for larger volumes of drugs to be injected. IP injections are not without risk and should have limited applications in pet medicine. Care must be taken not to puncture any abdominal organs. IP injections in rats require injecting into the left caudal quadrant, rather than the right, as in gerbils, mice, and hamsters (Figure 13.18). The rat's cecum is located in the right caudal quadrant. Slight resistance may be felt as the needle penetrates the abdominal muscles.

For IP injection:

1. Assemble the following supplies: 21– to 27-gauge needles, syringes, chlorohexidine, and alcohol swabs.
2. Restraining the animal in one hand by scruffing the loose skin over the back of the neck and shoulders is required. The little finger of the same hand can be used to keep the tail pressed against the palm of the hand.
3. The animal's head should be tilted lower than the rest of the body to cause the abdominal organs to fall forward.

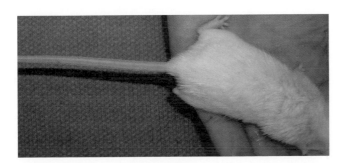

Figure 13.17. Dorsal tail artery on a mouse; note tail injections and blood venipuncture are performed via the tail vein, located bi-laterally on the tail.

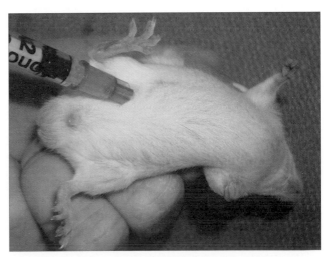

Figure 13.18. IP injection in a mouse. Note that for the mouse it is injected from the animal's right and in rats it is injected from the animal's left.

4. The needle should be inserted, bevel up, at an angle of about 20 degrees into the right caudal quadrant unless it is a rat, in which case use of the left caudal quadrant is required.
5. The syringe should be aspirated to ensure no organs have been punctured with the needle. If any yellow or greenish-brown fluid or any blood is aspirated, the needle and syringe should immediately be withdrawn and discarded. The procedure should be attempted again with a new needle and syringe, and the animal should immediately be started on parenteral antibiotics.
6. The needle should be disposed of in a puncture-proof biohazard container.

SQ

Larger drug volumes can also be given subcutaneously (1 to 3 ml in mice, up to 5 to 10 ml in rats). The injection can be given under the skin along the flank, or in the loose skin of the neck, which is simultaneously being scruffed for restraint purposes.

For SQ injection:

1. Assemble the following supplies: a 22- to 25-gauge needle for mice, 20-gauge needle for rats, syringes.
2. The animal's loose skin over the neck should be scruffed. This is the best area for SQ injections.
3. The needle should be inserted into the tented skin between the fingers. It is often easier to position the syringe over the animal's head and point the needle toward its hindquarters if doing this alone.
4. Aspirate prior to injecting the medication to ensure proper placement.
5. The needle should be disposed of in a puncture-proof biohazard container.

Oral Administration

Unprofessionally compounded medications mixed into food or water can affect the taste, leading to the animal's refusing to eat or drink. Liquid medications can be more accurately administered to awake animals by gavage, or slowly and carefully by tuberculin syringe. Gavage needles have ball-like tips to prevent trauma to the animal, and may be straight, curved, or bent (depending on the operator's preference). Professionally compounded medications can be made up without flavor, color, or odor, or they can be made up in the flavor, color, and odor of the rodent's own pelleted diet. These two options increase palatability and decrease stress because the animal can receive its medications in its own food or water and not know it.

Gavaging

For gavaging:

1. Gather the following supplies: a gavage needle of appropriate gauge and length attached to a syringe large enough to hold the entire dose of medication.
2. The top of the gavage needle should be lined up with the animal's nose, and the ball of the needle lined up with the animal's last rib to gauge depth of gavage needle insertion.
3. Wetting the ball of the needle with water may help it slide down more easily.
4. The animal should be restrained by scruffing the loose skin over the back of the neck, tucking the tail under the little finger. The animal should be held vertically with the head up.
5. The gavage needle should be inserted into the space behind the incisors, and the needle gently pushed into the animal's mouth, allowing it to follow the curve of the mouth down into the esophagus.
6. If any resistance is felt, or the animal becomes cyanotic (indicating you are probably in the trachea),

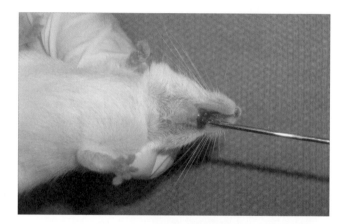

A

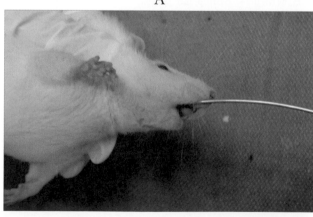

B

Figure 13.19. (A) Gavaging a mouse. (B) Gavaging a rat.

immediately remove the needle, put the animal on oxygen, treat with parenteral antibiotics, and repeat if the animal fully recovers.

7. When inserted to the level measured in step 2, inject the contents of the syringe and withdraw the gavage needle (Figure 13.19).

Blood Collection

In all rodents, except the hamster, blood can be collected from the tail veins located laterally on the tail. It is recommended that no more than 0.14 ml of blood be collected from mice, 0.3 ml collected from a gerbil, 0.65 ml from a hamster, and 1.3 ml from a rat (Quesenberry and Carpenter 2003, Hillyer and Quesenberry 1997). The saphenous vein is another option and works quite well in rodents.

To collect blood:

1. Assemble the following supplies: 23– to 27-gauge needles, tuberculin syringes or 3 cc syringe if a rat, chlorohexidine and alcohol swabs, restraint device if available (rodent restrainers that leave the tail free are commercially available and work quite well).

2. Have an assistant restrain the animal if no restraint device is available.

3. Warming the tail with a warm water compress or low-wattage light may help to visualize the vein and will cause vasodilation.

4. Pressure must be applied proximally to the venipuncture site, and can be accomplished using a rubber band and hemostats.

5. The needle should be inserted bevel up into the vein and gently aspirated to prevent collapsing the vessel.

6. After blood collection, apply pressure to the venipuncture site as the needle is withdrawn to prevent hematoma formation (Figure 13.20).

Blood can also be collected retro-orbitally by puncturing the venous sinus or plexus with a microhematocrit tube or a beveled micropipette tip inserted into the medial canthus of the eye. This procedure requires the animal to be anesthetized briefly with isoflurane (Figure 13.21). There is a risk of causing damage to the eye, so this procedure should only be performed

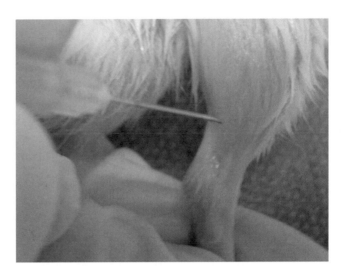

Figure 13.20. Blood collection from the saphenous vein in a rat. Note that sterile KY lubrication is used to part the fur and enable drop blood collection into the collection tube.

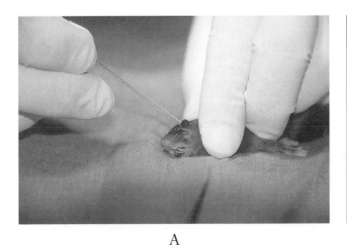

A

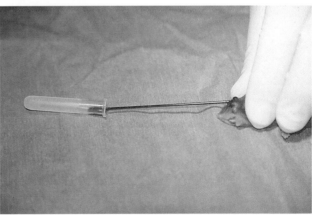

B

Figure 13.21. Blood collection from the venous sinus. (A) Restraint of a mouse during the initial insertion of a microhematocrit tube into the medial canthus. (B) Blood collection after successful puncture of the venous sinus with the microhematocrit tube.

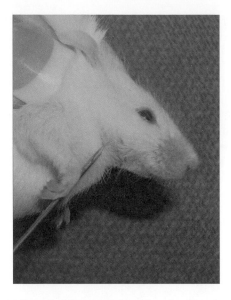

Figure 13.22. *Submandibular blood collection in a mouse.*

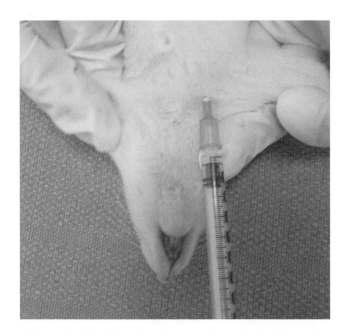

Figure 13.23. *Blood collection from the jugular vein of a rat.*

by highly skilled personnel and never with the owner present. Alternatively, submandibular bleeds can be performed on the mouse and the rat (Figure 13.22). This method is easier and safer. It also enables more blood to be collected and is best performed without anesthesia.

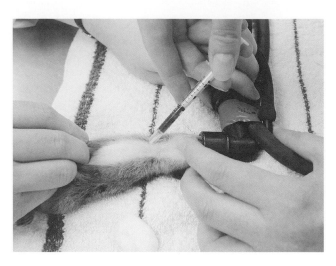

Figure 13.24. *Blood being drawn from a rat using the cranial vena cava, an uncommon route.*

To collect blood at the medial canthus of the eye:

1. Assemble the following supplies: microhematocrit tubes or beveled micropipette tips, gauze sponges, ophthalmic ointment, isoflurane machine.
2. Insert the microhematocrit tube into the eye at the medial canthus, rotating the tube gently to puncture the sinus.
3. Blood will fill the tube by capillary action.
4. Following the collection of blood, the tube should be removed, excess blood wiped from the site, and the eyelids gently held shut until hemostasis occurs.
5. Apply a sterile ophthalmic ointment into the eye (Quesenberry and Carpenter 2003, Hillyer and Quesenberry 1997).

The jugular vein is the preferred and recommended site for venipuncture and blood collection in rats (Figure 13.23). While not a common venipuncture route, blood can be drawn from the anterior vena cava in rats. Further, anesthesia is required for venipuncture of the anterior vena cava, the method has inherent risks, and is generally highly discouraged (Figure 13.24). Additional information about venipuncture using the anterior vena cava can be found in the technique section of Chapter 11.

EUTHANASIA

As with any pet, the owner may request to be present during the euthanasia procedure. An overdose of isoflurane is effective. If the induction chamber is relatively large, pre-fill it with the anesthetic to decrease the amount of time it will take before having the desired effect. Staff members not fond of rodents must keep in mind that pet rodent owners can be just as emotionally attached as the more familiar dog and cat owner can. Remains should be treated with the same respect afforded to all deceased pets.

Dr. Romagnano would like to express gratitude to James B. Nichols, DVM, MS, for his critical review of the chapter and his expertise. She is also grateful to Shannon Sunday, CVT, SRA, LAT, for her critical review of the chapter and expertise, and would like to thank both Shannon and Raul Ortiz-Umpierre, DVM, for taking pictures for the chapter. She would like to thank Dr. Tarah Hadley for the picture conversion.

ADDITIONAL READING

Bechtold S, et al. 2007. Laboratory Animal Technician: LAT Training Manual. American Association for Laboratory Animal Science (AALAS).

Bratcher C, et al. 2008. Laboratory Animal Technologist Training Manual. American Association for Laboratory Animal Science (AALAS).

Harkness JE, Wagner JE. 1989. The Biology and Medicine of Rabbits and Rodents. 3rd ed. Philadelphia: Lea and Febiger. 2–179.

Harkness JE, Wagner JE. 1995. The Biology and Medicine of Rabbits and Rodents, 4th ed. Philadelphia: Williams and Wilkins. 28–34.

Hillyer EV, Quesenberry KE. 1997 Ferrets, Rabbits and Rodents: Clinical Medicine and Surgery. Philadelphia: W.B. Saunders Co. 296–389.

Plunkett SJ. 1993. Emergency Procedures for the Small Animal Veterinarian. Philadelphia: W.B. Saunders Co. 177.

Quesenberry KE, Carpenter JW. 2003. Ferrets, Rabbits, and Rodents: Clinical Medicine and Surgery. 2nd ed. St. Louis: Sauders.

CHAPTER FOURTEEN

Chinchillas

Trevor Lyon and Bonnie Ballard

TAXONOMY/COMMON SPECIES SEEN IN PRACTICE

The chinchilla is classified as a rodent and is most closely related to the guinea pig. There are three subspecies of chinchilla; *Chinchilla langier* is the most commonly available in the pet trade. These animals inhabit the Andes Mountains of South America and are adapted well to living on cold and rocky slopes. Their average life span in captivity is ten years but they can live to the age of twenty. Because they are closely related to the guinea pig, similarities in their physiology, care, and treatment will be apparent.

ANATOMY AND PHYSIOLOGY

External Anatomy

There are two distinctive features in the external anatomy of the chinchilla. The first is the very dense fur that covers the entire body. It is so dense, in fact, that up to ninety individual hairs can come from each root (Hayes 2000). The second is the locomotory apparatus, which can be compared to the rabbit but is closer to that of the nutria. Chinchillas have very short front legs that are used for support and to hold food. These small legs have four digits (numbers 2, 3, 4, and 5; digit 1 is lost). The rear legs, however, are very large and powerful. Designed for jumping, they have three digits varying in size (numbers 2, 3, 4). The first and fifth digits are rudimentary only.

Digestive Tract

The mouth is largely filled by the tongue. The two lateral areas of the tongue are wider than the dorsal side, giving it an unusual shape.

The adult chinchilla has four incisors and sixteen molar-type teeth. The upper incisors usually have a right angle indentation, while the lowers are ground down to a point. Only about one third of the incisors protrude from the jaw. The grinding and cutting teeth have open roots, which means that they are growing continuously. Therefore, the correct positioning of each tooth is crucial because it assures that each tooth is being constantly ground down. There may be slight differences in dentition among the different species. The most distinctive part of the mouth is the palatal ridges. Each chinchilla, no matter how closely related, has palatal ridges that distinguish it from any other chinchilla (Kraft 1987). Their dental formula is 2(I1/1 C0/0 PM1/1 M3/3 = 20. (Quesenberry and Carpenter 2004)

The stomach is located in the abdominal cavity behind the diaphragm. It is similar in shape to that of a horse or pig. The duodenum has several afferent ducts from the pancreas as well as the bile duct. The longest portion of the small intestine is the jejunum and in conjunction with sections of the large intestine, it takes up a large portion of the abdominal cavity. The ileum is the shortest section of small bowel that makes up the transition to the cecum. The cecum in chinchillas is similar to that in other rodents; it is located on the left side of the abdomen and under normal conditions, its contents are of liquid consistency. The cecum and the ascending colon help to fill the remainder of the abdomen, as it is the segment with the greatest volume. The ascending portion of the colon is also the longest section of the large bowel. The descending portion of the bowel and the rectum are usually filled with compact fecal matter and can be easily palpated if the animal is relaxed. It is difficult to determine the end of the colon and the beginning of the rectum. The end of the rectum widens slightly before reaching the anus. The posterior end of the rectum is surrounded by glandular packets; these packets in females appear to be thicker ventrally. In males, these packets are twice the circumference of the females' packets. The skeletal anatomy is shown in Figure 14.1; the visceral anatomy is shown in Figure 14.2.

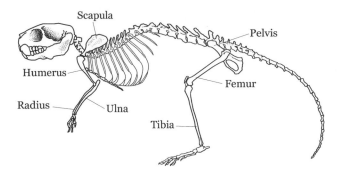

Figure 14.1. Skeletal anatomy. (Drawing by Scott Stark.)

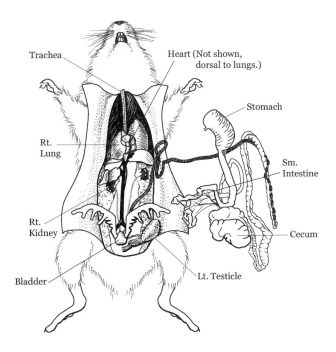

Figure 14.2. Visceral anatomy. (Drawing by Scott Stark.)

Liver

The liver is located between the diaphragm and stomach. There is very little lobulation visible and the gallbladder is located between the right and median sides. In the adult chinchilla, the liver weighs about 8 to 10 g (Kraft 1987).

Pancreas

In the chinchilla, the pancreas can be difficult to locate because it has many lobes. In addition, the surrounding fatty tissue and lymph nodes can make it difficult to distinguish with the naked eye.

Spleen

The spleen is of similar shape and location of other rodents. It is triangular in cross section and in the shape of an "L." The bottom of the "L" is located near the last rib on the left side.

Respiratory Tract

Starting with the head of the chinchilla, the first portion of the respiratory tract visualized are the nostrils. To the outside of each narrow nostril is a "false" nostril. The nasal cavities arch upward and are interconnected along the upper portion. The chinchilla's nasal cavity is very large for an animal of this size. The trachea is dorsoventrally compressed as it moves down toward the lungs. The trachea splits at the level of the fourth and fifth vertebrae, descending toward the lungs. The right lung has four distinct lobes and the left only three.

Reproductive Organs

Female sex organs (ovaries) are located just below each kidney and are very small, about the size of a grain of rice. As the female reaches maturity, small lumps appear on the ovary, giving it an unusual shape. These lumps are caused by eggs migrating to the surface of the ovary. Several eggs mature at the same time, which means that several eggs can be fertilized at the same time. Unlike other mammals, as the eggs migrate down the oviduct they do not go into the ovarian pouch. They remain in the wall of the pouch where they are fertilized. After fertilization, the eggs move via peristaltic action to the uterus. The reproductive tract ends with the vagina, which becomes very visible when the animal is in heat. It is visualized as a horizontal slit between the anus and the urethra. Unlike many other mammals, the urethra of the female chinchilla terminates outside the vagina. There are no labial folds present.

The male sex organs are somewhat different from most other mammals. The testicles do not descend down into the scrotum and are considered incomplete. Only the epididymis is located outside the abdominal cavity and there is no scrotum. The sperm cells mature in the epididymis before they move to the sperm duct, and from there, they move across the mesentery of the urinary bladder. The sperm ducts open right next to each other into the urethra, along with the openings of the other sex glands. The penis is S-shaped when in the normal resting position, with the glans penis terminating below the anus. Because the foreskin extends all the way to the anus, the actual opening is very narrow. A small bone about 1 cm long supports the penis during copulation. As blood fills the penis, pushing the tip forward, small backward facing spines can be seen. These assure better attachment during copulation.

Urinary Tract

The chinchilla's urinary system is similar to that of other mammals, in that it has two kidneys, two ureters, a bladder, and a urethra.

Anal Sacs

Located just inside the lower corner of the anal slit is a yellow nodular anal sac. Similar to dogs and cats, the chinchilla can expel the contents of this sac. It is a foul-smelling substance, which is probably used as a defense against natural enemies.

REPRODUCTION

The following are average numbers for the different species of chinchillas:

First "heat": Three to four months of age
Gestation period: 110 to 138 days
Number of young: One to three per pregnancy
Number of litters: One to two per year
Young: Born precocial

The female returns to heat every twenty-five to thirty-five days if she does not conceive. The most reliable method of determining if the female is in heat is the behavior of the male (Johnson-Delaney 1996, Kraft 1987).

HUSBANDRY

Because the chinchilla's normal habitat is the Andes Mountains in South America, it does not tolerate heat or humidity. Therefore, they should not be housed in a location where there is no protection from the heat. The enclosure should be large and made of material that they cannot chew through. The enclosure must have ample hiding places because chinchillas in the wild live mostly in caves. It is in their nature to jump, so it is recommended that the enclosure have multiple levels. Small platforms on which they can perch are also helpful. All items should be made of materials that are easily cleaned.

Suitable bedding includes aspen shavings, newspaper, or recycled newspaper products. Because of their aromatic oils, pine and cedar shavings are not recommended and can lead to respiratory problems (Mitchell

and Tully 2009). Chinchillas are much easier to keep than guinea pigs or rabbits because they seem to defecate and urinate less, so the cage stays cleaner. However, the cage should be cleaned at least once a week.

The teeth of the chinchilla grow constantly, so they need ample objects for gnawing. Branches, wood blocks, pumice stones, and salt blocks are all good choices.

The most specific requirement for chinchilla care is making a "dust bath" available on a daily basis. This helps to keep the coat and skin healthy. There are several commercial dust baths on the market; however, they can be made by using cornstarch or unscented talc powder mixed with sand. Diatomaceous earth can be used in place of sand. The bath mixture should be dry before allowing the chinchilla to use it. The mixture of choice should be placed about one to two inches deep in the bottom of a litter box, large bowl, or glass jar (one gallon or larger).

NUTRITION

Chinchillas are herbivorous and because their digestive tract is similar to that of the horse, they need large amounts of roughage. As in other rodents, chinchillas are coprophagic. In captivity a diet of hay supplemented with a good quality pelleted diet should be offered. Pellets that have 16% to 20% protein, 2% to 5% fat, and 15% to 35% bulk fiber should be obtained for feeding (Quesenberry and Carpenter 2004). If the amount of hay is inadequate, the low amount of fiber may lead to enteritis. The quality of the hay must be monitored closely. Small amounts of fruits, veggies, seeds, and grains may be offered as treats. Finally, as with all animals, fresh water must be made available at all times. Chinchillas, because they are so active, can be messy when it comes to water bowls. They will either knock them over or manage to get substrate in them. A water bottle is a preferable way to provide water, because it keeps the water and cage cleaner (Quesenberry and Carpenter 2004).

COMMON AND ZOONOTIC DISEASES

Dental Diseases

A common problem in chinchillas is "slobbers," or malocclusion (Hayes 2000). This can occur in the incisors, premolars, or molars. As the teeth overgrow, they cause ulcers of the buccal mucosa and the tongue. Clinical signs may be drooling, pawing at the mouth, weight loss, anorexia, and decrease in stool volume. Malocclusion can be caused by hereditary factors or a lack of objects in the environment to gnaw on. Routine teeth trimmings may be necessary in cases of hereditary problems.

Skin Diseases

Husbandry issues are the leading cause of skin disorders in chinchillas. Bite wounds, traumatic injuries, fur chewing, and unthrifty coat can all occur when the environmental conditions are poor. These disorders can appear rapidly if chinchillas are housed in a cage that is too small or if two incompatible animals are housed together. The animals may chew on themselves or their cage mates, which may lead to other injuries. Inadequate access to a dust bath may also cause a poor coat quality.

Dermatophytosis is a disease usually caused by the introduction of contaminated hay or bedding to the chinchilla's housing. As in other species, scaly, circular areas of hair loss around the face, feet, and ears are the most common presentation. A fungal culture should be done to confirm the diagnosis. This disease has zoonotic potential.

Gastrointestinal Diseases

Choke

Like rabbits and rats, chinchillas cannot vomit, so esophageal choke can result if the animal ingests an object too large to swallow. The most common objects are bedding and treats. The animal usually presents with excessive salivation, dyspnea, and anorexia. The object may be palpated on physical exam or diagnosed with radiographs.

Bloat

Bloat can occur for many reasons, as in other species. The chinchilla presents similarly to other animals with a distended and painful abdomen, dyspnea, and reluctance to move. Many treatments are recommended, from exercise in mild cases to decompression by transabdominal trocar.

Hairballs

Hairballs are as common a problem in chinchillas as they are in rabbits. They are usually caused by excessive fur chewing in combination with low dietary fiber. The animal usually presents with lethargy, reluctance to move, and anorexia. The hairball may be palpated on physical exam or diagnosed with contrast radiographs. Treatment protocols are similar to those for rabbits: fluid therapy, feline laxatives, increased dietary fiber, and proteolytic enzymes (pineapple juice) (Hayes 2000). If the animal is anorectic, then force-feeding may also be necessary.

Enteritis

Proper diet for chinchillas is one of the most important factors when discussing their care. An improper diet can be one of the most likely causes of enteritis, although a sudden diet change may also be a factor (Hayes 2000, Kraft 1987, Ritchey et al. 2004). If the animal is not offered hay, the hay is of poor quality, or the animal is eating a large amount of pellets or fruit and green vegetables, this may cause a change in the normal flora and fauna of the gastrointestinal tract. The motility of the gut and the fermentation process may also be altered, leading to an overgrowth of pathogenic bacteria. Other less common causes of enteritis are parasitic infection and prolonged or inappropriate use of antibiotics (Hayes 2000, Lightfoot 1999). Animals may present with anorexia and bloating. Those who have had chronic enteritis may present with constipation, impactions, intussusceptions, and rectal prolapse.

Determining the cause may be difficult because of the multiple factors involved. Radiographs, fecal floatation for parasites, and fecal cultures may be needed to determine an etiology. Symptomatic treatment is usually best with fluid therapy, antibiotics, and antiparasitics given as indicated.

Constipation

As mentioned above, improper diet is one of the most common problems associated with caring for a chinchilla. In most cases owners feed a diet of pellets almost exclusively, which can lead to many of the problems mentioned before. The pelleted diets are high in protein as well as calories, but are low in fiber. This low-fiber diet can also lead to constipation, which may be seen more often than diarrhea (Hayes 2000, Kraft 1987, Johnson-Delaney 1996). Clinical signs are straining to defecate and fecal pellets that may be small, hard, and in some cases, bloodstained. Treatment involves slowly increasing the amount of fiber in the chinchilla's diet by feeding a small amount of fresh vegetables or good quality hay.

Respiratory Diseases

Chinchillas are susceptible to pneumonia; however, these cases usually occur when there are large numbers of animals housed together and the husbandry is poor (Kraft 1987). Most pet owners should not have any problems in this area. Clinical signs include depression, dyspnea, and a nasal discharge. The treatment protocol includes antibiotics administered by nebulization if conditions allow.

Neurologic Diseases

Chinchillas are highly susceptible to *Listeria monocytogenes* infection; however, it is unlikely that pet chinchillas would be exposed (Hayes 2000). Ataxia and circling are usually followed by convulsions and death. Treatment protocols have been ineffective once clinical signs are noticed.

Heat Stroke

Chinchillas are very prone to heat stroke and should not be housed in temperatures over 80°F with high humidity. A chinchilla's cage should be away from windows that provide direct sunlight as well as heater vents. Just as with any other pet, they should never be left in a car during hot weather. The treatment for this condition is the same as would be given to a dog or cat (Quesenberry and Carpenter 2004, Mitchell and Tully 2009).

Zoonotic Diseases

Pet chinchillas may be exposed to *Baylisascaris procyonis* in contaminated hay (Ness 1999). This nematode infects the cerebrospinal fluid, causing ataxia, torticollis, and paralysis. There is no treatment for this condition and there is zoonotic potential for anyone handling the contaminated bedding and feed. Strict hygiene practices, including wearing gloves and washing hands, should be followed.

While not common, dermatophytosis has been diagnosed in chinchillas. It is treated with oral or topical medications just as in dogs and cats. And also just as in dogs and cats, this disease poses a zoonotic risk for the owner. Owners should be instructed to wear gloves when treating their pet and cleaning its cage. Children should not handle their pet during treatment.

Salmonellosis has occurred in fur production herds of chinchillas, but healthy chinchillas have had *Salmonella* isolated from them as well. It is not recommended that clinically normal chinchillas be treated, but owners should practice strict hygiene when handling them (Mitchell and Tully 2009).

BEHAVIOR

Chinchillas are usually nocturnal, but may be active during daylight hours. They have become popular as pets because of their curious personality, gentle nature, and the fact that they rarely bite. They are very entertaining pets to watch because they are very athletic and if given the materials to do so, will jump high in the air to reach a ledge or run around the walls of their enclosure. Their level of activity does not seem to diminish with age. Because by nature their means of defense is flight, they are very fast on their feet. If a chinchilla is allowed to get loose in a house, it will be a challenge to catch it.

TAKING THE HISTORY AND PERFORMING THE PHYSICAL EXAM

An accurate history is vital when working with chinchillas, because husbandry is often the most significant factor. These animals can be difficult to handle, because they are very quick and agile, and in most cases do not want to be touched. A good preliminary exam should be done prior to actually handling the animal. A visual exam may be performed if the owner has brought the pet in a wire cage. If not, then placing the chinchilla on the floor of the exam room and allowing it to move around normally is the best option. Be sure that all doors are closed, because they are very curious about their surroundings. A healthy chinchilla should be alert with bright eyes and a twitching nose. It may breathe rapidly, but it should not open-mouth breathe. The tail should be erect and its hair coat should be thick, soft, and smooth.

HANDLING AND RESTRAINT

Chinchillas can be very difficult to restrain and should be handled with care. Because they are very excitable and nervous, handling a sick or debilitated patient can pose a challenge. A chinchilla should never be scruffed. The base of the tail and hind legs should be held gently with one hand while the other hand supports the chest and shoulders (Figure 14.3). Some patients may be easier to handle if allowed to hide their face in the bend of the handler's elbow. Making the patient feel secure is of the utmost importance; if not, it may attempt to jump from the handler's grasp. If this is the case, sitting on the floor while completing the exam may be necessary. This allows for better support and if the chinchilla does get away, it will not fall and sustain a traumatic injury. If the patient is frightened while being restrained, it may release a large portion of fur in areas where it is being held. This is called a "fur-slip" (Lightfoot 1999). This can also occur due to rough handling. Great care should be taken while handling chinchillas, because no one wants to have a hairless patient leave the facility.

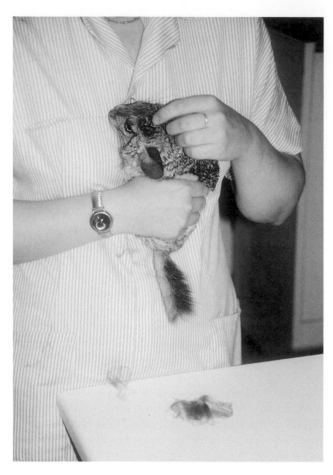

Figure 14.3. *Restraint of a chinchilla. (Photo courtesy of Dr. Stephen J. Hernandez-Divers, University of Georgia.)*

Once the patient is comfortably restrained, the examination can begin. The average weight of a chinchilla is 400 to 600 g, with the male usually being smaller than the female (Johnson-Delaney 1996, Lightfoot 1999). The temperature can be taken rectally, although chinchillas may object to this procedure. The normal temperature is 97°F to 102°F (Johnson-Delaney 1996, Lightfoot 1999). The heart rate and respiratory rate can be obtained by normal means. The normal HR is 200 to 350 beats/minute and the normal RR is 40 to 80 breaths/minute (Johnson-Delaney 1996, Lightfoot 1999).

RADIOLOGY

If the circumstances allow, radiographs are most easily obtained if the animal is anesthetized, because the chinchilla may be difficult to restrain. The most notice-

able difference on a radiograph is the very small thorax in comparison to the abdomen.

ANESTHESIA AND SURGERY

Very few surgical procedures are commonly performed on chinchillas. However, on occasion there may be need to neuter a male chinchilla to allow it to be housed with others. With this procedure and some of the others listed above, isoflurane or sevoflurane gas is the preferred anesthetic agent. A face mask or induction chamber should be used to administer the anesthetic gas. Intubation is not recommended because blind intubations can cause trauma, which can lead to epiglottal edema and dyspnea.

Injectable anesthetics can be used such as acepromazine, butorphanol tartrate, and ketamine hydrochloride in combination with diazepam or xylazine. However, gas anesthesia such as isoflurane or sevoflurane is highly preferred for surgical procedures, venipuncture, radiographs, and catheter placement

PARASITOLOGY

Fecal flotations and direct smears should be performed, although intestinal parasites are uncommon in chinchillas. Depending on the organism, the patient may be asymptomatic or present with diarrhea. Protozoal infestations by *Trichamonas* spp., *Balantidium* spp., Cryptosporidium, and *Eimeria chinchillae* may occur. The latter is the chinchilla coccidian that has been shown to be transmissible to other rodents. Nematode infestations by Physoloptera and *Haemonchus contortous* have been reported. It is also possible for chinchillas to have flea infestations, so they may also have tapeworms, usually *Hymeolepsis nana* (Ness 1999). One unusual aspect of the life cycle is that the same animal can be the intermediate and permanent host.

URINALYSIS

Normal urine values are as follows:

Color: Yellow to slightly red
Turbidity: Most often cloudy
pH: 8.5
Protein: Negative to trace
Glucose: Negative
Ketones: Negative

Bilirubin: Negative
Urobilinogen: 0.1 to 1 ng/dl
Nitrates: Negative
Blood: Negative
Specific gravity: Usually > 1.045

During a urine sediment examination of a normal chinchilla, some calcium carbonate crystals may be found along with amorphous debris. Casts, bacteria, erythrocytes, and leukocytes are rare in a normal patient, but occasional squamous epithelial cells are common (Ness 1999).

EMERGENCY AND CRITICAL CARE

Most of the diseases and ailments discussed previously are not considered emergencies. However, in the case of an emergency with a chinchilla, protocols similar to those of other small mammals should be followed. For example, an IV catheter can be very helpful in an emergency as well as in a critically ill patient. Once the patient has been stabilized, a calm and quiet environment is also very important for the recovery process.

SEX DETERMINATION

Determining the sex of a chinchilla can be very difficult, especially in young animals. The testicles can be visualized in adult males but the lack of a scrotum can make this more of a challenge. The fact that the clitoris, because of its size and shape, can often be mistaken for a penis, provides another obstacle when sexing chinchillas. The location of the penis versus the clitoris can often be the determining factor because the distance from the rectum to the penis is greater than that of the clitoris.

TECHNIQUES

Venipuncture
For a procedure of this nature, it is preferable to have a chinchilla anesthetized. There are several sites for venipuncture; the jugular vein being the most common site, and it allows larger blood volumes to be obtained. There are five other sites for venipuncture: the cephalic, saphenous, femoral, lateral abdominal, and tail vein (Figure 14.4).

The process for collecting blood from the jugular is as follows (Ness 1999):

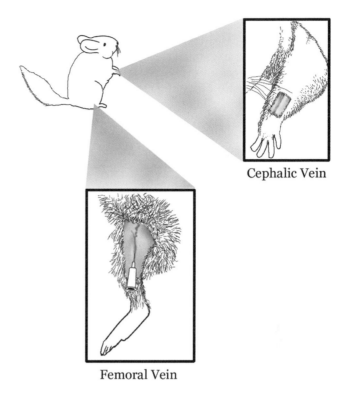

Cephalic Vein

Femoral Vein

Figure 14.4. Venipuncture sites. (Drawing by Scott Stark.)

1. Place the patient in sternal recumbency.
2. Extend the head and neck to make the lateral aspect of the lower cervical region accessible.
3. Apply gentle pressure to one side of the thoracic inlet to occlude the vessel.
4. Wet the area with an alcohol swab and visualize the distended vein.
5. Using a 23– to 25-gauge needle attached to a 1– to 3-ml syringe, insert the needle into the vein at approximately a 45 degree angle.
6. Draw back slowly if using a 3-ml syringe so as not to collapse the vein.

A 25– to 27-gauge needle on a 0.5– to 1-ml syringe should be used to collect samples from the other sites mentioned above. The femoral and cephalic veins are the most commonly used of those mentioned.

Intravenous Catheter Placement
The cephalic vein is the most common site used for catheter placement. The procedures are the same as in any other small animal. See Chapter 11 in the Technique section for ferrets. Note that a small cutdown may not be necessary.

Intraosseous Catheter Placement

While in most cases the chinchilla's peripheral veins are readily accessible, in an emergency it may be necessary to place an intraosseous catheter. In critical patients, sedation or anesthesia is not usually required for this procedure. The steps for placement are as follows:

1. Locate the site for placement of the catheter. The two sites used in chinchillas are the femur or tibia. The femur is preferred due to its size and location, so this one will be discussed.
2. Locate a syringe needle or catheter stylet of the largest bore possible for the patient (usually 22-gauge is sufficient). A spinal needle may also be used. A syringe of heparinized flush will also be needed.
3. Clip and surgically prep the site.
4. Once the site has been prepped, the greater trochanter should be palpated and stabilized for insertion of the needle. The needle is then inserted and with a gentle twisting motion, advanced slowly. The needle should continue to be advanced through the bone and into the marrow cavity. Aspiration with the flush syringe until blood is visualized in the hub should be performed. It should be flushed quickly because the marrow can clog the needle.
5. The needle should be secured with tape and in some cases, it may need to be sutured in place to provide more stability.
6. This catheter may be used for up to seventy-two hours, after which a replacement in another location will be required.

Once the catheter is in place, great care must be taken to maintain it. Its location may inhibit normal movement and cause some discomfort. This in turn may cause the patient to attempt to remove the catheter by chewing or rubbing.

Administration of Medication

In the event that medications need to be given, there are several routes of administration. As with many other exotics, one must make sure to downsize the equipment and the volume of medications used.

Per os: Medication is usually liquid and can be given by needleless syringe in the side of the mouth just behind the incisors.

Subcutaneous: 23– to 25-gauge needle under the skin in the flank or neck area.

Intravenous: 25– to 28-gauge needle, preferably an insulin syringe in the lateral saphenous or cephalic.

Intramuscular: 23– to 25-gauge needle with no more than 0.3 ml/site. Recommended sites include the semimembranosus, quadriceps, and semitendinosus muscles (Ness 1999).

EUTHANASIA

As with most other small animals, the preferred method of euthanasia is lethal injection. If an IV catheter has been placed in the cephalic vein, it can be used for administration of the euthanasia solution. If a catheter is not available, either an IV or intracardiac injection (after anesthetized) with a syringe can be used. It is frequently easiest to first use isoflurane or sevoflurane to anesthetize the patient and then follow up with injectable euthanasia solution.

REFERENCES

Hayes PM. 2000. Diseases of Chinchillas. Philadelphia: W.B. Saunders Company.

Johnson-Delaney CA. 1996 Exotic Companion Medicine Handbook for Veterinarians. Lake Worth: Wingers Publications.

Kraft H. 1987. Diseases of Chinchillas. Neptune City: T.F.H. Publications.

Lightfoot TL. 1999. Clinical Examination of Chinchillas, Hedgehogs, Prairie Dogs, and Sugar Gliders. *Veterinary Clinics of North America: Exotic Animal Practice* 2(2): 447–54.

Mitchell M, Tully T. 2009. Manual of Exotic Pet Practice. St. Louis: Saunders.

Ness RD. 1999. Clinical Pathology and Sample Collection of Exotic Small Animals. *Veterinary Clinics of North America: Exotic Animal Practice* 2(3): 591–619.

Quesenberry K, Carpenter J. 2004. Ferrets, Rabbits, and Rodents: Clinical Medicine and Surgery. St. Louis: Saunders.

Ritchey L, Cogswell EL, Cogswell M. 2004. Joy of Chinchillas. Self published.

CHAPTER FIFTEEN

Guinea Pigs

Anne Hudson and Maria Crane

COMMON TYPES

The domestic guinea pig, *Cavia porcellus*, also referred to as a cavy, has been raised as a meat animal in South America. Guinea pigs are considered rodents, despite several differences between guinea pigs and other common pet rodent species. They are grouped as hystricomorphic rodents along with porcupines and chinchillas. Male guinea pigs are called boars, and females are called sows. The American or English variety, the Abyssinian, and the Peruvian are the most commonly seen in companion animal practice. English cavies have short, smooth hair coats. Abyssinians have a rougher coat that looks swirled; the hair is described as growing in rosettes. Peruvian guinea pigs have long hair coats that require grooming to maintain good condition. Guinea pigs are available in a wide variety of colors and combinations of colors.

BEHAVIOR

Guinea pigs are docile animals that rarely bite. They are sociable and will share housing with another if introduced at an early age; however, crowded animals or breeding animals may fight. Cages with tops are not needed if the sides are eight to ten inches high because jumping seldom occurs.

A wide variety of vocalization patterns have been demonstrated, and cavies will vocalize in response to hearing their food being prepared, lights being turned on, and so forth.

They are neophobic animals, mistrusting any new foods or changes in their normal routine. Therefore, it is important to gently handle young animals on a regular basis and to expose them to a variety of certain foods. Trying to change feed types for a mature animal is nearly impossible. When frightened, guinea pigs may "stampede" in an effort to escape, bolting around the cage. Another typical response is to suddenly freeze and remain immobile for a brief period of time.

ANATOMY AND PHYSIOLOGY

Guinea pigs have short, stocky, tailless bodies with one pair of inguinal teats. The legs are short, and the front feet have four toes and the rear feet have three toes. Like all rodents, they have open rooted incisors. Guinea pigs also possess open-rooted premolars and molars, and malocclusions seem to occur more frequently with these teeth than the incisors. The dental formula is 2 (I—1/1, C—0/0, P—1/1, M—3/3) (Harkness and Wagner 1989).

The soft palate is continuous with the base of the tongue, forming a membranous covering of the posterior pharynx. Food, water, and air pass through an opening called the palatal ostium. The cecum in the guinea pig is very large, occupying a large portion of the abdominal cavity.

Male guinea pigs have open inguinal canals, allowing them to retract their testicles into the abdominal cavity, and an os penis. Females have two uterine horns and a single cervix. A thin membrane covers the vagina except for during estrus and parturition. The symphysis pubis of the guinea pig is fibrocartilaginous and is capable of separating during parturition. Failing to breed a female prior to six months of age may lead to dystocia because the symphysis will be less able to separate. Physiological data are contained in Table 15.1.

BIOLOGIC AND REPRODUCTIVE DATA

Guinea pigs reach breeding age at approximately three months of age. Females housed with other females will mount each other if in heat. It is possible to keep breeding pairs together long term; breeding may take place during the postpartum estrus. Evidence of breeding is finding a copulatory plug in the bedding of the cage. This plug is an accumulation of secretions that falls from the vagina shortly after breeding takes place.

Table 15.1. Physiological data for the guinea pig.

Lifespan	5–7 years
Average adult weight (M/F)	900–1,200 g/700–900 g
Puberty	45–70 days
Breeding age	3–4 months
Estrous cycle length	15–17 days
Gestation period	63–68 days
Litter size	2–5 pups
Weaning age	21 days
Respiratory rate per minute	70–130
Heart rate	230–300
Rectal temperature °F	99–103.1

Harkness and Wagner 1989 (21), Hillyer and Quesenberry 1997 (248).

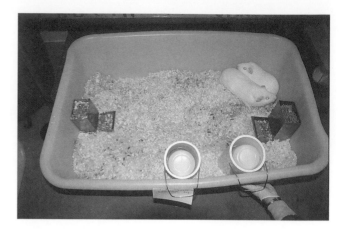

Figure 15.1. An appropriate housing set-up for guinea pigs. (Photo courtesy of Ryan Cheek.)

Sows do not build nests like other rodents, and young are born precocious. Litters of two to five pups are typical, although larger litters are possible (Hillyer and Quesenberry 1997). Pups are born fully furred, with eyes open, all teeth erupted, and able to walk. Within a few hours, pups can begin eating from a bowl.

HUSBANDRY

Guinea pigs can be messy, often tipping over food crocks and scattering food throughout the cage. They defecate throughout the cage as well. Water should be provided in a bottle with a sipper tube. Fresh water may need to be provided more frequently than for other rodents due to the guinea spitting food particles into the bottle, and their tendency to play with the sipper tube. The bedding must be changed and the cage surfaces cleaned more frequently as well.

Cages do not need lids if the sides are tall, unless the owner has a dog or cat; a secure lid would then be a requirement. Solid flooring is preferable to wire mesh to prevent trauma to the feet. Wire cages with deep solid bottoms are nice because the tray contains scattered bedding material, and the open sides allow the guinea pig to see out and observe what is going on around it. Nonaromatic wood shavings or shredded paper can be used as bedding material (Queensberry et al. 2004).

Guinea pigs are comfortable at a normal room temperature of about 70°F. Good ventilation is essential to help prevent respiratory diseases. Owners should be cautioned to keep cages away from drafty areas, windows, and home heating sources (Figure 15.1).

Abyssinian and Peruvian guinea pigs benefit from gentle grooming. Fecal pellets may become stuck in the longer fur of these animals. If needed, they can be bathed with a mild shampoo as long as they are dried carefully and not subjected to chilling.

NUTRITION

A variety of food items, including commercial pellets and some fresh vegetables, must be offered from an early age to prevent rigid food preferences from forming. Guinea pigs are herbivores. The daily recommended diet for guinea pigs is a good quality grass hay (offered at all times), a commercial guinea pig pellet, fresh vegetables, and a limited amount of fresh fruits. Vegetables and fruits should be washed thoroughly prior to feeding to remove any pesticide residue. The fruit and vegetables should be removed from the cage after a few hours to prevent spoilage. Pellets are a good source of crude protein and fiber and they also help wear down the teeth through chewing activity.

Like primates, guinea pigs cannot synthesize vitamin C and must be supplemented with this nutrient. Reputable brands of commercial guinea pig pellets are fortified with vitamin C or ascorbic acid; however, most of the vitamin C is oxidized or lost by ninety days of manufacturing. Therefore, pellets should not be relied on as the sole source of vitamin C. Fresh vegetables such as dark leafy greens, red and green peppers, and broccoli, and small amounts of fresh fruits such as kiwi, oranges, and tomatoes are good sources of daily supplements. Another route for supplementation of vitamin C is in the water. One gram of vitamin C/l of water mixed fresh daily is recommended. (Quesenberry and Carpenter 2004). However, vitamin C in water begins to break down within twenty-four hours and must be changed daily to ensure adequate intake. Pregnant animals have a higher (30 mg/kg/day) vitamin C requirement than nonbreeding adults (5 mg/kg/day) (Harkness and Wagner 1989).

COMMON AND ZOONOTIC DISEASES

Stress is a major factor in developing illness. Poor diet or sudden dietary changes, overcrowding, and failure to maintain clean caging all result in stress.

Failure to receive adequate vitamin C supplementation may result in the development of scurvy, a musculoskeletal disease. Guinea pigs with scurvy are lethargic, anorexic, and may actually bite due to painful joints. Diarrhea and weight loss may also be evident. Supplementation with appropriate amounts of ascorbic acid, (50 to 100 mg/animal, PO, SC every 24 hours) (Quesenberry and Carpenter 2004) coupled with good supportive care usually result in a rapid recovery.

Common respiratory diseases seen in guinea pigs include those caused by *Bordetella bronchiseptica* and *Streptococcus pneumoniae*. Transmission is via aerosolization, fomites, direct contact with another sick guinea pig, or in the case of *Bordetella*, any animal capable of carrying the bacteria: dogs, cats, rabbits, and nonhuman primates. Signs of respiratory disease include anorexia, ocular-nasal discharge, dyspnea, and death. Treatment with antibiotics and increased vitamin C, as well as supportive care, is needed. The animal may also require force feeding.

Guinea pigs may contract salmonellosis and clostridial infections through fecal contamination of food. Signs include rough hair coat, weight loss, lethargy, and diarrhea. Again, treatment involves antibiotics, based on culture and sensitivities, and good supportive care.

Swellings on the neck are usually due to inflamed or abscessed lymph nodes caused by *Streptobacillus spp.* or *Streptococcus spp.* infection. Cervical lymphadenitis, or "lumps" as it is commonly called, may result from a bite wound, abrasion from bedding or caging equipment, or trauma from malocclusion. Abscesses are usually drained and flushed, followed by systemic antibiotic therapy. Contact with the drainage will infect any other guinea pigs housed with the affected animal so isolation is necessary until wound healing has occurred.

Pododermatitis is often associated with animals housed on wire flooring. The surfaces of the feet become irritated, thickened, and ulcerated. A secondary staphylococcal infection may ensue. The animal will vocalize and be unwilling to move due to pain. Treatment consists of appropriate antibiotics, surgical debridement, topical cleaning, and appropriate analgesic therapy. This painful disease is best prevented with clean flooring that is non-abrasive. If wire flooring is used, provide some solid areas of flooring or bedding so that the animals can move to softer areas.

Antibiotic therapy in guinea pigs must be undertaken with great care, because many of the antibiotics effective against Gram-positive organisms, such as penicillin, can lead to enterotoxemia.

The significant reproductive problems in guinea pigs are dystocia, common if females are not bred prior to reaching six months of age, and pregnancy ketosis. Obesity also puts the female at risk for problems during parturition. Straining, abnormal vaginal discharge, depression, and/or failure to produce a pup within thirty minutes after onset of contractions are all indications of dystocia (Hillyer and Quesenberry 1997). Cesarean sections are often necessary. Ketosis is most commonly associated with obesity and stress. Rapid onset of signs, including anorexia, dyspnea, convulsions, and death, may occur. The problem is easier to prevent through proper diet and husbandry than to treat.

Zoonotic diseases include salmonellosis, sarcoptic mange, ringworm, and lymphocytic choriomeningitis.

HISTORY AND PHYSICAL EXAMINATION

Questions to ask when interviewing a client are the basic signalment questions asked with all species:

- The chief complaint
- Where the owner obtained the pet and how long she has owned it
- The owner's past experience, if any, in keeping guinea pigs

Ideally, the pet is brought into the clinic in the cage it is normally housed in, allowing staff to see what type of bedding and equipment the patient is exposed to. When scheduling appointments, advise the owner not to clean the cage prior to the appointment.

Information about appetite, type of diet, fecal pellet production and quality, and overall attitude should be obtained. Observe the animal in its cage; healthy guinea pigs are active and vocal. The patient should be weighed on a gram scale, and while gently restraining the guinea pig, a rectal temperature can be obtained with a standard rectal thermometer. The technician must restrain the guinea pig so the veterinarian can

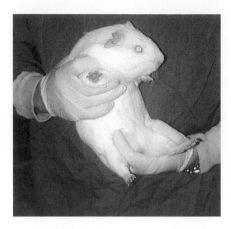

Figure 15.2. Proper guinea pig restraint. (Photo courtesy of Ryan Cheek.)

examine the mouth and teeth, and should be prepared for the patient to squirm and vocalize its objection to the exam.

RESTRAINT

Guinea pigs respond well to gentle restraint; inappropriate handling stresses the animal and can cause damage to the internal organs. Always use two hands to restrain a guinea pig (Figure 15.2).

To properly restrain a guinea pig:

1. Gently place one hand under the thorax of the guinea pig, just caudal to the front limbs.
2. Support the hindquarters of the patient with the other hand.
3. The guinea pig may also have the dorsal thorax supported in one hand in a cradling fashion while supporting the hind limbs with the other hand. This placement may be more comfortable for pregnant animals because it avoids any pressure on the abdomen.

Restraint for jugular venipuncture is similar to that used on cats in that the animal's forelegs are extended over the edge of a table while the head is gently extended up. Stop the procedure immediately if the animal becomes stressed (Hillyer and Quesenberry 1997).

RADIOLOGY

Whole body studies are common in guinea pigs, and may require anesthesia to prevent movement during exposure. Exposure times of 1/60 of a second or less are necessary. Masking tape can be used to secure the sedated animal in position. For ease in tabletop technique, taping the animal to a small sheet of Plexiglas rather than directly to the cassette prevents having to retape the patient each time cassettes are changed (Imaging Resources 1995). The references listed at the end of this chapter have excellent recommendations for radiology techniques.

ANESTHESIA AND SURGERY

Guinea pigs should be fasted for one to two hours prior to surgical procedures. Induction with isoflurane gas via face mask is recommended, and the animal can be maintained on gas administered by face mask and a nonrebreathing circuit (Hillyer and Quesenberry 1997).

Depth of anesthesia in most rodents can be evaluated partially by pinching the toes or gently pinching the ear for reaction to pain; however, there has been concern that pedal reflexes may not be reliable depth indicators in guinea pigs and may actually indicate the animal is too deeply anesthetized (Plunkett 1993).

Doppler monitors and pulse oximeters are helpful in monitoring the patient in addition to watching the chest wall for movement related to respiration. Take care to keep the animal warm perioperatively, and turn the animal from side to side every fifteen to thirty minutes to prevent fluids from pooling on the dependent side. Once fully recovered, ensure the client keeps the cage and bedding fresh and clean to prevent any surgical wound contamination.

PARASITOLOGY

Guinea pigs may be parasitized without showing any clinical signs. *Crypto sporidium wrairi*, an intestinal protozoan parasite, may result in diarrhea, weight loss, and death. Immunocompromised animals and weanlings are most susceptible. The protozoan can be seen on fecal examinations and there is no proven treatment. Animals generally recover on their own after a period of weeks and tend to be resistant to reinfection. (Quesenberry and Carpenter 2004). There is a zoonotic risk from this parasite so owners should be cautioned.

Fleas, mites, and lice are ectoparasites that can infest guinea pigs, causing intense itching, alopecia, and excoriation of the skin. Humans may be affected by the sarcoptic mange mite, *Trixacaruscaviae*. The

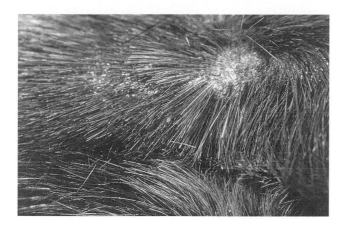

Figure 15.3. A guinea pig with mange. (Photo courtesy of Dr. Chris King.)

veterinarian may treat the guinea pig by prescribing ivermectin or topical pyrethrin products safe for use in cats (Figure 15.3).

URINALYSIS

Because of the potential of urinary calculi and cystitis in the guinea pig, the veterinarian may request that a urine sample be obtained by cystocentesis to perform a urinalysis. The technique is like that used in other small animals, except a 25-gauge needle should be used and anesthesia may be required (Hillyer and Quesenberry 1997).

EMERGENCY AND CRITICAL CARE

Pregnancy toxemia may occur in later days of gestation and does not respond well to treatment. The condition is usually fatal (Plunkett 1993).

Dystocia is an emergency that usually requires an immediate cesarean section. If the animal had several successful litters previously, demonstrating the pelvic canal is capable of separating, the veterinarian may try oxytocin prior to surgery (Plunkett 1993).

SEX DETERMINATION

Anogenital distance is not a reliable method for sexing animals. To sex a guinea pig, gently restrain the animal and examine the external genitalia. In the female, the genital area has a "Y" shape. The male appears to have more of a straight slit. Applying gentle pressure cau-

dally and cranially to the genitals causes the penis of the male animal to extrude.

TECHNIQUES

Techniques for administration of medication, venipuncture, catheter placement, bandaging, and wound care are discussed in this section (Lawson 2000).

Administration of Medication

Subcutaneous, intramuscular, or intraperitoneal administration of drugs is often used due to the difficulty of administering drugs intravenously. Many drugs given intramuscularly may lead to irritation of the tissue surrounding the injection site (Hillyer and Quesenberry 1997). Exercise caution when administering IP injections to avoid damaging internal organs.

SQ

Subcutaneous injection of medications allows for slightly larger volumes (5 to 10 ml) to be administered than with IM administration. Fluid therapy may also be administered via the subcutaneous route. Most guinea pigs will rest on the exam table and can be restrained by cupping your hands around them. A towel placed on the table gives the animal some traction.

For SQ injection:

1. Use a 20-gauge or smaller needle.
2. Tent the skin away from the underlying muscles over the scruff of the neck.
3. Insert the needle into the tented area at a slight angle, being careful not to pass all the way through the other side of the skin.
4. Administer the medication.
5. A butterfly catheter may be easier to use if the animal is very active.
6. Dispose of the needle into a puncture-proof biohazard container.

IM

Intramuscular injections are usually given in the large muscles of the hind limbs, such as the gluteal muscles. To avoid tissue damage, use needles less than 21 gauge, and do not inject volumes of greater than 0.3 ml into any one site.

For IM injection:

1. Place a towel on the table and gently restrain the animal or restrain it with your hands, being sure to support the hind end.

2. It may be helpful to "pinch" the muscle tissue with one hand while administering the injection with the other hand.
3. Aspirate the syringe prior to injection to avoid injecting into a blood vessel.
4. Administer the medication.
5. Dispose of the needle in a puncture-proof biohazard container.

IP

For IP injection:

1. Place the guinea pig gently on its back, supporting the animal in one hand.
2. Tilt the animal's head down and insert the needle at an approximate 45 degree angle into the lower right quadrant of the abdomen.
3. Aspirate prior to injection to ensure you are not in the bladder or digestive tract. If any blood or fluid enters the syringe, withdraw and discard the syringe before starting over.
4. Administer the medication.
5. Dispose of the needle in a puncture-proof biohazard container.

IV

Intravenous injection is difficult; the saphenous vein is the easiest to use.

For IV injection:

1. Use a needle size of 23 gauge or smaller.
2. Shave the area and clean with alcohol or other antiseptic solution.
3. Applying a low-watt light bulb (such as a penlight) or a warm-water compress to the area prior to the procedure may help to distend the vein slightly.
4. Apply pressure proximal to the injection site to distend the vein.
5. Aspirate prior to injection to ensure proper placement.
6. Inject medications slowly after releasing proximally applied pressure.
7. Apply direct pressure to venipuncture site as the needle is withdrawn to prevent formation of a hematoma.
8. Dispose of the needle in a puncture-proof biohazard container.

Venipuncture

Small quantities of blood can be taken from the ear veins or saphenous veins (Figure 15.4). Larger amounts of blood can be obtained using jugular venipuncture, extending the guinea pig's forelegs over the edge of an exam table as you would a cat. Jugular venipuncture can be stressful and should not be performed on very ill animals. The amount of blood that can safely be collected from guinea pigs is approximately 0.5 to 0.7 mL/100 g body weight (Hillyer and Quesenberry 1997).

For venipuncture:

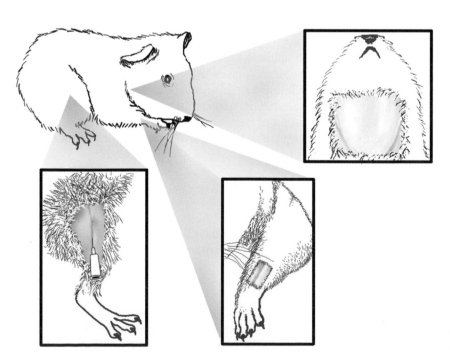

Figure 15.4. Venipuncture sites on a guinea pig. (Drawing by Scott Stark.)

1. Use a 23-gauge or smaller needle attached to a tuberculin syringe, or a 3-mL syringe if performing jugular venipuncture.
2. Shave the proposed venipuncture site and prep with alcohol to make it easier to visualize the vein.
3. Applying a low-watt light bulb (such as a penlight) or a warm-water compress to the area prior to the procedure may help to distend the vein slightly.
4. Apply pressure as described above for IV administration of medications; however, maintain pressure to keep the vessel distended.
5. After collecting the sample, withdraw the needle as you apply pressure to the venipuncture site.
6. Dispose of the needle in a puncture-proof biohazard container.

Catheter Placement

Intravenous catheterization in guinea pigs is difficult, and is more commonly performed in a research setting. Indwelling catheters meant for long-term use may need to be surgically placed under anesthesia. Catheter supplies are available from Harvard Apparatus. Intraosseous administration of medications can be performed; the technique is the same as for a chinchilla (see Chapter 14).

Bandaging and Wound Care

Minor wounds are best cleaned as thoroughly as possible during initial treatment to avoid repetitively stressing the animal. The risk of wound infection is decreased if the patient's caging receives regular bedding changes. External sutures and bandages are not usually well tolerated; subcuticular sutures and surgical glue are better alternatives (Hillyer and Queensberry 1997).

To treat a wound:

1. Keep the animal as comfortable as possible.
2. Gently clip hair from around the wound and clean with an antiseptic solution.
3. The wound can be temporarily covered with a sterile dressing until surgically closed.

More serious wounds and fractures can be quite difficult to manage.

EUTHANASIA

Guinea pigs can be euthanized using an overdose of barbiturate anesthesia administered intraperitoneally as described above.

REFERENCES

Harkness JE, Wagner JE. 1989. The Biology and Medicine of Rabbits and Rodents. 3rd ed. Philadelphia: Lea and Febiger. 21.

Hillyer EV, Quesenberry KE. 1997. Ferrets, Rabbits, and Rodents: Clinical Medicine and Surgery. Philadelphia: W.B. Saunders Co. 248–386.

Imaging Resources, Inc. 1995. An Overview of Small Animal Radiology. 3rd ed. Corvallis State: Imaging Resources.

Lawson PT, ed. 2000. American Association for Laboratory Animal Science; LAT and LATG Training Manuals. Memphis: AALAS.

Plunkett SJ. 1993. Emergency Procedures for the Small Animal Veterinarian. Philadelphia: W.B. Saunders Co.

Queensberry KE, Carpenter J. 2004. Ferrets, Rabbits, and Rodents: Clinical Medicine and Surgery. St Louis: Saunders.

Queensberry KE, Donnelly TM, Hillyer EV. 2004. Biology, Husbandry and Clinical Techniques of Guinea Pigs and Chinchillas. In: Ferrets, Rabbits, and Rodents: Clinical Medicine and Surgery, 2nd ed., edited by Quesenberry KE and Carpenter JW. Missouri: Saunders, Elsevier.

CHAPTER SIXTEEN

Hedgehogs

Michael Duffy Jones

TAXOMONY, ANATOMY, AND PHYSIOLOGY

Hedgehogs belong to the order of Insectivora, which includes the most primitive of all living placental mammals today (Storer 1994). There are many different species of hedgehogs, including the European, African, Pruner's, Algerian, long-eared or Egyptian, and Ethiopian or desert hedgehog. There are slight differences between these species, including ear size and times of hibernation. For the most part, the various species can be treated medically in a similar way. The Egyptian hedgehog is noted for its surly disposition (Lightfoot 1997). African hedgehogs are slightly different from their European cousins in that they do not hibernate (Storer 1994).

Hedgehogs' brains are small and primitive and are smooth, not fissured. The sensory parts of the brain, including the olfactory and tactile areas, are very well developed. They have vibrissae, which are long, stiff hairs around the mouth and nostrils that are used for their sense of touch (Storer 1994).

Their digestive tract consists of a simple stomach and not cecum. The transit time averages twelve to sixteen hours (Johnson 2004).

Most species of hedgehogs have five toes on each foot, except for the four-toed hedgehog, which only has four toes on the back feet (Storer 1994). They have very strong legs that are used for digging, and they have a nonexistent tail.

The urogenital opening of females is not connected to the anus but is directly anterior (toward the animal's head). The male's penis is more anterior than the female's genitalia (Storer 1994) (Figure 16.1). The males have a prominent penis sheath. The testes are intraabdominal and not readily visible. Pressure can be placed on the abdomen to push the testes into the inguinal area. Internally, males also possess complex accessory reproductive glands, which may account for as much as 10% of body weight during the breeding season (Johnson 2004).

Pregnancy detection is often accomplished by monitoring body weight. Typically if a female gains more than 50 grams within three weeks of being with a male, then she is considered pregnant. During pregnancy and lactation nutritional demands my increase up to threefold. The female may cannibalize, kill, or abandon her newborn young if she is stressed or disturbed. Therefore, the male must be removed before parturition and the mother should be not be disturbed for five to ten days after parturition (Johnson 2004). Dystocia is rare and passive transfer of immunity occurs through colostrum in the first twenty-four to seventy-two hours of life. Orphaned young can be raised on puppy or kitten milk replacer (Johnson 2004).

Dentition in these animals is unique because they are insectivores (Figure 16.2). The top row of teeth includes three incisors, one canine, three premolars, and three molars on each side, and the bottom consists of two incisors, one canine, two premolars, and three molars, for a total of thirty-six (Storer 1994, Johnson 2004). The incisors are sharp, the canines are small, and the molars and premolars are broad and flat for grinding. The first set of incisors has a large gap for appending and killing insects. Hedgehogs' teeth are very small and sharp. The baby teeth erupt at about twenty-three days and permanent teeth erupt at seven to nine weeks (Storer 1994). The skeletal anatomy is shown in Figure 16.3.

Hedgehogs' senses, including smell and hearing, are very developed. Their eyesight is of moderate ability with limited color vision. They are highly resistant to many toxins (Storer 1994).

Their face, underbody, and legs are covered with cream- to brown-colored soft hairs. The rest of the body is covered with quills (also called spines). Each quill is connected to a small muscle, which can help pull the quill erect. When the animal is frightened, the

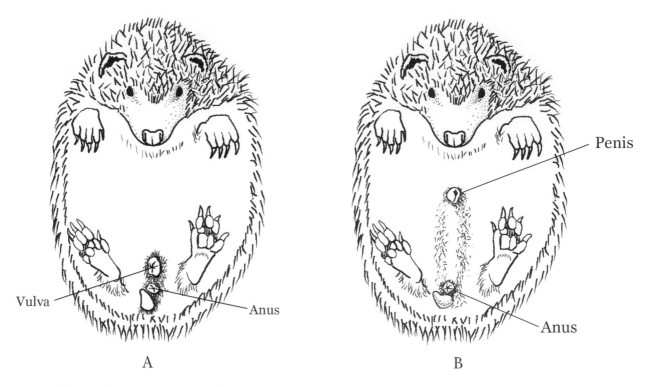

Figure 16.1. *Sex determination in a hedgehog. (A) Female. (B) Male. (Drawing by Scott Stark.)*

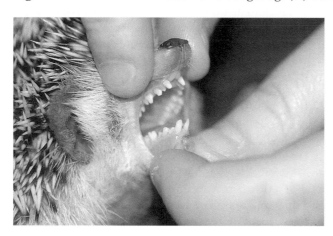

Figure 16.2. *Dentition. (Photo courtesy of Ryan Cheek.)*

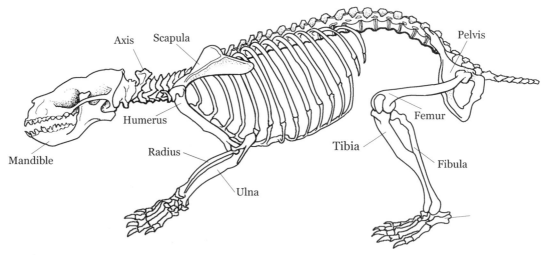

Figure 16.3. *Skeletal anatomy. (Drawing by Scott Stark.)*

Table 16.1. Biologic and reproductive data.

Sexual maturity	3–9 months (Storer 1994, 53)
Litter size	2–6 (Storer 1994 53)
Gestation	32–48 days (Storer 1994, 53)
Weaning	5–6 weeks (Storer 1994, 53)
Breeding	1–2 times/year spontaneous ovulates, but depends on environmental conditions (Storer 1994, 54)
Lifespan	3–4 years in the wild (Gregory 1992, 63)
WBC	5.8–21 × 103/ml (Ness 1999, 596)
Neutrophils %	49–70
Lymphocytes	22–38
Monocytes	0
Eosinophil	2–11
Basophils	0–5
Hematocrit	28–38
Hemoglobin	9.9–13.1
RBC (×106/ml)	4.4–6
MCV (fL)	60–67.4
MCHC (g/dl)	25.1–48.3
Platelets (×103/ml)	200–412
MCH (pg)	21.2–23.4
ALT (IU/L)	39.7–68.9 (Ness 1999 2:3, 600)
T. Bill (mg/dl)	0–0.1
T. Protein (g/dl)	5.3–6.3
Albumin (g/dl)	2.6–3.4
Glucose (mg/dl)	81.5–116.1
BUN (mg/dl)	21.3–32.9
Creatinine (mg/dl)	0.2–0.4
Calcium (mg/dl)	9.5–10.9

quills are erect and crossed, making a very formidable barrier (Storer 1994).

Hedgehogs are mostly terrestrial. They tend to walk slowly, looking for food, but can scurry at about six feet/second (four miles/hour). They can also use their spines as a cushion for rolling or dropping from high places (Storer 1994, Johnson 2004).

BIOLOGIC AND REPRODUCTIVE DATA

Table 16.1 includes biological and reproductive information. Clinical pathology data are also included.

BEHAVIOR

Hedgehogs are usually solitary animals and they can be aggressive when housed together. However, captive animals can become quite tame over time (Storer 1994).

Typical defense postures include rolling into a ball with erect spines. Hedgehogs will hiss and spit to try and scare off potential predators. The spines will stay erect and will vibrate, in an effort to try and drive the spine into anything that touches it. This posture makes it very difficult for hedgehogs to be picked up either by a human or another animal (Storer 1994).

Hedgehogs are also good at wedging themselves into very small places. This can make it difficult to examine these pets. It is a good idea not to have owners bring them in balls or other transport apparatuses that will make it difficult to remove them if they become frightened.

Hedgehogs can become excited when encountering smells or substances. They will engage in a behavior that is called self-anointing. When they encounter a small animal or substance they can become stiff, and they make licking motions with their tongues (which are very long). They can start to bite or tug and start producing large amounts of saliva. They can then get into extremely contorted positions by stiffening their front legs and pinning their heads back between their shoulder blades. This behavior can look much like a seizure, and can continue for a long period of time. There is much controversy about this behavior, and most people believe that it may be a sexual reaction or a self-defense behavior (Storer 1994).

HUSBANDRY

The optimal temperature is between 65°F and 90°F, with the best temperature at 80°F. If the temperature is too low, these pets may start to hibernate, and if too high, they can have significant health problems related to heat stress. Hedgehogs can tolerate temperatures of 100°F for short periods of time (Storer 1994, Johnson 2004).

It is best to keep adults in individual cages because they can become aggressive if housed together. Plastic or fiberglass crates are good due to ease of cleaning. Aquariums make great housing, but care must be taken to monitor for overheating. Twenty-gallon aquariums are of adequate size and can be purchased with wire covers. Recycled/shredded paper or aspen shavings are a very good substrate, and should be changed twice a week (Storer 1994). Litter box training is possible and hedgehogs tend to use the bathroom in one area of the cage. Once that area is found, a small litter pan can be placed in the cage. Dust-free litter seems to work best because these pets roll and scratch the litter (Storer 1994). Self-clumping litter can pose a problem for hedgehogs, because if they become wet for any reason, the litter can stick in the spines and be very difficult to remove. They should be kept on a twelve-hour light cycle (Johnson 2004).

Hedgehogs like security and they feel quite secure if they have a place to hide. A piece of PVC piping can be used for sleeping quarters. One side of the tube can be capped off, providing a small and secure place for them to sleep. However, should more than one hedgehog be housed together, the tube should not be capped, because they may pile on top of one another and become trapped inside (Storer 1994).

Regular rabbit or guinea pig water bottles work well. Bowls or saucers are potentially hazardous, because hedgehogs may climb inside and could drown.

Solid surface exercise wheels designed for hedgehogs can be used (Johnson 2004).

NUTRITION

Hedgehogs are insectivores, which means that they have a high-protein diet (Storer 1994). For nonbreeding hedgehogs, feeding live food is acceptable. Crickets, mealworms, grasshoppers, snails, slugs, pinkie mice, and small nontoxic frogs are good sources. Small amounts of fruit may also be fed. Feeding live food can also add interest to their lives (Johnson 2004). The dietary calcium : phosphorus ratio should be 1.2–1.5 : 1 (Carpenter 2002).

Nonbreeding hedgehogs can become fat on regular diets, so care must be taken with the quantity that is fed. Kitten food (wet or dry) may be used, as well as high-quality dog food mixed with cottage cheese in a 5 : 1 ratio (Storer 1994). Chopped meat or hard-boiled eggs can be given as an occasional treat.

COMMON DISEASES

Lameness

Often hedgehogs are presented for reluctance to move or weak gait. There are many causes of lameness, including overgrown toenails, constriction of toes with foreign material, fracture of long bones from trauma, and even neoplasia. Systemic disease causing weakness can be perceived as lameness (Lightfoot 1999).

Wobbling hedgehog syndrome is a demyelination neurologic condition of African hedgehogs. It is characterized by progressive ataxia and weight loss, eventually leading to paralysis and death. The age of onset is typically eighteen to twenty-four months. It starts in the hind legs and gradually ascends until only the head

can move. The progression can occur over weeks to months. There is no definitive treatment and no etiological agent has been found (Johnson 2004).

Anorexia

Because hedgehogs do not have continuously erupting teeth, malocclusion is a problem that is seldom seen. However, gingival and periodontal disease does occur in older hedgehogs. Gingivitis may improve with ascorbic acid (50 to 200 mg/kg PO, SC every 24 hours) (Johnson 2004). Husbandry problems, such as changing food, are often the cause of anorexia. If this does not seem to be the case, then blood work may be needed to determine whether there are any significant liver problems such as hepatic lipidosis or neoplasia (Lightfoot 1999).

Diarrhea

Diarrhea can be caused by many types of problems from husbandry, parasites, bacterial infection, and even salmonellosis. After reviewing correct feeding techniques and food with the owner, other appropriate diagnostics, such as fecal floats, should be taken. Other systemic illnesses can present with diarrhea as well.

Salmonella infections are well documented in hedgehogs. Symptoms include anorexia, mucoid diarrhea, dehydration, and weight loss. Treatment is supportive care (Johnson 2004).

Dermatologic Problems

Many forms of diseases can cause problems with skin or quill loss (Figure 16.4). The problems can range from ectoparasites, hypersensitivity, dermatophytosis, and neoplasia. Fungal infection can be found with normal fungal culture techniques and is most likely to be Trichophyton or Microsporum (Lightfoot 2000,

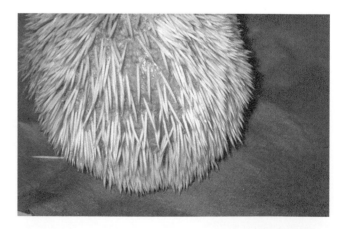

Figure 16.4. Mange. (Photo courtesy of Dr. Sam Rivera.)

Johnson 2004). Zoonotic transmission has been documented (Johnson 2004).

Generalized infections are characterized by crusting around the base of the spines. They can be treated with either griseofulvin (25 to 50 mg/kg by PO every 24 hours for thirty days) or ketoconazole (10 mg/kg PO every 24 hours for six to eight weeks) (Johnson 2004). If one hedgehog in a group is diagnosed, the entire group should receive treatment (Johnson 2004).

Ectoparasites are also common in the African Hedgehog. Mite infestations with Caparinia or chorioptes species are routine (Johnson 2004).

Neurological Problems
Progressive paralysis has been noted in hedgehogs. A viral encephalopathy has been noted in European hedgehogs (Ness 1999). Nutritional deficiencies can also cause many of the same signs. Rabies as well as Baylisascaris migration and polioencephalomyelitis are among the causes of neurologic disease.

Ophthalmologic Trauma
Due to the fact that these pets ball up, eye problems are usually associated with trauma and are not noticed until later in the course of the disease. These pets are also very difficult to treat. Enucleation is common and they do quite well with only one eye (Lightfoot 2000).

Liver Disease
Liver disease also occurs. Fatty liver disease and hepatic adenocarcinoma are two of the most common. Anorexia can be the only sign of liver disease (Johnson 2004).

Renal Disease
Tublointerstitial nephritis is the most common type of kidney disease found. Lethargy, weight loss, and polyuria and polydipsia may occur (Johnson 2004).

Internal Parasites
Hedgehogs are susceptible to internal parasites such as nematodes, cestodes, and protozoa. Isopora and Eimeria species coccidia can cause diarrhea. Lungworm infections can also occur and result in bronchopneumonia or even death. Internal parasites are diagnosed by fecal floatation and direct smear (Johnson 2004).

Respiratory Disease
Hedgehogs are susceptible to respiratory pathogens such as pasteurella, bordetella, and corynebacterium. Nasal discharge and sneezing may result. Diagnostic procedures include radiographs and culture and sensitivity. Treatment should be supportive and include antibiotics, fluid therapy, bronchodilators, and nebulization if needed (Johnson 2004).

Neoplasia
Neoplasia in hedgehogs is common. They can develop a wide range of tumors. Specific neoplasms reported in the hedgehog include squamous cell carcinomas, cutaneous mast cell tumors, mammary gland tumors, cutaneous hemangiosarcoma, alimentary lymphosarcomas, and plasmacytoma (Carpenter 2002).

OBTAINING A HISTORY AND PHYSICAL EXAMINATION

It is important to obtain as much information as possible about the pet before any actual handling takes place. Because hedgehogs are frightened very easily, it is better to observe the pet while taking a thorough history, including what the pet eats and drinks, its cage environment, or any other significant finding. Much of the physical examination must be performed under anesthesia to prevent the pet from balling up.

Hedgehogs can be difficult pets to pick up, but an object such as a spoon or litter box scooper can be used to pick them up. Be very gentle and make sure that a finger does not get caught if the pet is trying to ball up.

There are many techniques to get hedgehogs to unroll. One method is to hold the hedgehog over a flat surface with the head pointing downward. With time, the hedgehog will unroll and reach for the table. Once the pet has unrolled, gently grab the back legs and hold the animal suspended by the back legs over the table (Gregory 1992). If this fails, anesthesia is necessary. Isoflurane is very well tolerated by these pets (Lightfoot 1999). A mask or tank is the most effective way to administer anesthesia. Salivation is often encountered with isoflurane.

Hedgehogs have a wide variety of squeals, snuffling, and sneezes that should not be confused with abnormal respiratory sounds (Johnson 2004).

RADIOLOGY

Anesthesia is needed for accurate radiographs. Positioning is similar to that of other small animals.

ANESTHESIA AND SURGERY

Anesthesia is an important part of the physical exam (Figure 16.5). Isoflurane is well tolerated and is best

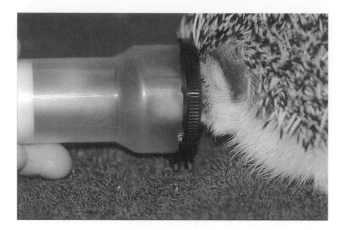

Figure 16.5. Anesthesia is maintained after initial induction by placing the patient in a face mask. (Photo courtesy of Ryan Cheek.)

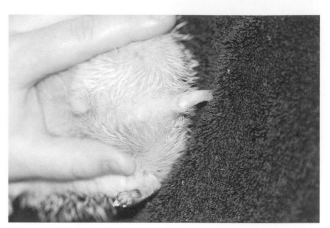

Figure 16.6. Male hedgehog. (Photo courtesy of Ryan Cheek.)

accomplished by using a large dog mask and removing the diaphragm. Place the entire mask over the hedgehog and then wait for sedation to occur. Once the hedgehog uncurls, it is preferable to switch to a smaller mask (Lightfoot 1999. Atropine (0.4 mg/kg SC, IM) can be given to help reduce hypersalivation. Injectable anesthetics are less reliable and seldom indicated. Supplemental heat is essential (Johnson 2004).

The most common surgical procedure is toe amputation, secondary to a foreign body that cuts off circulation. However, routine procedures are also performed including castration and ovariohysterectomy (Johnson 2004).

URINALYSIS

Extensive analysis of the urine of the African hedgehog has not been done but extrapolations can be made from research on the European hedgehog. Research showed that the urine was negative for glucose, acetone, and acetoacetic acid. Albumin was present in about half of the animals (Ness 1999).

PARASITOLOGY

Mites are a common problem with hedgehogs. The two major parasites commonly seen are the Caparinia and Chorioptic species. Caparinia is usually distributed over a significant portion of the body, and it may suddenly appear that entire hedgehog's skin is moving. Ivermectin is commonly used, but must be used with proper shampoos as well. The Chorioptic species usually presents as a moderate to severe skin infection around the face and ears. Ivermectin is very effective (Lightfoot 2000).

Dermatophytes are also common causes of quill loss. Trichophyton is the most common dermatophyte found.

A variety of nematode, cestode, and protozoan parasites have been found in hedgehogs. Coccidia is present in as much as 10% of wild hedgehogs (Ness 1999). *Crenosoama striatum* is a common lungworm of the wild hedgehog.

EMERGENCY AND CRITICAL CARE

Many of the same techniques used in small mammals can be used in hedgehogs; however, with hedgehogs, anesthesia is still needed to perform a good physical examination. Intraosseous catheters are very useful in these small patients. Many must be monitored carefully because they will start to curl up and make further diagnostics quite difficult.

SEX DETERMINATION

Figure 16.6 shows the reproductive anatomy of the hedgehog (also see Figure 16.1). Note that the distance from the penis to the anus is much greater than the distance from the vulva to the anus.

TECHNIQUES

Venipuncture

Venipuncture is next to impossible in the awake hedgehog. Supplies needed include a large face mask (diaphragm removed), small face mask; anesthesia machine; 1-ml, 25-gauge needle syringe; 3-ml, 22-gauge needle syringe; and blood collection tubes (preferably small tubes). The technique for a jugular venipuncture is as follows:

1. A large anesthetic face mask with diaphragm removed is obtained.
2. The patient is placed under the face mask with the opening of the face mask tight against the table.
3. Oxygen and anesthetic gas are turned on.
4. Wait for the patient to become anesthetized.

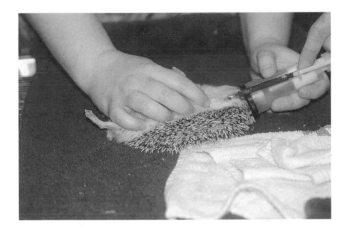

Figure 16.7. Jugular venipuncture. (Photo courtesy of Ryan Cheek.)

5. Once the patient is asleep the face mask is changed to a smaller one.
6. The patient is placed in dorsal recumbency.
7. Gentle pressure is applied to the thoracic inlet.
8. A 3-cc, 22-gauge or 1-cc, 25-gauge needle is inserted into the jugular vein caudally and directed cranially to the point of the jaw. Alternately, the needle could be inserted into the proximal vein with the needle directed caudally (Figures 16.7, 16.8). Gentle negative pressure is applied until blood is seen. **Note:** Many of these patients are obese so this technique is performed blindly.

TPR
Much of this information can be obtained while looking at the patient before it is handled; however, many times anesthesia is required. A large face mask with the diaphragm removed is placed over the patient and held tight to the table. Once the patient is anesthetized, a small face mask can be applied. The TPR can then be obtained along with a physical examination.

Urine Collection
The patient is anesthetized as described for the previous techniques. The patient is placed in dorsal recumbency once it is anesthetized. The bladder is palpated and stabilized while a 3-cc, 22-gauge needle is placed through the skin and body wall and then into the bladder. Once the sample collection is complete the needle and syringe are withdrawn.

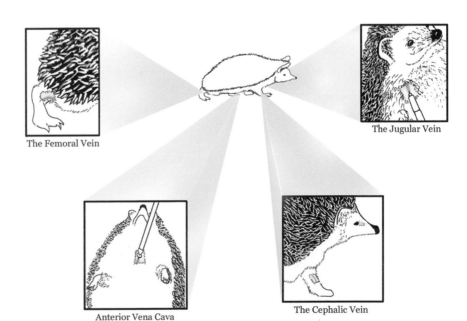

The Femoral Vein

The Jugular Vein

Anterior Vena Cava

The Cephalic Vein

Figure 16.8. Venipuncture sites. (Drawing by Scott Stark.)

Administration of Medications

Administration of fluids can be difficult. When hedgehogs are older they do not take to oral fluids easily, and they must be eating well if moistening the food is considered. Some oral medications can be injected into food but it must be certain that the patient is eating.

Injectable medications are tolerated well by these pets. Medications can be injected into the quill area subcutaneously (Lightfoot 2000). This is a high fat area of the hedgehog but absorption is sufficient.

Subcutaneous injections can be made in the rear legs or back. This is performed by carefully picking the patient up. A 25-gauge needle with a syringe is inserted between the quills and then under the skin. The medication is injected and then the needle and syringe removed.

Intravenous catheter placement can be done with the cephalic vein, but can be very difficult due to the size of the patient. When the pet awakens from anesthesia, it may curl up and cause the catheter to function improperly.

Bandaging and Wound Care

This is very difficult in these pets and one must be aware of what will happen to the bandage as the pet curls up. Anesthesia is required and normal bandaging techniques are used.

In general, many of the techniques used in small animal medicine can be used in hedgehogs; however, one must always consider the possible complications if the animal should curl up.

REFERENCES

Carpenter J. 2002. Diseases and Medicine of the African Hedgehog. Tufts Animal Expo.

Gregory M. 1992. Hedgehogs. In: Manual of Exotic Pets, edited by Beynon P, Cooper J. Gloucestershire: British Small Animal Veterinary Association. 63.

Johnson D. 2004. Diagnosing and Treating African Pygmy Hedgehogs. Atlantic Coast Veterinary Conference.

Lightfoot T. 1997. Clinical Techniques of Selected Exotic Species: Chinchilla, Prairie Dogs, Hedgehogs, and Chelonians. *Seminars in Avian and Exotic Pet Medicine* 6(2): 96–105.

Lightfoot T. 1999. Clinical Examination of the Chinchillas, Hedgehogs, Prairie Dogs, and Sugar Gliders. *Veterinary Clinics of North America Exotic Animal Practice* 2(2): 447–69.

Lightfoot T. 2000. Therapeutics of African Pygmy Hedgehogs and Prairie Dogs. *Veterinary Clinics of North America Exotic Animal Practice* 3(1): 155–72.

Ness R. 1999. Clinical Pathology and Sample Collection of Exotic Small Mammals. *Veterinary Clinics of North America Exotic Animal Practice* 2(3):591–620.

Storer P. 1994. Everything You Wanted to Know About Hedgehogs But You Didn't Know Who to Ask. Columbus, TX: Country Store Enterprises. 14–96.

CHAPTER SEVENTEEN

Skunks

Samuel Rivera

INTRODUCTION

Skunks are commonly kept as pets. They belong to the family Mustelidae. Other members of this family are ferrets, weasels, badgers, mink, and otters. The striped skunk (*Mephitis mephitis*) is the most common species found in the pet market. It is native to North America, ranging from southern Canada into the United States and northern Mexico. The most popular color pattern is brown fur with white stripes along the dorsum. The skunks in the pet market are usually descented at two to four weeks of age. Contrary to popular belief, skunks are usually not neutered at an early age. They have extremely sharp teeth and their bite can cause severe injuries.

Skunks adapt well to life in captivity and can be litter box trained and harness or leash trained. They are nocturnal animals but can adjust to a diurnal cycle. Even though they have poor sight, their hearing and sense of smell are very good. In the wild, skunks do not undergo true hibernation.

Skunks have unique health and dietary needs. Furthermore, there are limited resources describing their health and nutritional needs. In many states it is illegal to keep skunks as pets and it is essential for all the veterinary personnel to be familiar with the state and local regulations on keeping them as pets.

ANATOMY AND PHYSIOLOGY

The anatomy and physiology of skunks are similar to that of other carnivores. One difference is the highly developed anal sacs, which can eject their contents for a distance of three meters (Fowler 1986).

Biologic Data

Average lifespan: 10–12 years
Body temperature: 102°F (38.9°C)
Heart rate: 140–190 beats per minute
Respiratory rate: 25–50 breaths per minute
Average body weight: 4.5 kg
Gestation: 63 days
Litter size: 4–10
Urine pH: 6.0

HUSBANDRY AND NUTRITION

In the wild, adult males are solitary except during the winter months, when they may share a den with several females (Wallach and Boever 1983). Young skunks can be housed together, but as they get older they should be kept in separate enclosures. The cage should have a nest box and a litter box. Skunks have a natural instinct to dig and should be closely monitored when outside the cage.

Wild skunks are omnivores. Their natural diet consists of insects, rodents, small vertebrates, fruits, green vegetables, and grain. In captivity, skunks have been fed a variety of diets. To date there is not a formulated diet specifically designed for skunks. Light dog food or a zoo omnivore diet supplemented with fruits and vegetables has been recommended. A varied diet consisting of fruits, vegetables, eggs, a small amount of dog and cat food, yogurt, cottage cheese, mice, cereal, and insects should be provided. It is important to remember that skunks will eat anything in sight and as a result become obese. Dairy products are a good source of calcium but should be fed in limited amounts because they can cause gastrointestinal upset. Skunks tend to gain weight in the fall and are less active during the fall and winter months. Feeding an adequate diet will decrease the development of obesity and the associated health problems.

COMMON HEALTH PROBLEMS

Obesity
This is the most common clinical presentation and the leading cause of morbidity in skunks. Most pet skunks

are kept inside and fed an inadequate diet that leads to obesity. In some cases, correction of the diet and adequate husbandry practices can help to maintain a skunk at an ideal body weight.

Hepatic Lipidosis

This disease is caused by an increased accumulation of triglycerides in the liver, which is due to an increased mobilization of fat from the body stores and the inability of the liver to process it expeditiously. The end result is the buildup of fat within the hepatocytes leading to compromised normal function. There is a close relationship between obesity and the development of hepatic lipidosis. Clinical signs include prolonged anorexia, lethargy, vomiting, weight loss, and jaundice. The presumptive diagnosis of hepatic lipidosis is based on the history, physical exam findings, and serum chemistry abnormalities. A definitive diagnosis is based on the cytological evaluation of a liver fine-needle aspirate or biopsy. The treatment primarily involves supportive care.

AMYLOIDOSIS

This disease is characterized by the buildup of insoluble fibrillar proteins (amyloid) in multiple organ systems, leading to compromised function. The clinical signs are nonspecific and vary depending on which organ system is affected. The diagnosis is based on a histopathological evaluation of the affected tissue. There is no treatment reported in skunks.

Cardiomyopathy

Cardiac disease is commonly seen in obese skunks. The clinical signs are exercise intolerance, weight loss, dyspnea, lethargy, anorexia, coughing, ascites and/or edema, pale mucous membranes, and cold extremities. The diagnosis is based on radiographs, electrocardiogram, and echocardiogram. Cardiomyopathy is treated the same as in ferrets.

Dental Disease

The dental formula of skunks is 2(I3/3, C1/1, PM3/3, M1/1). Common dental conditions seen in skunks are advanced periodontal disease and fractured teeth. Common clinical signs are change in eating habits, halitosis, pawing at the mouth, hypersalivation, or facial swelling. Periodontal disease is usually a result of a poor diet. Treatment involves dental cleaning, antibiotics, and diet correction where appropriate.

Dermatitis

Skin problems are common in skunks, particularly in those that are obese. Some of the most commonly seen lesions are dry, scaly skin; alopecia; papules; pustules; and excoriations. Dermatitis can be caused by nutritional deficiencies, ectoparasites, and fungal or bacterial infections.

Canine Distemper

Canine distemper has been reported in the ferret, skunk, mink, badger, weasel, sable, and grison (Wallach et al. 1983). The clinical signs are fever, hyperemia of the face and ear, scleral inflammation, ocular discharge, depression, anorexia, diarrhea, dyspnea, hyperkeratosis of the foot pads, and neurologic signs. The incubation period is five to seven days for the acute phase. The diagnosis is based on clinical signs and serologic testing. Treatment involves mostly supportive care. Fluid support and broad-spectrum antibiotics should be initiated. Unvaccinated skunks that contract canine distemper have a poor prognosis.

Feline Panleukopenia

Feline panleukopenia has been reported in several mustelid species (Wallach et al. 1983). This is an acute viral disease that can lead to high mortality in skunks. The clinical signs are hemorrhagic enteritis, anorexia, and depression. Death usually occurs within three to five days after the onset of the clinical signs. A presumptive diagnosis is based on the characteristic clinical signs accompanied by a low white blood cell count. The best treatment is supportive care.

ZOONOTIC DISEASES

Baylisascaris columnaris is a roundworm found in skunks. This parasite can cause serious visceral larva migrans in humans. The usual contamination is through the fecal-oral route. Strict hygiene to decrease exposure to contaminated material is the best prevention.

Rabies is a serious human health problem. The rabies virus can be transmitted to humans through bites from infected skunks. In North America, the wild striped skunk is the most important wildlife reservoir of rabies (Drenzek and Rupprecht 2000). The clinical signs of rabies in skunks are varied. Generally, any behavior considered abnormal for the particular animal should be considered suspicious. The incubation period for rabies is from two weeks to six months. In the furious form of the disease, the virus can be shed in the saliva one to six days prior to death.

The diagnosis of rabies is based on the identification of viral antigen and/or characteristic lesions in the brain. Public health officials do not accept vaccination against rabies in pet skunks and the animal may need to be euthanized and tested for rabies if it is involved in a biting incident. Even though rabies is a concern in the wild skunk population, the disease is relatively rare in pet skunks. Pet skunks, as any other pet, can become infected with rabies if exposed to a reservoir in the wild.

PHYSICAL EXAMINATION

A healthy skunk should have a glossy, thick coat and bright, clear eyes. Yellow coloring of the white fur is considered abnormal. The stools should be formed. Obesity or an underweight patient should raise a red flag as to the health status of the pet.

Signs of illness in a skunk include change in stool consistency; dry, dull hair coat; yellowing of the white fur; obesity; dry, cracked feet; ocular or nasal discharge; coughing; sneezing; and bad breath.

VACCINATIONS

Pet skunks should be vaccinated against canine distemper, feline panleukopenia, and rabies (Miller 1995). There are no vaccines licensed for use in skunks. However, vaccines licensed for use in ferrets can be used in skunks. It is important to remember that if a skunk bites a person, public health officials will not accept rabies vaccination and the animal may need to be euthanized and tested for rabies.

RESTRAINT

Skunks can be restrained in a manner similar to cats. One difference is that many skunks lack a significant scruff, making scruffing behind the neck difficult and painful to the skunk. Most tame skunks can be picked up by placing one hand on each side of the body caudal to the axillary region. The animal can be restrained in this manner for taking the temperature or clipping the nails. The skunk's primary defense is the expression of its anal sacs; therefore, they tend to be less likely to bite as their primary means of defense. Leather gloves can be used for handling fractious animals, but remember that skunks have sharp teeth that can bite through leather gloves, causing severe injuries. Many fractious skunks need chemical immobilization prior to handling.

RADIOLOGY

The radiographic techniques and positioning are similar to those used in domestic animals. Many skunks require sedation to obtain good quality radiographs.

ANESTHESIA

Gas anesthesia is most commonly used in skunks. Sevoflurane and isoflurane are among the safest anesthetic agents used. The skunk can be anesthetized by placing it in an induction chamber. The animal can be maintained on gas anesthesia via a face mask or endotracheal intubation. Fractious animals that are difficult to handle can be anesthetized with parenteral drugs. If the animal cannot be safely contained, it can be transferred to a squeeze cage for intramuscular injection. Ketamine and medetomidine are commonly used together for induction of anesthesia.

PARASITOLOGY

Skunks are susceptible to a variety of parasites including roundworms, tapeworms, and coccidia. Roundworms and tapeworms are managed similar to an infestation in domestic animals. Coccidiosis can cause severe disease in skunks. The clinical signs commonly seen are diarrhea, weight loss, anorexia, dehydration, and depression. The diagnosis is based on the identification of oocysts in the feces. Treatment involves the administration of antiprotozoal agents similar to those used in domestic species.

Toxoplasmosis has been reported in skunks, ferrets, and weasels. The clinical signs are fever, lymphadenopathy, splenomegaly, myocarditis, pneumonitis, hepatitis, hydrocephalus, encephalitis, dermatitis, and enlarged lymph nodes. The antemortem diagnosis is based on serologic testing. Antiprotozoal drugs are used to treat toxoplasmosis.

The lungworm *Crenosoma mephitidis* is a parasite that can affect the lungs of skunks. The clinical signs are coughing, dyspnea, depression, anorexia, and depression. The diagnosis is based on the identification of the infective larvae in the feces.

CLINICAL TECHNIQUES

Blood Collection
Blood sampling is an important diagnostic tool, particularly when assessing a sick skunk. The sites most

commonly used are the jugular, cephalic, lateral saphenous, and femoral veins. Manual restraint for blood collection is appropriate for tame skunks used to handling or with extremely debilitated animals. Fractious animals need sedation for safe venipuncture. Remember that skunks have sharp teeth and can cause severe damage when they bite. The supplies needed include 25- to 22-gauge needles, 1- to 3-ml syringes, 70% isopropyl alcohol, and blood collection tubes. The size of the needle used depends on the size of the animal and the vein used.

Jugular vein: Skunks usually resist restraint for jugular venipuncture more than they do for cephalic or lateral saphenous collection. The restraint is similar to that used for cats. The animal should be restrained in sternal recumbency, with the front legs held over the edge of the table (Figure 17.1). The assistant can hold the head with one hand extended by holding the head from the dorsum; use the thumb and fingers and wrap the head in the palm, placing the thumb and fingers on opposite sides of the head under the temporomandibular joint. Gentle pressure is applied at the thoracic inlet lateral to the trachea. The needle is inserted bevel up at a 25 degree angle into the vein. After the sample is collected, pressure is released, the needle is withdrawn, and digital pressure is applied at the venipuncture site for thirty seconds.

Cephalic vein: The animal is restrained in sternal recumbency (Figure 17.2). An assistant should restrain the head by the scruff of the neck with one hand and the fore limb extended by the elbow. Alternatively, the head can be restrained as described for jugular venipuncture. Pressure is applied with the thumb around the elbow, rotating gently laterally. The limb is held with a free hand and the thumb is used to stabilize the

vein. The needle is inserted at a 20 to 25 degree angle. Once the vessel is entered, gentle suction is applied until the desired amount is obtained. Too much suction can cause collapse of the vein. Once the needle is withdrawn, gentle pressure should be applied to the venipuncture site.

Lateral saphenous vein: This vein is located in the lateral aspect of the hind limb. This is the third option if the other two vessels are not accessible. This vein is small and often yields a small volume of blood. The assistant can hold the skunk in lateral recumbency by holding the scruff of the neck with one hand and the venipuncture leg with the other hand. The leg is held around the stifle with the leg extended. The leg is grasped around the tarsus and the skin gently pulled to stabilize the vein. The needle is inserted at a 20 degree angle and the blood sample is collected. Digital pressure is applied for thirty seconds afterward to prevent hematoma formation.

Femoral vein: The femoral vein is located in the medial aspect of the thigh. Collection from this vein is performed similar to the cat. In obese skunks the femoral vein can be very difficult to find.

Urine Collection

Urinalysis is an important part of the health assessment in skunks. The techniques to collect urine are similar to those used in dogs and cats.

Voided urine: Urine can be collected from the bottom of the cage using a syringe. The disadvantage of this technique is that fecal and litter contamination affects the results.

Manual expression: With the animal sedated, transabdominal pressure is applied to the urinary bladder to overcome the sphincter pressure. The urine can be

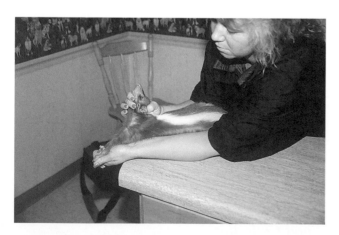

Figure 17.1. *Restraint for jugular venipuncture of the skunk. (Photo courtesy of Ryan Cheek.)*

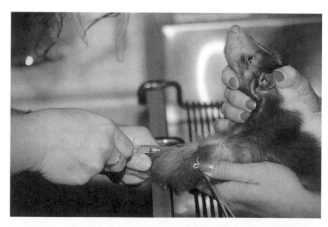

Figure 17.2. *Cephalic venipuncture in a skunk. (Photo courtesy of Ryan Cheek.)*

collected into a sterile container or from the tabletop.

Cystocentesis: With the animal sedated, the bladder is gently isolated. A 25- to 22-gauge needle on a 3- to 5-ml syringe is inserted into the bladder and the urine collected. This is the preferred method when performing a culture and sensitivity on the urine.

Fecal Analysis
The flotation and direct fecal smear techniques are the same as for domestic species.

ADMINISTRATION OF MEDICATIONS

There are several routes for administration of medications.

Oral route: Liquids or powders mixed with food are the most common forms of oral medications. In many cases the skunk's sharp teeth preclude the use of tablets. Liquid medications can be placed in the side of the mouth with a syringe. Powder medications can be mixed with a favorite treat or a small amount of soft food such as yogurt or cottage cheese.

Intramuscular route: Parenteral medications can be given in the thigh musculature or the biceps.

Subcutaneous route: This site is most commonly used for the administration of fluids to sick animals. The intrascapular and lateral flank regions are the best sites for the administration of subcutaneous fluids.

Intravenous route: The cephalic, jugular, and saphenous veins can be used for the administration of medications. In most cases the skunk must be sedated to facilitate intravenous medications, unless the animal is severely debilitated.

REFERENCES

Drenzek CL, Rupprecht CE. 2000. The rabies pandemic. In: Kirk's Current Veterinary Therapy XIII, edited by Bonagura JD. Philadelphia: W.B. Saunders Co.

Fowler ME. 1986. Descenting carnivores. In: Zoo and Wild Animal Medicine, 2nd ed., edited by Fowler ME. Philadelphia: W.B. Saunders Co.

Miller E. 1995. Immunization of wild animal species against common diseases. In: Kirk's Current Veterinary Therapy XII, edited by Bonagura JD. Philadelphia: W.B. Saunders Co.

Wallach JD, Boever WJ. 1983. Diseases of exotic animals: medical and surgical management. Philadelphia: W.B. Saunders Co.

CHAPTER EIGHTEEN

Sugar Gliders

Samuel Rivera

INTRODUCTION

Sugar gliders (*Petaurus breviceps*) are small marsupials native to Australia and New Zealand (Figure 18.1). They are nocturnal arboreal animals. In the wild, sugar gliders live in groups of up to twelve individuals (Booth 2000). They are very social animals that are best kept in pairs or small related groups, and they require a large enclosure with branches, nest boxes, and hiding areas. Proper husbandry and diet are essential for a healthy pet. During extreme weather conditions or food shortages, sugar gliders conserve energy by going into torpor for up to sixteen hours per day (Booth 2000).

ANATOMY

Sugar gliders have blue-gray fur with a dark line extending from the nose to the lower back. Each foot has five digits. The second and third digits of the hind feet are partially fused. They do not have the eupubic bones that support the pouch characteristic of marsupials. Sugar gliders have a membrane (the pet-agium) that extends from the lateral aspect of the fore limb to the tarsus. This membrane allows the sugar glider to glide a fair distance. Males have frontal, sternal, and urogenital scent glands. The females have a pouch and urogenital glands. Scent glands are also found on the paws, corners of the mouth, and external ears. The scent glands are used for marking territory and members of the same group (Smith 1984). The males have a pendulous scrotum located cranial to the penis. The female have a ventral abdominal pouch that opens cranially. Sugar gliders have a cloaca where the gastrointestinal, urinary, and reproductive tracts empty. They have a large cecum that may assist in digestion of the sap eaten in the wild (Henry and Suckling 1984).

Sugar gliders have a short gestation period with a longer development within the pouch.

Biologic Data

Weight range: 95–160 grams
Body length: 16–21 cm
Heart rate: 200–300 beats per minute
Respiratory rate: 16–40 breaths per minute
Rectal temperature: 96.5°F–97.9°F (35.8°C–36.6°C)
Gestation 15–17 days, young leave the pouch at 70 days
Weaning age: 110–120 days
Lifespan: 9–12 years

HUSBANDRY AND NUTRITION

Sugar gliders need a lot of room. The larger the enclosure, the better for the animal. An enclosure measuring 2 × 2 × 2 meters is adequate for housing up to six animals (Dunn 1982). A nest box for sleeping and hiding must be provided. The nest box can be lined with a piece of cloth, shredded bark, or dried leaves, and should be changed weekly. Newspaper and pine or cedar wood shavings are not recommended. Sugar gliders are arboreal animals; therefore, branches for

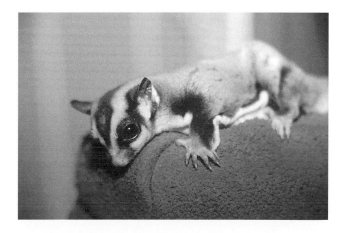

Figure 18.1. Sugar glider. (Photo courtesy of Ryan Cheek.)

climbing are essential. A pair is the minimum number to keep together.

The environmental temperature should be between 64°F and 75°F (18°C to 24°C). They can withstand temperature in the mid to high 80s but higher temperatures can predispose them to hyperthermia.

In the wild, sugar gliders eat sap and gum from eucalyptus and acacia trees, nectar from eucalyptus blossoms, and a variety of insects (Henry and Suckling 1984). The diet in captivity consists of a variety of fruits, commercial sugar glider pellets, commercial insectivore diets, insects supplemented with vitamin and minerals, nectar, and small invertebrates. They are mainly insectivores but also eat sugar-containing sap from several sources. Food and water should be provided in an elevated location. Nectar should be provided in covered feeders to keep the nectar from getting on the fur. The ideal amount of food to offer is 15% to 20% of their body weight (Booth 2000).

COMMON DISEASES

Nutritional Osteodystrophy
This is one of the most common diseases seen in captive sugar gliders (Pye and Carpenter 1999). The clinical signs include acute onset of hind limb paresis or paralysis. This disease is believed to be caused by feeding an inadequate diet low in calcium and vitamin D_3 and high in phosphorus. Too much fruit and muscle meat can predispose animals to this disease. The diagnosis is based on a thorough history and radiographs. The treatment includes cage rest, parenteral calcium, diet correction, and calcium and vitamin D_3 supplementation.

Trauma
Trauma is most common in wild sugar gliders. In captivity the most common cases of trauma involve cat and dogs attacks. Some of the common injuries are lacerations, pneumothorax, hemothorax, spinal trauma, and ocular trauma.

Dental Disease
Tartar buildup associated with periodontal disease is often seen. This has been associated with feeding carbohydrate-rich diets (Booth 2000). The teeth can be cleaned as needed. Feeding insects with a hard exoskeleton can help minimize tartar buildup.

Obesity
Obesity is seen in sugar gliders fed an inadequate diet. Diets high in fat and proteins predispose animals to obesity. Lack of exercise can also contribute to obesity. Obese animals are predisposed to cardiac and hepatic disease.

Stress-related Disease
Animals under constant stress are prone to developing behavioral problems. Some of the clinical signs of stress-related disorders include alopecia, self-mutilation, coprophagia, hyperphagia, polyuria, pacing, and cannibalism. The source of the stress must be identified and eliminated to help correct the problem.

Neoplasia
Neoplastic disease is relatively common. Lymphoid neoplasia is the most common type of tumor reported (Booth 2000). Other tumors reported include mammary gland tumors, bronchogenic carcinoma, and chondrosarcoma.

Malnutrition
Malnutrition is frequently seen in sugar gliders fed an inadequate diet. As a result, malnutrition leads to hypocalcemia, hypoproteinemia, and anemia. The clinical signs of malnutrition are nonspecific and include lethargy, weakness, dehydration, pale mucous membranes, cachexia, and in some cases seizures and pathologic fractures. The owner should be educated about the appropriate diet. Treatment involves correction of the dietary inadequacies and supportive care.

PHYSICAL EXAMINATION

Sugar gliders can be challenging to examine without sedation. A thorough history should be taken first. Ask about the number of animals kept and the enclosure size. The diet should be recorded. The owner should be asked whether there are other pets in the household, and where the animal was obtained. While taking the history, the animal's motor function and disposition can be observed. If a weight is needed, many times the owners can place the animal on the scale and then the weight can be recorded. If the animal is fractious, the weight can be obtained by placing the animal in a cloth bag.

RESTRAINT

The best way to restrain sugar gliders is by holding the head between the thumb and middle finger and using the index finger to restrain the top of the head. The body is then placed in the palm of the restrainer's hand. Fractious animals can be restrained using a cloth bag. To accomplish this the owner should place the animal in a small enclosure (scale basket or nest box). Then a cloth bag is placed over the hand that will grasp the animal. The animal is then grasped and the bag slipped over the whole body. Once in the bag one can gently expose the head and restrain it. It is important to keep the seam of the bag toward the outside to keep the animal from injuring itself with the small threads.

RADIOLOGY

The radiographic techniques are similar to those used in other domestic animals. Because of their small size, high-definition radiograph film offers the best detail.

ANESTHESIA

Gas anesthetics such as sevoflurane and isoflurane are most commonly used. Induction can be accomplished by either face mask or chamber induction. A large face mask can be used as an induction chamber. The animal can be maintained via a face mask.

PARASITOLOGY

Coccidia and *Giardia spp.* have been identified in captive sugar gliders (Ness 1999). The diagnosis is based on the identification of the oocysts or trophozoites in the fecal sample. There is limited information on the incidence of gastrointestinal parasites in sugar gliders.

CLINICAL TECHNIQUES

Blood Collection
The blood volume that can be safely collected is up to 1% of the body weight. Because of their active nature, sugar gliders often require sedation for blood collection, unless the animal is severely debilitated. They can be sedated using isoflurane or sevoflurane via a mask or chamber induction.

Supplies needed include 27– to 30-gauge needles, 0.5– to 1-ml syringes, and 0.5-ml collection tubes.

Jugular vein: The animal is placed in dorsal recumbency and the fore limbs are aimed caudally. Gentle pressure is applied in the thoracic inlet. The fur is moistened along the jugular groove to allow better visualization. The needle is then inserted at a 30 to 45 degree angle in the jugular groove. Negative pressure

is applied as the needle is advanced. The syringe will fill with blood as the jugular vein is entered.

Cranial vena cava: The animal is placed in dorsal recumbency. Both fore limbs are extended caudally. The needle is inserted at the angle formed by the manubrium and the first rib. The needle is aimed toward the contra-lateral hip joint at a very shallow angle. Suction is applied as the needle is advanced. It will fill with blood as soon as the vessel is entered. It is important not to reposition the needle in an attempt to find this vessel. If the vessel is missed, the needle should be withdrawn and another attempt made. Other vessels and nerves can be damaged inadvertently by excessive manipulation of the needle.

Medial tibial artery: The hind limb is held in the extended position with the medial aspect exposed. The fur is slightly moistened with alcohol. The artery runs superficially from the stifle to the tarsus. The vessel should be visualized and the needle then inserted at a 30 degree angle. After the blood is collected, gentle pressure should be applied to the site to avoid hematoma formation.

Other sites for blood collection include the cephalic, lateral saphenous, femoral, ventral coccygeal, and lateral tail veins. The main disadvantage is that only very small amounts of blood can be collected from these sites due to their small size. In some cases, a small-gauge heparinized needle can be inserted into the vein and the blood collected directly from the hub using small collection containers or capillary tubes.

Urine Collection
Urinalysis is an important part of the health assessment in sugar gliders. The techniques to collect urine are similar to those used in dogs and cats.

Voided urine: Urine can be collected from the bottom of the cage using a small syringe. The disadvantage of this technique is that fecal and litter contamination affects the results.

Manual expression: With the animal sedated, gentle transabdominal pressure is applied to the urinary bladder to overcome the sphincter pressure. The urine can be collected into a sterile container or from the tabletop.

Cystocentesis: With the animal sedated, gently isolate the bladder. A 27- to 25-gauge needle on a 0.5- to 1-ml syringe is inserted into the bladder and the urine collected. This is the preferred method when performing a culture and sensitivity on the urine.

Fecal Analysis
The flotation and direct fecal smear techniques are the same as for domestic species.

REFERENCES

Booth RJ. 2000. General husbandry and medical care of sugar gliders. In Kirk's Current Veterinary Therapy XIII, edited by Bonagura JD. Philadelphia: W.B. Saunders Co.

Dunn RW. 1982. Gliders of the genus Petaurus: their management in zoos. In: The management of Australian mammals in captivity, edited by Evans DD. North Melbourne, Australia: Ramsay Ware Stockland.

Henry SR, Suckling GC. 1984. A review of the ecology of the sugar glider. Possums and gliders, edited by Smith PA, Hume ID. Australian Mammal Society. Sydney, Australia.

Ness RD. 1999. Clinical pathology and sample collection of exotic small mammals. *The Veterinary Clinics of North America Exotic Animal Practice*, edited by Reavill DR, 2(3): 591–620.

Pye GW. 2001. Marsupial, insectivore, and chiropteran anesthesia. *The Veterinary Clinics of North America Exotic Animal Practice*, edited by Heard DL, 4(1):211–37.

Smith MJ. 1984. The reproductive system and paracloacal glands of *Petaurus breviceps* and *Gymnobelideus leadbeateri* (*Marsupalia: Petauridae*), edited by Smith PA, Hume ID. Australian Mammal Society. Sydney, Australia.

CHAPTER NINETEEN

Prairie Dogs

Samuel Rivera

INTRODUCTION

The black-tailed prairie dog (*Cyonomys ludovicianus*) is a rodent native to North America, more specifically to the western plains of the United States. Over recent years prairie dogs have become common in the pet trade. Prairie dogs are diurnal, social animals that live in large groups in the wild. The ownership of wild-caught prairie dogs should be discouraged due to serious zoonotic potential. It is important to be aware that owning prairie dogs is illegal in certain states.

ANATOMY AND PHYSIOLOGY

The anatomy and physiology of prairie dogs are similar to that of other rodents of comparable size. They are hindgut fermenters. The male has a prominent scrotum and the penis is relatively easy to exteriorize. The female has a short distance between the anus and the vaginal groove. Prairie dogs have a characteristic set of scent gland papillae that can be visualized on the anal margin when the animal is stressed.

Biologic Data

Average weight: 0.5–2.2 kg
Average lifespan: 6–10 years
Temperature: 95.7°F–102.3°F (35.4°C–39.1°C)
Heart rate: 83–318/minute
Respiration: 40–60/minute
Gestation: 30 days

HUSBANDRY AND NUTRITION

Prairie dogs are very social animals that are best kept in pairs or more. Prairie dogs require adequate room for digging. The enclosure should be made of heavy-gauge wire or stainless steel. It is important to provide a thick layer of substrate to allow the animals to burrow. Adequate bedding includes recycled paper, nonaromatic wood shavings, and hay. The larger the enclosure, the better. The enclosure should include a suitable hiding box and it should also be well ventilated.

Prairie dogs are not true hibernators. When exposed to low ambient temperature they may undergo torpor, a state in which the body's physiological activities are greatly reduced to conserve energy. The environmental temperature should be kept between 69°F and 72°F (20.5°C to 22°C) and the humidity at 30% to 70% (Johnson-Delaney 1996).

Prairie dogs are mostly herbivores. They should be fed high-quality grass hay ad lib, supplemented with a commercially formulated diet. Fresh water must be provided on a daily basis.

COMMON AND ZOONOTIC DISEASES

Barbering
This condition often presents as areas of abnormal fur appearance with underlying healthy skin. It can be caused by the animal or a cage mate chewing the fur. It is often related to stress, and husbandry practices must be evaluated to help minimize fur barbering.

Obesity
Obesity is commonly seen in prairie dogs. As with other unusual pets, this condition is often due to inadequate diet and lack of proper exercise. Diets high in fat, such as seeds and nuts, lead to obesity and should be avoided. Obesity predisposes prairie dogs to other conditions such as heart, respiratory, and liver disease.

Nasal Dermatitis
This is a common condition in captive prairie dogs. It is most often due to rubbing the face on the cage wire. This results in abrasions and inflammation leading to secondary bacterial infections.

Dermatomycosis (Ringworm)

Prairie dogs are susceptible to *Microsporum canis* and *Trichophyton mentagrophytes*. The most common clinical sign is alopecia. The diagnosis is based on a positive fungal culture. The treatment is similar to that of domestic animals and involves the administration of systemic antifungal drugs in addition to topical antifungal treatment.

Respiratory Disease

Respiratory disease is relatively common in prairie dogs. Obesity and poor ventilation are two common predisposing factors. Cedar bedding contains aromatic oils that can lead to irritation of the respiratory tract. Nasal foreign bodies (cage litter, hay, carpet fibers) are common presentations. Overgrowth of the maxillary incisor teeth roots can lead to increased pressure and irritation in the nasal sinus passages. Pneumonia is often associated with bacterial and viral agents. The clinical signs of respiratory disease are similar to those seen in dogs and cats. They include dyspnea, nasal or ocular discharge, cyanosis, anorexia, and lethargy. The treatment includes appropriate antibiotic therapy and supportive care. Appropriate husbandry is important in the prevention of respiratory disease.

Odontomas

This is a common cause of upper respiratory symptoms in captive prairie dogs (Phalen 2000). Odontomas are caused by an inflammation of the periodontal bone as a result of dental disease or trauma. This inflammation leads to narrowing of the nasal passages. The diagnosis is based on radiographic abnormalities of the incisor's root and surrounding soft tissue. Treatment involves removal of the affected teeth and debridement of the abnormal tissue.

Heart Disease

Obesity is a predisposing factor for the development of heart disease. Clinical signs are lethargy, syncope, cyanosis, dyspnea, and cold extremities. The diagnosis is based on auscultation, radiography, echocardiography, and ultrasonography.

Pododermatitis (Bumblefoot)

This condition is usually the result of poor husbandry. Animals kept on wire-bottom cages can develop small ulcers on the footpads that become infected. The infection results in severe swelling and abscess formation in the affected foot. In severe cases tendinitis and osteomyelitis can develop. Bumblefoot is treated by debriding the affected lesions in conjunction with topical and systemic antibiotics. Correction of the underlying husbandry problem is essential for resolution and/or prevention of bumblefoot.

Zoonotic Diseases

Prairie dogs, particularly wild-caught animals, can be reservoirs of *Yersinia pseudotuberculosis*, *Yersinia pestis*, and *Baylisascaris procyonidae*. *Yersinia pseudotuberculosis* can cause severe illness in humans. Affected humans can develop acute mesenteric lymphadenitis, fever, anorexia, vomiting, enteritis with diarrhea, and dehydration. This bacteria is transmitted to humans through the ingestion of contaminated material. *Yersinia pestis* is the causative agent of Sylvatic Plague in humans. This bacteria is transmitted to humans through the bite of fleas from carrier prairie dogs. Humans can also contract the infection from handling tissues from affected animals during necropsy. Flea control is essential to eliminate the human risk of exposure.

Baylisascaris procyonidae can cause serious visceral larva migrans in humans. This parasite is transmitted to humans through the ingestion of contaminated material or contact with open wounds on the skin.

Monkeypox is a zoonotic viral disease found primarily in wild mammals and people in the central and western African rainforests. The first report of this illness was in monkeys in 1958, hence the name, but many other mammals are susceptible to the virus. Monkeypox virus belongs in the Orthopoxvirus group. The majority of the viruses in this group can cause systemic disease characterized by fever and rashes and may be fatal in some species. In June 2003, an outbreak of monkeypox in people and pet prairie dogs occurred in the United States, primarily in the states of Illinois, Indiana, Kansas, Ohio, Missouri, and Wisconsin. These people began contracting monkeypox after handling sick pet prairie dogs. Transmission of the virus can occur through animal bites or direct contact with the animal's blood, body fluids or lesions. It can also spread from person to person. Traceback investigations conducted by the Centers of Disease Control and Prevention revealed that the sick prairie dogs had been exposed to the virus through a pet distributor prior to sale. The prairie dogs had been kept in close proximity to imported African rodents. Laboratory testing revealed that some of those African rodents (Gambian giant rats, dormice, and rope squirrels) were also infected with the monkeypox virus.

Monkeypox is not a typical zoonotic disease associated with prairie dogs in the United States. However, this outbreak is a good example of how important it is for veterinary staff and pet owners to be aware of the risk of disease that can exist with pet ownership.

The potential of acquiring a zoonotic disease depends on many factors. What is the origin of the animal (captive-born or wild, domestic, or imported)? How much contact with other animals did it have during shipping or in the pet store or with breeder? Is it housed outdoors and exposed to wild animals? These are only a few of the factors to consider when evaluating the potential of a zoonotic disease in a sick pet. Veterinarians and veterinary technicians should strive to remain informed and proactive with their pet owners so that appropriate information can be shared and actions taken in maintaining good health for the pet and its owners (CDC monkeypox website; CDC 2003).

RESTRAINT

Prairie dogs are difficult to restrain. Animals that are accustomed to frequent handling can be quite tame and examined awake. However, in many cases sedation is needed to perform a thorough physical exam. Prairie dogs do not have much loose skin around the neck, making it difficult to scruff. Prairie dogs have sharp claws and teeth that can cause severe wounds to the handler. Tame animals used to being handled can be restrained by placing one hand around the chest and supporting the hind end with the other hand. Alternatively, the animal can be grabbed at the base of the tail and lifted gently with the forelimbs resting on a flat surface. The free hand is used to grab the animal on the back of the neck. This technique can be used to move the animal or to perform minor procedures such as nail clipping. Additionally, a thick towel can be used to wrap the animal. This allows for closer examination of the head and the administration of intramuscular injections in the hind limbs. The towel also protects the handler from been scratched.

RADIOLOGY

The radiographic techniques and positioning are similar to those used in domestic animals. Prairie dogs, unless severely debilitated, require sedation to obtain good quality radiographs.

ANESTHESIA

Sevoflurane and isoflurane gas are the most commonly used anesthetic agents. Induction can be accomplished by chamber induction. Tracheal intubation is difficult in prairie dogs. As a result, the animal can be main-tained via a face mask. When the animal is anesthetized, its anterior end should be kept slightly elevated so the extensive viscera do not put excessive pressure on the diaphragm.

CLINICAL TECHNIQUES

Venipuncture
Many animals require sedation for blood collection. The jugular vein is the preferred site for blood collection. In obese prairie dogs this vein can be difficult to visualize and is often approached blindly. The sedated animal is restrained in dorsal recumbency. The animal is kept with the anterior end elevated to facilitate breathing. In prairie dogs the pressure from the abdominal organs on the diaphragm can compromise respiration. With the animal in dorsal recumbency, the fore limbs should be extended caudally. Gentle pressure should be applied at the thoracic inlet. The fur along the jugular groove should be moistened. A 23- to 25-gauge needle in a 1- to 3-ml syringe should be used. The needle should be inserted at a 45 degree angle and suction applied as the needle is advanced forward. In some cases the needle may need to be redirected to either side to find the vein. Blood will immediately fill the syringe as the needle enters the vein.

Venipuncture from the cephalic and lateral saphenous veins is done similar to the way blood is drawn in other animals of comparable size. The cephalic vein is located on the dorsal aspect of the front leg and the lateral saphenous vein is located in the lateral aspect of the hind limb, just above the tarsus.

Urine Collection
Urinalysis is an important part of health assessment in sick prairie dogs. The techniques to collect urine are similar to those used in dogs and cats.

Voided urine: Urine can be collected from the bottom of the cage using a small syringe. The disadvantage of this technique is that fecal and litter contamination affects the results.

Manual expression: With the animal sedated, gentle transabdominal pressure is applied to the urinary bladder to overcome the sphincter pressure. The urine can be collected into a sterile container or from the tabletop. Excessive pressure should not be applied because this can lead to rupture of the urinary bladder.

Cystocentesis: With the animal sedated, gently isolate the bladder. A 27- to 25-gauge needle on a 0.5- to 1-ml syringe is inserted into the bladder and the urine collected. This is the preferred method when performing a culture and sensitivity on the urine.

Fecal Analysis

The flotation and direct fecal smear techniques are the same as for domestic species.

Administration of Medications

There are several routes for administration of medications.

Oral route: Liquids are the most common forms of oral medications. The prairie dog's small mouth and sharp teeth preclude the use of tablets. Liquid medications can be placed in the side of the mouth with a syringe.

Intramuscular route: Parenteral medications can be given in the thigh musculature or the biceps.

Subcutaneous route: This site is most commonly used for the administration of fluids to sick animals. The intrascapular and lateral flank regions are the best sites for the administration of subcutaneous fluids.

Intravenous route: The cephalic, jugular, and saphenous veins can be used for the administration of medications. In most cases, the prairie dog must be sedated to facilitate intravenous medications, unless the animal is severely debilitated.

REFERENCES

CDC Monkeypox website: http://www.cdc.gov/ncidod/monkeypox/

Centers for Disease Control and Prevention (CDC). 2003. Multistate outbreak of monkeypox—Illinois, Indiana, and Wisconsin, 2003. *MMWR Morb Mortal Wkly Rep.* Jun 13:52(23): 537–40.

Johnson-Delaney CA. 1996. *Exotic companion medicine handbook for veterinarians.* Lake Worth: Wingers Publishing.

Phalen DN, Atinoff N, Fricke ME. 2000. Obstructive respiratory disease in prairie dogs with odontomas. *The Veterinary Clinics of North America Exotic Animal Practice*, edited by Phalen DN, 3(2): 513–17.

Section 6
Wildlife Rehabilitation

CHAPTER TWENTY

The Role of the Veterinary Technician in Wildlife Rehabilitation

Melanie Haire

INTRODUCTION

Wildlife rehabilitation is the process of rescuing, raising, and treating orphaned, diseased, displaced, or injured wild animals with a goal of releasing them back to their natural habitats. For rehabilitation to be deemed successful, these released animals must be able to truly function as wild animals. This includes being able to recognize and obtain the appropriate foods, select mates of their own species and reproduce, and show the appropriate fear of potential dangers (people, cars, dogs, etc.) (Pokras 1995).

The veterinary technician is on the front line for receiving injured and/or orphaned wildlife. A background in veterinary medicine and animal husbandry makes veterinary technicians perfect candidates for this rewarding endeavor. In fact, the general public often assumes that the veterinary technician is knowledgeable about all species. This assumption could be detrimental to the wild animal's welfare if the technician does not have access to the proper instruction, facilities, and materials needed to care for these unique individuals.

This chapter is a compilation of pertinent information to provide the veterinary technician with the resources and guidelines needed to provide temporary care for many of the wildlife species that are encountered in veterinary hospitals today. It includes charts, instructional articles, networking contacts, product sources, suggested readings, and references taken from numerous literary sources on the topic of rehabilitation of North American wildlife. Interested technicians should note there are many books, seminars, web groups, and related organizational memberships available for anyone interested in quality wildlife care and a list of a suggested few is provided in Appendix 11.

The information in this chapter is primarily to be used as a starting reference point for the wild animal care technician working in a small animal clinic. It provides immediate information that can be used until more detailed information is obtained or the animal is transferred from the veterinary clinic to a licensed rehabilitator for long-term care and release.

GETTING STARTED

For a veterinary technician, the level of involvement in wildlife rehabilitation can range from the care of an occasional orphan discovered by a hospital client to a career on staff at a wildlife center. The technician can rehabilitate wild animals as a full-time occupation, as a volunteer at a wildlife center, on the job at a veterinary clinic, or at home in addition to a separate career. Many zoological parks and aquariums also provide care to injured and orphaned wildlife and have separate facilities and staff designated for such activity.

Although the numbers and types of animals received by different wildlife technicians varies, legal obligations are relatively consistent. To keep or possess in captivity any sick, orphaned, or injured wildlife, one must first obtain a wildlife rehabilitation permit from the state and/or federal government. Everyone, including the veterinarian, must have his or her own permit or be listed on someone else's permit to rehabilitate wildlife. Each state has its own laws and requirements but most require a permit to work with any indigenous species. A federal permit is required in addition to a state permit to work with migratory birds. A list of governmental departments that issue applications and permits is provided in Appendix 1. The permitee is responsible for knowing which species are covered on the permit and their individual regulations. The rehabilitator is responsible for keeping records on each animal and knowing its current listed status (non-threatened versus endangered).

It is very important for anyone doing rehabilitation to build a reference library. The collection should contain literature on three basic topics: natural history, wildlife rehabilitation, and veterinary medicine as rehabilitation, which is a combination of all three. The veterinary technician should always keep in mind, when reading articles and talking to other rehabilitators, that there is more than one way to do things. New information is always coming out and it is the veterinary technician's responsibility to keep current as well as to learn to recognize which techniques might work better in different situations. Common sense and experience are the best ways to sort out contradictory suggestions and inaccurate information.

Networking with other rehabilitators is one of the most important sources for information. A list can be obtained from your state's special permits department with the names and contact numbers of all the rehabilitators in your state. These contacts can prove helpful for answering questions as they arise, helping to place animals that aren't covered by your permit, placing animals when the clinic has reached a full capacity, and building a network team to help with long-term animal care and releases.

REHABILITATING WILDLIFE IN A SMALL ANIMAL VETERINARY HOSPITAL

If the staff at a veterinary practice is interested in wildlife rehabilitation, it needs to establish a set of protocols. To accomplish this, the staff needs to first understand all that is involved. Rehabilitation can be both expensive and time-consuming. Profit making is not a valid or realistic reason to do rehabilitation. Currently there is no monetary assistance provided by any governmental departments to cover or reimburse rehabilitators for the costs of wildlife care.

Another crucial and difficult point that needs to be understood and accepted is that half of the animals that come in for rehabilitation will die or need to be euthanized. This is often extremely taxing emotionally on veterinary personnel, people who chose their profession to save lives. Deciding to euthanize an animal that could otherwise be saved but not returned to the wild with a good quality of life (such as releasing a one-legged hawk) may just be too hard for some individuals. Euthanasia is never an easy choice but keeping a wild animal alive because one "cannot handle" putting it to sleep is selfish and inhumane. Occasionally, nonreleasable wildlife can be placed in appropriate educational facilities but quality of life should always be the highest priority.

Another issue concerns zoonotic diseases and learning to recognize them. Injured wildlife may expose hospital staff and animals to new risks. Proper personal hygiene as well as facility disinfecting techniques and protocols are critically important. Separate housing areas and separate clothing available for these areas provide safeguards against infectious or zoonotic cases. One method is to always treat the sick animals last so as not to transmit diseases to any other patient.

Hospital staff that has any contact with the wildlife should consider having the appropriate prophylactic vaccinations, such as tetanus and rabies, to protect them. Consultation with a personal physician is recommended.

Despite these cautions, there are many reasons to consider this volunteer work. It generates good clinic PR, provides a valuable service to the community and the clinic's clientele, is a kind act of giving something back to nature, and offers a personal reward for giving a living creature a second chance that it otherwise may not have had. Veterinarians benefit by gaining skill at performing new procedures (i.e. IM pin in an owl) by first learning on wildlife patients. Veterinary technicians can gain valuable experience in exotic animal handling from wildlife work such as restraint, anesthesia, blood collecting, bandaging, radiology, and necropsy.

CLINIC PROTOCOLS

Selecting Types of Wildlife to Care For
If the decision is made to rehabilitate, clinic procedures and protocols must be written and clear. Among the decisions to make are the types and number of animals the practice can reasonably take in. Taking in more animals or more species than personnel are prepared to properly and safely handle can easily overwhelm a clinic. One way to set limits is to specialize in a particular species or area (i.e. only birds of prey or injured wildlife, no orphans, etc.) and refer the other calls to another qualified recipient.

Above all, the motto "Do no harm" should always be remembered when working with animal patients, and wildlife is no exception. Wildlife rehabilitation should not be attempted at a clinic without sufficient staff to do the feedings, treatments, cage cleanings, and so forth, because the animals will be the ones that suffer. The ability to realize one's limits shows professionalism. Hospital managers and owners need to make a clear decision about animal limits based on costs and expenses. Staffing and other business costs are very real factors that should be discussed ahead of time to help avoid staff "burn out" or resentment.

Stabilization or Long-Term Rehabilitation—An Important Decision

Temporary stabilization verses long-term care should be determined by examining the layout of the buildings and grounds, available facilities, and the number and experience of participating staff. Barking dogs, staring cats, ringing phones, and exposure to people are unacceptable conditions for long-term rehabilitation. A treatment room might be a marginally acceptable area to keep an orphaned two-week-old squirrel (both eyes and ears are closed at two weeks) but not a high-stress, imprintable, or easily habituated animal such as a deer fawn or raptor. Very few veterinary hospitals have flight cages of appropriate sizes and materials to adequately recondition a red-tailed hawk for release. Wildlife must be respected as wild and provided with suitable housing to reduce additional stress and fear and to promote natural behaviors that are necessary for successful release.

If there is no dedicated space for the animals, the clinic should provide temporary care only until they are stable and can be safely transferred to another rehabilitator. Veterinary hospitals without adequate facilities for rehabilitation can still perform a vital function for wildlife by becoming a drop-off and/or referral site for the public. This arrangement can benefit both the animal, by providing it with proper temporary care away from the well-intentioned but often detrimental handling of the rescuer, and the rehabilitator by providing a valuable time-saver of a one-stop pick-up location.

Often the single most crucial role for the technician in a veterinary practice is simply to give the public accurate names and phone numbers of appropriate rehabilitators. Putting the public in direct communication with the rehabilitation facility that will provide long-term care can eliminate the sometimes-fatal animal stress and delay of using the hospital as a drop-off site. This system allows the rehabilitator to be the clearing point and advise the finder about how to return the animal if care is not truly needed or have the caller transport the needy animal directly to the appropriate care provider. If the caller is willing to bring the animal to the clinic, chances are the caller will be willing to transport the animal directly to the rehabilitator. This method promotes the best use of time for both the veterinary staff and rehabilitators, thus allowing the medical personnel to best use their valuable expertise by caring mainly for the injured wild patients that must receive immediate medical attention.

Whether a hospital chooses to be a drop-off site, a referral center, or both, a current list of participating rehabilitators' names, locations, phone numbers, and species covered under each permit is a prerequisite. A prearranged plan for informing rehabilitators when a pick-up or transport needs to be scheduled is a must to prevent unnecessary and often detrimental delays before an animal can receive adequate care.

On the other hand, if the practice can provide adequate staff time and housing for the wildlife patients, then the hospital can consider becoming more involved in longer-term care such as surgery, wound care, emaciation, and hand rearing.

Choose your hospital's role wisely, putting the animal's best interest foremost in the decision-making process.

Euthanasia

Before receiving animals, the hospital must have a clear euthanasia policy, including who will make the decision and do the actual procedure, what techniques will be used, and what criteria are used. There is a section on nonreleasable criteria and euthanasia later in this chapter to help with this difficult topic.

Phone Protocols

So often overlooked, one of the most important areas in which the wildlife veterinary clinic personnel must be trained is the telephone procedure. Posting a clear protocol for handling wildlife calls near every phone helps to ensure that the information received is accurate and consistent. The development of a wildlife phone call protocol should be a combined effort between the veterinary staff and the participating wildlife rehabilitators. Many animals come into rehabilitation that never should have been removed from the spot in which they were found. Educating the public is part of the responsibility of anyone participating in wildlife rehabilitation. Taking proper animal history information before the animal is even touched drastically reduces the number of "orphans" that are kidnapped and end up needing to be hand raised, thus reducing wasted time, money, and energy.

The caller should be asked if the animal appears to be orphaned or injured. What brought the finder to this conclusion? Many times it turns out that a little education in animal natural behavior can turn a "needy" or "nuisance" animal call into a lesson in living with wildlife. If the animal does appear to need assistance and the caller cannot handle it, advise the person to bring it in. One should never instruct or allow the caller to take care of the foundling himself. If the caller cannot bring the animal to the clinic, he should be provided with phone numbers from the contact list for a rehabilitator, rescue volunteer, or wildlife center in his area.

Handling Phone Calls

In most instances, if an adult wild animal can be caught and picked up by a person, then it has sustained some type of injury, is in shock, or is sick and needs some type of rehabilitation.

Conditions that require immediate medical attention include:

- Unconsciousness
- Bleeding
- Cold body temperature
- Open fracture
- Weakness, inability to stand (emaciated)
- Head swelling
- Head/eye twitching
- Eyes closed or matted shut
- Shock
- Puncture wounds from cat/dog bite
- Broken bones
- Flies, fly larva, or eggs present

If the animal found is an infant, have the caller describe the baby and its condition. It should be determined if the animal is truly an orphan. If warm, strong, and apparently healthy, the baby is probably not an orphan and every attempt should be made to return it to its mother or nest. If the baby is cold, weak, or emaciated, or if there are dead siblings nearby, the animal is probably orphaned. Mother animals do not abandon their young because humans have touched them.

Baby Songbirds

If the bird is naked or has a few body feathers but no tail feathers, the baby should be put back in the nest if at all possible. If the nest cannot be reached, instruct the caller to hang a homemade nest made from a basket or container near the old nest. The "surrogate" nest should be placed up off of the ground and protected from direct sunlight and rain. If the mother does not return by dark, advise the caller to bring the baby in to the clinic.

If the bird has body feathers with one inch or longer tail feathers, is hopping around and chirping, it is probably a fledgling. These youngsters have left the nest but the parents are still providing them with food. Instruct the caller to look around for a parent bird. If the baby is picked up and it vocalizes and attracts an adult bird's attention, leave it alone. If there are no parent birds in sight, the bird should be left and checked several hours later. It may take three to four days for a "grounded" fledgling to learn to fly but a healthy one should be active, very mobile, and left where it was found.

Baby Raptors

If the nestling has closed eyes or has no feathers, return it to the nest if at all possible or make a surrogate nest. If the juvenile is hopping around or perching, has wing feathers and a short tail, it should be left alone. "Branchers" are young raptors that have left the nest but cannot yet fly. Both parents are still providing care to these birds on the ground or in low trees and shrubs. The only time to bring in a nestling raptor is if the caller cannot return it to its nest or secure a surrogate nest to the nesting tree. Refer the caller to a raptor rehabilitator for further instructions on how to replace a baby in its nest or make a surrogate one.

Baby Squirrels

Young squirrels are independent when they are about half the size of the adult and have bushy tails. If the baby does not yet have a fluffy tail, is crying, or is cold, it might be orphaned. Mother squirrels often move their babies from nest to nest so a baby found at the base of a tree is not automatically an orphan. Even if there is no adult squirrel visible but the caller can stay nearby and watch for the mother, leave the baby unmoved. If the caller cannot watch, advise the caller to tie a small basket or box up off of the ground, with the baby inside, onto the possible nest tree out of reach of ground predators. The caller or someone must check the nest before dark and make sure that the infant has been reclaimed. If it is still in the box by dark, have the caller bring it in. Infant squirrels make a very high-pitched squeal or "chirp" when they are frightened, hungry, or cold, and the mother can hear it from quite a distance.

Baby Rabbits

Baby cottontail rabbits should be left alone if uninjured and found in the nest. Even if the nest has been disturbed, the mother will usually come back. The deciding factor seems to be the extent of the nest disturbance. If the nest has sustained minimal disturbance of the nesting material, the babies should be covered back up and left alone. If the nest site has been destroyed or dug up by a predator, the mother may not come back. An attempt can be made to put the nest back together and a string placed on top of the nest. If, by morning, the string has been disturbed and the babies are warm and plump, the mother has come back to feed them. However, if the string is undisturbed or the babies are cold or look thin, they should be brought in. If the location of the nest is unknown and the baby's eyes are closed, it should be brought in. But if the young rabbit's eyes are open and its ears are upright and capable of rotating, they should be left undisturbed. Mother rabbits will not pick up and carry a baby back to the nest. Infants only feed at dusk and dawn and the mother will leave the nest in between feedings but stay nearby. Due to rabbits' secretive nature and infrequent visits to their nests, one should not automatically assume the babies are orphaned.

Baby Opossums

If an infant opossum is found that is less than six inches long and alone advise the caller to bring it in. Baby opossums that are old enough to leave the mother's pouch should cling to the mother's coat or follow along behind her. If they fall off or cannot keep up, they are sometimes left behind.

Baby Deer

Fawns should be left alone unless injured. The doe often leaves the fawn alone for hours at a time while she feeds.

Baby Raccoons

Baby raccoons are usually on their own by the time they are four to five months old and weigh eight to twelve pounds. If a younger raccoon is discovered alone, the caller should leave the youngster where it was found and check on it periodically. Although nocturnal, the mother raccoon will look for her missing infant during the daytime as well as during the nighttime. If twenty-four hours pass with no sign of the mother, the licensed rabies vector rehabilitator should be called for instructions. Be careful in advising the public to handle any rabies vector species.

Reuniting Mother and Baby

Reuniting diurnal species' (active during the day) babies during the daylight hours and nocturnal species' (active at night) babies during the night should be practiced. If the infant gets cold while waiting for the parent, a warm water bottle should be provided and placed with the baby. It may take several hours for a mother to reclaim its baby. If a diurnal species is found at night, it may be worth a try in the morning to reunite it with its parent.

Orphans that are brought to the hospital probably need to be taken home at night by a caretaker and brought back in the morning to provide the young animals with enough nourishment.

Callers Who Want to Care for Animals

If the caller wants to try to take care of the animal herself, explain why that is not in the animal's best interest. Some points to argue this point include:

1. The problems of imprinting—the rehabilitators probably have more infants of the same species that they can put with the caller's animal and raise together as siblings.
2. The possibility of zoonotic or infectious diseases.
3. It is illegal for the caller to care for the animal without a permit.
4. Using the wrong formula or feeding technique can cause harm to the animal, or even death.
5. Hand raising is very time-consuming. Give the caller an idea of how often the animal needs to eat and how long the care time may be.
6. Acquiring and preparing the proper foods may be difficult, expensive, and sometimes unpleasant (mealworms, grubs, mice that must be killed, etc.).

If the caller has a raccoon, fox, bear, bobcat, owl, hawk, or any rabies vector species, or potentially dangerous animal, the name and phone number should be taken immediately in case he decides to keep it and not bring it in. This information should then be turned over to the appropriate authorities (county game protector, federal wildlife agent, etc.).

INTAKE PROCEDURES

Under no circumstances should animals be handled or looked at in between the necessary feedings and treatments intervals. This rule needs to begin in the reception room with the arrival of the animal. Without lifting the lid or opening the transport cage, the receptionist should immediately transport the animal to the examination area while the rescuer fills out an intake form. This form should include the rescuer's name, address, phone number, animal type and numbers, and finally the animal's circumstances for needing care. A detailed account of how, when, and where the animal was found can help determine the nature of the animal's problem. Also, information should be recorded about how long the rescuer had the animal and if she attempted to medicate or feed the patient. This helps the caretaker to investigate what happened to the animal and determine the correct form of treatment. This form should be used as a pet's chart would be, with the recording of physical exam findings, treatments, observations, and final disposition. The state and/or federal permit issuing departments also require this information. A copy should be made and given to the rehabilitator who receives the animal to provide the new caretaker with all the available information. The original should be filed at the facility and used to help make the end-of-year report required by most states (Appendix 2).

Meanwhile, back in the treatment room, the animal should have a quick visual exam to check for emergency conditions such as shock, hypothermia, or bleeding. If the animal appears stable and is not in a critical position, it should be allowed a little time to calm down from the previous handling and car ride before pulling it out of the box.

ETHICAL CONSIDERATIONS AND REDUCING STRESS IN CAPTIVE WILDLIFE

"It is incumbent upon a person who takes the responsibility of manipulating an animal's life to be concerned for its feelings, the infliction of pain, and the psychological upsets that may occur from such manipulation" (Fowler 1986).

The wild nature of these animals should always be respected and sensitivity shown for the unique needs of these unusual patients. Stress is the number one reason that wild animals under human care die. All sick or injured animals need their strength to recover and cannot afford to use it up in attempts to escape from captive stress. Learning to recognize signs of early stress, with each species as well as between individuals, may possibly prevent or at least reduce such fatalities. Many birds have a natural escape pattern of moving up and away from danger and they feel threatened if they are housed down low and looked at from above. Typically, they are calmer if their cage is placed at or above human eye level.

All prey animals fear direct eye contact or being stared at or even looked at. Consider the animal's viewpoint: typically the first thing a predator does while hunting is keep its eye on the prey and then move directly toward it. When humans do this, they mimic the predator's behavior and frighten the animal. It is a good idea to look in another direction when walking past wildlife cages.

Housing for different species is discussed further in each of their sections but a note on stress-reducing environmental factors should be mentioned here. Within each animal's enclosure, using something natural and familiar to the patient will help decrease stress. Housing away from sight or sound of predators (humans, domestic animals, wild predators; i.e. avoid housing hawks and cottontails in the same room) is of foremost importance. Second, providing something of a natural setting is calming to many species of captive wildlife. Many bird species need to feel hidden or protected from view by vegetated plant cover. Cutting a few small leafed branches off of a nearby tree or shrub and placing them inside the animal's enclosure (preferably before placing the animal inside) can provide naturalistic hiding places for the recovering patient. Animals such as rabbits, squirrels, opossums, and chipmunks seek refuge by hiding under or inside something that cannot be seen through. Providing these types of patients with a nest box, hollow log, plastic tube, or even layers of cloth that they can burrow in increases their sense of security and well-being as well as the chance of keeping them alive. Animals also equate having choices with comfort. Offering a bird several perches provides them with the opportunity to feel as if they have some control in their strange, new, captive world.

INITIAL EXAM

The visual exam is the first part and perhaps one of the most important parts of the examination. Before even touching the patient, observe its posture, color, behavior, and stool quality. Look for discharges, level of alertness, body conditioning, head tilts, nystagmus, limping, or wing droops. Record all observations either on the intake sheet or the examination form (whichever one the hospital's wildlife protocol calls for). An example of each form is provided in Appendix 2. Many of these signs are not as obvious once the animal has been picked up and held in an unnatural position. Also, an animal will try its best to conceal these "signs of weakness" to a predator if it knows it is being watched, so try to be sly about the visual exam. Sometimes using binoculars and watching from across the room gets the best results.

When performing the hands-on part of the examination, the examiner should be swift and thorough, reducing the handling time and the animal's psychological stress. Restraint should be performed on the animal quickly and with confidence, without a lot of repositioning. Prey animals view a predator's grip as fatal, and frequent shifting of the animal's position only draws out the suffering.

Use of a systematic approach when doing exams ensures that no area gets overlooked. Even though it may be obvious that the patient has a wing injury, the exam should be performed in a systematic manner and all the animal's systems evaluated in order. The animal's eyes, ears, mouth, nose, skin turgor, limbs, body condition, and reflexes should be checked. Respiratory sounds should be observed and noted as well as any signs of bleeding. All anticipated supplies and medications must be ready before handling the animal so the patient does not have to wait unnecessarily. It is not uncommon to find secondary problems days later because they were initially overlooked due to the examiner's mistake of starting right at the big problem and then forgetting to follow through with the rest of the exam.

Restraining and examination techniques should be practiced as often as possible because this is the only way to become fast and efficient. Examine healthy live animals whenever possible to become familiar with "normals" in order to recognize the "abnormals." Information obtained from examining dead animals should not be underestimated. Restraint positions, palpation, injection training, IO or IV catheter placement, bandaging, tube feeding, necropsy, and even surgical techniques can be practiced on deceased patients.

CHOOSING TREATMENT ROUTES

When choosing appropriate treatment regimens, take into consideration the differences between the wild animal patient versus the domestic animals that are more routinely seen in the office. Domesticated animals can withstand more extensive procedures done with manual restraint alone. On the other hand, the use of anesthesia (i.e. isoflurane) should be considered when obtaining quality radiographs or performing even minor but painful procedures on wildlife.

Routes and frequencies of medication need to be carefully compared as well. Oral medications should be chosen, when appropriate, that can be injected into food items and fed to the patient. For example, enrofloxacin can be injected into a cricket and fed to a blue jay, or into a minnow and fed to a heron. Every effort should be made to weigh the stress of handling and administering treatments against the benefits they provide. Although the first treatment of choice may recommend BID-TID treatments, realize that with wildlife this may not always be practical or possible. Wildlife medicine is a balance between what is effective and what the patient can tolerate.

This sometimes calls for some creative medicine delivery ideas. Raptors can receive treatments of dexamethasone, LRS, vitamins, or antibiotics injected into a small or pinkie mouse that the bird can swallow whole at its normal eating time. Some pediatric suspensions have a more palatable taste and may be more readily eaten either right out of the medicine dropper or when mixed in with a favorite food item (i.e. Clavamox drops mixed in with fruit yogurt offered to an opossum). Another option is to have frequently used oral medications specially flavored or concentrated at a compounding pharmacy. Banana-flavored dewormers, meat-flavored antibiotics, alfalfa-flavored anti-inflammatories, just to name a few, have been very useful in both zoological and wildlife medicine.

Animals that do not swallow their food whole or eat food items in which medications are not easily hidden (i.e., adult squirrels, rabbits) may need to be hand injected. In these cases, effective medications with the longest action time to reduce multiple daily "catch ups" should be chosen. Ideally, medications that need to be given only once daily should be sought.

In conclusion, it is not the role of veterinarians to know the best way to rehabilitate every wild animal. Veterinarians' expertise is in anatomy, surgery, diagnostics, and treatment, not necessarily the natural history and behavior patterns of a southern flying squirrel. To assist the veterinarian in making more informed decisions, the technician should collect as much information as possible pertaining to the types of wildlife that the clinic decides to work with. Teamwork is crucial and the combined efforts of many individuals make up the best rehabilitation team. Each wildlife technician needs to form good working relationships with several veterinarians. One veterinarian cannot be expected to look at every baby squirrel, but can advise on general treatment regimes and drug dosages.

A technician should always realize his limitations and should never feel as if networking makes him look incapable. Using the experience of others is the best way to learn and can also prevent animals from suffering unnecessarily. No one should ever reinvent the wheel at the animal's expense. Always remember that the ultimate goal is to release the animal back into the wild with the best possible chance of survival. A technician can offer this to each and every animal that he works with if he learns to recognize when someone else may be more qualified. This may even mean transferring the animal to another person who may have a better rehabilitation setup, more experience or time, animal conspecifics, or better release sites.

While wildlife rehabilitation can be difficult, time-consuming, expensive, and many times downright frustrating, the benefits and personal rewards gained from this unselfish kind deed can be life changing.

RELEASE CRITERIA VERSUS EUTHANASIA

Some animals arrive at the clinic with injuries that warrant euthanasia. Other injuries and illnesses may not present themselves as life threatening but in fact are just as profound in terms of release and survivability in the wild. The veterinary technician should learn to recognize these less-obvious conditions that will ultimately lead to death of the animal if released back into the wild.

Merely saving a life for survival in captivity is not the goal. The animal must be capable of recognizing, obtaining, and processing food; recognizing and evading or defending against predators; acquiring shelter; acquiring and defending territories; performing normal seasonal movements and dispersal; and be capable of normal socialization with conspecifics (Diehl and Stokhaug 1991). Each type of animal, depending on its natural history and what it needs to do to survive, has different criteria, so a handicap considered relatively minor for one species may be life threatening to another.

For instance, a bird of prey must be capable of hunting and catching prey animals that may be as quick and fast as they themselves are. If a Cooper's hawk was released with any degree of flight defect, it would not be able to obtain prey that is often caught in midair. On the other hand, a mallard duck with a slight wing defect but flight capability may be considered for release because it acquires its food while swimming and dabbling in the water, breeds in the water, and can also escape predators by diving as well as flying. Furthermore, in some areas mallards do not have to migrate so the need to fly great distances is also reduced.

Another example would be an animal with impaired vision. An animal that does not depend on excellent sight to obtain food and avoid predation could also be considered releasable. For instance, a one-eyed, adult opossum might be considered releasable because in the wild it has few predators and relies on its sense of smell to find food items (carrion, insects, vegetation) that do not require a great deal of visual acuity to acquire. However, a fox needs perfect vision to obtain its mainstay diet of live and very quick prey animals such as mice, chipmunks, birds, and rabbits.

The species of the animal involved should also be considered. An opossum with a fractured limb has a good chance for recovery. Opossums tend to tolerate bandages and splints well, plus they are relatively inactive, which provides for optimal recovery. A deer with a fractured limb, on the other hand, is a challenge.

Many hospitals or centers do not have the facilities to deal with an injured deer. At best, these animals, even with adequate facilities, are difficult to maintain in captivity and they tend to further injure themselves trying to escape.

The potential for current handicaps to create new problems for an animal must be considered. For example, is a one-footed bird likely to develop bumblefoot or frostbite on the remaining foot? The bottom line is that the animal must have enough of the equipment and capabilities necessary to survive by means natural to its species if it is to be released (Diehl and Stokhaug 1991).

Being a careful observer, understanding the animal's natural history, performing a thorough physical exam, and knowing the release requirements could spare an animal hours or days of suffering. Each animal deserves a careful and unbiased evaluation. If the releasability is in question, contact a rehabilitator immediately so a speedy decision can be made and the animal can begin to receive the treatment it deserves, whether it turns out to be freedom by release or euthanasia.

Situations that may require euthanasia include:

- Compound or open fracture more than forty-eight hours old. These old injuries rarely can be properly repaired and the animal would lose full function of the limb, making the animal nonreleasable.
- Complete loss of sight or hearing in any animal.
- Impaired vision in both eyes. Depending on the species, some animals can be considered for release if only one eye is affected.
- Nocturnal owls with hearing impairment.
- Amputated wings or legs. "Any birds that have sustained injuries requiring amputation of a wing at the elbow (humero-ulnar) or above, a leg or a foot … should be euthanized" (U.S. Fish and Wildlife—Rehabilitation regulation 50 CFR 21.27 #8). No animal should be put through the stress and pain of surgery only to be euthanized later because it can never be released.
- Raptors need unimpaired function of their feet to grasp, kill, and carry prey; therefore, any injury involving the unilateral loss of both the hallux (digit 1) and digit 2 on the same foot or the bilateral loss of both hallux.
- Fractures involving the wing or leg joints (or very near the joint) will never heal sufficiently enough for the animal to have normal use of the limb. The joint will heal by fusing in place and not allow for normal movement, thus preventing the animal from flying or walking.

- Fractures with a significant piece of bone missing.
- Some wing fractures can heal out of alignment and result in a wing droop. Although flight may be possible, the wing cannot be allowed to drag on the perch or ground. The feather tips will become damaged and soiled and over time the bird may become nonflighted or develop an infection in the damaged follicles.
- Head trauma that results in abnormal posture in any animal.
- Back injuries that have resulted in loss of limb function in any animal.
- Animals imprinted on humans should never be released. These animals are not able to behaviorally fit into their own natural population and they could be dangerous to the public.
- Animals that have a highly incurable infectious disease.
- A rabies vector species from a rabies endemic area (follow current state guidelines) should never be released.
- Mammals with two or more nonfunctional legs.
- Rodents or rabbits with a fractured jaw or any facial injury leaving permanently unaligned incisors. (Opposing incisor teeth must be able to be normally worn down or they will overgrow and eventually kill the animal.)

Nonreleasable animals can sometimes be placed in an approved educational research program or breeding facility. There are now several nonreleasable animal placement programs designed to help place these animals. Do not euthanize an endangered species without first contacting your local and federal authorities for authorization.

"We look to wildlife for the rules that we follow. Wildlife leads a life of quality, or it isn't alive—it's one or the other for wildlife" (Moore and Joosten 1995a).

IMPRINTING AND TAMING

Imprinting

The veterinary technician's code of ethics to "do no harm" could not be more pertinent to this subject. Understanding the definitions and what these two things mean to a wild animal under a technician's care can make the difference between life and death.

Imprinting is a socialization process by which an individual animal learns to identify itself with a species. This is a natural psychological process, which occurs early in life, during a restricted period of time called a critical period. Once this has occurred, the animal then identifies with the adult of its own species and learns by imitation and observation the methods for acquiring shelter, food, mates, and proper behaviors.

The route in which a mammal, bird, or reptile imprints is different and still not completely understood. In the area of wildlife rehabilitation, imprinting is probably only relevant to birds. The critical periods for most species of birds have not yet been determined. With ducks and geese it occurs within the day of hatching and with smaller raptor species between days eight and twenty-one after hatching. Larger raptor species usually imprint between days twelve and twenty-eight. The variations of days between species are largely due to their different rates of development. The most important period seems to be when the bird's visual focus develops. Before their eyes open, neonates also imprint on their parents' calls and vocalizations.

What this all means for the wildlife caregiver is that the animal could be improperly imprinted on humans if a great deal of care is not taken. Imprinting is not believed to be reversible so if the process is transferred to a person the animal will have a poor chance to survive. Birds that do not imprint on their own species will lack the survival skills they need, will not reproduce in the wild, and are often killed outright by their own species. A bird that has imprinted on a human is not releasable and will probably need to be euthanized.

To reduce the chances of improper imprinting, the baby should be returned to its nest and/or parents if at all possible. Sometimes orphans can be placed in foster nests and raised with like species of similar age. Many rehabilitation centers have nonreleasable surrogate parents (most commonly birds of prey) that raise same species' orphans that are not their own. If that is not possible, care should be taken to be sure all animals are raised with at least one other member of the same-aged species. Rehabilitators and nature centers that have permanent nonreleasable raptors can also house the young beside the adults to allow the juveniles a chance to observe, listen, interact, and possibly imitate the same species adult. With some birds, a mirror may be helpful if the baby has no nest mates.

Birds (especially raptors) should be fed during their critical period from behind a curtain-type blind or while wearing a hooded poncho with a mask to hide the human shape. By also using a hand puppet shaped like the head of the adult to feed raptor chicks, the young do not associate food with humans. Wildlife should be handled as little as possible, with limited talking, and housed out of sight or sound of humans, dogs, cats, and pet birds.

Taming

Taming is the process of an animal becoming socialized to humans by association with foods or other comforts over a prolonged period of time (Beaver 1984). Baby animals in a wide range of species are especially easy to tame. These tame animals have properly imprinted and identify with their own species but socialize with humans. Taming differs from imprinting in that the bond to humans is not as strong, takes longer to establish, and is more readily lost once human contact no longer occurs (Klinghammer 1991).

The lack of fear tame animals show toward humans often leads to their deaths. These animals often get shot or trapped because few people trust a "friendly raccoon" and often misinterpret it to be diseased or rabid. Tame game species are often easy targets for hunters and trappers. Tame animals are also unsuitable for release due to possible dangerous encounters with humans. This process is usually reversible but should be done by a person other than the one who caused it before the animal is released. Taming can be avoided by minimizing human contact, especially human-associated positive stimuli such as food (Diehl and Stokhaug 1991). Wild animals no longer requiring hand-feeding should never be fed by hand. Food should be scattered around the enclosure when animals are sleeping and not likely to see the provider (i.e. feed opossums and flying squirrels one to two hours before dark when they are still asleep and out of view).

It is critical that the distinction be made between a true human imprint and a tamed animal with regard to the release potential. The animal's history must be traceable from the day it came in. Again, good record keeping is essential because it will help determine if improper imprinting is even a possibility. If the animal can be proven to be tame but not imprinted on humans, it may still have a chance to be released.

TRANSPORTING WILDLIFE

A variety of containers can be used to transport wildlife. The two main considerations for choosing the appropriate transport container are the animal's safety and comfort. If a caller asks for advice on how to bring an animal in to the clinic, he should always be asked for information about the animal such as what type of animal is it, whether it is conscious, and whether it is a baby or adult. Each call should be taken on a case-by-case basis to determine the safest way to capture and transport each animal. After determining that the animal needs assistance, it should also be determined whether the caller has the tools on hand to safely get the animal into the transport container, such as gloves, a blanket, or a broom. The caller's confidence and experience level should be ascertained before even suggesting that he attempt to handle a potentially dangerous animal. Human safety comes first. If in doubt, referring the caller directly to the rehabilitator may be the safest thing to do.

After capture an animal should be placed in a suitable container with holes and a lid and kept in a quiet area before and during the transport. Unnecessary talking or playing the radio in the vehicle during transport should be avoided. Extreme temperatures should also be avoided by providing ventilation, shade from the sun, or extra heat if needed. Cardboard boxes make good temporary cages and can be quickly altered to suit many different types of animals. Ideally, the size of the container should be just large enough for the animal to comfortably fit into but not large enough for a great deal of activity. Cardboard boxes and pet carriers make the best types of transport containers because they offer solid sides and tops, which reduce visual stress for the patient and are also disposable after use. Placing wildlife in a clear aquarium or plastic tote should only be done if there is a towel or blanket available to cover the enclosure to block out light and remove visual stimuli.

Proper nonslip material should be placed on the enclosure bottom to ensure proper footing and reduce stress as a result of slipping and sliding during the transport. The cage should be secured so it does not slide or flip over. No food or water should be provided during the time of the transport because the animals are usually too stressed to eat and the bowls often end up tipping over and spilling their contents, getting the animal wet or dirty.

Adult Birds

Open-wire bird/rodent cages are not advisable for transporting because they need to be covered with a towel and the wire can be very damaging to the flight feathers. Songbirds can be placed in a wide open paper bag with the top rolled tightly shut and clipped with a paper clip or clothespin. Several pencil-sized air holes should be provided in the bag for fresh air and ventilation. Plastic pet carriers work well for waterfowl, raptors, and the larger songbird species (i.e. blue jays, robins), but care should be taken with the smaller species (i.e. wrens, warblers) that can fit through the holes on the cage door. Appropriate sized cardboard boxes work equally well for small sparrows on up to large herons.

Carpet pieces, paper towels, or cloth towels serve as good cage flooring. Newspaper is too slippery, as is the plain plastic bottom of a pet carrier. Alert and standing adult birds might use a perch to stand on if it is securely fastened and proportionate to the bird's foot size. Tightly wedging a tree branch down low inside of a box before placing the bird inside can give the animal an option to perch. Raptors need a branch about two to three inches in diameter to properly perch on.

Provide soft material (i.e. rolled towel) to prop the animal on if it is not capable of standing on its own.

If the rescuer describes a heron-type bird, warn her of the dangers of the spearlike beaks and advise her not to go near the bird without eye protection such as safety glasses.

If the caller describes a bird of prey, first warn her about the dangerous talons. It may be best to refer the caller directly to a raptor rehabilitator for an on-site rescue.

Baby Birds

Young featherless birds need supplemental heat and can be transported using a warm water bottle or a zip-lock bag (double bagged to prevent leaks) filled with warm water placed under or next to the baby's enclosure. The nestling bird can be placed in a small box, berry basket, or any plastic margarine-sized container lined with nonscented toilet or facial tissues as nesting material. The artificial nest, not the infant itself, should be placed on the heat source to prevent the chance of skin burns. Keep in mind that these types of portable warming devices stay warm for only thirty to sixty minutes. Covering the nest or carrier with a light cloth reduces drafts and helps hold the warmth inside. These young animals need to be transferred as quickly as possible to prevent chilling or further dehydration.

If the baby's nest also fell, advise the rescuer against bringing it with the baby due to the strong possibility of unwanted parasites living in the nest.

Adult Mammals

A wire cage or live trap is suitable to transport an adult squirrel, raccoon, opossum, fox, or groundhog, to name a few. Most of these animals can chew out of cardboard or plastic kennels in a surprisingly short period of time. The transporter's safety is of foremost importance so do not advise him to put himself at risk over the animal. Also be informed as to the status of rabies in the caller's area and of the vector species that carry the disease so the caller can be warned of any potential danger.

Injured medium to large mammals such as deer, coyotes, and bobcats may need chemical immobilization and special capture equipment, such as punch poles, dart guns, and snare poles, to prevent injury to the animal or the handler.

Flying squirrels and chipmunks are escape artists and need to be contained in a box or solid sided container with the lid taped or snapped shut. Instruct the caller to make the air holes on the lid only and no larger around than a pencil or they could chew and enlarge the air holes to escape through them.

The cage bottom should be lined with ravel-free cloth and the entire cage draped for privacy. The cloth inside the cage provides better footing and a layer to hide under, which greatly reduces stress. The transporter can be advised to protect the vehicle's floor or seats by placing an old blanket down first before setting the cage inside. The rescuer should be warned to use caution when handling these potentially dangerous animals and their cages.

Baby Mammals

Cardboard boxes and pet carriers work well to transport these animals. Soft, ravel-free cloth should be placed inside the cage and a heat source (warm water bottle) provided for hairless babies or those whose eyes are closed. The heat source should never go directly against the baby's skin but rather under the cage to warm up the cage bottom.

Turtles

Cardboard boxes or plastic buckets work for transporting these animals. Do not transport water turtles in a container filled with water because the turtle will bump against the sides of the container as it is moved about.

Snakes

Snakes are best transported in a pillowcase with the opening tied in a knot. The bag can then be placed into a box, cooler, or bucket. The handler should carry the bag by the tip of the knot because the snake could bite through the cloth bag. Snakes can also be gently swept with a broom into a lidded box or small trash can. Unless the caller has experience in identifying venomous snake species from nonvenomous ones, care should be taken in advising anyone to handle any snake. This may be a job for animal control or a reptile rehabilitator.

See Appendix 3 for additional information on handling and restraint of wildlife species.

RAPTOR CARE

Birds of prey include eagles, falcons, condors, vultures, harrier, hawks, kites, osprey, owls, and the caracara. Raptors are legally protected by a number of federal acts such as the migratory bird treaty act of 1918, bald eagle protection act of 1940, and endangered species act of 1973. Many federal bird rehab permits do not automatically include birds of prey due to the special training and housing needed to work with these animals.

Raptor Handling

When handling any of these species of birds always keep in mind that their first line of defense is their talons. Be careful to safely secure the raptor's feet and legs before attempting to pick up or move the bird. Heavy gauntlet-type welding gloves, such as the type used for restraining aggressive cats, should be worn to catch a medium to large raptor. Small raptors such as screech owls and kestrels can be caught up using leather work gloves.

If a raptor feels trapped, it may either roll onto its back with feet up and talons ready or make a bold dash at its restrainer. A gloved hand should be kept ready at all times to deflect or grab such a bird in midair. If the bird flips onto its back, a rolled towel or a spare glove can be handed to it to grab with its feet and distract it long enough to allow a gloved hand to slip under the barrier and grab the animal by its legs.

To remove a raptor from a cage, one gloved hand should be used to block the bird from darting out around the other gloved hand while reaching in. It is often helpful to drape a towel over the door to prevent the bird from seeing a "get away" space around the restrainer's body. With medium and large birds of prey, it is best to grab both legs, up high against the bird's body, with one hand keeping a finger between the birds legs. Once the legs are both contained, the wings can be folded up against the body with the other hand as the bird is pulled out. Every attempt should be made to avoid allowing the bird to beat its wings against the cage as it is extracted through the door.

When only one leg is grabbed, the natural reaction of the raptor is to grab back at the handler with its free foot. If the raptor manages to talon and hold onto a glove either the restrainer or someone else must first fully extend the leg in order for the toes to be opened back up. Then one by one, each nail is removed with care taken to locate each of the other needle-sharp talons. It is very difficult to open up a foot on a raptor with a flexed leg.

Some birds also attempt to bite, so securing the head or covering it with a towel may be necessary. The head must be secured when the eyes, mouth, nares, and ears are being examined. The handler needs to distract the bird with one hand and quickly grasp the head from behind with the other. Head restraint is accomplished by firmly holding the head between the thumb and index finger at the articulation of the mandible. Covering the bird's eyes also tends to relax many raptor species and allows minor procedures to be more easily accomplished (giving injections, weighing, taking radiographs, or collecting blood). The use of an orthopedic stockinet to cover the head and body is another useful technique for raptor restraint when weighing. A Velcro strip can be used as leg restraints by first attaching around one leg, just above the feet, then wrapping around both legs.

If the bird is on the ground or in a large open-top box, a towel, blanket, or net can be draped over the bird and then the bird picked up after first feeling for and securing the legs through the draped material with a gloved hand (Figure 20.1).

Raptor Initial Exam

Birds of prey are most commonly brought into veterinary hospitals with wing and/or leg fractures due to their frequency of colliding with motor vehicles. These birds tend to survive many of these collisions, and due to their large size are more easily noticed alongside the road and thus rescued by passing motorists. Two other common presentations are head or eye injuries.

Some of these animals, when presented to the hospital, may be in shock and need to be treated accordingly. Usually dexamethasone and lactated Ringer's solution is the treatment of choice but only after first checking with the veterinarian. During the initial examination of any wild animal, be quick but thorough. A systematic method of examination that covers the patient from head to toe in the shortest time possible should be developed. Decreasing the handling time dramatically reduces the bird's stress and increases its survival chances. Any cold bird should be placed on or under heat to allow the body temperature to reach a normal range (98°F–102°F) before continuing with the exam.

Because raptors receive most of their water intake from the prey they eat, they easily become dehydrated when they are undernourished. Signs of dehydration include sunken eyes and thick, cloudy strands of mucous in the mouth. These birds should to be immediately treated with warmed lactated Ringer's solution by the oral, subcutaneous, intravenous, or intraosse-

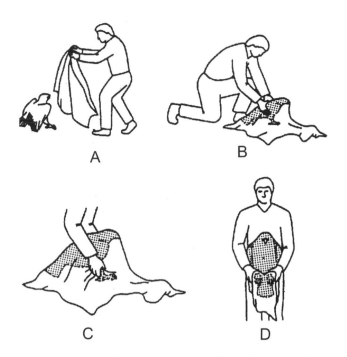

Figure 20.1. Picking a raptor up from the ground. (A) Blanket technique used to cover and catch a raptor. (B) The covered raptor is initially grasped with both hands over back shoulders. (C) Both hands secure the legs just above the feet. (D) Restrain and carrying method with the raptor held between the arms against the handler's body. (Permission for drawing use granted by the National Wildlife Rehabilitators Association)

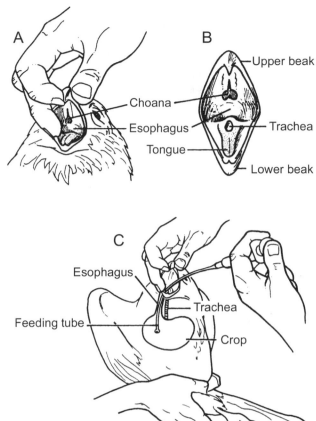

Figure 20.2. Anatomy of the avian oral cavity and technique for assisted feeding in birds. (A). The beak is held open by placing a finger in the corner of the mouth. (B) Close-up view of oral anatomy showing the esophagus at the back of the throat and trachea at the base of the tongue. (C) Proper placement of feeding tube in crop. (Permission for drawing use granted by the Georgia Department of Natural Resources and Branson Ritchie, DVM, MS.)

ous routes. One method is to tube feed small amounts of lactated Ringer's solution with 5% dextrose into the bird's crop every fifteen minutes for the first hour or two (Figure 20.2).

Next, the bird should be examined for fractures by palpation and radiology. Many raptors will tolerate a quick radiograph without sedation if properly held to the table with a combination of manual and paper tape restraint. Any potentially repairable broken limbs should immediately be stabilized with the proper splints or bandages. A bandage should be chosen that immobilizes the joint above and below the fracture site. The figure-eight bandage is good for immobilizing the wing and then can be wrapped to the body to eliminate joint movement (Figure 20.12).

If there is a fracture found in or very near any limb joint or if any two or more limbs contain a break, euthanasia should be strongly considered. These types of injuries often result in a nonreleasable animal and immediate euthanasia is the most humane treatment. If the veterinarian is unsure of the releasability of any

injured raptor, a raptor rehabilitator should be called first to help make the decision.

The bird's feather and muscle condition are two clues that are useful in determining the reason why the bird may have come in. Ragged and soiled feathers are evidence that the bird has probably been "grounded" for a long period of time, so any injury is not likely to be fresh and wounds should be examined for fly eggs or larva. Any raptor that has been on the ground for several days or more will be dehydrated and potentially emaciated because these birds are unable to acquire live prey without flight. Dark green mutes (feces) are another sign of starvation. The bird's keel (sternum) can be palpated with the fingertips to help assess the bird's level of health. A thin or emaciated bird's keel feel "sharp" to the touch, meaning that the keel bone is prominent and the breast muscles are atrophied (Figure 20.3). Use a combination of physical condition, body weight, and degree of muscling on the keel to evaluate the bird.

Another all too common reason birds of prey end up in rehabilitation is gun shot injuries. Poisoning, whether intentional or unintentional, is also worth mentioning here because the veterinarian can sometimes determine toxicities with specific blood tests. Due to the nature of a raptor's eating habits, these birds may end up consuming a rodent or bird that ate poisoned bait and thus become secondarily poisoned. Emaciated juvenile birds often end up in hospitals and wildlife care centers during their first winter due to their inexperienced hunting skills and the difficulties of surviving without an established hunting territory in the months when prey is most scarce.

Once the bird has been examined, it should be weighed (ideally in grams) so the medication, fluids, and food dosing will be accurate. The animal's weight is often the best indicator of how it is doing overall after being admitted for medical care. Good medical records that include all procedures, treatments, food intake, and weights should be maintained daily. A copy of these records can be made to give to the rehabilitator when the bird is transferred.

All treatments should be done as quickly as possible and with minimal talking. If any food, fluids, or medications need to be given orally, this should be done last after everything else has been done (injections, radiographs, venipuncture, etc.) to lessen the chances of regurgitation.

IM injections can be given in the leg or breast muscle. SQ fluids can be administered in either the

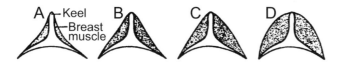

Figure 20.3. Subjective evaluation of a bird's condition based on pectoral muscle mass. (A) Severe muscle atrophy indicating a substantial amount of weight loss. (B) Moderate weight loss. (C) Severe weight loss, mild muscle atrophy. (D) Excellent condition with no detectable muscle atrophy. (Permission for drawing use granted by the Georgia Department of Natural Resources and Branson Ritchie, DVM, MS.)

axilla (wing web), lateral flank, or inguinal areas, with the doses divided into several sites, to provide maintenance or mild dehydration fluids. Intraosseous (IO) fluids are most often delivered via sterile catheter placed into the hollow cavity of the distal ulna or tibia for severe dehydration. This technique is described in Chapter 2 in this text. IV injections are given in the medial metatarsal or the right jugular vein. Once the patient is self feeding, many medications can be injected or pilled into a food item that the bird can swallow whole, such as a pinkie or small mouse, and offered as part of the daily meal.

Raptor Caging

Most veterinary clinics can do short-term convalescent care with birds of prey but do not have the proper facilities for any long-term care or housing. All housing for raptors, as well as all wildlife, should be separate from the domestic patients and in a quiet area away from people and animal traffic.

Feathered healthy birds can be comfortably maintained at 60°F–85°F. Cages should have solid sides such as the stainless sterile hospital rack cages or a large plastic pet kennel. A towel should be draped over the inside of the door opening to provide a complete visual barrier for the patients and to prevent them from catching their wings on the vertical door bars. The cage size should be large enough to allow the bird of prey to stand, turn around, and step up on a perch without touching its head or tail feathers, yet not so large that the bird can fly within it and potentially further injure itself. Newspapers are adequate for lining the bottom of the cage.

Proper perching should always be provided for rehabilitating birds. Perches need to be of appropriate size and well secured to the floor or cage sides. Large wooden tree branches or small logs can be used if the bird is only staying for several days. A cage perch can be made by combining PVC pipes into a "T" shape and then mounting it to a block of wood. These plastic perches should be wrapped with outdoor carpet or Astroturf and can be cleaned and reused. Raptors that require longer-term hospital stays should have padded perches to stand on to reduce foot injuries caused by the pressure of standing for long periods of time. The technician can wrap the perches with Vetrap to add cushioning and provide an easy gripping surface. The perches should be secured at a height to prevent the bird's tail from dragging on the cage bottom but low enough to be easily stepped up on to.

The nature of the bird's injury should determine perch placement. No high perches should be available to a bird with a limb injury. To avoid any additional trauma, the perch should be six to twelve inches off the ground to begin with and gradually raised as the bird learns to step up and hop down from the perch. Ramped perches can cause problems if the injured bird climbs up to the top but "forgets" its handicap and jumps off. Most raptors never learn to descend from these learning perches the same gentle way they climbed up them.

A towel should be provided for padding to protect the bird's sternum if it is unable to stand. A rolled-up towel can be used to prop a weak bird up on its stomach at a 45 degree angle. The head should be level to prevent any fluids from the bird's nose or mouth from draining down into the lungs. Another caging method used for birds too weak to stand or with fractured legs is to place them in a box half full of shredded newspapers. This material not only supports the bird's body but also allows the feces to fall away from the bird.

The importance of keeping the feathers in good condition cannot be stressed enough. Wing and tail feathers, especially, are easily damaged if the birds are improperly housed. Even if the clinic is only holding the bird for a day or two, housing the bird in any cage in which the feathers or feather tips can stick out will do some degree of damage. It only takes two or three broken flight feathers to deem an otherwise fit bird temporarily nonreleasable. If the damage in any way interferes with normal mobility, the bird must remain in captivity until it undergoes a molt and replaces the broken feathers with new ones. This is a normal process but may take up to a year to naturally occur.

In addition to proper housing, a tail guard can be easily applied. Some rehabilitation centers and veterinary clinics wrap tails as a common intake procedure. See Appendix 4 for a tail-wrapping method that is reprinted with permission from the North Carolina Raptor Center in Charlotte, North Carolina.

Raptor Feeding

As with any animal, the bird should be warm and hydrated before solid food is offered. If the bird appears in good condition and is not emaciated, it can be offered a natural prey item for its diet. Healthy diurnal birds of prey (hawks, falcons) need to be fed once a day during the daylight hours. Nocturnal birds (owls) should be fed once a day but only in the evening.

These birds eat a variety of rodents, birds, rabbits, fish, insects, and snakes in the wild but in short-term hospitalization, fresh-killed or thawed adult mice will do. In some cases it may take the new patient several days to accept the new surroundings and food. As long as the bird came in at a good weight this should not be a problem and the bird will start to eat when it gets really hungry. The food presentation may also confuse the bird and it may not recognize a dead white lab mouse as a food item. Offering brown or black mice sometimes helps, as well as cutting open the mouse cavity to reveal the organ tissue, which often stimulates the bird's appetite.

Occasionally a raptor needs a little help with one or two hand-feedings to get started. A mouse may need to be cut into small bite-size pieces depending on the size of the bird. The pieces can be offered from a hemostat while leaving the bird inside the cage. Be quiet and do not stare at the bird or make sudden movements. The food should be slowly held up to and allowed to touch the bird's beak. Sometimes the bird will bite at the food defensively and accidentally take the offering. Stay still until the bird swallows it, which could take a minute or two for the first bite. This can be repeated several times, and then the remaining part of the meal can be left inside the cage with the bird. If the bird will not swallow the food or is too aggressive and tries to foot and bite the feeder, then it may need to be force fed.

With the bird wrapped securely in a towel and properly restrained, the beak should be opened and pieces carefully placed one by one into the back of its mouth (past the glottis) with fingers or blunted hemostats. The bird needs to be allowed to swallow each bite one at a time. Care should be taken to open the beak at the base and not the biting curved tip. Once the beak is open, it can be kept open long enough to place the food by wedging a finger inside at the extreme base of the mouth. Always remember that these birds can be dangerous and will foot or bite at any given chance. Once a stubborn raptor swallows several pieces of delicious rodent, even if it is a white one, it usually gives the bird incentive to start self feeding.

If the bird is emaciated, dehydrated, or too weak to eat solid whole items, then tube feeding may be needed. Start first with SQ LRS fluids and then switch to the oral route once the bird has stabilized. Continue with liquid formula feeding (such as Emeraid II or Isocal) until the bird has gained strength. Next, bites of skinless and boneless pieces of muscle or organ meat such as raw beef liver or muscle meat from a cut-up mouse or rat can be offered. Only after the bird has recovered its strength, which can take up to three to four days, should it be offered solid whole foods. Table 20.1 provides feeding guidelines for birds of prey.

Raptor Orphan Initial Care

The intake of many raptor "orphans" into the veterinary hospital can often be prevented by good phone

Table 20.1. Recommended feeding guidelines for birds of prey.

Species	Average male/female weight (g)	Food type	Amount
American kestrel	M-111 g/F-120 g	1 mouse	25 g
Bald eagle	M-4,123 g/F-5,244 g	2 rats	200–300 g
Barn owl	M-442 g/F-490 g	2–3 mice	50–75 g
Barred owl	M-632 g/F-801 g	2–3 mice	50–75 g
Broad winged hawk	M-420 g/F-490 g	2 mice	50 g
Cooper's hawk	M-349 g/F-529 g	2–3 mice	50–75 g
Great horned owl	M-1,318 g/F-1,769 g	3–5 mice or 1/2 rat	75–125 g
Peregrine falcon	M-611 g/F-952 g	4 mice	100 g
Red-tailed hawk	M-1,028 g/F-1,224 g	3–5 mice or 1/2 rat	75–125 g
Rough-legged hawk	M-1,027 g/F-1,278 g	4 mice	100 g
Saw-whet owl	M-74.9 g/F-90.8 g	1 mouse	25 g
Screech owl	M-167 g/F-194 g	1 mouse	25 g
Sharp-shinned hawk	M-103 g/F-174 g	1–2 mice	25–50 g
Red-shouldered hawk	M-475 g/F-643 g	2–3 mice	50–75 g
Turkey vulture	1,467 g	6–8 mice or 1 rat	150–200 g

(Information in part from Engelman 1993)

protocols and animal history taking. Raptors have a stage of development between the nestling and fledgling stages referred to as "branching." At this age, young birds are feathered, still being fed by the parents, and have left the nest, but are not flighted. Well-meaning people often discover these birds and believe them to be orphaned or injured because they will not fly away and there is no nest in sight. Because these birds are so easily captured, they are usually first picked up before the rehabilitator is notified. By asking the right questions, many of these "kidnapped" birds can be returned to the founding sight before any harm is done. If the clinic receives these calls, the best thing to do is to instruct the caller to leave the bird where it is and have the person call one of the raptor rehabilitators (on the referral phone list) to determine if the bird is truly orphaned or not.

Raptors are hatched with down but unable to leave the nest (semi-altricial). While hawks are born with their eyes open, owls are born with eyes closed. Hatchling- and nestling stage babies found on the ground should be replaced into the nest if at all possible. Some rehabilitators, nature centers, or wildlife agencies may have individuals to help with this process. If returning to the original site is not possible, the orphan should be temporarily cared for until a foster nest or captive foster parent can be found. Many of the larger wildlife rehabilitation centers have permanent foster parent birds that willingly feed many orphans each year.

Initial temporary care of orphaned raptors is similar to that of all animal species (make sure they are warm and hydrated). The chick should first be provided with heat if it is not old enough to regulate its own body temperature. One accepted rule for raptor brooding temperature is:

- Unfeathered birds should be kept at an ambient temperature of 85°F to 90°F.
- Downey chicks with quills present can be kept at 80°F to 85°F.
- Birds with feather quills and small feathers should be kept at 75°F to 80°F.

Estimating actual raptor-chick age is beyond the scope of this chapter due to the sheer number of species and classifications of birds of prey. The raptor rehabilitator can be called with the bird's description and weight for age estimate and feeding instructions. After the chick is warm and active, provide hydration fluids orally by carefully placing two to four drops of solution into the throat beyond the glottis every fifteen to twenty minutes until the bird becomes active.

Raptor Orphan Feeding
If the chick's transportation cannot be arranged before it needs to eat, the technician can offer it small pieces of rodent from tweezers or hemostats. Caution should be taken to avoid improper imprinting from the chick watching hand feeding (refer to imprinting section). Imprinting within raptors occurs anywhere between five and fifteen days of age. Raptor chicks do not gape for food like songbird babies do, but they readily take food with the tips of their beaks and sometimes even

nibble on the feeding tool as they would their parent's beak.

If the chicks eyes are closed, it is safe to hand-feed by touching the bird's beak with the feeding instrument containing small bites of food and trying to imitate the parents' feeding calls by whistling or chirping quietly. Because the chicks cannot see the person feeding it, the only concern is the chicks' not hearing the person talking.

If the bird's eyes are open and it demonstrates no fear or aggression, it is within the dangerous critical imprinting period and much care should be taken to prevent the youngster from seeing or hearing a human or any animal in the hospital. Some centers feed these birds with gloves and ski masks to partially hide the human shape or better yet feed with a hand puppet of a raptor-type bird (rubber bird hand puppets can sometimes be found at gift shops of nature stores and zoos) (Figure 20.4). Another option is to hang a towel, sheet, or curtain, to serve as a kind of blind, in front of the infant and feed by reaching around and peeking through a hole in the blind. These animals must never be available for "show and tell," and should be dis-

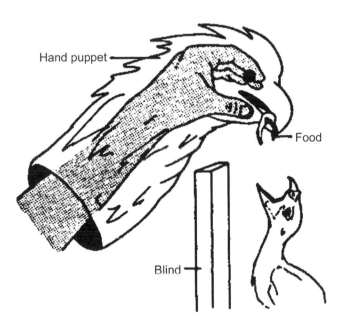

Figure 20.4. A hand-feeding puppet used for feeding neonates. During critical imprinting periods, hand-feeding puppets should be used in conjunction with blinds to prevent a young animal from associating food with humans. (Permission for drawing use granted by the Georgia Department of Natural Resources and Branson Ritchie, DVM, MS.)

turbed only for care-taking until they can be transferred to the rehabilitator.

A juvenile raptor that shows fear or aggression is beyond the critical imprinting stage and, one hopes, has properly imprinted on its own species by now. These birds may also be capable of self-feeding, so try placing small pieces of food in with the bird. If it refuses to pick up the food on its own after several feedings, refer to the above section on feeding adult raptors for hand-feeding ideas.

Raptor Orphan Food

Young raptors eat enormous amounts of food and often three to four times the amount of an adult. Weigh the chick in the morning before feeding and then feed 8% to 10% of body weight. The first few meals should be less to allow the digestive tract time to adjust to the changes. The crop should be allowed to fully empty before offering the next meal. Unlike hawks, owls do not have crops but tend to turn away from food when full (Crawford 1988).

Very young chicks, zero to seven days old, should eat just the soft muscle organ meat of prey foods dipped into vitamin water. Initially the parents would remove all skin, fur, and bones from the meals. These young raptor chicks should eat, until they are satisfied, every three to four hours. Feed them until the crop is half to three-quarters full but not so full that it feels hard or extended. Meals should not be skipped, and birds should be fed for a twelve-hour day.

Once the birds are seven to ten days old, small amounts of moistened hair, skin, and small bones can be introduced into the diet, which will serve as roughage and later be casted up.

Around days ten to twenty, the chicks can be fed larger moistened pieces of meat with bones, skin, and fur for three feedings a day. Starting at three weeks of age, the young should be able to eat the entire mouse cut into three to four pieces and will start to pick these up on their own.

Feed the three-week-olds to fledge twice a day and offer whole-prey items for them to tear on their own. Continue to hand-feed them until it is certain that they are picking up enough food on their own to sustain themselves. Once fledged, these birds can be fed once daily (owls in the evening, hawks in the morning).

Whether the baby is staying at the veterinary hospital for one meal or many, it is the clinic's responsibility to NOT allow this animal (or any wild animal) the opportunity to improperly imprint on human beings. If this is allowed to occur, the raptor will be deemed unreleasable and usually will need to be euthanized.

Raptor Orphan Housing

A small cardboard box lined with cloth works well for a very young raptor (Figure 20.5). A twisted towel made into a circle with the baby placed inside the "doughnut" serves well for support. Walls may need to be covered or cleaned daily because hawks and eagles tend to shoot when they excrete feces. Use of an incubator, heat lamp, or heating pad to provide external heat for the very young (two weeks old or younger) is necessary. Healthy raptors do not need as much heat as other birds, but if they seem lethargic or shiver, they may be cold. A panting chick is too warm. Housing temperatures are outlined below in the initial care section.

As the young become more active, pieces of branches can be placed on the nest bottom to provide the birds with foot-gripping exercise, which is necessary to develop coordination and strength.

When raptors fledge, they need a larger enclosure with stable perches that are larger around than the bird's grip. The enclosure should have solid sides to prevent the flight feathers from sticking out and becoming damaged. The growing chick now needs room to hop and flap its wings.

Misting these newly feathered birds daily with water helps stimulate them to preen and activate their uropygial gland for waterproofing. Once they are eating on their own, acclimated to the outside, and waterproofed, juvenile raptors are ready for outdoor flight caging. By now the bird should be transferred to a raptor rehabilitator to be trained to catch live food and prepared for release.

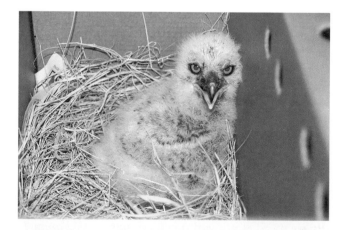

Figure 20.5. Baby hawk. (Photo courtesy of Melanie Haire.)

ALTRICIAL ORPHAN SONGBIRDS

Basic Care

This section is to be used for general information only. Remember that every bird is slightly different in development and behavior. These guidelines are to be used by the veterinary technician until the bird can be transferred to a licensed rehabilitator.

Altricial birds are those that are hatched blind, naked, unable to control body temperature, and completely helpless (blue jays, robins, mockingbirds).

Development

The development of the altricial bird is generally five stages. All species follow these stages but at different rates, depending on their natural history.

1. Hatchling: Zero to four days old, newly hatched, no voice, eyes closed, naked, or sparsely downy
2. Nestling: Five to ten days old, eyes open, partially feathered, feeding call
3. Fledgling: Eleven to fourteen days old, almost fully feathered, can perch, hop, first attempts to fly, ready to leave the nest, able to thermoregulate, frequently preening, wing stretching, short tail feathers
4. Juvenile: Fully grown, defensive, independence begins, lasts until sexual maturity
5. Adult: Sexually mature

Initial Care

An animal should never be fed until it is warm. Use an incubator, brooder, heat light, or heating pad to warm up a chilled infant and keep the baby on heat until it is feathered. Altricial baby birds' temperature guidelines are:

Hatchlings: Should be kept at 80°F–90°F
Nestlings: Should be kept at 80°F–85°F
Fledglings: Should be kept at 70°F–80°F

Once the bird is warm, it should be hydrated by offering drops of Pedialyte or lactated Ringer's solution orally every five to ten minutes until the baby passes a normal fecal sac. For most birds this should consist of a dark solid part (stool) and a milky white softer part (urates) contained within a clear sac.

The baby bird should be examined for injuries, bruises, puncture wounds, bites, mites, and so on. The species must be identified to determine the proper diet and feeding schedule. Begin offering the infant hand-rearing formula.

Identification

A bird rehabilitator should be called for help in identifying the bird. Also refer to Appendix 5.

Information should be obtained about where and how the bird was found from the person who found it. These details not only help identify what type of bird it is, but also may help determine if the bird needs further help or if it can be returned to its parents.

The following items help to identify altricial nestling species:

1. Mouth color: The inside membranes of the mouth are usually brightly colored to attract attention from the feeding parent bird.
2. Gape flanges color: The fleshy "lips" that edge the mouth may be a different color than the inside of the mouth.
3. Beak: The length and shape of the beak helps identify a species by what it eats. Insect eaters tend to have long, slender beaks and seed eaters tend to have thick, short, and conical shaped beaks.
4. Skin color or color of down: Presence or absence of down, natal down, and skin color are also species specific.
5. Vocalizations: Many songbird species have unique feeding calls.
6. Location baby was found: Was the baby found in a tree cavity (woodpeckers, nuthatches), a fireplace (chimney swifts), hanging planters (wrens, finches)?
7. Body size: When the tail feathers emerge from their sheaths, a baby bird has reached its full body size.

Housing Nestlings

The baby bird should be placed in a homemade nest constructed of a berry basket, small plastic bowl, or margarine tub lined with unscented toilet or facial tissues.

A cuplike cavity with the nesting material can be constructed so the baby can nestle down but still receive support from all sides. The baby could develop leg problems if not properly supported during the nesting stage. For extra support, a paper towel can be rolled (snakelike) and coiled around the inside of the nest, and then the tissue placed over the top.

If the tissue is piled high enough (within one-half inch of the nest container top), the baby can defecate over the side of the nest and help keep the inside clean. Replace the tissue as it gets soiled.

Do not use the old natural nest because it may contain parasites and is too difficult to clean. Do not line the artificial nest with fresh grass because it is too cold and damp.

If the baby bird is very young, it may be necessary to use an incubator with a wet sponge or other source of moisture for humidity. A homemade incubator can be made out of a small plastic tote with air holes in the lid. Care should be taken to provide enough ventilation that the humidity does not build up and allow moisture to collect on the inside of the container, which in turn allows rapid growth of pathogens. Instructions for how to make a homemade incubator are available on the International Wildlife Rehabilitation Council (IWRC) web page: www.iwrc-online.org.

If an incubator is not used, the nest should be placed inside a safe container such as a lidded box or basket to prevent any unfortunate mishaps from babies falling out or pets getting into the nest. This especially applies to the technician who has the babies at work in a busy veterinary practice.

The nest should be kept on a heating pad or under a heat lamp at all times to keep the baby from chilling. A thermometer should always be used to monitor the ambient air. The warmth should circulate around the infant (Figure 20.6). A tissue or soft wash cloth should be draped over the top of the baby to hold in the warmth and simulate the security of a brooding parent. Baby birds can usually come off the heat when they feather out, as long as they are active and healthy.

Housing Fledglings

The babies will require a larger cage once they are ready to leave the nest. The nest can be placed inside a small flight cage so the youngsters can hop in and out of their nests until they no longer return to it. The cage should be large enough to allow the birds to take

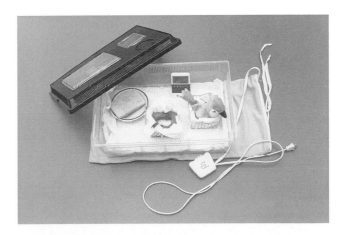

Figure 20.6. *Baby bird incubator with a hygrometer, wet sponge, nest with facial tissues, and heating pad. (Photo courtesy of Melanie Haire.)*

short flights and hop from perch to perch, but small enough to be easily carried inside and out.

The sides should be constructed out of or lined with soft netting or nylon mesh to prevent injury to the bird or its feathers. Reptariums—affordable, commercially available soft-sided mesh cages—can be successfully used to house fledgling and injured adult songbirds. These cages are available in different sizes and are easy to clean because the mesh zips off the plastic frame and can be machine washed.

Wire bird or mammal cages should never be used. If the feathers stick out from between the cage bars they will fray, break off, and possibly become too damaged to support flight. At best these birds with damaged plumage will have to be held over until they molt out a new set of flight feathers, which may take up to a year for many songbird species. Occasionally these birds develop permanent feather follicle damage and need to be euthanized.

The cage bottom can be lined with paper towels and should be changed daily. Several secured low branches should be included to allow for landing and perching practice.

If the weather is mild, the cage should be moved outside during the day but brought inside at night to start acclimating the birds to outdoor temperatures, sights, and sounds.

In addition to introducing the young bird to natural temperatures, the sunlight will provide vital and accurate doses of vitamin D_3. Birds require a proper balance of calcium and phosphorus in their diet for the development of normal, healthy bones. Vitamin D_3 is necessary to ensure that the body can absorb the dietary calcium; otherwise the bones and the bill can become rubbery and soft. This deficiency, called metabolic bone disease, results in bone deformities or even stress fractures that are difficult at best to treat. Prevention is the best medicine, and a combination of thirty minutes a day of direct daylight or thirty to sixty minutes a day with artificial full-spectrum light plus a balanced diet meets the requirements.

Plastic and glass filter out the necessary ultraviolet light so sunlight coming through a window or aquarium does not provide adequate light. The entire cage should never be placed in direct sunlight. The babies can quickly overheat if a shaded area is not easily accessible. Ultraviolet rays from the sun are still available on cloudy days and in the shade.

The enclosure should never be left unprotected from possible predators. A screened porch or a fenced yard is no protection from a stray cat or hungry raccoon. Predator-proof caging can be affordably built but is not be discussed in this chapter.

All hand-raised wild bird releases should be done by a licensed bird rehabilitator. Many of the rehabilitation manuals listed on the source pages have instructions for building pre-release and release caging.

Feeding Methods

There are many feeding methods in practice for feeding wild baby birds (Figure 20.7). Blunt forceps, tweezers, pipettes, syringes, eyedroppers, small artists' paint brushes, Popsicle sticks, blunted toothpicks, and fingers are just some of the tools that can be used for administering food. A discussion of feeding techniques with a local avian rehabilitator will aid in choosing the best method. Many of these feeding implements only work with certain types of formulas, and sometimes a combination works well. Often the thickness of the formula depends on the age of the bird, so feeding several birds of different ages may require the use of more than one tool.

Many healthy nestlings and fledglings gape readily and hungrily, making feeding time for the caregiver much easier. These willing participants will continue to gape, for the most part, until their crops are full. Care should be taken to avoid over filling the crop. If the bird is slow to swallow or flings food, it might be full or too dehydrated.

If the baby is hesitant to gape, it may be dehydrated or otherwise ill, not hungry, too frightened, or nervous, or it may not recognize the gesture as a feeding attempt. Tap on the side of the nest and whistle softly in an attempt to imitate the parent bird's arrival to the nest. This may require patience and several tries with different chirping sounds. Gaping nest mates often help stimulate gaping in all individuals, including newcomers.

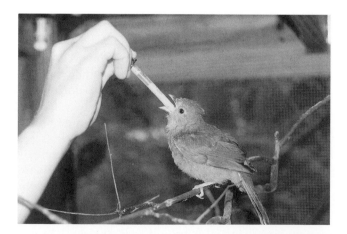

Figure 20.7. *Hand-feeding a baby cardinal. (Photo courtesy of Melanie Haire.)*

If the baby is hydrated and healthy but still will not gape, gently prying the beak open with fingers and placing a small amount of food toward the back of its mouth may be necessary. Some birds get the picture quickly and only need one or two force feedings to understand that they are being offered food and will not be harmed.

Once birds imprint on their parents and are old enough to have developed fear of humans in the wild, they become more difficult to hand feed and may need to be force fed until they become self feeding. Introducing a bowl of food into their cage for this older fledgling group may be the answer.

Several altricial species of baby birds (i.e. some swifts, swallows, nighthawks, pigeons, and all doves) never gape, and knowing the identification of these species will save a lot of time and frustration. These individuals must be fed in a different manner. Fledgling or juvenile swifts, swallows, and nighthawks are examples of birds that will probably need to be force or tube fed until release. Hatchlings and nestlings may adjust to hand feedings but need to be fed by holding the food up to the bird's beak.

Pigeon and dove babies do not gape but they do beg. They naturally feed by sticking their beaks inside their parent's mouth, which is the opposite position of many songbirds, and thus the concept of willingly opening their mouths to the sight of an eyedropper full of food has no meaning to them. These birds must be tube fed until they self feed. Once the birds are seven days old or older, a feeder can be made that resembles the feeding technique naturally used by this group.

Pigeon and Dove Feeder

A 12- or 20-cc syringe casing can be filled with a balanced parakeet seed mix (small seeds without a lot of hulls or shelled sunflower seeds) and tightly wrapped with Vetrap over the opened bottom of the case to keep the seeds in. A quarter- to half-inch slit is then cut in the center of the Vetrap (long enough for the bird's beak to fit through but not too big to allow seeds to spill out around beak). Next, the bird's beak can be inserted into the slit in the Vetrap, and while holding the back of the bird's head to keep it from pulling out of the dispenser, the syringe can be tapped to simulate the movement of the parent bird (Figure 20.8). It will take several attempts to get the bird to quit struggling and pulling away from the feeder. Once the baby swallows some seeds (probably by accident the first time), it will quickly start self feeding right out of the dispenser. Then, in addition to tube feeding into their crop with a hand-rearing formula, the baby can be

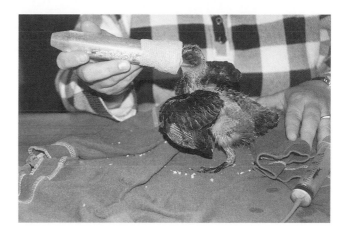

Figure 20.8. Pigeon feeder. (Photo courtesy of Melanie Haire.)

offered the feeder several times a day to facilitate the self feeding and weaning process.

A size 10 or 12 red rubber catheter cut to about three inches in length can be used to crop tube feed pigeons and doves. Exact, Pretty Bird, and Emeraid are examples of quality hand-rearing powdered diets commercially available at pet stores or veterinary clinics.

Food Prep

The bird formulas ideally should be made fresh daily and refrigerated until use. Each feeding should be allowed to warm to room temperature before feeding it to the bird.

The consistency varies depending on the diet and the age of the bird. Most diets are thick like oatmeal when hand mixed but can be blended to a slurry that can be pushed through a syringe or dropper. Some formulas tend to thicken over the day during refrigeration, and a little water may need to be added to keep it at the proper consistency. Remember that baby birds need as many calories as possible so do not thin formulas down more than absolutely necessary. Runny or drippy formulas should never be fed because the food could drip down into the trachea and cause aspiration pneumonia.

Many diets can be made in batches and stored in the freezer for short periods of time. Making a week's worth of food at once and freezing it in ice cube trays can save a lot of time. Then as many cubes are needed for the day can be thawed, and a back-up supply is available if more babies are received. It is important to know about nutrition because some ingredients lose dietary value when frozen or stored for long periods of time. Always start with fresh, good quality ingredients.

Feeding Frequency

Feeding frequency should follow this guideline:

Hatchling: Feed every ten to twenty minutes (6 a.m. to 10 p.m.)

Nestling: Feed every twenty to thirty minutes (6 a.m. to 10 p.m.)

Fledgling: Feed every forty-five to sixty minutes (7 a.m. to 10 p.m.)

Juveniles: Feed every two hours (7 a.m. to 9 p.m.)

In the wild, baby birds are fed from sunup to sundown. A technician should not make the mistake of thinking that baby birds can be fed enough calories in a 9:00–5:00 work day. Hand-raising a baby bird is not a part-time responsibility. If the bird cannot be transferred over to a rehabilitator the same day, feeding arrangements must be made for the baby for a full twelve- to fourteen-hour day. The biggest single mistake made by well-meaning people who hand rearing baby wild birds is underfeeding them. The caretaker cannot make up for several missed feedings by feeding larger volumes at the next couple of feedings.

The only flexibility a caretaker has is to pick when the twelve to fourteen hours begin and end. By covering the cage and making it dark or leaving the lights on in the nursery past sundown, the "daytime" can be slightly altered if need be. This is not recommended for the long term or with older juvenile birds because they need to develop a sense of natural time.

Diets

It is ideal to feed the same diet that the rehabilitator will use to prevent the stress of change to the baby's gastrointestinal tract. The recipes and ingredients should be on hand prior to the start of baby season in order to be prepared. All too often the babies seem to come in at 10 p.m. on a Sunday night, just as the pet stores close.

Proper bird species identification is necessary to choose the best diet recipe. Read as much natural history information as is available to learn about food preferences, feeding methods, food presentation, and normal behavior.

The following are some examples of passerine hand-rearing formulas used at rehabilitation centers:

1 part soaked Hill's Science Diet Feline Growth
1 part Gerber's High Protein Cereal
1 tsp. bone meal
Water to proper consistency (Evans 1986)

1 cup soaked puppy chow
1 T baby food beef
1 T hard-boiled egg yolk
3 to 4 drops balanced avian vitamins (Avitron)
1/2 tsp. ground egg shell (Johnson 1991)

1 cup soaked Hill's Science Diet Feline Growth (original recipe only)
1/2 cup chick starter added to 1/2 cup boiling water
3 to 4 drops balanced avian vitamins (Avitron)
1/2 tsp. Rep-cal (calcium with vitamin D_3, phosphorus-free)
1 tsp. powdered Benebac
Mix cat food and hot chick starter together in blender. Add other ingredients after mix cools (Ivie 1999). Note: Science Diet Feline Growth original recipe only is advised due to avian digestive problems associated with the other flavors.

These sample diets can be fed to a wide variety of species with the exception of doves and pigeons. These diets are a balanced base. Depending on the bird species, food items can be added to more closely match their natural diet.

- Insectivorous birds such as woodpeckers, swifts, and wrens should have insects added to the base. Mealworms, wax worms, crickets, and freeze-dried insects are examples of supplements that should make up to 50% of the diet.
- Frugivores such as waxwings and orioles should have chopped fruit added.
- Birds with a tendency to develop a calcium deficiency, such as mockingbirds, thrashers, and kingbirds, should have food items rich in calcium or a calcium supplement added to the diet.
- Doves and pigeons, which are strictly seed and grain feeders, can be tube fed with a commercial brand of baby bird food formulated for psittacines. These powdered diets, which are ready to use after adding water, are available in most pet stores.
- Hummingbirds need a commercial nectar such as Nekton or Roudybush. Pet store or homemade sugar-water diets (although good for providing energy) only provide calories and will not keep a hummingbird alive long term.

Additional Information

Avoid allowing formula to dry on the baby's beak, nares, or feathers. Remove any spilled food while it is still moist and easier to remove. Food that is allowed to dry on feathers may cause feather loss or a skin infection. Use a damp cotton swab to clean food off of the baby; wiping should be in the direction of the feather growth.

Always try to house single baby birds with conspecifics. The rehabilitator should be contacted to help place the baby with other same-species orphans or, even better, into a foster parent situation. Arrangements should be made to get them together as soon as possible. The benefits of orphaned animals being raised with natural or foster siblings are immeasurable. They learn critical behavioral and social skills from interacting with the correct species.

Never forget that the goal of wildlife rehabilitation is to provide temporary care with the goal of releasing the animal with its best chances to survive. Technicians must above all do no harm and never release an animal that cannot properly care for itself. To achieve this goal:

- Limit talking around wildlife.
- Avoid improper imprinting.
- Keep adequate notes that can be used as reference material later. Good record keeping may also prevent mishaps due to shift changes in caregivers.
- Limit handling and activity to feeding and cleaning time only.
- Never house wild birds near domestic pets, especially pet birds.
- Clean all food containers and tools with hot soapy water after each use and allow them to air dry or towel dry them before the next use. Dip feeding instruments in 5% diluted bleach or soak in 10% diluted Nolvasan for thirty minutes once daily.

CARING FOR ADULT PASSERINE (SONG) BIRDS

Initial Care

The bird's history should be obtained on the intake form to help diagnose why the bird came in to the clinic. The rescuer might know for certain that it was hit by a car, flew into a window, or was caught by a cat. If no cause is known, good "investigative" questions should help find the answer. If the bird was found in the driveway, ask if there is a nearby garage with windows it might have collided with. If the bird was found under a bird feeder and has had its tail feathers pulled out, the rescuer should be questioned about the possibilities of outdoor cats in the area.

After the history taking, a visual exam should be performed first before touching the bird. The bird should be observed for signs of disease or illness such

as ruffled feathers, squinted or closed eyes, sneezing, clicking, mouth breathing, dull feathers, lethargy, diarrhea, squatting instead of standing, and wing droops.

Next, a physical examination should be performed, looking for obvious wounds and fractures along with more subtle signs of shock and dehydration. (See the section on performing the physical exam under "Initial Exam," above). Body and feather condition should be checked and noted. The keel should be palpated to determine if the bird is thin or emaciated. When checking for lacerations or bruising, feathers can be blown out of the way to better visualize the skin underneath.

Restraint for adult songbirds is relatively easy. Pressure should not be placed on a bird's sternum because it breathes by expanding its chest and abdominal cavities. Using the "bander's" hold enables the examiner to check the bird thoroughly while keeping a secure yet gentle hold on the patient (Figure 20.9). This hold should be used for any handling, medicating or force feeding procedures.

An accurate weight in grams should be obtained and monitored every twenty-four to forty-eight hours. The bird should be kept warm and hydrated before attempting to feed it. If the bird feels thin; has bright green stools, sunken eyes, wrinkled skin; or is weak and lethargic, it should be offered two to four drops of rehydrating solution orally by placing the drops behind the glottis into the throat every fifteen minutes for the first one to two hours.

Dehydrated birds can receive SQ fluids injected into their wing web or into the loose medial skin folds where the legs join to the body. Injecting fluids, although more painful than delivering oral fluids due

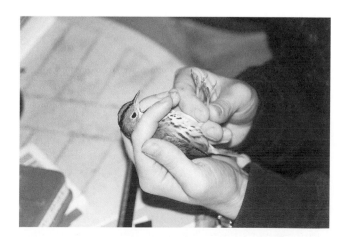

Figure 20.9. Bird bander's hold. (Photo courtesy of Melanie Haire.)

to the needle prick, ultimately may be less stressful due to the larger volume that can be given at one time, which decreases the number of times the bird must be restrained.

Immobilizing Fractures

Immobilization of any fractures should be performed as soon as possible so the bird does not further injure itself. The wildlife veterinary technician should know how to apply all of the following bandages. The veterinarians may not be able to look at every bird that comes in with a fracture, but if the proper stabilizing wrap is applied, the fracture may have all it needs to heal properly. Do not allow a bird with a fractured bone to sit in the hospital without a proper bandage. Waiting one or two days to apply the wrap could be too late.

If the bone needs more than a bandage to properly mend (long bones on larger birds such as ducks, owls, and hawks), the wrap should still be applied until the veterinarian can schedule the bone surgery procedure.

If the lower leg (tibiotarsus or tarsometatarsus) is fractured on a small bird, a tape splint usually works well (Figure 20.10). The leg is held in a natural "perch" position and tape is placed on each side of the leg. Seal the tape firmly to the leg by pinching it with a pair of hemostats. The more tape applied, the more stable the splint, but remember the weight of the apparatus versus the small size of the patient. The bird should be able to stand and perch with this type of bandage if it is properly trimmed.

A fractured femur needs more than tape. Cast padding and a splint (made of toothpicks, tongue depressors, halved syringe case, etc.) covered in Vetrap, depending on the size of the bird, are needed. The joint above and below the fracture site must be covered. If this is not possible, it is best not to bandage at all and arrange to have the bird transported to an experienced avian veterinarian or rehabilitator immediately.

Any leg bandage applied too tightly will prevent blood flow from leaving the foot, and the foot and toes may swell. The toes must be evaluated daily for swelling, loss of function, or discoloration.

Foot injuries can be bandaged several different ways. In small songbirds, toes can be taped down individually onto a cardboard "snowshoe." In larger birds, a padded ball bandage can be made to keep the toes aligned and the talons from puncturing the footpads (Figure 20.11). A circular piece of cardboard is cut to fit in the bottom of the bird's foot and is padded with cotton. The pad is taped in place by wrapping the cotton padding with Vetrap between the bird's toes. The toe tips should be

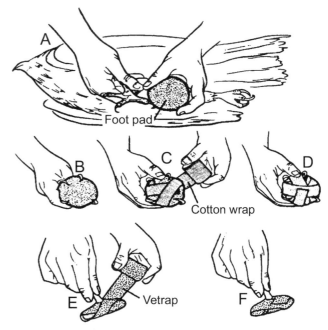

Figure 20.11. *A padded bandage used in avian foot and leg injuries. (A) A cardboard plate is cut to fit the foot and padded with cotton wrap and covered with tape. (B) The foot pad is placed against the bottom of the foot with the toes properly positioned and in extension. (C and D) The foot pad is wrapped in place with cotton padding. (E) Cotton padding is covered with Vetrap. (F) Completed bandage. (Permission for drawing use granted by the Georgia Department of Natural Resources and Branson Ritchie, DVM, MS.)*

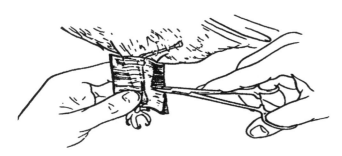

Figure 20.10. *Tape splint used for fracture immobilization in the lower leg bones of small birds. Tape is placed on each side of the leg with the sticky sides facing each other. The tape is pressed together with hemostats. (Permission for drawing use granted by the Georgia Department of Natural Resources and Branson Ritchie, DVM, MS.)*

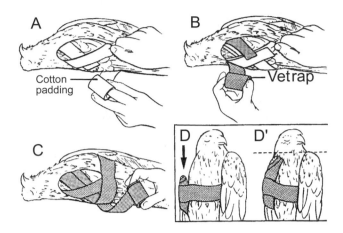

Figure 20.12. Figure-eight bandage used for the immobilization of the avian wing. (A) Cotton padding is wrapped from the carpus to the humerus and back to the carpus. (B) The same pattern is repeated with the Vetrap. (C) The Vetrap is passed around the midbody and taped in place. (D) A properly bandaged wing should be held at the same level as the normal wing. (D′) If the wing drops below the level of the normal wing, the bandage should be removed and reapplied. (Permission for drawing use granted by the Georgia Department of Natural Resources and Branson Ritchie, DVM, MS.)

slightly visible so they can be checked for bandage tightness. The bandages should be kept as clean and dry as possible because replacing the wrap before the bone is healed will delay or prevent healing.

For wing fractures, as with all fractures, the joint above and below the fracture site should be immobilized. The figure-eight bandage holds the wing closed in a natural position and is adequate to immobilize a fracture on any portion of the wing as well as reduce the weight of the wing on the shoulder. If the fracture involves the humerus, continue the wing bandage around the body to immobilize the shoulder joint (joint above the fracture).

If using the body wrap, be sure to pass the tape under the good wing on the opposite side and across the body on the upper keel (Figure 20.12). The fit should be snug but not tight enough to interfere with respiration or circulation. When this bandage is properly applied, the bird should be able to stand and perch while holding the wing in a normal anatomic position. All wing feathers should be in alignment as well. If the bandage pulls the wing in an abnormal position, the bandage should be removed and reapplied.

Bird bones heal much more quickly then mammal bones do, so bandages usually only have to remain on

for two to three weeks, as long as the bird is confined to strict cage rest for several days after the bandage is removed. After this cage-rest period, the bird should have manual limb massage and gradual limb extensions. After a good callus is formed, the bird can be placed in a flight cage.

Housing Adult Birds

Make sure the housing is as stress free as possible. Cover the fronts of all bird caging and if possible give the bird natural materials to hide in. Reptariums (See mesh cages in Appendix 10) and the collapsible framed, mesh laundry hampers (available at discount stores) make excellent injured adult bird caging due to their soft-sided, feather protecting material and light weight. Reptariums are machine washable. Perching of various heights should be provided if the bird is capable of standing.

As soon as its hospital stay is over, the patient should be transferred to the rehabilitator to be housed in an appropriate aviary.

Feeding Adult Birds

Adult birds should be encouraged to eat on their own by providing natural food items that they may recognize. Use whole berries, millet sprays, seed mixes, and live insects along with grains, cracked corn, bran, and chopped fruits. A stressed bird usually will not eat, so noise, bright lights, visual disturbances, and extreme temperatures should be reduced to allow the avian patient to settle down and eat.

If after one day the bird has not eaten, it must be force fed at least four times a day. This can be performed by gently placing a thumb and forefinger at the corners of the mouth and pressing it to open or by using the other hand to open the mouth and placing food carefully down the throat behind the glottis. Most birds will swallow when food is placed far enough back. Use one of the homemade diets in the nestling care section for hand feeding or Lafeber's Emeraid Psittacine (powdered diet for debilitated birds) for tube feeding. For prey eating birds, powdered diets such as Emeraid Carnivore or Oxbow Critical Care for Carnivores are good products for tube feeding.

Sometimes force feeding a bird several times is all it takes to get it to start self feeding. Make sure it is eating enough and maintaining a healthy weight.

Live insects (wax worms, mealworms, and crickets) should be "gut-loaded" with healthy, nutritionally rich ingredients and not fed off the shelf from a bait store. When insects are purchased, they usually have eaten much of the food that was in the container they have been living in, so they need to be provided with nutrition for at least twenty-four hours before feeding them to wildlife patients. Mealworms can be put into a plastic tub with a ventilated lid at room temperature with coarsely ground whole grains such as corn meal, rolled oats, wheat bran, or game bird starter. For moisture, a cut-up potato can be added to the top of the mixture. Crickets and wax worms can also eat this mixture. Fresh-dug earthworms are also good to offer to insectivorous or omnivorous birds, especially robins, thrashers, ducks, thrushes, jays, and mockingbirds.

See Appendix 6 for the average weight of selected North American songbirds (Dunning 1984).

PRECOCIAL BIRD BASIC CARE

At hatching, precocial birds are covered in feather down, self feeding, ready to leave the nest, and can see, hear, run, and swim. These baby birds have no flanges on the sides of the mouth and have small, developed wings. The eggs of the precocial bird contain more nutrients and require more time to hatch, but the chick hatches out fully developed.

These birds (ducks, geese, killdeer, pheasant, quail, woodcock, and other shorebirds) have different dietary and housing needs than altricial birds.

Initial Orphan Care
Never feed any animal until it is warm. An incubator, brooder, or heat light should be used to warm a chilled infant. Despite their downy covering, precocial chicks need to be kept at slightly warmer ambient air temperature than altricial chicks. Temperature guidelines are:

Newborn chicks (zero to seven days): 90°F to 95°F
Chicks developing quills: 85°F to 90°F
Birds with quills and developing feathers: 60°F to 85°F

These chicks, if healthy, usually eat readily and drink on their own. They are social and eat better in groups of similar species and ages. If the chick is not eating, its dehydration and temperature should be checked. Some chicks can be quite nervous, and covering the box or cage with a towel may help them to eat.

If the bird is dehydrated, it can be offered drops of Pedialyte every fifteen minutes for the first several hours or until it passes a normal stool. The fluid may have to be placed into the throat beyond the glottis if the baby is weak and dehydrated.

The bird should be examined for injuries, cuts, mites, or wounds. The species should be identified to determine its proper diet and feeding schedule. Begin offering the infant hand rearing formula.

Identification
A bird rehabilitator should be contacted to help identify the species. Field guides may also be helpful. Ducks and some dabbling water birds have webbed feet or toes. Hatchling wood ducks have a visible egg tooth on the tip of the bill. Most shore birds have very long legs and can run quite fast. Be sure to look at the beak shape. Ducks and geese have wide, flat bills, whereas the killdeer have thinner, tapered beaks (Figure 20.13). Quails and pheasant have short, sturdy, conical beaks.

Housing
A box or plastic tote lined with newspaper covered with paper or ravel-free cloth towels will do. The container should be covered with a screen top because some ducks (wood ducks) can jump very high. These birds are messy and cardboard will become soiled and need to be replaced often.

A wild bird should never be housed in a wire pet bird or mammal cage. A ceramic brooder-heating element or a brooder heat light can be hung in one half of the cage, making sure the enclosure is large to allow the birds to move in and out of the heated area.

It is very important to provide these birds with hiding places, such as a small box on its side. A feather duster can be hung down inside the cage so babies can snuggle up under it for security, shelter, and comfort. All these cage items will get soiled and need to be cleaned and kept as dry as possible.

Waterfowl splash in the water bowl and then seek the heat lamp to dry off underneath. As the birds grow

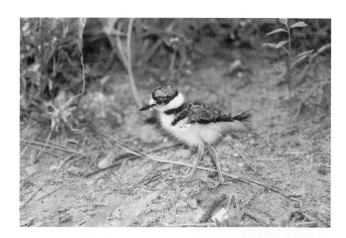

Figure 20.13. *One-week-old killdeer. (Photo courtesy of Melanie Haire.)*

feathers and spend less time under the lamp, it can be gradually raised up until the birds are weaned off of the supplemental heat.

Do not provide waterfowl with a pool unless directed to do so by an avian rehabilitator. Baby ducks and geese should never be left unattended during swimming time. If instructed to provide "swim time," a painter's roller tray can be used to provide a ramp and shallow swimming area.

These young chicks need appropriate shelter and a quiet room to prevent stress that can oftentimes be fatal.

As they grow, so should their housing. Older juveniles and adults need to have a large outside predator-proof pen with a pool. This type of setup cannot usually be provided at a veterinary clinic or at most people's homes, so transferring the birds to the rehabilitator or wildlife center is recommended.

Feeding

Food and water bowls should be placed on the side away from the heat. Caution must be used with the selection of the water bowl to prevent babies getting soaked and chilled. Using a Mason jar filled with water and inverted over a shallow lid or a commercial chicken waterer (available at most feed and farm stores) works well. A small water bowl filled three-fourths full with rocks or marbles also provides a readily available drinking source and keeps the babies from jumping into the water.

Food varies slightly between species but most do well on crumbled, unmedicated chicken starter. Some food can be sprinkled on the cage floor, as well as in a food bowl.

A very young, single chick may be unsure how and what to eat. It learns these skills by watching and imitating its mother. Contact other bird rehabilitators so another chick can be placed with it. Sometimes these birds need to be force fed until placement can be found. In the meantime, try to teach the youngster by "pecking" at the food with a finger. Food in motion also seems to help stimulate feeding behavior, so the grain can be gently rolled around and tiny live mealworms, earthworms, or crickets offered to inspire the infant to begin to peck. In addition, floating chopped greens and small amounts of chick starter on water tends to stimulate unsure waterfowl.

The food should be changed twice a day, and small, live mealworms, chopped greens and berries, cracked corn, and crickets can be offered as the babies grow. Fresh food should always be available, because the birds eat free choice.

ADULT PRECOCIAL BIRDS (INCLUDING WATERFOWL AND WADING BIRDS)

Identification of the species and familiarity with its natural history, food preferences, and habitat is required. An examination for injuries should be performed.

Care must be taken with the water birds with long, pointed beaks. Herons, cranes, kingfishers, loons, and egrets will stab at faces and eyes when they feel threatened. Smaller birds such as grebes, coots, gulls, and rails can strike very quickly with short sturdy beaks and give quite a pinch as well. Coots kick and use the spurs on their legs to defend themselves. Ducks, geese, and swans can be difficult to restrain due to their strength and size. These birds will bite and twist with their powerful bills and will beat at their restrainer with their very powerful wings. Take precautions, wear goggles, secure their heads, and work in pairs when restraining these animals. Even the small species are surprisingly strong and difficult to restrain.

Examination, body temperatures, hydration, and treatments are similar to other adult birds. See Chapter 2, "Psittacines and Passerines."

These species are particularly susceptible to lead poisoning (from ingesting fishing sinkers and lead bird-shot used for duck hunting), fish hook ingestion, monofilament entanglement, and botulism due to their aquatic nature.

Diving birds (grebes, some sea ducks, loons, etc.) are built for floating, swimming, and diving, but not walking, so many times these birds are presented with "broken legs" because they will not or cannot stand. The legs on these birds are positioned far back on the body, for propelling through the water, instead of underneath the body, for walking. Many times these birds get tired during migrational movements and come down for a rest. If a loon lands on a wet pavement or parking lot thinking it looks like water, it has no way to take off again. Many times these birds just need a few meals and to be placed on a large body of water to allow for takeoff. This is a good example of why learning about a patient's natural history is so important.

Housing

A plastic pet kennel works well if a water bird needs to be housed. Keeping the pen clean can be challenging due to the large volume of liquid stool these birds produce. If the bird is too weak to hold itself upright or has a fractured leg, placing it in a box half filled with shredded newspapers makes a good body support setup and also allows the feces to drop away from the bird, which keeps the feathers and vent clean.

Water birds must keep their feathers in perfect condition and naturally do so by constant preening and bathing. If the birds are strong enough and do not have a bandage on, they can be provided with a bath water source either in the enclosure or in a sink or tub to allow them to bathe and keep their feathers waterproof. Caution should be used with pools because even ducks can drown, especially if they are weak or not waterproof. It may be best to transfer these birds out as soon as possible and allow the rehabilitator to do this process.

Many water-type birds do not have feet designed for long-term perching. A kennel, box, or mesh cage can have a flat "shelf-type" perch or a split log available to those that feel comfortable standing up off the ground.

These adult birds, especially the herons, rails, and egrets, are quite nervous and will pace and wear themselves out trying to escape if they do not feel secure and hidden. These birds should be provided with the quietest place possible with covering on all sides of the caging.

Feeding

Although the commercial game bird grain mixes are sufficient in nutrition for short-term care of many of these species, getting them to eat it is the biggest challenge. These birds, with the possible exception of some ducks and geese, tend to be very difficult captive feeders. One problem is that many are normally used to feeding in or while on the water. Sitting on a towel in a box is too unnatural, and they don't understand the concept of eating with a bowl of food in front of them. Due to their nervous nature, they might not ever feel secure enough to eat.

Often these species need to be tube fed or force fed while they remain in captivity. Kingfishers, herons, and gulls must be fed fish, insects, and/or mice. To force feed a fish, be sure to insert the fish headfirst into the bird's mouth and gently push it down the throat until the bird swallows. Holding the head in an upright position for several moments after feeding each fish may help prevent the bird from regurgitating the meal.

Several tube feeding formulas that can be used depending on the diet requirements of the species include Emeraid II, infant bird hand rearing powdered diets, Clinicare (liquid diets made for debilitated dogs or cats), ground game bird pellets mixed with water, or blended fish.

All of the medical procedures, cleaning, moving, and so on should be done before feeding is attempted.

Feeding should always be the last procedure done on any animal and should be immediately followed by low stress, quiet, and privacy to aid the animal in the digestion process. Sudden loud noises or big movements may cause the animal to regurgitate the food and possibly even aspirate it.

Some fish eaters can learn to fish live minnows or goldfish out of a pan or bucket. Ducks, geese, coots, shorebirds, and similar species may eat live insects and chopped greens if provided in addition to the grain diet. Another hint is to float grain, insects, and greens on top of a dish of water. Sometimes this more natural presentation stimulates the birds to stab or dabble at the groceries.

GENERAL ORPHAN MAMMAL CARE

What to Do First

Never feed any animal until it is warm and hydrated. Use a heat lamp, heating pad on low and always under the cage (not inside), or a warm water bath to warm up a cold baby. Once the baby is at normal body temperature, it can start to be rehydrated. Oral fluids such as lactated Ringer's solution (LRS) or Pedialyte are the preferred method of rehydration for infants. Subcutaneous fluids (LRS) can be used if the animal is moderately dehydrated. Consider all animals that come into rehabilitation to be dehydrated to some extent. Fluids should always be warmed first before administering, regardless of route.

The infant should be weighed and fluids provided at the rate of 40 to 50 ml/kg over a twelve- to twenty-four-hour period or until hydration is complete. See the fluid chart in the glossary in Appendix 9 under "Dehydration."

Introducing Formula

Once the baby animal is warm and properly hydrated, formula can begin to be fed gradually. It should be introduced slowly to prevent digestive problems. Never start an animal on full-strength formula. It should take twenty-four to seventy-two hours to introduce a milk formula, depending on the degree of initial dehydration. A severely dehydrated animal's digestive tract cannot handle full-strength or solid foods. Feeding these food items prematurely could prove to be fatal. The following dilution procedure should be followed:

Day 1: 25% full-strength formula/75% water or Pedialyte
Day 2: 50% full-strength formula/50% water or Pedialyte

Day 3: 75% full-strength formula/25% water or Pedialyte, OR 100% full-strength formula if no diarrhea develops and the infant remains hydrated

If diarrhea or bloating develops, at any stage, the concentration of formula should be reduced or replaced entirely with Pedialyte until the situation clears up. Veterinary advice should be sought if problems persist for more than twenty-four hours.

If bloating occurs, gently message the infant's abdomen while submerging the bottom half of its body in a warm water bath. Also consider giving oral simethicone drops for gas relief if the massaging is not completely effective. Using a probiotic (Lactobacillus) product, such as Benebac, can be helpful to reduce stress to the babies' intestinal tract and help prevent or treat diarrhea.

If the neonate regurgitates formula, feeding should be discontinued and that feeding skipped altogether. At the next feeding, the formula can be thinned with water by half and the volume reduced. Seek veterinary advice if the vomiting continues.

Preparing Formulas

Milk formulas should be mixed according to the label's instructions using warm water to help dissolve the powdered milk. Ready to use liquid formulas are also available, but they tend to be more expensive. Once the can is opened, unused milk must be discarded after seventy-two hours, making this sometimes wasteful (Figure 20.14). Enough milk formula should be made up to last for twenty-four hours and kept refrigerated. When ready to feed, only enough should be heated for

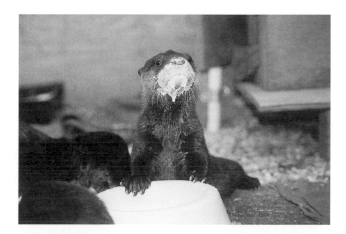

Figure 20.14. Three-month-old river otter enjoying a bowl of Esbilac milk formula. (Photo courtesy of Melanie Haire.)

one feeding (100°F to 102°F; warm but not hot on a wrist). One way to warm formula is to drop formula-filled syringes into a mug of warm water. Using an electric coffee mug warmer may be helpful to keep multiple syringes warm. Also, remember to cap syringes or milk will leak out and mug water will refill the syringes, resulting in diluted formula.

Do not use the microwave to heat formula. This method tends to cook the milk and leaves the contents unevenly heated.

The infant should be weighed and the species care pages in Appendix 7 used to determine the quantity of food intake.

Some infants prefer to be stimulated to urinate and defecate prior to feeding. Use of a cotton ball or soft facial tissue dipped in warm water to lightly wipe the babies' abdomen and genitals will suffice. This process also seems to stimulate the nursing reflex in some species.

Selecting Milk Formulas

Many brands of milk replacers are available, and there are as many variations of how to use them. Again, this is when it becomes critical to contact a local rehabilitator. The importance of using the correct diet cannot be stressed enough. Do not try to switch formulas unless the baby is having trouble digesting the milk replacer that has been chosen. The animal transfer process will be much easier on the infant if the same formula that the rehabilitator will be using is chosen.

Of the many commercial formulas available, no one milk substitute meets the needs of all species. Substitute domestic animal milk formulas for puppies, kittens, lambs, and foals have been used successfully. Recently a commercial line of milk replacers, formulated for wildlife, has become available. Due to space limitations, this chapter does not cover detailed wildlife nutritional requirements and comparisons. Refer to the species care sheets in Appendix 7 for general diet guidelines. Good reference articles and books are available through the National Wildlife Rehabilitators Association (NWRA) and International Wildlife Rehabilitation Council (IWRC) on wildlife nutritional requirements. The company Pet-Ag has been manufacturing milk replacer products since 1930 and most of the wildlife nutritional studies have been done on their products (e.g. Esbilac, KMR, Multi-Milk, Zoological Milk Matrix). Homemade formulas are sometimes used but these rarely meet the complete nutritional requirements for wildlife. Cow's milk is not compatible with the natural milk of most wild animals and tends to cause gastrointestinal problems.

Syringe Feeding

Use the smallest syringe that will hold the needed volume of formula. This provides the most accurate measurement of the animal's formula intake and the best flow control.

Many animals resist the first few feeding attempts due to the newness of the plastic feeder and the taste of the formula. However, after several feedings, they begin to accept their foster care.

Use of a soft rubber nipple (Catac) or silicone nipple (Mothering Kit) on the end of the syringe often helps facilitate the feedings. To help keep the nipple from slipping off the syringe tip, remember to wipe the syringe's slip tip dry and roughen the surface slightly with a hemostat before slipping the nipple on. Make sure that an overeager youngster does not pull the nipple all the way off and choke on it. It may be necessary to discontinue the nipple use once rodents' incisors appear, due to their ability to chew the tip off and possibly ingest it.

In the case of tiny neonates (i.e. newborn chipmunks, flying squirrels, mice), a handmade "preemie nipple" can be made from two common veterinary supplies. A size 16 gauge intravenous indwelling catheter cut off about one-half inch from the end can be used as the base for the nipple apparatus because it fits onto any slip-tipped syringe. The nipple is made from the rubber sleeve that covers the needle of a multiple-sample blood collection needle used to draw blood. First, the rubber sleeve should be pulled down and punctured with the collection needle to make the nipple hole. Then the sleeve is pulled off of the blood collection device and slipped over the cut catheter. A size 16 gauge catheter provides a snug fit for the nipple, and the apparatus is ready to attach to the feeding syringe (Figure 20.15).

Other feeding syringe attachment examples are tomcat catheters, feeding tubes, or teat infusion cannulas. Any slip-tip syringe will work but the O-ring type syringe is much smoother, and the rubber plunger doesn't stick and wear out as quickly as the regular plungers do. (See the suppliers list in Appendix 10.)

Slow and steady pressure on the base of the syringe should be used to allow infants to drink small amounts at a time. Some species will nurse (i.e. squirrels, chipmunks, raccoons, and beavers), while others may lap (i.e. cottontails, opossums, and mink) at the tip of the nipple or syringe. Use the following methods to help control the formula flow rate.

To increase flow rate:

- Apply more pressure on the syringe.
- Allow air into the syringe.

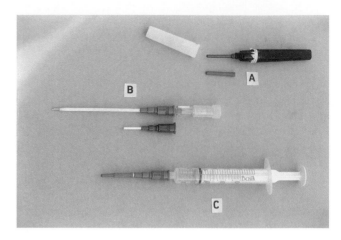

Figure 20.15. "Preemie" feeding nipple. (A) A multiple sample collection needle. (B) A 16-gauge IV indwelling catheter. (C) Assembled. (Photo courtesy of Melanie Haire.)

- Enlarge the opening of the syringe tip or nipple.
- Thin the formula.
- Use a smaller size syringe.

To decrease flow rate:

- Hold back on the syringe plunger.
- Remove air from syringe.
- Use another nipple with a smaller hole.
- Add rice baby cereal to thicken the formula.
- Use a larger size syringe.

Each animal is different and several different syringes and nipple combinations may need to be tried, even when feeding litter mates (Figure 20.16). Individual infants may drink too quickly regardless of what is done and the syringe will have to be moved away every few seconds to reduce the chance of the baby choking or aspirating formula.

Other Feeding Implements

Bottle feeding can be used for some species of animals. Pet nursers and puppy and kitten bottles are sometimes used with small wildlife such as squirrels and rabbits. Human baby bottles and nipples work for such species as large felids, canids, older raccoons, and otters. Neonatal carnivores should be started out on a human premature-infant-sized nipple. Hoofstock prefer a goat/foal-type nipple and bottle due to the size and shape of their mouths. This method offers a faster formula delivery system but less control over milk flow speed and quantity.

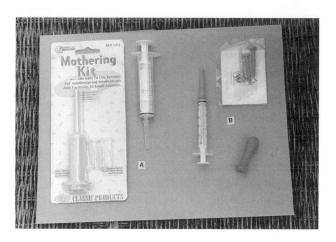

Figure 20.16. (A) Mothering Kit silicone feeding nipples. (B) Catac rubber feeding nipples. (C) Pet nurser nipple tip tied to a catheter tip syringe. (Photo courtesy of Melanie Haire.)

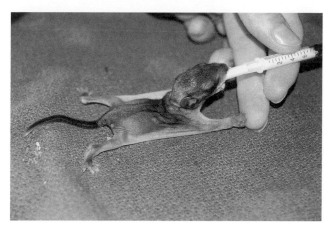

Figure 20.17. Three-week-old flying squirrel being fed with a silicone nipple and syringe. (Photo courtesy of Melanie Haire.)

Remember to make the size of the nipple hole appropriate for the animal. Holes can be made in the nipple by several methods. By cutting the tip off with scissors or cutting an "X" into the tip, different flow patterns are created. To create a very small round hole, an appropriate-sized gauge needle is heated with the beveled tip in the flame. When the needle tip is hot, allow it to melt through the center of the end of the nipple. With the needle still in place, the entire apparatus should be placed in cold water until cool. Once the needle is removed, the hole remains approximately the same size as the needle gauge.

Eyedroppers can be used for hand-feeding but tend to produce air bubbles and make the milk flow difficult to control.

Gavage feeding, or stomach tubing, is another option for difficult feeders, such as armadillos, opossums, and nervous cottontails, who do not suck or drink consistently from other implements.

Stomach tubing can also be a lifesaving technique used with older juveniles and adult mammals but can also be the most difficult to do correctly and safely. When using the stomach tube method, never feed more then the calculated stomach capacity volume. Remember that an emaciated animal's stomach capacity may be reduced by as much as 50%. Due to space limitation of this chapter, the gavage technique is not covered here. This method is covered in Chapter 9 under "Techniques."

Feeding Procedure

Infant mammals should be fed in an upright position on a soft, warm surface. Some babies like to feel secure and be wrapped in a cloth. They should never be fed on their backs because this could result in aspiration of the formula (Figure 20.17).

Mammals should be fed their calculated amounts until their stomachs are rounded but not tight. Never overfeed a baby because it can lead to diarrhea, bloating, and perhaps death. Even with every effect made, occasionally babies will aspirate formula and get milk in their nose or lungs. If this happens, feeding should immediately be discontinued, and the baby should be turned nose down and lightly tapped on its back. Any bubbles or drops should immediately be wiped off as they come out of the infant's nose or mouth to prevent reinhalation.

Once fed, all formula must be wiped off of the mammal. Allowing the milk to dry on the skin or hair of an infant can result in hair loss or skin infections. If the baby was not stimulated to eliminate before the feeding, this should be done afterward. Gently stroke the belly and anal area with a warm, moist cloth until the flow stops. After about a minute, stimulation should be discontinued whether the baby has defecated or not. Stimulation can be discontinued when the infant's eyes are open and there is evidence that it is eliminating on its own. Any uneaten formula should be thrown away; reheated milk should never be saved.

All feeding implements should be cleaned with hot, soapy water after each feeding and a bottlebrush used to remove milk residue from hard-to-reach places inside the syringes/bottles. Syringes, bottles, and nipples should be disinfected once daily by soaking in an appropriate cleaning solution such as diluted 10% Nolvasan or 5% bleach for ten to fifteen minutes, followed by a thorough rinse.

All items should be allowed to completely dry before each use to reduce the chance of bacterial overgrowth. Once they are cleaned and rinsed, feeding materials should be stored on an absorbent material such as a clean hand or paper towel or in a drying rack until the next feeding.

Orphan Mammal Housing

Most eyes-closed mammal infants can be housed in an incubator generally kept at 85°F to 95°F. A set of plans to make an incubator is available at the IWRC web site: www.iwrc-online.org. A homemade incubator can be made from a plastic tote with a lid and ventilation holes. Some rehabilitators use glass or plastic aquariums, cardboard boxes, plastic pet carriers, or laundry baskets, of appropriate height and size, for this stage. A heating pad set on low, placed a quarter of the way to halfway under the tote, can provide the heat, and a water-soaked sponge placed in a plastic container with holes for evaporation can provide the humidity. Make sure that moisture does not collect on the inside of the incubator by providing enough ventilation. A heat lamp can be used in place of a heating pad but both should never be used at the same time (Figure 20.18). A soft, ravel-free cloth such as cotton T-shirt, sweatshirt, or flannel or fleece material can be considered for bedding. Terry cloth should never be used because fingers, toes, and nails are too easily caught and twisted in the loops.

Once their eyes are open, baby mammals tend to become more active and they begin to explore their surroundings. When the mammals become more active, they can be placed in a larger enclosure to allow for more room to exercise, dig, or climb. Be careful

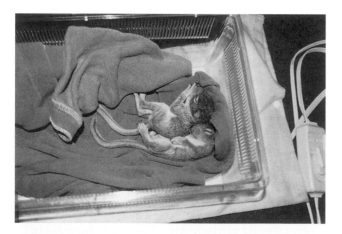

Figure 20.18. Two four-week-old gray squirrels on supplemental heat. (Photo courtesy of Melanie Haire.)

that the adventurous youngster cannot escape out of kennel door holes that are too large or unsecured cage lids. The supplemental heat and humidity can be removed when the baby is furred and able to thermoregulate, and spends most of its time away from the heat. This time varies from species to species and even from individual to individual.

Once the heat is no longer needed, begin to acclimate the babies by placing their cage outside for short periods of time at first and then gradually lengthening the time. Caution and common sense should be used with the placement of the cage, shade should be provided, and monitoring should be done for predators and sudden inclement weather. Acclimating usually can wait until the animal has been transferred to the rehabilitator's facility. Features such as nest boxes, hammocks, shelves, and natural items can be added to the cage at this stage.

The next phase usually begins once the mammals are weaned, eating natural foods, acclimated to the outside temperatures, and grown out of their cage. Preparing them for release by placing them in the large prerelease cages should be done at the rehabilitator's facility.

Recommended housing materials, sizes, and standards are also available at www.iwrc-online.org.

SPECIES CARE SHEETS

The species summary sheets provided in Appendix 7 are meant for quick reference only. Entire books have been written on the care of each of these species and, whenever possible, more than one source should be consulted for more complete and detailed care. The charts are included to serve as a summary of age determinators and growth characteristics to provide the technician with enough general information to accurately confirm age and thus temporarily care for the most common species. Due to regional variations, standardized weights and infant developmental patterns are difficult to predict. Factors such as geographic location, subspecies, weather, season, and quantity and quality of food are just a few things that determine how fast or large an animal can grow. The species care sheets in Appendix 7 should only be referred to after reading the general orphan mammal care section. See Appendix 10 for a list of products mentioned in this chapter.

ACKNOWLEDGMENTS

Avian illustrations (Figures 20.2, 20.3, and 20.4): Illustrated by Linda A. Orebaugh, MS, AMI, from the Care and Rehabilitation of Injured Native Wildlife training manual. Permission for use granted by the Georgia Department of Natural Resources and Branson W. Richie, DVM, MS.

Raptor tail wrap procedure (Appendix 4): From Raptor Rehabilitation, A Manual of Guidelines Offered by the Carolina Raptor Center. Permission to use granted by Mathias Engelmann and Pat Marcum.

State and federal wildlife permit offices lists (Appendix 1): International Wildlife Rehabilitation Council Membership Directory 2001. Names and numbers are likely to change.

Raptor restraint illustration (Figure 20.1): Illustrated by George Carpenter. Raptor Restraint, Handling, and Transport Methods by Terry A. Schulz from the NWRA Volume 8 Symposium Proceedings. Permission for use granted by the National Wildlife Rehabilitators Association.

Photos: By Melanie Haire.

Admission, examination, and animal care record forms (Appendix 2): By Janet Howard.

Handling and Restraint of Wildlife Species paper: By Florina S. Tseng, DVM, from IWRC 1991 Conference Proceedings. Permission granted for use by the International Wildlife Rehabilitation Council.

Guide to Identification of Hatchling and Nestling Songbirds (Appendix 5): By Marty Johnson from NWRA Principles of Wildlife Rehabilitation, The Essential Guide for Novice and Experienced Rehabilitators. Permission granted for use by the National Wildlife Rehabilitators Association.

Special thanks: To Michael Haire, Veola Herron, Michael Ellis, Mike Fost, and Sue Barnard for all their help.

REFERENCES

Beaver P. 1984. Imprinting and Wildlife Rehabilitation. Suisun, CA: International Wildlife Rehabilitation Council.

Crawford WC. 1988. Hand Rearing Birds of Prey. In: *IWRC Proceedings*, Suisan, CA: International Wildlife Rehabilitation Council. 1–6.

Diehl S, Stokhaug C. 1991. Release Criteria for Rehabilitated Wild Animals. *Symposium Proceedings*, St. Cloud: National Rehabilitators Association. 159–81.

Dunning JB. 1984. Body Weights of 686 Species of North American Birds. Suisun, CA: IWRC.

Engelman M, Marcum P. 1993. Raptor Rehabilitation, A Manual of Guidelines Offered by the Carolina Raptor Center. Charlotte: Carolina Raptor Center.

Evans RH. 1986. Care and feeding of orphan mammals and birds. In: Current Veterinary Therapy IX, edited by Kirk RB. Philadelphia: W.B. Saunders Co.

Fowler ME. 1986. Zoo and Wild Animal Medicine. 2nd ed. Philadelphia: W.B. Saunders Co.

Ivie D. 1999. Individual bird rehabilitator. Personal communication.

Johnson V. 1991. Wild Animal and Rehabilitation Manual, Kalamazoo Nature Center. Kalamazoo: Beech Leaf Press.

Klinghammer E. 1991. Imprint and Early Experience: How to Avoid Problems with Tame Animals. *Symposium Proceedings*. St. Cloud: National Wildlife Rehabilitators Association.

Moore AT, Joosten S. 1995a. Euthanasia—The three stages of euthanasia. In NWRA—Principles of Wildlife Rehabilitation, The Essential Guide for Novice and Experienced Rehabilitators. St. Cloud: National Wildlife Rehabilitators Association.

Pokras M. 1995. NWRA—Principles of Wildlife Rehabilitation, Introduction. St. Cloud: National Wildlife Rehabilitators Association.

Section 7
Hematology

CHAPTER TWENTY-ONE

Avian and Reptile Hematology

Denise I. Bounous

INTRODUCTION

Birds and reptiles are not so different as one may suppose. Phylogenetically, these species emerge closer to each other than to mammals (Gauthier et al. 1988). Hematology of both is similar, in that they have nucleated erythrocytes that develop and mature in the bone marrow sinusoids, unlike mammalian erythrocytes, which migrate into the sinusoids and into vessels after developing into mature anucleate erythrocytes (Campbell 1967). However, these nucleated erythrocytes present problems for complete blood analysis. Automated hematology instruments do not accurately count nucleated erythrocytes. The morphology of blood cells may vary, not only between animal groups of birds and reptiles, but also between species within a group (e.g. iguanas and chameleons or boas and rat snakes). Additionally, there are variations in the white blood cell differential among the different genera of birds and reptiles. In some snakes, such as the boidae family (e.g. boa constrictors, pythons), the predominant leukocyte is the azurophil, whereas other snakes, such as rat snakes, have predominantly heterophils.

Morphology of peripheral blood constituents can also vary. Thrombocytes of some birds and boid snakes are elongate and easily differentiated from small lymphocytes (Color Plate 21.1), but thrombocytes of the rat snake are small and round, very similar to lymphocytes (Bounous et al. 1996) (Color Plate 21.2). When performing a differential leukocyte count on birds or reptiles, it is advisable to scan the smear, examining each cell type and identifying the characteristics that can be used to classify the cell types before actually starting the count.

BLOOD COLLECTION

Avian and reptilian blood volume is approximately 10% and 5% to 8% of body weight, respectively, and approximately 10% of blood volume can be taken from a healthy bird or reptile with no ill effects (Mader 2000, Campbell 1995). Therefore, approximately 3.5 mL can be withdrawn from an Amazon parrot weighing 350 grams, but only 0.35 mL from a budgerigar weighing 35 grams. Thus, it is necessary to prioritize which assays are to be performed when only small volumes are available.

Blood for hematologic procedures must be collected in anticoagulant. Potential anticoagulants include EDTA (ethylenediaminetetracetic acid), heparin, or sodium citrate. Heparin can interfere with staining of blood cells, and using sodium citrate causes dilution of the blood, resulting in incorrect cell counts. Comparison studies with the three anticoagulants show that citrate causes significant changes in PCV as well as increased cell lysis.

Samples for hematology that are collected into any of these anticoagulants should be evaluated within twelve hours of collection for best results, because greater than 50% lysis can occur at twenty-four hours.

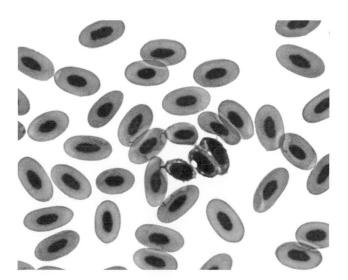

Plate 21.1. Blood smear from an owl: cluster of elongate thrombocytes. (Wright stain, EDTA, original magnification × 100.) (See also color plates)

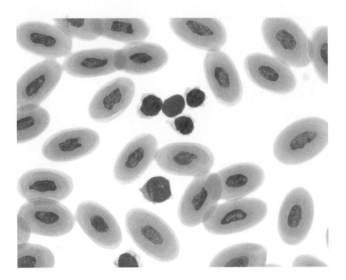

Plate 21.2. Blood smear from a rat snake: cluster of small round thrombocytes, one lymphocyte. (Wright stain, EDTA, original magnification × 100.) (See also color plates)

Heparin is frequently used as the anticoagulant for avian and reptile blood samples only because it allows both hematology and biochemistry analysis to be performed on the same sample tube. Blood for biochemical analysis can be collected into lithium heparin or into "serum" tubes without anticoagulant. However, glucose, potassium, and chloride concentrations were shown to change significantly at twenty-four hours in python samples collected in lithium heparin (Davidson et al. 2002). When possible, EDTA is the optimal anticoagulant for hematology analysis and serum for biochemistry; however, the volume of blood that can be removed from birds and reptiles frequently limits this optimization. Blood collected for biochemistry into heparin or into tubes without anticoagulant should be separated immediately to prevent artifactual changes.

BLOOD SMEAR AND ASSESSMENT

Smears should be made as soon as possible after blood collection to avoid any deterioration of the cells. Methods for making smears include (1) using a spreader slide across the slide containing the drop of blood, and (2) placing a cover slip on top of another cover slip containing a blood drop, then pulling the two cover slips apart. The cover slip method requires extra care in staining and must be fixed to a regular glass slide to evaluate microscopically. Blood smears are stained with classical Romanowsky-type stains, containing the dyes azure A, azure B, methylene violet, and methylene blue (e.g. Wright's stain, Giemsa stain,

or rapid stains such as Diff-Quick or Accustain). A properly made smear can be used to assess the number of leukocytes and platelets, as well as evaluate erythrocyte morphology.

LEUKOCYTES

Total Leukocyte Count

Leukocytes from birds are classified as heterophils, eosinophils, basophils, monocytes, and lymphocytes (Campbell 2000). Reptiles have an additional leukocyte, the azurophil (Hawkey and Dennett 1989, Frye 1991). In general, electronic counters cannot be used for avian and reptilian leukocyte counts. Avian and reptilian leukocytes are best enumerated using a hemocytometer. Various stains have been reported for use in differentiating and counting types of leukocytes from thrombocytes and erythrocytes. Using the Natt and Herricks staining method, all leukocytes and thrombocytes stain varying degrees of a blue-violet color. One must be able to identify thrombocytes from leukocytes in the hemocytometer to calculate the leukocyte count.

Use of the Unopette #5877 eosinophil system containing phloxine B, which stains avian granulocytes (heterophils, eosinophils, basophils), is an indirect method for leukocyte counting. This procedure requires an accurate differential to calculate the number of leukocytes. After counting the number of cells staining an orange-red color on both sides of the hemocytometer chamber, the count is corrected for all leukocytes (to include monocytes, lymphocytes, and azurophils) based on the differential as follows:

Total WBC =

$$\frac{\text{\# of cells stained in the chamber} \times 1.1 \times 16}{\text{\% granulocytes}/100}$$

$$\text{Example:} \frac{300 \times 1.1 \times 16}{0.60} = 8,800 \text{ cells/}\mu l$$

Estimating the leukocyte count is highly variable and not very accurate. A "guestimate" of the number of leukocytes/μl blood can be made from a well-made smear by counting the number of leukocytes per high field (40 × objective) in ten fields, taking the average of the ten and multiplying by 1,500.

Heterophils

Heterophils are functionally similar to the mammalian neutrophil. Heterophils are usually the most numerous leukocytes in pet bird blood (Color Plate 21.3). They

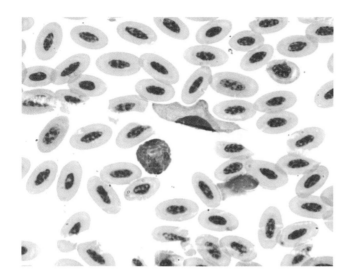

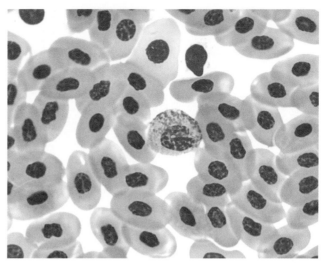

Plate 21.3. Blood smear from a hawk: heterophil, erythrocytes containing hemoparasite, Leucocytozoon. (Wright stain, EDTA, original magnification × 100.) (See also color plates)

Plate 21.4. Blood smear from a tortoise: heterophil with band-shaped nucleus and area of basophilic cytoplasm. (Wright stain, EDTA, original magnification × 100.) (See also color plates)

are round cells with clear cytoplasm and prominent eosinophilic, rod-shaped to oval granules, which may partially obscure the nucleus. The nucleus of a mature heterophil usually has two to three lobes containing coarse, purple-staining chromatin. Immature heterophils are rarely present in peripheral blood of birds or reptiles, and usually are associated with inflammation (Bounous et al. 1989). The nuclei of these immature cells (toxic heterophils) have fewer lobes and may appear mononuclear with more basophilic cytoplasm and less mature granules (Color Plate 21.4). Very early granulocytes may be so poorly differentiated that granules are round and exhibit staining characteristics of both eosinophilia and basophilia (Color Plate 21.5).

Heterophils of reptiles are similar to those of birds, with some subtle differences. This cell can account for approximately 30% to 45% of leukocytes in reptiles. Mature heterophils of reptiles contain an oval-to-lenticular nucleus that can be eccentrically located in the cell with a chromatin pattern similar to that of birds. The nuclear color may range from more light blue in lizards to purple in other reptiles. The reddish-orange granules can be pleomorphic across the species, ranging from needlelike to oval and from large to small (Color Plate 21.6). Heterophil cytoplasm of reptiles can frequently have a foamy appearance. As in birds, immature heterophils in the peripheral blood of reptiles indicates an increased demand for heterophils, such as in conditions of inflammation (Mateo et al. 1984).

Heterophilia, an increase in the number of circulating heterophils, is usually a response to stress or

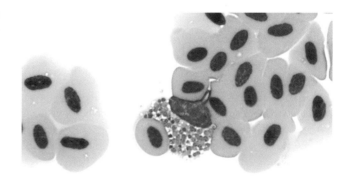

Plate 21.5. Blood smear from an owl: toxic mononuclear heterophil with eccentric nucleus and both basophilic and eosinophilic granules. (Wright stain, EDTA, original magnification × 100.) (See also color plates)

inflammation. Heteropenia may also occur with severe inflammation that exceeds or affects bone marrow production.

Eosinophils

Eosinophils are uncommon to few in the peripheral blood of birds and reptiles. They are round, peroxidase-positive cells, with pale basophilic cytoplasm and many spherical reddish-orange cytoplasmic granules (Color Plate 21.7). Eosinophil granules from birds may appear brighter than heterophil granules. The nucleus is eccentrically located, and nuclear lobulation is less than in heterophils. Reptilian eosinophil size varies with species; snakes have the largest cells, turtles and

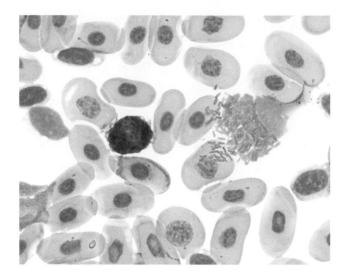

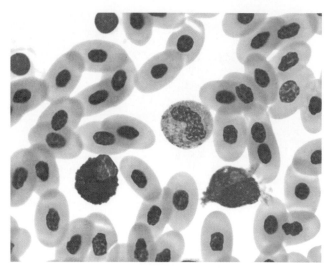

Plate 21.6. *Blood smear from a tortoise: basophil with granules obscuring the nucleus, ruptured heterophil with loose granules. (Wright stain, EDTA, original magnification × 100.) (See also color plates)*

Plate 21.8. *Blood smear from a lizard: basophil, band heterophil, monocyte. (Wright stain, EDTA, original magnification × 100.) (See also color plates)*

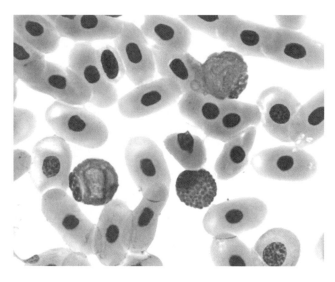

Plate 21.7. *Blood smear from a tortoise: heterophil with ill-defined rod-shaped granules, eosinophil with round distinct granules, heterophil. (Wright stain, EDTA, original magnification × 100.) (See also color plates)*

crocodilians have intermediate-sized cells, and lizards have the smallest eosinophils. Eosinophils can make up from 7% to 20% of the leukocytes in healthy reptiles. Increased eosinophil numbers in pet birds have been associated with parasitism (Campbell 1994).

Basophils
Basophils are uncommonly seen in the peripheral blood of birds and most reptiles. Depending on the

species, they may compose from 0% to 40% of the leukocytes in reptiles, with turtles having the highest percentage. Basophils are easily identified because of their large, round, deeply basophilic granules. The round to oval nucleus is centrally or eccentrically located and frequently obscured by the granules (Color Plates 21.6 and 21.8). Reptilian basophils, as mammalian basophils, appear to be involved in processing immunoglobulin and histamine release (Sypek and Borysenko 1988).

Lymphocytes
Lymphocytes occur in different sizes and somewhat different morphology. They are round or oval mononuclear cells with variation in the appearance of the nucleus and cytoplasm. Most are small to medium sized (5 to 10 μm) round cells with a centrally located nucleus containing densely aggregated chromatin. The nuclear shape is usually round to indented, and cytoplasm is pale blue. The nuclear to cytoplasmic ratio of small lymphocytes is high. Larger lymphocytes (15 μm) can have larger nuclei with more dispersed or reticulated chromatin and more cytoplasm, so that the N:C ratio is less. Lymphocytes may have cytoplasmic blebs and sometimes deeper blue staining cytoplasm at the periphery of the cytoplasm. Occasionally a few azurophilic granules may be present. Lymphocytes may occasionally appear to be indented by surrounding cells on the smear. In some parrots (e.g. Amazons, Eclectus), lymphocytes are reported to be the most common leukocytes in peripheral blood. Reptilian

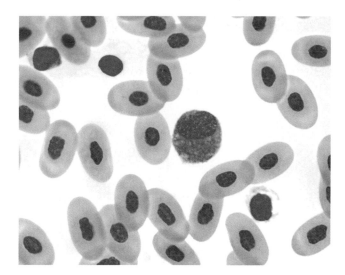

Plate 21.9. Blood smear from a lizard: monocyte with gray-blue cytoplasm and oval nucleus. (Wright stain, EDTA, original magnification × 100.) (See also color plates)

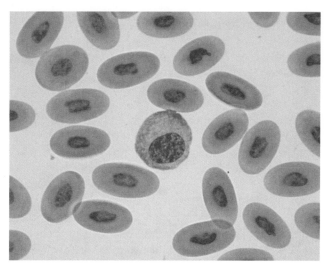

Plate 21.10. Blood smear from a rat snake: azurophil with granules at cytoplasmic periphery instilling a pinkish-purple hue. (Wright stain, EDTA, original magnification × 100.) (See also color plates)

lymphocytes are similar, and can compose as much as 80% of the circulating leukocytes (Color Plate 21.2).

Reactive lymphocytes are larger cells with large nuclei containing dispersed chromatin and deeply basophilic cytoplasm. Reactive lymphocytes may result from antigenic stimulation of the immune system due to infection or inflammation. Lymphocytosis in reptiles can occur with viral diseases, inflammation, wound healing, and certain parasitic infections (Campbell 1996).

Monocytes

Monocytes are large mononuclear cells found less commonly in the peripheral blood of birds and reptiles than lymphocytes. These cells are more variable than most other types of leukocytes. They can be round to oval to rhomboid shape. The nucleus may be small or large and round, indented, bilobed, or U-shaped. Monocytes may appear similar to large lymphocytes, but with finely granular cytoplasm that is blue-gray, and may also occasionally contain vacuoles. Monocyte nuclear chromatin is usually less clumped when compared to lymphocytes (Color Plate 21.9). Monocytosis in birds can occur with chronic illness, such as tuberculosis, chlamydia, and aspergillosis.

Azurophils

Azurophils are unique cells identified only in reptiles. (These cells eventually may be determined to be a type of monocyte.) They are similar in size to heterophils with abundant cytoplasm that is finely to coarsely

granular and may sometimes contain vacuoles. Granules may impart a purplish hue to the cytoplasm, particularly to the outer region (Color Plate 21.10). Occasionally azurophils are observed with vacuolated cytoplasm (Dotson et al. 1995).

ERYTHROCYTES

Early erythrocytes are round with round nuclei. The cells and nuclei become more oval, and the nuclear chromatin becomes increasingly condensed as the cell matures. Mature avian and reptile erythrocytes appear oval to elliptical on the blood smear with a centrally located nucleus that is also oval. It is not unusual for the erythrocyte nucleus to be irregularly shaped in some reptiles (Color Plate 21.11). The cytoplasm of the early erythrocyte is basophilic, becoming polychromatic, and then pale orange to pink when the hemoglobin and cell is mature.

The change in color from basophilic to eosinophilic as the erythrocyte matures parallels the maturation of hemoglobin in the cell. The mature erythrocyte varies in size, and to some degree, in shape, depending on the species of bird or reptile. A slight variation in the size of erythrocytes is normal. Polychromatophilic erythrocytes make up less than 5% of erythrocytes in the peripheral blood (Color Plate 21.11). These cells can be identified and enumerated as reticulocytes by staining with a supravital stain, such as new methylene blue.

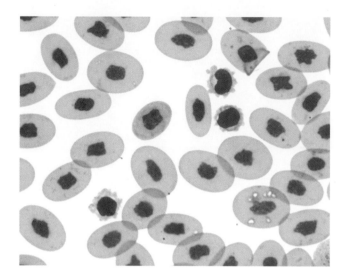

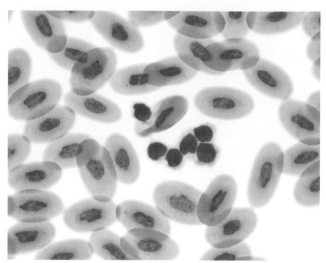

Plate 21.11. Blood smear from a lizard: basophilic erythrocyte in the center, two thrombocytes. Note the irregularly shaped erythrocyte nuclei, tiny cytoplasmic vacuoles in erythrocytes. (Wright stain, EDTA, original magnification × 100.) (See also color plates)

Plate 21.12. Blood smear from a rat snake: cluster of thrombocytes. (Wright stain, EDTA, original magnification × 100.) (See also color plates)

The variation in size of erythrocytes and number of reticulocytes can be used to classify anemia. A greater degree of anisocytosis in the presence of increased polychromasia is indicative of responsive anemia. A large number of hypochromatic erythrocytes is associated with an erythrocyte disorder such as iron deficiency anemia. Marked poikilocytosis may indicate a maturation dysfunction. Occasionally erythrocytes of reptiles may contain small, clear cytoplasmic vacuoles that are not associated with any pathology (Color Plate 21.11).

THROMBOCYTES

Mature thrombocytes in birds and reptiles are round to oval with a round to oval nucleus containing clumped chromatin. Their shape can vary from one species to another, but the cytoplasm is colorless to pale gray. Thrombocytes frequently contain a few small azurophilic granules. In some animals, thrombocytes are difficult to discern from small lymphocytes. Thrombocytes occasionally occur in closely associated groups in the smear, and this characteristic can be helpful in identifying thrombocytes from small lymphocytes (Color Plate 21.12). Thrombocytes have been reported to have potential phagocytotic capabilities, but in general function as do mammalian platelets (Bounous et al. 1989).

REFERENCES

Bounous DI, Dotson TK, Brooks RL Jr, Ramsay EC. 1996. Cytochemical staining and ultrastructural characteristics of peripheral blood leukocytes from the yellow rat snake (*Elaphe obsoleta quadrivitatta*). *Comp Haematol Int* 6:86–91.

Bounous DI, Schaeffer DO, Roy A. 1989. Diagnosis of a coagulase negative *Staphylococcus* sp. septicemia in a lovebird. *J Am Vet Med Assoc* 195:1120–22.

Campbell F. 1967. Fine structure of the bone marrow of the chicken and pigeon. *J Morphol* 123:405–40.

Campbell TW. 1994. Hematology. In: Avian Medicine: Principles and Application, edited by Ritchie BW, Harrison GJ, Harrison LP, Lake Worth: Wingers Publishing Inc. 176–98.

Campbell TW. 1995. Avian Hematology and Cytology, 2nd ed. Ames: Iowa State University Press.

Campbell TW. 1996. Clinical pathology. In: Reptile Medicine and Surgery, edited by Mader DR, Philadelphia: W.B. Saunders Co. 248–57.

Campbell TW. 2000. Hematology of Psittacines. In: Schalm's Veterinary Hematology, edited by Feldman BF, Zinkl JG, Jain NC, 5th ed., Baltimore: Lippincott Williams and Wilkins. 1155–60.

Davidson D, Harr K, Raskin R. Hematologic and biochemical changes caused by commonly used anticoagulants on Burmese python (*Python molurus bivittatus*) blood over time. *Vet Pathol*, in press.

Dotson TK, Ramsay EC, Bounous DI. 1995. A color atlas of blood cells of the yellow rat snake. *Compend Contin Educ Pract Vet* 17:1013–17.

Frye FL. 1991. Hematology as applied to clinical reptile medicine. In: Biomedical and Surgical Aspects of Captive Reptile Husbandry, edited by Frye FL. 2nd ed. Malabar: Krieger Publishing Company.

Gauthier J, Kluge AG, Rowe T. 1988. The early evolution of Amniota. In: The Phylogeny and Classification of the Tetrapods, edited by Benton MJ, Volume 1: Amphibians, Reptiles, Birds. Oxford: Clarendon Press.

Hawkey CM, Dennett TB. 1989. Color Atlas of Comparative Veterinary Hematology. Ames: Iowa State University Press.

Mader DR. 2000. Normal hematology of reptiles. In: Schalm's Veterinary Hematology, edited by Feldman BF, Zinkl JG, Jain NC, 5th ed., Baltimore: Lippincott Williams and Wilkins. 1126–32.

Mateo MR, Roberts ED, Enright FM. 1984. Morphological, cytochemical, and functional studies of peripheral blood cells of young healthy American alligators (*Alligator mississippiensis*). *Am J Vet Res* 45: 1046–1053.

Sypek J, Borysenko M. 1988. Reptiles. In: Vetebrate Blood Cells, edited by Rowley AF, Ratcliff NA. Cambridge: Cambridge University Press.

State/Federal Wildlife Permit Offices

STATE AND U.S. TERRITORY WILDLIFE PERMIT OFFICES

Listings are alphabetical by state or territory.

Chief of Law Enforcement, Division of Wildlife/ Freshwater Fisheries, PO Box 301456, Montgomery, AL 36130-1456; 334-242-3467; Craig.hill@dcnr. alabama.gov

Director of Wildlife Conservation, Department of Fish and Game, PO Box 115526, Juneau, AK 99811-5526; 907-465-4148

Wildlife Building Coordinator, Arizona Game and Fish Department, 2221 W. Greenway Rd., Phoenix, AZ 85023-4312; 623-582-9806

Karen Rowe, Wildlife Permit Officer, Arkansas Game and Fish Commission, 31 Hallowel Lane, Humphrey, AR 72073; 870-873-4302; krowe@agfc.state.ar.us

Nicole Carion, California Department of Fish and Game, 601 Locust St., Redding, CA 96001; 530-357-8690; ncarion@dfg.ca.gov

Wildlife Permit Officer, CDOW/Special Licensing, 6060 Broadway, Denver, CO 80216; 303-291-7143; kathy.konishi@state.co.us

Wildlife Permit Officer, Department of Environmental Protection, Wildlife Division, 79 Elm St., Hartford, CT 06106-5127; 860-424-3011, 860-424-4078 fax; laurie.fortin@po.state.ct.us

Kenneth Reynolds, Program Manager, Division of Fish and Wildlife, 4876 Hay Point Landing Rd., Smyrna, DE 19997; 302-653-2883, 302-653-3431 fax; Kenneth.reynolds@state.de.us

Wildlife Permit Officer, Florida Fish and Wildlife Conservation Commission, 620 S. Meridian St., Tallahassee, FL 32399-1600; 850-488-6253

Wildlife Permit Officer, Georgia DNR, Wildlife Resources Division, 2065 US Hwy 278 SE, Social Circle, GA 30025; 770-761-3044, 706-557-3060 fax; todd_nims.dnr.state.ga.us

Administrator of Forestry and Wildlife, 1151 Punchbowl St., Honolulu, HI 96813; 808-587-0166

Chuck Harris, Department of Fish and Game, PO Box 25, Boise, ID 83707-0025; 208-334-2920

Permit Officer, Department of Natural Resources, 1 Natural Resources Way, Springfield, IL 62702-1271; 217-782-6431; bclark1@dnrmail.state.il.us

Linnea Petercheff, Wildlife Permit Officer, IN DNR, 402 W. Washington St. #W273, Indianapolis, IN 46204-2212; 317-233-6527, 317-232-8150 fax

Daryl Howell, Iowa DNR, Wallace State Office Bldg., 502 E 9th St., Des Moines, IA 50319-0034; 515-281-8524, 515-281-6794 fax; daryl.howell@dnr. state.ia.us

Wildlife Permit Officer, Kansas Department of Wildlife and Parks, 512 SE 25th Ave., Pratt, KS 67124-8174; 620-672-5911, 620-672-2972 fax; kenb@ wp.state.ks.us

Permit Officer, Department of Fish and Wildlife Resources, #1 Game Farm Rd., Frankfort, KY 40601; 502-564-7109

Nongame Biologist, Louisiana Department of Wildlife and Fisheries, Natural Heritage Program, PO Box 98000, Baton Rouge, LA 70898-9000; 225-763-3557

Susan Zayac, Department of Inland Fish and Wildlife, 284 State St, Station #41, Augusta, ME 04333-0041; 207-287-5240

Mary Goldie, DNR 580 Taylor Ave., Tawes State Office Bldg., Annapolis, MD 21401; 410-260-8540; mgoldie@dnr.state.md.us

Tom French, Asst. Dir. Division of Fisheries and Wildlife, Rte. 135, Westboro, MA 01581; 508-792-7270 ext. 163

Dennis Knapp, DNR, Box 30031, Lansing, MI 48933; 517-241-0330

Nancy Huonder, WL Rehab. Program Coordinator, DNR Sect. of Wildlife, 500 Lafayette Rd., Box 25, St. Paul, MN 55155-4025; 651-259-5108; nancy.huonde@dnr.state.mn.us

Richard G. Rummel, Department of Wildlife, Fish and Parks, Mississippi Museum of Natural Science, 2148 Riverside Dr., Jackson, MS 39202-1353; 601-354-7303, 601-354-7227 fax; richardr@mmns.state.ms.us

Lynn Totten, Department of Conservation, PO Box 180, Jefferson City, MO 65102-0180; 573-522-4115 x3322

Stella Capoccia, Montana Fish, Wildlife and Parks, 23 S Rodney, Helena, MT 59601

Nebraska Game and Parks Commission, 2200 N 33rd St, Lincoln, NE 68503-1417

Law Enforcement, Nevada Division of Wildlife, 4600 Kietzke Lane D-135, Reno, NV 89502; 775-688-1500

Attn: Lt. Bruce Bonenfant, New Hampshire Fish and Game Department, 11 Hazen Dr., Concord, NH 03301; 603-271-3127

Amy Wells, NJ Division of Fish, Game and Wildlife, PO Box 400, Trenton, NJ 08625-0400; 609-292-2965; amy.wells@dep.state.nj.us

New Mexico Department of Game and Fish, Special Use Permits Program, Law Enforcement Division, PO Box 25112, Santa Fe, NM 87507; 505-476-8064

Patrick P. Martin, NYS Department Env. Con., 625 Broadway, Albany, NY 12233-4752; 518-402-8985; pxmartin@qw.dec.state.ny.us

Daron Barnes, 1722 Mail Service Center, Raleigh, NC 27699-1722; 919-707-0060

Sandra Hagen, North Dakota Game and Fish Department, 100 N Bismarck Expressway, Bismarck, ND 58501; 701-328-5382

Carolyn Caldwell, Asst. Administrator, Wildlife Management and Research, Division of Wildlife, 2045 Morse Rd. Building, Columbus, OH 43229-6693; 614-254-6300; carolyn.caldwell@dnr.state.oh.us

Law Enforcement Division, Department of Wildlife Conservation, PO Box 53465, Oklahoma City, OK 73152-3465; 405-521-3719

Carol Turner, Oregon Department of Fish and Wildlife, 3406 Cherry Ave. NE, Salem, OR 97303-4924; 503-947-6318; carol.d.turner@state.or.us

Jason DeCoskey, Pennsylvania Game Commission, 2001 Elmerton Ave., Harrisburg, PA 17110-9797; 717-783-8164

Wildlife Permit Officer, Division of Fish and Wildlife, 277 Great Neck Rd, West Kingston, RI 02892; 401-789-0281; lori.gibson@dem.ri.gov

Wildlife Permit Coordinator, Sandhills Research and Education Center, PO Box 23205, Columbia, SC 29224-3205; 803-419-9645

Wildlife Permit Officer, Game, Fish and Parks Department, Division of Wildlife, 412 West Missouri, Suite 4, Pierre, SD 57501; 605-773-4191

Captive Wildlife Coordinator, TWRA/Law Enforcement Division, PO Box 40747, Ellington Ag Center, Nashville, TN 37204; 615-781-6647

Jennifer Blecha, Nongame Permits Specialist, 4200 Smith School Rd., Austin, TX 78744-3291; 512-389-4481

DNR Division of Wildlife Resources, 1594 W. North Temple, Suite 2110, PO Box 146301, Salt Lake City, UT 84114-6301; 801-538-4701

Law Enforcement Assistant, Agency of Natural Resources, Fish and Wildlife Department, 103 S. Main St., 10 South, Waterbury, VT 05671-0501; 802-241-3727

Diane Waller, VA Department of Game and Inland Fisheries, PO Box 11104, Richmond, VA 23230-1104; 804-367-9588

Judy Pierce, Division of Fish and Wildlife, 6291 Estate Nazareth 101, St. Thomas, VI 00802-1104; 340-775-6762

Peggy Crain, Department of Fish and Wildlife, 600 Capitol Way N., Olympia, WA 98501-1091; 360-902-2513, crainpsc@dfw.wa.gov

Wildlife Permit Officer, Division of Natural Resources, Wildlife Resources, 1900 Kanawha Blvd., Bldg. 3, Rm. 816, Charleston, WV 25305; 304-558-2771

Wildlife Veterinarian Liaison DNR, Box 7921, WM/6, Madison, WI 53707-7921; 608-267-6751, Jennifer.haverty@dnr.state.wi.us

WL Law Enforcement Coordinator, Game and Fish Department, 3030 Energy Lane, Casper, WY 82604; 307-233-6413

UNITED STATES MIGRATORY BIRD PERMIT OFFICES

The following list includes only the US Fish and Wildlife Service Migratory Bird Permit Offices.

Region 1: CA, HI, ID, NV, OR, WA

Tami Tate-Hall, US Fish and Wildlife Service, Migratory Bird Permit Office, 911 N.E. 11th Ave., Portland, OR 97232-4181; 503-872-2715; tami_tatehall@fws.gov

Region 2: AZ, NM, OK, TX

Kamile McKeever, US Fish and Wildlife Service, Migratory Bird Permit Office, PO Box 709, Albuquerque, NM 87103-0709; 505-248-7882, 505-248-7885 fax; kamile_mckeever@fws.gov

Region 3: IL, IN, IA, MI, MN, MO, OH, WI

Andrea Kirk, US Fish and Wildlife Service, Migratory Bird Permit Office, Region 3, 1 Federal Dr., Fort Snelling, MN 55111; 612-713-5449 (direct office), 612-713-5436 (general line), 612-713-5393 fax; andrea_kirk@fws.gov

Region 4: AL, AR, FL, GA, KY, LA, MS, NC, SC, TN

Carmen Simonton, US Fish and Wildlife Service, Migratory Bird Permit Office, PO Box 49208, Atlanta, GA 30359; 404-679-7049

Region 5: CT, DE, ME, MD, MA, NH, NJ, NY, PA, RI, VT, VA, WV

David Dobias, Migratory Bird Permit Office, PO Box 779, Hadley, MA 01035-0779; 413-253-8643

Region 6: CO, KS, MT, NE, ND, SD, UT, WY

Janell Suazo, US Fish and Wildlife Service, Migratory Bird Permit Office, PO Box 25486 DFC 60154, Denver, CO 80225-0486; 303-236-8171 x630

Region 7: AK

Meg Laws, US Fish and Wildlife Service, Migratory Bird Permit Office, 1011 E. Tudor Rd., Anchorage, AK 99503; 907-786-3693

Wildlife Admission/Exam/Care Forms

Admission Form
Clinic Name • Address • Phone Number

Date Admitted: _____ / _____ / _____   Case No. _____

Time Admitted: _____ AM / PM

Rescuer Information

Name: _____

Address: _____

City: _____ State: _____ Zip _____

Phone: _____

Do you wish to be contacted via email about the animal's status?   □Yes   □No

Email Address: _____

Animal Information

Species: _____   □ Young   □ Adult

Date and time found: _____ / _____ / _____   Time: _____ AM / PM

Have you fed or medicated the animal? □No   □Yes, I gave it _____

Location Found:

_____

Describe circumstances found:

_____

Was anyone bitten or scratched by the animal ? □ Yes   □No

Did you come in contact with blood/urine/feces/saliva? □ Yes   □No

Other treatment/ comments:

_____

Condition (Mark all that apply):

Cause of Admission:
(circle one)
- □ Cat / Dog Attack
- □ Hit by car
- □ Found on ground
- □ In road
- □ Abused
- □ Exposed to Chemicals
- □ Disease suspected
- □ Nest disturbed
- □ Hit window
- □ Shot
- □ Other: _____

Observations:
- □ Easy to catch
- □ Limping
- □ Can't stand
- □ Can't walk
- □ Panting
- □ Bleeding
- □ Wet
- □ Oiled
- □ Cold
- □ No apparent injury
- □ Other: _____

Describe condition: _____

_____

Disposition:

Date: _____ / _____ / _____

Circle One: R   TR   TD   TE   P   DOA   DIC   EOA   E

Location: _____

□ US F&WS Notification (Illegal activity, E/TH species, B/G eagle) Date: _____

Examination Form
Clinic Name • Address • Phone Number

Case No.: _____
Date: _____ / _____ / _____   Time: _____ AM / PM

Basic Information:

Species: _____   Age: _____
Sex: ☐ Male ☐ Female   Weight: _____

Visual Observation:

Weight Distribution: ☐ Even ☐ Abnormal   Notes: _____
Movement/Attitude: ☐ Walks in circles ☐ Head tilt Notes: _____
Alertness: ☐ Comatose ☐ Lethargic ☐ Normal ☐ Excitable   Notes: _____
Body Condition: ☐ Emaciated ☐ Underweight ☐ Normal ☐ Overweight

Temp: ☐ Hypothermic ☐ Cool ☐ Normal ☐ Warm ☐ Hyperthermic
Hydration: ☐ Severely dehydrated ☐ Moderate dehydration ☐ Normal

Mouth: ☐ Normal ☐Plaque/lesions ☐ Cap refill _____ seconds
   Notes:_____
Eyes: ☐ Follows movement ☐ Proper dilation ☐ Abrasions/Cuts ☐ Consensual
                                                            response
   Notes: _____
Ears: ☐ Normal ☐ Parasites ☐ Discharge/bleeding   Notes: _____
Nose: ☐ Normal ☐ Discharge/bleeding ☐ Cuts/abrasions Notes: _____
Fur/Skin: ☐ Cuts/wounds ☐ Abrasions ☐ Bald spots ☐ Parasites Notes: _____

Gastrointestinal: ☐ Normal ☐ Mouth odor ☐ Vomiting ☐ Blood
Urogenital: ☐ Normal ☐ Discharge ☐ No urine/stool
Notes_____
Anal Area: ☐Normal ☐ Clogged ☐ Loose ☐ Parasites Notes: _____
Abdomen: ☐ Normal ☐ Bloated ☐ Painful ☐ Cuts/abrasions Notes: _____

Cardio/Pulmonary: ☐ HR _____/min. ☐ RR _____/min.
         ☐ Cough ☐ Chest sounds Notes: _____
Muscular/Skeletal: ☐ Swelling ☐ Lameness ☐ Fractures/dislocation ☐ Pain
                                                            response

401

Animal Care Record

Clinic Name • Address • Phone Number

Case No.: _____

Species: _____   Description: _____

Weight Record

Date	Weight	Date	Weight	Date	Weight	Date	Weight

Feeding Chart

Date	Food Description	Amount per feeding	# Feedings Daily	Feeding Frequency	Comments

Treatment

Date	Medication/ Treatment	Comments/ Observations

Veterinary Care

Date	Description

Handling and Restraint of Wildlife Species

Florina S. Tseng, DVM
HOWL Wildlife Center, P.O. Box 1037, Lynnwood, WA 98046

INTRODUCTION

Wildlife rehabilitation involves the care of sick, injured, and orphaned wildlife. These animals, while in captivity, require special husbandry practices—they must be transported, housed, and fed. When they are ill, they must be examined and treated. In addition, it is sometimes necessary to relocate "nuisance" wildlife to more appropriate locations. All of these situations necessitate the handling and restraint of wildlife species.

CONSIDERATIONS

Restraint can be as direct as holding the animal in your hands or as indirect as restricting an animal's movement by fencing. The responsibility for the animal's welfare is in the hands of the rehabilitator. The amount of restraint on the animal should be as minimal as possible, yet enough to accomplish the purpose of the restraint and afford the handler maximum safety.

There are four basic considerations in the selection of a restraint technique:

A. Human safety: Human safety always comes first in the execution of any capture or restraint plan. If a person is injured during an attempt to handle the animal, all attention is focused on the care of that person and the capture will be unsuccessful.
B. Animal safety: If the animal is hurt or dies during the capture/handling, you will not have achieved your goal.
C. Technique: Choose the proper technique to accomplish the desired result. Have you chosen a technique that is likely to work given the environment and the expected behavior of the species?
D. Observation: Can the animal be observed during and after the procedure? Observation of the animal during and after capture/handling and transport

allows you to act in a timely manner if problems arise, e.g. breathing difficulties, hyperthermia etc.

In addition to the basic considerations above, there are also environmental, behavioral, and humane factors in handling and restraint. A major environmental consideration should be the possibility of hyperthermia generated during the capture procedure. An animal usually must be chased and caught before it can be restrained, which means increased muscle activity for the animal. This, in turn, translates into heat generation, especially if the air temperature and humidity are high. Smaller species tend to overheat faster than larger species because they have a higher metabolic rate. Therefore, keep these factors in mind when planning restraint, e.g. try to plan activities for cooler times of the day, if possible, and try to work quickly and efficiently if it is necessary to work during the hotter times of the day.

Animals dissipate heat by a variety of methods, including excretion of moisture via evaporation, urine, feces, etc. Moisture can be evaporated from the skin (as long as the relative humidity is not too high) and the skin can become wet from sweat glands, from the animals' licking themselves, etc. Evaporation also takes place from the lungs of all breathing animals, so panting serves to increase cooling from the respiratory tract. Be aware of restraint techniques that inhibit heat dissipation—e.g. a stockinette placed around a bird's body prevents it from spreading its wings to allow convection cooling, wrapping a mammal in a heavy towel decreases evaporative cooling, and taping a beak shut inhibits the ability of the bird to pant.

Clinical signs of hyperthermia include increased heart and respiratory rates, open-mouth breathing, and increased salivation/sweating in those species that are capable of sweating. These signs may, in turn, lead to dehydration and subsequent loss of cooling ability, weakness, depression, and incoordination. If the temperature rises above 108°F, eventually convulsions, collapse, and death will occur.

The converse side is hypothermia, or low body temperature. This occurs while working outdoors in cold temperatures, or when animals are housed in outside areas on cold concrete or other surfaces. It may also occur when in a weak or sedated animal that has lost the ability to shiver and generate heat. Be wary of placing these animals on a cold exam table because their body temperature will quickly drop.

Be aware of the immediate surroundings in which you are working. You may be able to use the physical environment to your advantage in capturing an animal. For instance, herding an animal by using portable barriers (plywood) into a large pen or shed or against a fence or cliff wall will make the final capture much easier. Also be aware of physical hazards in the environment that the animal may encounter during a capture episode.

The physical environment can be used to decrease the animal's sense perceptions. If, for instance, the animal is nocturnal, try to capture it during daylight hours. Conversely, if it is diurnal, try to work at night or dim the lights during the capture attempt.

There are also behavioral considerations in the decision regarding capture technique. You must know the natural history of the species: nocturnal or diurnal, breeding season, when its young are raised, food habits, habitat, etc. These factors will aid in your decisions; for instance, if you capture an adult of the species, will you potentially leave young behind?

Animals have a natural fear of predators; this fear is what drives the flight or fight response. As you approach an animal, its first response will be to flee, if possible. If this is not possible and/or you come within a critical distance of the animal, the fight response will then be initiated. You may be able to use long-handled nets, poles, or projectiles to extend the effective range of capture by staying outside of this critical distance until the animal is effectively restrained.

Know what the animal's fight response will be. Wild felid kits respond to being grabbed by the nape of the neck much as domestic kittens do. However, this is not true of adults. Raccoons will turn and bite if they are held in this manner. Knowing the behavior of the species helps determine what an animal will do next. Buteo hawks use their feet more than their beaks, whereas falcons use both feet and beaks. Eagles are perfectly willing to bite, too, whereas vultures regurgitate. Pigeons and waterfowl beat their wings when alarmed, etc. An understanding of behavior allows you to give more complete and better care to your patients.

Never underestimate the power of confidence on your part. Your voice, eye contact, and body language can all be used to psychologically restrain an animal or, conversely, will let the animal know that you are afraid. Be sure of yourself, but never let yourself become overly confident.

"Every restraint procedure should be preceded by an evaluation as to whether or not the procedure will result in the greatest good for that animal" (Fowler 1985). Finally, consider the most humane method of capture. Try to reduce stress to the animal as much as possible during the capture. These stressors include visual, auditory, olfactory, tactile, or psychological factors. Be sensitive but do your job. This means being prepared ahead of time so you can work as quickly as possible. In addition, try to minimize exacerbating any preexisting injury or condition during the capture and handling episode.

PREPARATION

Try to work in pairs whenever possible—having a back-up person ensures the safety and efficacy of the plan. Next, decide on the technique you'll use beforehand. Talk it through to make sure that everyone understands their role. Be prepared for all eventualities, especially the worst case scenario. Then, make sure all necessary equipment is ready and in working order before you attempt the capture. Protective clothing, such as long pants, long-sleeved shirt, boots, gloves, and goggles, is helpful in most situations.

TOOLS OF RESTRAINT

The first tool of restraint is psychological restraint—have confidence in your abilities. Everyone is aware that animals can sense when a person is afraid of them and react accordingly. Next, consider diminishing sensory perceptions. The more you can decrease or eliminate visual, auditory, or other sensory stimuli during the restraint episode, the easier it will be on both humans and animals.

Physical barriers, such as shields made of plywood, Plexiglas, blankets, etc., can be used to herd animals from one area to another and provide a protective barrier between the handler and the animal. Confinement techniques include the use of squeeze cages, restraint bags, plastic tubes for holding snakes, etc.

It is also possible to use equipment to act as extensions of your arms, for example, nets, snares and tongs.

Nets: These come in all sizes and shapes. Many manipulative procedures, such as injections, examinations, or obtaining samples for blood work, can be carried out by placing a net on the animal. Hoop nets with long handles are commonly used. Be aware that the hoop edge can injure the animal. It is better to allow the animal to enter the net than to swing the net at the animal. The net should be sufficiently deep to allow the hoop to be twisted, trapping the animal in the bottom of the net. If it is too shallow, the animal will be able to climb out. Placing the net on the ground or against the wall will help to restrict escape. Birds with talons or animals with claws are difficult to handle in large mesh nets. They may poke their limbs through the netting, possibly causing feather damage and fractured bones.

They may also cling to the netting with their talons, making it difficult to extract them. Try to use smooth netting for birds. If the mesh is too large, the animal may force its head through the mesh and strangle. Know the characteristics of the net's construction materials. Nylon, cotton, and manila all withstand different degrees of stretch and wear. Inspect nets for flaws before using them.

Rectangular nets can be placed in the path of various types of animals. As the animal runs towards it, the net is extended, then dropped over the animal. Mist nets are used to capture small birds and bats. Cannon nets are shot over the top of the animal or herd. Nets can also be suspended over feeding areas and dropped over the animal to entangle it.

Snares: Used carelessly, snares can cause unnecessary pain or strangle an animal. Commercial snares are designed with swivels for humane and effective manipulation. Quick-release snares (Ketch-all™) permit the animal to twist without being suffocated. Always try to include one front leg through the snare as well as encircling the neck to decrease any problems with twisting. Don't catch the animal around the chest or abdomen because you may cause crushing injuries to this part of the body. This also allows too much mobility of the head. Animals with good fore limb dexterity, such as raccoons, are sometimes difficult to catch with snares. Once you have the animal snared, grasp the tail and bring the animal taut to the pole, control the head, and remove the snare as quickly as possible.

Tongs: Vise tongs grasp an animal at the neck. They act like snares but do not completely encircle the neck; they clamp behind the back of the head. These are used for initial control.

The use of physical force involves using your hands to grasp the animal. You must know where and how to grasp, how much pressure to use, and how this varies from species to species. Your greatest protection is detailed knowledge of the animal. Gloves vary from thin cotton gloves to heavy, double layered, coarse leather gloves. Leather welder's gloves are good for general use. The thicker and heavier the glove, the less ability you have to determine how tightly you are grasping the animal or to feel the animal's response. Try to keep the glove loose on your hand so you can slip your fingers up or out of the way if teeth penetrate the leather. Gloves do not protect from crushing injuries! Chain mail gloves alone or within leather gloves offer more protection against the tearing effects of large canine teeth.

Finally, chemical restraint can be administered via injection, pole syringe, blow-dart, or pistol. These techniques and restraint drugs are further detailed in Restraint and Handling of Wild and Domestic Animals by Murray E. Fowler.

SPECIFIC TECHNIQUES BY SPECIES

Opossums
Danger potential: Sharp claws and 50 small, sharp teeth. Technique: Fortunately, opossums usually move slowly during the daytime and often "play possum" when stressed. Be careful if there are fetuses in the pouch; you may cause the fetuses to pull away from the nipples and they will need to be replaced right away. Opossums can be netted, snared, tonged, or manually handled by covering the head with a towel, grasping at the base of the tail, and supporting under the chest or grasping at the scruff of the neck.

Rabbits
Danger potential: Scratch with sharp claws and have powerful back legs. Technique: Be aware that rabbits can kick so strongly with their rear legs that they can fracture their spines. Grasp the loose skin over the back of the neck, lift the hind quarters with the other hand for added support, and cradle the animal against your body. Rabbits can be induced into a torpid state by placing and holding them on their backs for a few seconds or blindfolding them.

Rodents
Danger potential: The sharp incisor teeth especially adapted for chewing and gnawing, and sharp claws for burrowing. Technique: Be aware that rodents possess no specialized thermoregulatory mechanisms. They achieve homeostasis by a high level of behavioral activity. Therefore, rodents are predisposed to hyperther-

mia when handled and hypothermia when sedated or anesthetized.

Squirrels and Chipmunks

A fine mesh net can be used, though claws sometimes become entangled. You can use a towel and gloves (they can bite through gloves), and try to grasp behind the neck and one fore leg.

Beavers

Do not lift beavers by their tail. Doing so can cause spinal injuries because they are so heavy. Restrain a beaver with a snare or tongs around the neck, then lift up and hold it at the base of the tail. Some people feel that beavers don't have much in the way of a neck and prefer to wrap the animals in a blanket and just pick them up manually; they do not tend to be very aggressive.

Porcupines

Separate porcupines that are in a group before attempting to capture one; otherwise they may bump into one another, causing quill discharge and injury to one another. Approach from the rear when the porcupine is facing into a corner, reach under the tail and grab the underhairs, pull backward, and don't let the tail flip up or it will discharge quills into you. Then, slide your other hand beneath the tail and up under the body. You can also use a snare around the base of the tail and other snares on each foot to stretch the animal if you need to get a blood sample for any reason.

Carnivores

Danger potential: Teeth designed for grasping and tearing prey with well-developed jaw muscles. Claws can rip and tear. Technique: In general, control the head first then the body. Wear gloves to guard against scratches; most can bite through gloves.

Fox, Coyote, and Wolf

Smaller canids can be netted or grasped by the base of the tail, and then manipulated until the scruff of the neck can be grasped. Tongs can be used around the neck for initial control, and the animals can be muzzled for further control of the mouth (though muzzling decreases their ability to pant).

Bear

These animals have extremely powerful paws and limbs. Immature bears less than five months old may be hand-held or controlled with nets or snares. Mature bears can be handled only with squeeze cages and chemical restraint.

Raccoons

Use nets, squeeze cages, tongs, and snares. Raccoons have great forelimb dexterity.

Skunks

To restrain a skunk, use a shield of plate glass or plastic and wear goggles or protective clothing. Use a net to capture the animal, then sedate or anesthetize to handle it further.

Minks and Weasels

Minks and weasels can be restrained by using snares or manually grasping at the base of the tail, pulling up and out of the cage, then grasping behind the neck. You must move quickly. Sometimes it is best to simply try to pin them behind the neck, then sort out where the rest of the body is.

Otters

River otters can be netted or snared. Sea otters require specialized techniques. They are trapped in the wild using basket nets from beneath while the otters float on the surface of the sea. The net is closed with a drawstring, then lifted out of the water. They are extremely susceptible to stress and have no insulating blubber layer. They are protected from hypothermia by their dense fur coats. You must prevent soiling of the coat.

Cats

Infants are easily handled manually or wrapped in towels or canvas restraint bags. If the cat is under 30 lbs., it can be netted with a fine mesh net, snare, or tongs, then the tail grasped with a gloved hand. Squeeze cages can be used for the larger species. One of our secret techniques for luring them into cages is to use catnip.

Hoofed Stock

Danger potential: Antlers, sharp hooves. Technique: Small cervids without antlers can be handled manually. With one arm, hold the animal under the abdomen in front of the rear legs and with the other arm, hold it under the neck. Lift the animal up and away from the ground and point the legs away from the handler's body. Larger cervids usually need to be chemically immobilized to work on individual animals. For herding or transporting, be aware that deer do not recognize chain link or wire net fences as barriers; therefore, these should be draped with opaque plastic sheeting. You can also use plastic sheeting to herd deer toward a certain area. Most injuries occur during herding and transport. Try to arrange it so that you can funnel them via chutes into their new enclosure or a transportation crate. Select the correct sized crate—if it is too large, they may try to turn around and injure themselves. Capture myopathy is a big problem in cervids.

Birds

Waterfowl
Waterfowl can be captured manually or with nets or hooks. Drape a towel over the wings to hold the bird against the body, then grasp behind the head. To carry, support the body, restrain the head, and let the legs dangle.

Shorebirds
Shorebirds sill try to bite and stab with long, sharp bills. Protect your face with goggles if necessary. Shorebirds can be netted like gulls, or can have a towel placed over them. Control the wings first, then the head. Herons, cranes, etc. have long, thin legs that are easily broken by rough handling. They will aim for your eyes with their beaks and are fully capable of spearing an extremity. Exercise extreme caution and always control the head first.

Raptors
Beaks and talons are adapted for grasping and tearing flesh. Vultures will employ their beaks but have very weak feet. Wear heavy leather gloves, and use a hood or towel on their heads to decrease visual stimuli. If a bird is on the floor of an enclosure, throw a towel or heavy cloth over the bird, wrap it in the fabric, and then grasp the feet, then the head. Try to remove the gloves after the initial capture to facilitate handling. The feet should be grasped with one hand above the talons (but not too far above the foot or you will lose control of the talons) and with your finger between the two feet, the head should be grasped from behind without obstructing the trachea. If the bird is perched, it can be approached from the front or back. If approaching from the front, grasp the legs first, one in each hand, and then transfer the legs to one hand and grasp behind the head. If approaching from the back, grasp the wings, body, and legs together, then separate the legs in one hand and the head with the other hand.

Galliform Birds
These birds are usually docile but have claws, and some males have well-developed tarsal spurs. Do NOT grab them by the feathers, especially the tail feathers, because the bird will release them into your hand. Hold the wings close to the body and try to control the legs. Pigeons and doves do not scratch, don't peck, and have mild dispositions. They will attempt to beat their wings when alarmed. Grasp them from above and behind and press the wings close to their body.

Small Passeriformes
Capture small passeriformes with a net in the aviary, and hold them cupped in one hand with the fingers around the base of the head. Do not completely surround the sternum and interfere with respiration. Sometimes it helps to darken the room and approach from behind.

Reptiles and Amphibians

Chelonians
Small species can be handled manually. Hold them on either side of the carapace. It may be necessary to insert a finger between the carapace and plastron to prevent the shell from completely closing. Do not rapidly turn the animal upside down and then right side up again because it is possible to cause a torsion of the bowel with this sudden movement. Snapping turtles can inflict serious bite wounds. Grasp them at the base of the tail, them lift off the ground, and then grab the carapace just behind the head. You can turn them over onto the carapace; they usually relax in this position.

Snakes
Danger potential: Can bite, produce venom, or constrict. Technique: Grasp behind the head (if nonpoisonous), then support the body. If unsupported, the snake can thrash so much that it dislocates or fractures its vertebrae. Snake hooks can be used to pin the head to the ground. Snakes can be cooled for procedures that require only mild restraint but respiratory ailments are a possibility after prolonged chilling. Handling poisonous snakes is beyond the scope of this section. Suffice it to say that you must be extremely careful, always have antivenin on hand, and know what you are doing!

Amphibians
Danger potential: Toothless but can bite with hard-keratinized plates in the mouth. None are venomous. Technique: Amphibians can be netted. Then, surround the body with your hand (two fingers surround the neck and the rest of the hand encircles the body and back legs).

CONCLUSION

Just as there are a myriad of different animal species that the wildlife rehabilitator may be called upon to handle, there are similarly a wide variety of handling and restraint techniques that are available for use. Our job as knowledgeable rehabilitators should include familiarity with the proper techniques for each indi-

vidual animal in each individual situation. In this way, we will best serve the interests of our unique patients.

REFERENCE

Fowler ME. 1985. Restraint and Handling of Wild and Domestic Animals. Ames, Iowa State University Press. p. 5.

APPENDIX FOUR

Tail Wrapping

A. Standard wrap (to be used with tail feathers not in molt)
  1. Materials
      a. 1 to 2 tongue depressors
      b. Spray bottle with water (set on mist)
      c. Gummed paper packaging tape (sticky when wet)
      d. Used X-ray film or other plastic
      e. Scissors
      f. Stapler
      g. Adhesive tape
  2. Procedure
      a. Tear or cut off several strips of paper tape (2 to 3 inches long for American kestrel, 6 to 8 inches long for red-tailed hawk).
      b. Cut a strip of X-ray film about 1/3 the length of the tail and about the same width as the folded tail. Fold it in half and staple it at the fold.
      c. Gather all tail feathers fairly close together without bending them. The narrower the tail wrap, the stronger and less cumbersome it will be.
      d. Place the tongue depressor along the center of the tail so that one end is flush with the feather tips and the other end almost reaches the bird's body. You may have to trim the tongue depressor.
      e. Fit the X-ray "sleeve" over the tips of the tail and tongue depressor.
      f. Wet the first strip of paper and fold it around the end section of the tail, making sure no feathers are bent (Appendix Figure 4.1).
      g. Repeat with as many strips as necessary to cover the tail to the bare shafts, making sure that each strip overlaps the previous one; do not include tail coverts (downy feathers on the underside of the tail). Try to conform the

shape of the wrap to the natural curvature of the tail feathers.
      h. Finally, fold one long strip lengthwise around the tip of the tail wrap and press all strips firmly together, making sure they all stick well (Appendix Figure 4.2).
  3. Notes
      a. For long-tailed birds (Cooper's hawk, etc.), you may have to tape two tongue depressors together.
      b. For American kestrals, you may have to cut one off a little.
      c. Make the wraps as lightweight as possible.
      d. Press the edges together firmly and dry the tail wrap. A wet or loose wrap will slide off as soon as the bird is returned to its cage.

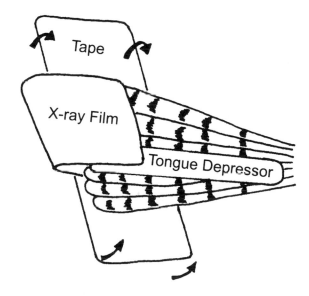

Figure A4.1. Wrapping the paper tape around the tail feathers.

Tail wrapping article reprinted with permission from the Carolina Raptor Center, www.birdsofprey.org, Raptor Rehabilitation, A Manual of Guidelines, pp. 30–31.

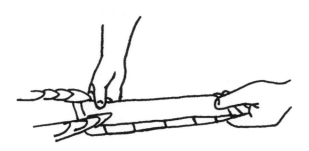

Figure A4.2. The completed tail wrap.

e. Tail wraps will have to be repaired or replaced periodically.

4. Tail wrap removal

a. Soak the whole tail in a pitcher or bucket filled with warm water. Gently begin separating the tape from the feathers with your fingers. After thirty to forty-five seconds, the whole wrap will often slide off in one piece. Do not try to cut or tear the wrap off dry—it will permanently damage feathers.

B. Modified wrap (To be used with tail feathers in molt)

1. Materials

a. Piece of used X-ray film or similar lightweight plastic

b. Masking tape

c. Stapler

2. Procedure

a. Cut a piece of plastic as long as the tail and twice as wide as the folded tail (not fanned out).

b. Fold this piece in half lengthwise so it now matches the shape of the folded-up tail fairly well.

c. Place a few staples along the long edge (where the two edges meet) and along one short edge. You should now have an "envelope" with one short side still open.

d. Carefully slide this sleeve over the folded-up tail.

e. Attach the sleeve to some of the downy coverts on the underside and backside with some strips of masking tape. Be sure not to cover up the oil gland or the feathers covering the vent area.

3. Notes

a. Depending on the material used, this wrap may be stiff enough without the addition of tongue depressors.

b. If the bird is active or when the masking tape wears out, this wrap will have to be repaired/replaced.

c. Standard-size sleeves can be prepared and kept on hand for quick applications.

Guide to Identification of Hatchling and Nestling Songbirds

Table A5.1. Yellow to Orange Mouth Birds. *

Species	Mouth color	Gape flanges	Beak contour	Down	Legs/feet	Approximate weight in grams			Feeding call	Feathers	Special features
						Hatchling	Nestling	Adult (F)			
Starling	bright yellow	bright yellow, very prominent, lower larger than upper	very wide	grayish-white, long and plentiful on head, back, and wings	long legs	5.5–30	40–60	80	hatchling—single squeaky note	gray-black	
Mockingbird	yellow	yellow	wide	dark gray, plentiful	long legs	5–18	20–32	43	hatchling—single, clear, piping note; then throaty bark	gray and white striped wings and tail	gray, irides., crescent marking on roof of mouth
Robin	yellow to yellow-orange	pale yellow	wide	sparse, cream on head, back, legs	long legs	5–35	40–60	77	hatchling—staccato trill	rust-tipped speckly chest	skin often yellowish
Black phoebe	bright yellow-orange	bright yellow	wide, flat, tapering to a point	gray and sparse	long, thin legs	2–5	7–15	18	peep-peep	brown-tipped black feathers	insect eater
Pacific slope flycatcher	bright yellow-orange	yellow	flat, wide, pointy tip, "arrowhead" look	white on head, back and wings in a "star" cluster	long, thin, delicate, dark blue-gray, white toenails	2–6	7–8	11	insistent—crowlike squawk, frog-like when older	buff abdomen, buff and white striped wings	insect eater
Cliff swallow	orange-yellow	flesh	very wide, flat, pointy beak	light gray head and back	short legs, small chubby feet	2–13	13–15	22	barking type chirp	nestlings—light tan on back by tail, otherwise adult	insect eater, cavity nest

Species											
Violet-green swallow	orange-yellow	cream	very wide, pointy beak	cream on head, shoulders, and back	short legs	1.5–8	8–10	14		white eyebrows	insect eater, cavity nest
California thrasher	orange-yellow	cream	curves down as nestling grows	dark gray on head, back, wings, thighs, plentiful	long legs	6–35	40–60	84		medium gray	
Chestnut-backed chickadee	orange-yellow	very yellow, prominent	flat, wide	gray on head and back	long, pale bluish-purple	1–4	6–8	10	squeaky cheep	buff abdomen, black head, buff-white circles on side of head circles	insect eater
Bewick's wren	orange	yellow	flat, wide, pointy	long, gray on head only	long, delicate	1–4	6–8	10		circles	
Bushtit	deep orange-yellow	yellow	short	none	long, delicate	1–3	3.5–4	5	3 syllable "locator" call, "mohawk" look	gray, first feathers on crown of head	females have blue eyes, cavity nesters yellow irides.
Wrentit	deep orange	yellow	pointy	none		1.5–6	7–11	14		gray-brown	

Source: Marty Johnson, Wildlife Rescue, Inc., Palo Alto, CA 94303, 1995.
*Bushtits, chickadees, creepers, dippers, flycatchers, mockingbirds, robins, shrikes, starlings, swallows, thrashers, thrushes, titmice, wrens, and vireos.

Table A5.2. *Pink to Red Mouth Birds.**

Species	Mouth color	Gape flanges	Beak contour	Down	Legs/feet	Approximate weight in grams			Feeding call	Feathers	Special features
						Hatchling	Nestling	Adult (F)			
House sparrow	pink	med. yellow, prominent	short, cone-shaped	none	short, chunky	2–13	14–20	27	melodic, single chirp	smooth, gray white chest dark back, white spots on wings and tail	
Rufous sided towhee	pink	pale yellow	conical and pointed	dark gray	long legs, big feet	3–18	20–29	39			
California towhee	pink to red	pale yellow, not prominent	conical and pointed	long, brown-gray on head, back, and wings	long legs, big feet	4–20	25–39	52	high-pitched repeated, like crickets, changes to single peep	brown	
Brown-headed cowbird	deep pink	white to cream not prominent	heavy, to a point narrower than a towee's	long, snow-white	long legs, big feet, black-tipped nails	2–20	25–30	39	continuous, high-pitched vibrating sound	breast yellowish when coming in	bald face, parasitic, often found in nests of towhees
Northern oriole	deep pink	pale yellow	long, pointed, narrow	long, white-light gray on back, wings, 2 rows on head	long, slate-gray legs	2.5–18	20–25	33	high, staccato, repeated notes, similar to blackbird	yellow breast, gray back, white wing bars	insect eater
Lesser goldfinch	red	pale yellow	similar to finch	grayish	short, pink, stubby	1–6	7–8	10	green to rust back, yellow abdomen	red dot at corner of gape flanges	

Red-winged blackbird	red	yellow, not prominent	long, pointed	scant, white on back, lower wings, and thighs	long legs	3–15	20–30	42		bald face, similar to cowbirds	
Brewer's blackbird	red	white, not prominent	long, pointed	blackish-gray, fairly plentiful	long legs, white toenails	3–15	20–30	42	raucous, repeated call, sounds like a rusty hinge	black	
Scrub jay	red	white, not prominent	long and wide	none	long legs, grabby feet, white toenails	6–30	35–70	87	hatchling-short repeated peeping, later a single squawk	ruddy skin furry gray head, blue wings and tail	
House finch	red	white to yellowish	short, conical	white, long and plentiful. 4 rows on head	short, stocky	1.5–8	10–15	21	none when newly hatched, then high-pitched peeping	stripey, gray	white chest
Crow	red	white	very long, large, heavy	sparse, gray-brown on head, underparts	long, heavy	18–70	70–328	438		black	ruddy skin

Source: Marty Johnson, Wildlife Rescue, Inc., Palo Alto, CA 94303, 1995.
*Blackbirds, cowbirds, crows, finches, goldfinches, grosbeaks, jays, orioles, sparrows, tanagers, towhees, and waxwings.

Average Body Weights of Selected North American Songbirds

Bird species	Weight range (grams)	Average weight (grams)
American robin		77
Bluebird, eastern		31
Cardinal	33.6–64	45
Carolina wren		21
Chickadee, black-capped	8.2–13.6	10.8
Crow, American		448
Dove, mourning		126
Duck, mallard	720–1,580	1,082
Finch, house	19–25.5	21
Flicker, yellow-shafted	130	106–164
Goldfinch, American	8.6–20.7	12.6
Grackle, common		115
Hummingbird, ruby-throated	2.4–4.1	3
Jay, blue	64.1–109	85
Mockingbird	36.2–55.7	49
Oriole, orchard	16–25.1	19.6
Pigeon		270
Purple martin		49.4
Sparrow, house	20.1–34.5	27.4
Swallow, barn	13.4–23.4	19
Thrasher, brown	57.6–89	69
Titmouse, tufted	17.5–26.1	21.6
Warbler, pine	9.4–15.1	11.9
Woodpecker, pileated		290
Woodpecker, red headed	56.1–90.5	72

(Information in part from Dunning 1984).

Species Care Sheets

RACCOONS

Raccoon Diet and Feeding

Formula: 1 part powdered KMR:2 parts water.

- Stomach capacity is 50 to 66 ml/kg (5% to 7%). Use 50 ml/kg to reduce chances of diarrhea (.05 × BW in g =_____ml.). There are 30 ml/fluid ounce.
- Do not allow free choice formula feeding because some raccoons overeat and develop diarrhea or bloat.
- Very young raccoons can be fed with a dropper, pet nurser bottle, or nipple attached to a syringe. The pet nurser has the least amount of flow control, so use it with caution.
- Older juveniles are often fed with preemie baby bottles and nipples. After bottle feeding always remember to burp the baby by patting firmly between the shoulder blades and down the infant's back.
- New incoming infants may take several days to become accustomed to the new diet and feeding instrument.
- Scratching the back of a raccoon's neck, while holding the nurser in its mouth, usually stimulates a suckling reflex.
- Once baby raccoons get the idea of bottle nursing, the rest of the feeding times are spent trying to slow them down. They tend to drink very fast and you must pull the bottle away after they have received the measured formula amount or they will swallow air.
- Stimulate before feeding until eyes open and self elimination is evident (four to five weeks).
- Add baby rice cereal to formula as a thickener to slow down overzealous nursers.
- Gradually begin introducing solid foods (applesauce, yogurt, baby foods, softened puppy food), either mixed in the formula or separate, once raccoons have their eyes open and begin to get teeth (four weeks).
- Once they have a taste for the puppy food in the formula, start offering it dry.

- Gradually decrease the bottle feeding until weaned (seven to twelve weeks).
- Begin to offer drinking water when raccoons begin to eat solid foods, but plan to refill the water bowl several times a day because they love to climb in and also dunk their food items in bowl.
- Some rehabilitators prefer to teach the babies how to lap formula out of a bowl. This method takes patience and a lot of wash cloths to clean up afterward.
- Raccoons may resist weaning and lose weight at first.
- Dry puppy food (Science Diet Canine Growth) should constitute 90% of the post-weaning diet.
- The remaining 10% of the diet should be apples, grapes, berries, eggs, vegetables, sweet potatoes, fish, worms, clams, small rodents, chicks, and crayfish.
- By the age of twelve weeks raccoons should be able to kill crayfish.
- By fourteen weeks raccoons should be able to kill young rats.
- Some individuals need to be fasted for twenty-four hours before they will try new foods.
- Use caution and protective clothing when handling raccoons because they are a rabies vector species.

Raccoon Housing

- From zero to five weeks of age, a cardboard box or pet carrier works best because it can be thrown out after it becomes soiled. Due to the zoonotic concern with the internal parasite *Baylisascaris procyonis*, any fecal-contaminated materials should be burned or thrown away. Never reuse any cages or caging materials used with raccoons with any other species because disinfectants are ineffective in killing the raccoon roundworm. Fresh feces are not infective, but become so in three to four weeks. The intake procedure for raccoons should include weekly dewormings of pyrantel pamoate suspension (4.5 mg/ml at 0.5 to 1 cc/lb).

- Use soft, ravel-free cloth as bedding. Do not use terry cloth because their fingernails get caught in the loops too easily.
- Provide supplemental heat until they are four weeks old.
- At six weeks provide the animal with a wire cage with logs, natural substrate, tree limbs for climbing,

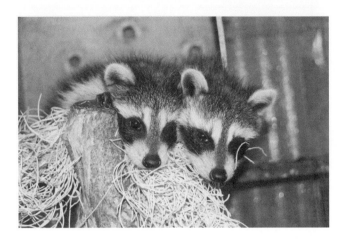

Figure A7.1. Raccoon babies.

and a hammock made from canvas or tight-weave netting, which should be hung near the top of the enclosure. The hammocks are a good substitute for wooden nest boxes because they can be changed and washed.
- By eight weeks, raccoons are very active and need a large cage with lots of natural items to help keep them from getting bored (i.e. hollow logs, rocks, live plants, dirt for digging, water bowls for dunking food, pine cones, small pool).
- Outdoor acclimation usually starts at six weeks and finishes by twelve weeks.

Raccoon Release
- The release age is four to five months, when they are self feeding and acclimated to the outdoors.
- This section does not cover raccoon release due to the regulations on possessing rabies vector species in many states and the numerous difficulties one can face with this procedure. Turning all raccoons over to a licensed rehabilitator, vaccinated against rabies, is recommended.

Table A7.1. Raccoon Care Sheet.

Age (weeks)	Weights (g)	Age determinates	Diet	Amount	Frequency
0–1	50–100	Faint tail rings and mask, very lightly furred, ears pressed against head	KMR	Volume by B.W.	q 3 hr, 1 PM feeding
1–2	100–150	Face mask furred, eye slit visible, crawling on belly	KMR		q 3.5 hr, 1 PM feeding
2–3	100–200	Ear canals open, 18–24 d eyes open	KMR		q 3.5 hr, no PM feeding
3–4	200–300	Fully furred tail rings, responds to sight and sound	KMR, add cereal		q 4 hr
4–5	175–300	Able to walk, eyes open but cloudy blue, deciduous teeth erupting	KMR, add soaked kibble		q 4 hr
5–6	300–400	Able to run and climb, eyes darken			QID
6–7	400–600	Adult pelage begins (ends 12–14 weeks)			TID
7–8	600–650	2nd & 3rd premolars erupt, full sight & hearing	Start weaning		TID
8–9	650–675	1st permanent incisors erupt	Start dish feeding		BID
9–10	675–700	1st premolars erupt	No bottle feedings		SID
10–11	700–775	Wean 10–12 weeks	Weaned		
11–12	775–825				
12–13	825–875	3rd permanent incisors erupt			
13–14	875–900				
14–15	900–1,100				

FLYING SQUIRRELS

Flying Squirrel Diet and Feeding

Formula: 1 part powdered Esbilac:2 parts water.

- Feed with a 1- or 3-cc O-ring syringe with silicone nipple.
- Flying squirrels have a good suckling reflex and the formula may need to be thickened to prevent aspiration.
- Gradually thicken formula with rice baby cereal starting at three weeks.
- Stimulate after each meal until the eyes are open and there is evidence of self elimination in cage.
- Once the eyes are open begin to introduce solid food items.
- Start decreasing the number of formula feedings as solid food is being consumed (four to five weeks).
- Wait at least four days between feeding reductions.
- A useful weaning tool is to add powdered rodent or primate chow to the formula starting at five weeks.
- Examples of weaning foods include dog chow, raw nuts, fresh corn on the cob, apple, grapes, rodent blocks, primate chow, seed mix, vegetables, sweet potatoes, carrots, broccoli, wheat germ, etc.
- Natural food items to offer include mushrooms, lichens, bark, buds, insects, acorns, hickory nuts, pine cones, beech nuts, berries, green buds, etc.
- The diet ratio of food groups should be: 80% rodent mix (dog, primate, rodent chow); 20% fruit and vegetable matter; one nut/squirrel/day; two to three insects/squirrel/day.
- Offering the squirrel "nutri-bites" (recipe under grey squirrel diet, below) until release will help assure proper nutrition.
- Provide drinking water in a bowl or water bottle when babies are weaned down to twice a day formula.
- Once weaned, feed the squirrels at night (they are nocturnal) and scatter food around the cage.

Flying Squirrel Housing

- Supplemental heat is needed until they are five to six weeks old. Using a heating pad under half of the enclosure is recommended.
- Masters of escape, flying squirrels need to be housed in a secure enclosure with a tight lid.

Table A7.2. Flying Squirrel Care Sheet.

Age (weeks)	Weights (g)	Age determinates	Diet	Amount	Frequency
0–1	3–6	Pink, no fur, eyes closed, few whiskers	Esbilac	0.2–0.3 ml	q 2 hr, 2 PM feeding
1–2	6–10	Short hairs appear, toes separate	Esbilac	0.3–0.6 ml	q 2 hr, 1 PM feeding
2–3	10–15	Downy hair darkens, able to right themselves, ear canals open, lower incisors erupt	Esbilac	0.6–1.0 ml	q 3 hr, no PM feeding
3–4	17–23	Lateral tail hairs develop, responds to loud noises	Esbilac, add cereal	1.0–1.5 ml	q 3 hr
4–5	25–30	Fur covers body, upper incisors erupt, days 28–32 eyes open	Esbilac, cereal, add solid food	1.5–2.0 ml	q 4 hr
5–6	30–38	Miniature version of adult	Weaning begins	2.0–2.5 ml	TID
6–7	38–43		Add rodent pellets	2.5–3.0 ml	BID
7–8	40–47		Add natural foods	3.0–5.0 ml	SID-BID
8–10	47–53		Wk 8–9 weaned		
12–14	60	Ready for release			

- One to four weeks in an aquarium or small box.
- Four to six weeks in a larger wire portable cage (begin to acclimate to the outdoors).
- Provide a nesting box because these squirrels live in tree cavities in the wild.
- Six to fourteen weeks in an outdoor pre-release pen (once acclimated). This pen needs to be large enough for the young flying squirrels to practice jumping and gliding. Minimum size of 6 feet H × 6 feet W × 8 feet L.
- The pen needs both horizontal and vertical branches to assimilate the trees.
- Flying squirrels move from tree to tree and rarely go to the ground.

Flying Squirrel Release

- Release age is fourteen to sixteen weeks.
- Release criteria: Fully acclimated to outdoors, nocturnal behaviors, running from humans, opening shelled nuts, and eating natural food items.
- Whenever possible, raise and release flyers with a group because these animals live in colonies. Also release in a well-wooded area where other flyers have been seen or heard.
- Release by closing animals inside their nest box one hour before dark outside (tape hole shut). Tie box to tree trunk (6 feet or higher up) and remove tape from nest box entrance at dusk. Flyers will exit the box and explore the tree tops, then sometimes return to the nest box until they find another cavity to sleep in.
- Supply back-up food by having a nearby feeding station or putting a bowl on top of the nest box.

Flying Squirrel Miscellaneous Information

- When startled, flying squirrels flip on their backs and box at the invader with all four feet. Wake the sleeping baby up slowly and gently to prevent this aggressive display.
- Do not worry if the infant does not eliminate each time it is stimulated. Discontinue stimulation after about a minute. As long as the squirrel has at least one bowel movement a day bloating should not occur.

OPOSSUMS

Opossum Diet and Feeding
Formula: 1 part powdered Esbilac:2 parts water
- Stomach capacity is 50 to 66 ml/kg or 5% to 7% of BW. (.05 × BW in g = _____ml).

- Opossums have a poorly developed suckling reflex, which makes gavage feeding the most effective method to feed young animals under 45 grams.
- Gavage tube size ranges from size 3-1/2 to 5 French feeding tube.
- Pinkies should be started on very dilute formula (1:5 with water) and gradually built up to full strength formula over three to five days. Until infant is on full strength, feed more often.
- Zero to seventy-five days: tube feed q 2 hours at 5% BW. Belly should be rounded but not tight after a feeding and a milk line in the stomach should be visible through the skin.
- By the time they weigh 50g, they do not tolerate tube feedings. Even before their eyes open, a jar lid of warm formula can be placed with baby opossums. By dipping their noses in the milk and allowing them to walk through the formula they will clean the milk off of themselves (and their litter mates) and learn to self-feed faster.
- When able to lap up formula out of bowl, start thickening with rice baby cereal.
- Foods to help facilitate the weaning process: fruit yogurt, meat baby foods, bananas, grapes, cooked sweet potatoes, and applesauce. These items can be mixed with milk formula in the bowl to encourage self feeding.
- By ten to twelve weeks gradually start adding puppy or cat chow to formula.
- By sixteen weeks opossums should be weaned and eating solid food items such as fresh carrion, live crickets, mealworms and earthworms, fruit and vegetables native to the area, raw eggs, dead minnows, and crayfish. Lightly sprinkle the diet with a calcium supplement. Offer food in the evenings.
- Make sure there is always fresh drinking water available during and after weaning. Opossums have a habit of defecating in their food and water bowls, so offer a water bottle to guarantee a clean water source.

Opossum Housing
- Housing: Small box or pet carrier with soft, ravel-free cloth, heating pad set on low, and a source of humidity until eight weeks old. Be careful to use cage lids and small (less than1/2 inch) ventilation holes due to the opossum's ability to easily escape.
- Maintain nest humidity at 70%.
- Move to1/4 inch to 1/2 inch mesh hardware cloth 2 feet × 2 feet × 4 feet cage at eight to ten weeks.
- Use a heating pad until ten weeks or 80 to 90g at external temperatures of 95°F.

Table A7.3. Opossum Care Sheet.

Age (weeks)	Weights (g)	Age determinates	Diet	Amount	Frequency
2		Whiskers start, blond nose hairs, pink skin	Tube—Esbilac	.50 ml	q 2 hrs, 24 hr
4	20	Blond belly hairs, pink skin	Same	1 ml	q 2–3 hr, 1 PM feeding
5–6	25–35	Slight bluish coloration, ears open	Same	1–2 ml	q 2–3 hr, 1 PM feeding
6–8	35–50	Furred, eye slits developed, mouth fully open	Same	2–3 ml	q 3–4 hr, 1 PM feeding
9	45–52	Eyes open, running around, lapping formula, teeth present, white-tipped guard hairs, ears erect	Bowl—Esbilac, add cereal	2.5–3 ml	QID
10–11	50–75	Self-defecating/urinating; 3–6″ excluding tail	Bowl—Esbilac, cereal, add cat or puppy chow	2.5–4 ml	QID
12	75–100	Thermoregulating; 4.5–6.5″	Start weaning	4 ml	TID
13–15	100–500	Actively climbing; 6–10″	Weaned, dry chow	5 ml	BID-TID
15–20	500–1,000	20 weeks—ready for release	Natural foods		BID

- At twelve weeks begin outdoor acclimation. Opossums need exercise and a daily dose of vitamin D$_3$, naturally provided by sunlight, to help prevent metabolic bone disease (MBD). Opossums are very prone to MBD and must receive daily dietary calcium in addition to thirty to sixty minutes of unfiltered U/V light.
- Use caution when putting animals in sunlight. Opossums are prone to overheating and can die quickly if not provided with some shade and proper ventilation. They do not need to be in direct sunlight to benefit from natural U/V, just placed outside during daylight hours. Beneficial U/V rays are blocked out by glass windows.
- Move to a release cage at four months.
- Opossums are becoming nocturnal and sleeping during the day by four months.
- Small groups of same age preweanlings can be housed together. Cannibalism can result when housing older juveniles together.

Opossum Release
- Consider release when the opossum is five months old and 8 to 10 inches in body length, 1.5 lbs., self-feeding, acclimated to weather and outside temperatures, and baring its teeth at the caretaker.
- If the cage is on a suitable release site, open the cage door one hour before dark and allow the opossum to come and go. Provide back-up food until the animal moves on.
- Some opossums will leave the cage and explore at night but come back to the nest box by morning and sleep until the next dusk.
- If the cage is not on a suitable site, be certain the animal is ready and release it near cover and trees right before dark.

Opossum Miscellaneous Information
- Opossums are sensitive to corticosteroids and Levamisole the is dewormer of choice.
- Opossums tolerate sutures, bandages, and splints well.
- Orphans have immature immune systems so wash hands before and after feeding.

GREY SQUIRRELS

Grey Squirrel Diet and Feeding
Formula: 1 part powdered Esbilac:2 parts water

- Stomach capacity is 50 ml/kg (.05 ml × BW in g = _____ ml).
- Use O-ring syringe with a silicone or Catac nipple to feed orphan squirrels.
- Stimulate after each feeding until five weeks.

- A healthy squirrel should gain 4 to 7 g/day once established on Esbilac formula.
- Squirrels should be fed lying on their stomachs with heads slightly raised.
- Add rice baby cereal to thicken formula at about three weeks.
- Add powdered rodent blocks to further thicken formula at about five weeks.
- When eyes open and the squirrel is eating rodent blocks or monkey chow, start offering self feeding diet items such as cracked nuts, small pieces of fresh corn on the cob, apple, grapes, broccoli stems, cauliflower, and rodent seed mixes.
- Start to wean at eight weeks and finish by ten to eleven weeks.
- The ratio of the diet offered should be 80% rodent/primate chow:20% other items. Do not allow the animal to "choose" a balanced diet for itself; stick with the ratio.
- Limit nuts to one nut/squirrel/day or they will not eat enough of the more nutritious foods.

- Make sure the squirrel is off milk and eating solid and natural food items for at least two weeks prior to release.
- Post-weaning foods: rodent blocks, high quality dog chow (i.e. Purina One, Proplan, Eukanuba), uncracked acorns, hickory nuts, pecans, buds, bark, pine cones, fungi, sunflower seeds, insects, fresh vegetables, and rodent seed mixes.
- Squirrel nutri-bites are a healthy weaning tool. The recipe is as follows:
  1-1/2 cups powdered rodent or primate chow
  1/3 cup powdered Esbilac
  2/3 cup warm water
  1/3 cup chopped pecans
  1/3 cup crushed cuttlebone, if needed.
  Mix together and roll into small meatball-size balls. Keep refrigerated up to three days or freeze for up to six months.
- These "squirrel nutri-bites" can be offered in place of a milk feeding and once the squirrels start eating them they can be offered free choice. Due to the

Table A7.4. Grey Squirrel Care Sheet.

Age (weeks)	Weights (g)	Age determinates	Diet	Amount	Frequency
0–1	15–25	Pink, no fur, eyes closed tight—bulgy	Esbilac	0.5–1.0 ml	q 2 hr, 1 PM feeding
1–2	25–35	Scant gray color to head, shoulder, and back Day 10—lose umbilical cord	Esbilac	1–2 ml	q 2 hr, 1 PM feeding
2–3	35–60	Scant grayish fur, ears unglued, eyes less bulgy; Day 21—lower incisors emerge	Esbilac	2–4 ml	q 2–3 hr, no PM feeding
3–4	60–90	Slick, shiny fur except under tail; ears open, eye slits relaxed and ready to open	Esbilac, add cereal	3–6 ml	q 3–4 hr
4–5	90–115	Downy white hair on belly, slight bush to tail, eyes open, may begin to walk	Esbilac, cereal, add rodent block	5–9 ml	QID
5–6	115–175	Thicker hair, tail curling over back, upper incisors emerge, sitting up	Same; keep thickening	5–12 ml	TID-QID
6–7	175–250	Furry all over, sleeping less, can sit up fruit	Add small pieces	9–15 ml	TID-QID
7–8		Bushy tail, back molars come in	Rodent blocks	15–20 ml	BID-TID
8–9		Looks like miniature squirrel	Begin to wean	20–25 ml	SID-BID
9–10		Furred on underside except for 1″ at base tail, tail bushy	Wean	20–30 ml	SID
10–11	300–425		Wean		
11–12		Tail completely furred	Weaned		
12–14		Ready for release			

milk content, do not leave them in cages long enough to spoil.

Grey Squirrel Housing

- From zero to four weeks: lidded box, cardboard pet carrier, plastic or glass aquarium with heating pad on low under one-half of the cage.
- Use soft, ravel-free cloth for bedding, such as cotton T-shirts, flannel, sweat shirts, fleece.
- At five to six weeks discontinue heating pad use.
- Around six to eight weeks move to a small wire flush bottom cage (1/2 inch × 1 inch mesh or smaller) with tree limbs for climbing, and provide a nest box inside cage.
- Start acclimating to outdoor temperatures by placing cage outside during warm days and bringing it back in at night. Gradually leave out for longer periods of time until the squirrel can comfortably be left out overnight. Baby squirrels do not have to be brought inside if a heat lamp can be provided near one of the nest boxes.
- At eight to twelve weeks move squirrel to large outdoor wire release cage (minimum size 4 feet × 4 feet × 6 feet); the larger the better. I should have a covered, waterproof roof, back, and one side. Hang a water bottle on the cage. Attach nest box to the top of the cage. Use natural substrate on the cage bottom and inside the nest box.
- House animals with similarly aged conspecifics.

Grey Squirrel Release

Release Criteria:

- At least twelve to fourteen weeks of age and acclimated to the outdoors for at least two weeks.
- Squirrels should hide at the sight or sound of approaching people and should not allow any handling, even from the hand raiser.
- Squirrels should be weaned for a minimum of two weeks, be building nests, eating natural food items, and able to crack open whole shelled raw nuts.
- If these criteria are met, open the cage door and allow the animal to come and go. Continue to supply food until squirrels move on or at least for three to four weeks.

COTTONTAIL RABBITS

Cottontail Rabbit Diet and Feeding

Formula: 1 part powdered KMR:2 parts water

- Feed with O-ring syringe and nipple or tube feed rabbits.

- Stomach capacity = 100 to 125 ml/kg (10% to 12.5%) of BW. Safer to use 100 ml/kg or .1 × BW in g = _____ml.
- Cottontails benefit by receiving daily Benebac to aid with digestion and diarrhea prevention.
- Rabbits can be fed with a syringe but they seldom suckle. Some will lick formula from the tip of the syringe drop by drop or swallow milk as it is dripped onto their lips.
- If your new cottontail refuses to eat, try a drop of Karo syrup on the end of the nipple or add a bit of baby food (no sugar added) applesauce to the formula. Another trick is to add orange flavored Pedialyte to the formula to enhance the flavor.
- Allow cottontails to drink as much formula as they want per feeding. It is better to feed these babies in as few feedings as possible. Twice a day is the goal as long as they get enough calories and are gaining weight.
- Gavage feeding is a faster method and ideal if there are many babies to feed or if the babies are frightened of handling and refuse to nurse. Be sure to watch a veterinarian or an experienced rehabilitator do this method before first trying it yourself. Although faster, tube feeding can be potentially lethal if done incorrectly. The rabbit's pallet skin is very fragile and can be punctured by the soft end of the feeding tube, resulting in SQ delivery of formula followed by death.
- Stimulate baby rabbits before feeding until their eyes open.
- Keep a secure hold on baby rabbits when handling. Rabbits have a habit of suddenly jumping out of your hands or off the table.
- When the eyes are open, start offering diced (easily done with scissors), fresh natural greens (clover greens and flowers, grass, dandelion leaves, alfalfa, privet) twice daily. No stems of plants should be given until rabbits are approximately three weeks old. Offer only a small amount at first and be sure the greens are clean and chemical free.
- Once they have adjusted to the new food items (three to four days after they begin to sample them), offer larger amounts. There should always be some left over. After a week of eating solid foods, discontinue dicing the greens and offer them whole.
- Remove uneaten greens as new greens are added. Greens and grasses wilt quickly, becoming undesirable to the rabbits, and they can mold in just a day or two.
- Provide drinking water in a shallow lid or a water bottle when young rabbits start to nibble on solid foods.

- Other solid food items include rabbit chow, rolled oats, wheat germ, corn, apple and carrot slivers, dry hay, or alfalfa fed free choice until released.
- Introduce new food items slowly and one at a time to allow the gut to adjust to the changes.
- Wean rabbits by three to four weeks.

Cottontail Rabbit Housing

- From zero to two weeks use a small cardboard box or aquarium with secure lid.
- Use a heating pad on low under one half of the cage or a heat light on one half of the cage.
- Supply soft, ravel-free cloth for bedding. Rabbits like layers to burrow into and they prefer to be covered up.
- Once weaned, remove the heating pad and cloth bedding. Instead, bed with natural substrates such as hay, grasses, leaves, or pine straw.
- At three weeks move to a large plastic pet carrier or enclosed rabbit hutch. Rabbits need solid sided cages and a quiet area to reduce stress.
- Do not overcrowd the cages.
- Litter mates can be housed together but be careful when mixing unrelated animals and do not mix different ages because they tend to fight and become stressed.
- Fatal enteritis can develop from environmental stress.
- Albon at 25 to 50 mg/kg PO SID × five to fourteen days given to all rabbits initially may help prevent enteritis caused by stress-induced coccidiosis flare ups.
- Be sure there are no holes in the cage or cage door larger than 1/2 inch square because infant rabbits can squeeze out of a 1-inch by 1-inch hole. Securely cover any questionable holes with burlap, netting, or screen.
- Acclimate to outside temperatures once rabbits are weaned.
- Provide hiding spots such as hay to burrow into, or a cardboard or wooden nest box.

Cottontail Rabbit Release

- Ready for release by the end of four weeks.
- Many rabbits do not do well in captivity past five to six weeks of age and should not be kept this long unless there is a medical reason.
- Rabbits ready for release should run and hide from all humans, pets, and noise.
- The Release weight is between 100–200 g, ideally about 150 g.
- Find a site with open fields or pasture with n earby cover for a release site. Open the cage door and allow rabbits to hop out by themselves or place them under cover and quietly leave the area.
- Cottontails do not need back-up food if released in a proper habitat, and they rarely return to the release site.
- Release at dusk or dawn in mild weather.

Table A7.5. Cottontail Care Sheet.

Age (weeks)	Weights (g)	Age determinates	Diet	Amount (ml)	Frequency
0–1	30–40	Pink, thin fur all over, eyes closed, ears flat and closed	KMR	0.5–1.5 ml	3–4 × /day
1–2	35–55	Fully furred, 7–10 days eyes open, greens ears erect	KMR, offer	2–6 ml	2–3 × /day
2–3	50–90	Ear length growth, 3 weeks self-defecating	Same	3–9 ml	1–2 × /day
3–4	60–120	Hopping, running, ears fully erect	Natural food; weaned		0–1 × /day
4–5	150–190	Release			

Biological Data of Selected North American Wild Mammals

Table A8.1. Biological Data.

Animal	°F body temp	Pulse rate/min	Respiration rate/min	Weight at birth (g)	Adult weight (kg)	Weaning age (weeks)	Feeding formula	Eyes open (days)	Release age (weeks)
Armadillo	84–92			51–150.3	5–6	8	Esbilac	birth	9–12
Badger	99–102			95	6–11	8–10	Esbilac	28–36	6–8
Bat (big brown)	95–102.2			3.3–4.0	11–16g	6–8	Mother's Helper K-9	Hrs after birth	
Bat (red)	97–98.6			1.5–2.0	10–12g	3–6		10	6–8
Bear (black)	100–102	60–90	15–30	170–227	90–214	22–26	Esbilac	35–42	1 yr.
Beaver	98–101	100	16	400–500	13–27	6–8	Esbilac	birth	10–12
Bobcat	99–102	110–140	26	283–340	6–15	8–9	KMR	3–11	16–20
Cottontail	100–103	130–325	32–60	35–45	0.9–2	2–3	KMR	6–8	3–4
Coyote	100–103	100–170		200–275	8.1–18	5–7	Esbilac	10–11	6 mo.
Deer (white tail)	101–102	70–80	16–20	2.5–4.0kg	M 34–180 F 22–112	8–12	lamb, doe, goat milk	birth	6–8 mo.
Fox (gray)	100–103			86	3–6	7–8	Esbilac	10–12	20
Fox (red)	100–103			71–119	5–7	8–10	Esbilac	8–9	24
E. Chipmunk	99–102	660–702		2.5–5.0	65–127g	5–6	Esbilac	30–33	8
Hare (black tailed jack rabbit)	99–102			60–180	1.8–3.6	3–4	KMR	birth	
Mink	99–103	250–300	18–20	6–10	0.5–1.4	5–8	Esbilac	21–30	8–10
Muskrat	98–101	148–306*	45	21	1–2	3–4	Esbilac	14–16	8–10
Opossum (Virginia)	90–99	120–140		.2	4–6	13–15	Esbilac	58–72	15
Otter (river)	99–102	130–178	20–60	132	5–11	12–16	Esbilac	21–35	9 mo.
Porcupine	99–100	280–320	100	400–500	5–12	3–5	Esbilac	birth	10–12
Raccoon	100–103	128–180	15–30	60–75	5–16	10–16	KMR	18–24	20
Skunk (spotted)	101–102			28	.340–1.2	6–8	Esbilac	28–32	
Skunk (striped)	101–102			33	3–6	6–8	Esbilac	14–28	9–12
Squirrel (S. flying)	98–102			3–6	50–79 g	8–9	Esbilac	29–40	12
Squirrel (fox)	98–102			14–18	0.5–1.4	8–9	Esbilac	28–35	12
Squirrel (grey)	98–102	390*		14–18	0.038–0.069	8–9	Esbilac	28–35	12
Weasel (least)	100–103	172–192		1.0–1.5	38–69 g	2–3		26–29	6–8
Wolf	100–102			454	23.5	6–8	Esbilac	11–15	
Woodchuck	99–100	180–264*		28.4–42.5	1.8–6.3	8–12	Esbilac	30	12

Source: Information in part from Evans (1987), Fowler (1979), Stokes (1986), and Schwartz (1974).
*Pulse rate under anesthesia.

Glossary of Medical Conditions and Treatments

Bloat: Causes of bloat include a change in diet, internal parasites, improper diet, feeding a cold infant, over-feeding, or constipation. If an infant bloats, hold its belly down on a heating pad and gently but firmly massage its side from top to bottom of the abdomen. Also use gas relief medications such as Di-gel, simethicone, activated charcoal, or powdered calcium carbonate dissolved in water orally in addition to warmth and massage. Long-term treatment is to eliminate the cause of the bloat.

Broken Blood Feathers: Feathers that are actively growing (pin feathers) contain a blood supply and when damaged may bleed. These feathers need to be removed by grasping the quill at the skin surface with hemostats, supporting the bone with the other hand, and pulling straight out. The entire feather must be cleanly removed from the follicle for the bleeding to stop.

Bumblefoot: A generalized inflammation of the foot that is most commonly seen in raptors but could occur in any bird. The condition usually starts out as a cut, puncture, swelling, bruising, crack, or abrasion on the bottom of the foot. Bacteria then enter the break in the skin and cause a generalized infection. The problem is often caused by improper or unclean perches and cages. Therapy must include topical cleaning and flushing of the wounds, proper bandaging, and often systemic antibiotics.

Constipation: In infant mammals, constipation may be due to over feeding, change in diet, internal parasites, dehydration, intestinal obstruction, or too long since stimulation. If increasing the fluid intake and stimulating for a longer than normal time does not work, remove impacted feces in the colon by a warm water or mineral oil enema. A couple of drops of mineral oil or Laxatone orally may help alleviate constipation.

Crop Stasis: "Sour crop" or crop stasis occurs when the contents of the crop fail to empty. This sometimes occurs when the food was fed too cold, the crop was overfilled, foreign bodies are present, or food was sour when fed. Crop infections such as trichomoniasis and systemic illness are other causes. Because the contents must be removed, administer a small amount of sterile water and gently massaging the crop. If the crop does not empty on its own within a few hours, the contents must be removed by drawing the material out with the tube and syringe used to feed the bird. Flush the crop with warm, sterile water. Possible treatments consist of antimicrobial therapy and correction of dehydration and nutrition.

Dehydration: Dehydration is the excessive loss of fluid from the body. It is life threatening and prevents every system in the body from functioning properly. The body cannot digest food, maintain body temperature, deliver proper oxygen or blood flow, or excrete toxins in a dehydrated state. The condition must be quickly assessed by determining the level of dehydration and the fluid treatment should be started immediately. Neonates need two to three times the fluid requirement of adults.

Maintenance: 50 ml/kg/day (OR) BW in g × .05 = daily mls fluids
Replacement: decimal value of % dehydration × BW in g = daily mls needed; 0.10 = 10% (replaces fluid loss volume for volume, e.g. diarrhea, hemorrhage)
Dehydration: 100 ml/kg/day (OR) BW in g × .10 = daily mls fluids (give 1/2 volume over two to six hours; then 1/2 volume plus maintenance over next twenty-four hours (OR) 50 ml/kg BID until rehydrated)
The daily volume must be divided by the number of times you wish to administer fluids. Use the least evasive method to resolve the dehydration. Oral is

Table A9.1. Method to determine degree of dehydration.

% Deyhdration	Skin turgor (in seconds)	Clinical signs
6%	1–2	Tented skin; slight loss of skin elasticity
8%	2–3	Eyes slightly depressed; slow CRT; dry, tacky mucous membranes
10%	3–5	Sunken eyes and cere; dry, tented, scaly skin; very slow CRT; wrinkling
12%	>5	Early signs of hypovolemic shock; easily collapsible peripheral veins

preferred for birds, provided the animal is conscious and its bowels are functional. IV therapy is mandatory in cases of dehydration and shock, comatose animals, and starvation.

Emaciation: Body weights and degree of muscle wasting are diagnostic. These animals should slowly be weaned onto solid food depending on category stage. First, offer a rehydrating solution such as LRS or LRS with 2.5% Dextrose orally. Then start with a diet such as Ultracal, Ensure, or Isocal. These liquid diets are high calorie, low volume, isotonic (requiring minimum energy for digestion) food sources that can be fed to birds or mammals. Probiotics should be offered to help reestablish normal healthy gut flora. When the animal is hydrated and passing normal looking stools, begin to offer diets for debilitated animals such as Clinicare, Hill's A/D, or Emeraid II.

The progression time period from fluids to solid foods varies from category to category as well as from patient to patient. Always slowly mix new foods in with the old diet to make the changes gradual (over several days) and easier on the animal. Meals should be small and as often as possible (weighed against frequent handling stress). These animals should be on vitamin supplementation to promote appetite. Supportive care should include heat and a stress-free environment.

Table A9.2. Method to determine degree of emaciation.

Category I	Category II	Category III
90–100% BW	75–90% BW	50–70% BW
Not eaten in 1 day	Not eaten in several days	Not eaten in 1 week
Hypoglycemic	Seizures	Near comatose
Mild muscle atrophy	Moderate muscle atrophy	Severe atrophy
Generally salvageable	Difficult to save	Few recoveries

Fleas, Ticks: Use VIP flea powder, 5% pyrethrin dust or powder safe for kittens and puppies. Manually remove ticks.

Glue Traps: Use a light sprinkle of cornstarch to neutralize the glue and prevent the animal from becoming more entangled. Cut away as much of the trap as possible. Warm canola oil to 102°F to 104°F and apply oil to stuck feathers or fur by gently working it in with your fingers. The warmed oil will soften the adhesive bond and after several minutes allow you to remove the animal from the trap. Work the soft, gummy substance that forms up and off of the animal without pulling on the feathers or fur directly. After several more minutes most of the glue should be soft enough to be removed or washed out. If the canola oil leaves a residue you may need to do a bath with Dawn dishwashing detergent and rinse as described under "soiled feathers."

Hyperthermia: Factors which predispose animals to hyperthermia, abnormally high body temperature, are fever, infection, excessive muscular exertion, or exposure to high ambient temperatures or high humidity. These patients need to be cooled quickly. Submerge animals in a cold water bath and perform cold water enemas. A circulating air fan helps provide evaporation cooling. The danger here is taking the body temperature down below normal levels, so be sure to discontinue cooling methods once the temperature nears normal.

Hypothermia: Animals suffering from hypothermia, abnormally low body temperature, must be warmed slowly. With temperatures 10° to 15° below normal, the animal is likely to become comatose and unable to respond or even shiver. At this point it is critical to understand why a heating pad will NOT be effective. Circulation is decreased to the peripheral parts of the body due to the its attempt to conserve blood for the vital organs, so contact heat from a heating pad is wasted. The body is not capable of carrying heat from the skin touching the warm pad into the rest of the body. The best sources of heat are from heat lamps, incubators, or a warm water bath that supplies radiant heat evenly over the entire body at one time. Warm water enemas are helpful as well. Gradually increase the temperature and make sure the animal does not burn or get heated up too fast, which is equally damaging.

Maggots: Maggots in small numbers are best removed manually. Heavy infestations may require flushing with peroxide to kill them. Applying cornstarch to the maggots dries them out and they often fall off. A dose of Ivermectin kills any remaining maggots and any eggs that may hatch. If the infestation is advanced and they have entered the body cavities, euthanasia is recommended.

Malocclusion: Improper tooth alignment is most critical with rodents and lagomorphs. These animals have two upper and two lower incisors that continue to grow throughout the animal's life. They normally wear down from chewing on hard objects and grinding teeth. Maligned incisors may continue to grow and overgrow, resulting in starvation (from not being able to chew food) or self-induced puncture wounds (from the lower teeth puncturing the roof of the mouth). The prognosis is poor with this condition, but manually trimming the teeth biweekly or so may allow the teeth time to grow back normally after the animal has healed from the fractured jaw or other facial injury that caused the trauma.

Mites: Dust baby and adult birds with an avian mite powder. Ivermectin applied to the back of the neck treats birds for mites, but be sure to accurately measure the dose by body weight, not just by applying "a drop." Ivermectin is effective against mites in mammals by injecting one dose SQ.

Ruptured Air Sac: A ruptured air sac, which appears like an air bubble under the bird's skin, is often caused by impact trauma such as falling from a nest. Small SQ pockets that do not interfere with the bird's mobility or breathing can be left to heal on their own. Otherwise, clean the skin over the bubble and make a small incision about 1/8 inch to 1/4 inch long with a sterile scissors to let the air out. Be sure to avoid the cutaneous blood vessels that can usually be seen through the skin.

Shock: The definition of shock is an acute failure of the heart to provide adequate blood flow to the tissues. Signs of shock include glassy eyes, fixed stare, unresponsive pupils, rigidity of the limbs, paleness of the gums, listlessness, decrease in blood pressure, increase in pulse, lower body temperature, or unresponsiveness to stimuli. Treatment is a combination of heat, fluids, medications, oxygen, and stress removal. Seek veterinary care for animals that come into the clinic in this condition.

Soiled Feathers (oil, tar, dirt): Feathers need to remain clean and waterproof to provide insulation and flight. If a bird comes in with soiled feathers or becomes soiled during rehabilitation, a warm water bath (103°F to 104°F) using Dawn dishwashing detergent followed by a clean warm water rinse will remove caked-on food, feces, oil, and glue. It is very important to keep the bird warm at all times until completely dry. Wash and dry under a heat lamp if possible. Fill a container with warm soapy water and dip the bird into the solution, carefully wiping with the grain of the feathers. Agitate the bird's body around in the solution, being careful to keep the animal's head dry. Then dip bird into warm, clean rinse water until all soap and residue are gone. Repeat if necessary until water beads on the feathers. This procedure is very stressful and should only be done on stable animals.

Wildlife Product Sources

Products	Manufacturer/Supplier	Products	Manufacturer/Supplier
Aviary netting	Cutler's Pheasant Supply www.cutlersupply.com Memphis Net and Twine Co., Inc. P.O. Box 80331 Memphis, TN 38108-0331 Phone: 888-674-7638 E-mail: www.memphisnet.net Sterling Net Co., Inc. 18 Label St. Montclair, NJ 07042 Phone: 800-342-0316 www.sterlingnets.com	Live insects: mealworms, crickets	Grubo, Inc. Phone: 513-874-5881 www.grubco.com Rainbow Mealworms Inc. Phone: 800-777-9676 www.rainbowmealworms.net Nature's Way Phone: 800-318-2611 www.thenaturesway.com discount to rehabilitators

Nipples "Catac" (Latex rubber nursing nipples, 3 sizes,) fits on slip tip or catheter tip syringes	Chris's Squirrels and More, LLC
	Phone: 860-749-1129
	www.squirrelsandmore.com
		Powdered egg whites
		
		Avimin®
		   (avian minerals)
		Avitron®
		   (avian vitamins)
			www.eggstore.com
			
			Lambert Kay
			www.lambertkay.com
			Pet stores

Nipples "Mothering Kit" (Silicone small tapered nipples fit on slip tip syringes) Catac nipples, Esbilac, KMR, Multi-Milk, Bene-Bac, plastic feeding cannula	Upco Phone: 800-254-8726 www.upco.com Discounts to licensed rehabilitators Chris's Squirrels and More, LLC Phone: 860-749-1129 www.squirrelsandmore.com Feed stores, pet stores	Esbilac, KMR, Multi-Milk, Benebac, Snuggle Safe (microwavable disks that stay warm for 12 hours), Nekton nectars, Zupreem Primate Diet, scales, homeopathy remedies, reference books	Chris's Squirrels and More, LLC Phone: 860-749-1129 www.squirrelsandmore.com
Feeding tubes, feeding catheters, flexible white syringe tips, pipettes	Chris's Squirrels and More, LLC Phone: 860-749-1129 www.squirrelsandmore.com	Syringes (O-Ring) for feeding	Chris's Squirrels and More, LLC Phone: 860-749-1129 www.squirrelsandmore.com
Dried insects	Oregon Feeder Insects, Inc. Phone: 866-641-8938 www.oregonfeederinsects.com Biconet www.biconet.com Hagen www.hagen.com Any good fish, reptile, or pet store		Medcare 246E. 131st Street Cleveland, OH 44108 Phone: 800-433-4550 www.medcareproducts.com
Soya Musca (powdered dried flies)	www.ladygouldianfinch.com		

Products	Manufacturer/Supplier	Products	Manufacturer/Supplier
Animals for food: Rats and mice Coturnix quail, eggs, chicks; Frozen: rats, mice, chicks, and live crickets	The Gourmet Rodent Bill and Marcia Brant Phone: 352-495-9024 www.gourmetrodent.com	Monkey Biscuits/Chow	Jeffers, Inc. Phone: 334-793-6257 www.JeffersPet.com Zupreem-primate chow
	Northwest Gamebirds 228812 E. Game Farm Rd. Kennewick, WA 99337 Phone: 509-586-0150 www.nwgamebird.com	Hummingbird nectars	Chris's Squirrels and More, LLC Phone: 860-749-1129 www.squirrelsandmore.com Guenter Enderle Enterprises, Inc. Nekton Clearwater, Florida Phone: 727-669-1030 www.nekton.de
	Perfect Pets, Inc. 23180 Sherwood Belleville, MI 48111 Phone: 800-366-8794 www.perfectpet.net		Roudybush Nectar Hummingbird nectars Phone: 800-326-1726 www.roudybush.com
Zoologic Milk Matrix products, Esbilac, KMR, Multi-Milk	Pet-Ag, Inc. Phone: 800-323-0877 www.petag.com	CliniCare® Canine/feline Liquid diet	Abbott Laboratories Animal Health Phone: 888-299-7416
Mesh cages (reptariums)	Chris's Squirrels and More, LLC Phone: 860-749-1129 www.squirrelsandmore.com	Isocal® Human liquid diet formula	Mead Johnson and Company Evansville, Indiana 47721 Order from local pharmacy
Wildlife-related book Sources: mail-order Catalogues, veterinary topics, specializing in: natural history books, field guides, rehabilitation manuals	Zoo Book Sales 403 Parkway Ave. N Mail To: P.O. Box 405 Lanesboro, MN 55949-0405 Phone: 507-467-8733 www.zoobooksales.com	Emeraid® Diets: (Psittacine) (Carnivore)	Lafeber Company Cornell, IL Phone: 800-842-6445 ext. 888 www.lafeber.com
	Wild Ones Animal Health Library P.O. Box 947 Springville, CA 93265 Phone: 800-539-0210 www.for-wild.org write or call for catalog	Carnivore Care® (raptors, carnivores), Critical Care® diets (herbivores)	Oxbow Pet Products 800-249-0366 www.oxbowhay.com
	National Wildlife Rehabilitators Association (NWRA) www.nwra.com	Rodent blocks	Kaytee Products, Inc. Chilton, WI phone: 800-KAYTEE-1 www.Kaytee.com
	International Wildlife Rehabilitation Council (IWRC) www.iwrc.com		Pet stores that sell Kaytee
	Wildlife Publications PMB 293 897 Oak Park Blvd. Pismo Beach, CA 93449 Phone: 805-489-0411 www.wildcare.com	Animal-related catalogues: Animal handling and restraint nets, traps, and Services, Inc. punch poles, animal handling gloves, blowpipes, darting equipment, Ketch-All poles, snake hooks	Aces Animal Care Equipment Phone: 800-338-ACES www.animal-care.com Tomahawk Live Trap P.O. Box 323 Tomahawk, WI 54487 Phone: 800-272-8727 www.livetrap.com
	Krieger Publishing Co. Natural Science and Veterinary Topics Catalog Phone: 800-724-0025 www.krieger-publishing.com		One Of A Kind Phone: 920-4854369
	Chris's Squirrels and More, LLC Phone: 860-749-1129 www.squirrelsandmore.com Wildlife Rehabilitation Information Directory www.tc.umn.edu/~devo0028/pub.htm		Ketch All Company Phone: 877-538-2425 www.ketch-all.com

Products	Manufacturer/Supplier	Products	Manufacturer/Supplier
Intensive care units, incubators	Thermocare Inc. P.O. Box 6069 Incline Village, NV 89450 Phone: 800-262-4020 www.thermocare.com Lyon Electric Company, Inc. Phone: 888-LYONUSA Lyonelectric.com	Animal caging Products: cages, wire, netting, latches, watering systems, cage building supplies, incubators, brooders, heat lights, etc.	Valentine Inc. Phone: 800-GET-STUFF www.valentineinc.com Stromberg's P.O. Box 400 Pine River, MN 56474 Phone: 800-720-1134 www.strombergschicken.com
Banding and tagging supplies	National Band and Tag Company 721 York Street P.O. Box 72430 Newport, KY 41072-0430 Phone: 859-261-2035 www.nationalband.com	Chicken/duck starter Crumbled balanced diet for growing ducks, chicken, geese	Feed stores and some larger pet stores
Pet Store Products: bowls, vitamins, foods, milk formulas, cages, water bottles, vaccines, Nutri-cal®, books, nest boxes, etc.	Upco Phone 800-254-UPCO www.upco.com That Pet Place Phone: 888-THAT-PET www.thatpetplace.com Pet Warehouse P.O. Box 310 Xenia, OH 45385-0310 Phone: 800-991-3299 www.petswarehouse.com R.C. Steele 1989 Transit Way P.O. Box 910 Brockport, NY 14420-0910 Phone: 800-872-3773 www.rcsteele.com	Falconry equipment, raptor books, raptor handling gloves Reptile equipment: Tongs, hooks, transport bags, heat lamps, U/V light bulbs, light stands, etc.	Northwoods Limited P.O. Box 874 Rainier, WA 98576 Phone: 800-446-5080 www.northwoodsfalconry.com Mid-West Products 14505 S. Harris Rd. Greenwood, MO 64034 Phone: 816-537-4444 www.tongs.com

For a listing of additional books, resources, supplies, links, and information for the rehabilitation professional: Wildlife Rehabilitation Information Directory, www.tc.umn.edu/~devo0028/index.htm.

APPENDIX ELEVEN

Additional Resources

NATURAL HISTORY: GENERAL

Peterson RT. 1980. Peterson Field Guides. Boston: Houghton Mifflin Company.

Rue LL, III. 1981. Furbearing Animals of North America. New York: Crown Publishers, Inc.

Stokes D, Stokes L. 1986. Stokes Nature Guides, A Guide to Animal Tracking and Behavior. Boston: Little Brown and Co.

Chapman JA. 1982. Wild Mammals of North America. Baltimore and London: Johns Hopkins University Press.

BIRDS

Campbell TW. 1995. Raptor Rehabilitation in the Private Veterinary Hospital. In: Exotic Animals: A Veterinary Handbook, Trenton: Veterinary Learning Systems Co., Inc. 121–25.

Eastman J. 1997. Birds of Forest, Yard and Thicket. Mechanicsburg, PA: Stackpole Books.

Eastman J. 1999. Birds of Lake, Pond and Marsh. Mechanicsburg, PA: Stackpole Books.

Eastman J. 2000. Birds of Field and Shore. Mechanicsburg, PA: Stackpole Books.

Ehrlich PR, Dobkin DS, Wheye D. 1988. The Birder's Handbook, A Field Guide to the Natural History of North American Birds. Fireside, Simon and Schuster.

Fox N. 1995. Understanding the Birds of Prey. Blaine, WA: Hancock House Publishers.

Johnsgard P. 1988. North American Owls, Biology and Natural History. Smithsonian Institution.

Morzenti A. 1998. Captive Raptor Management. Madison: Omnipress.

Sibley DA. 2001. The Sibley Guide to Bird Life and Behavior. National Audubon Society. New York: Chanticleer Press, Inc.

Stokes D, Stokes L. 1979. Stokes Nature Guides, A Guide to Bird Behavior. Volumes 1–3. Boston: Little Brown and Co.

Terres JK. 1980. The Audubon Encyclopedia of North America Birds. New York: Alfred A. Knopf, Inc.

Tyrrell EQ. 1985. Hummingbirds, Their Life and Behavior. New York: Crown Publishers, Inc.

RODENTS

Allen EG. 1938. The Habits and Life History of the Eastern Chipmunk (*Tamias striatus lysteri*). NY State Museum Bulletin.

Barkalow F, Shorten M. 1973. The World of the Gray Squirrel. New York: J.B. Lippincott Co.

Booth ES. 1946. Notes on the Life History of the Flying Squirrel. *Journal of Mammalogy* 27 (1): 28–30.

Costello DF. 1966. The World of the Porcupine. New York: Lippincott Co.

Hanes PC. 1988. Hand-Rearing Infant Tree Squirrels. *IWRC 1988 Proceedings*, Suisun, CA: International Rehabilitation Council. 77–93.

Nichols JT. 1958. Food Habits and Behavior of the Grey Squirrel. *Journal of Mammalogy* 39 (3): 376–80.

Rue LL, III. 1964. The World of the Beaver. Philadelphia: J.B. Lippincott.

Long K. Squirrels: A Wildlife Handbook. Boulder, Colorado: Johnson Nature Series, Johnson Publishing Co.

Long K. 2000. Beavers: A Wildlife Handbook. Boulder, Colorado: Johnson Nature Series, Johnson Publishing Co.

Wasserman J. 1988. Raising Orphaned Flying Squirrels. IWRC 1988 Proceedings. Suisun, CA: International Wildlife Rehabilitation Council.

LAGOMORPHS

Lockley RM. 1964. The Private Life of the Rabbit. New York: Macmillan Publishing Co., Inc.

OPOSSUMS

Keefe JF, Wooldridge D. 1967. The World of the Opossum. Philadelphia: J.B. Lippincott.

McManus J. 1974. *Didelphis virginian*. Mammalian Species, No. 40: 1–6.

Nave P, Lacy J. 1983. Rehabilitation notes: Opossum (*Didelphis marsupialis*). WRC J, Winter, 7–10.

CANIDS

Fox MW. 1971. Behavior of Wolves, Dogs and Related Canids. New York: Harper and Row.

Henry D. 1986. Red Fox, The Cat Like Canine. Smithsonian Institution Press.

Rue LL, III. 1969. The World of the Red Fox. Philadelphia: J.B. Lippincott.

Van Wormer J. 1964. The World of the Coyote. Philadelphia: J.B. Lippincott.

MUSTELIDS

Caine-Stage M. 1990. American River Otter, *Lutra canadensis*. *Wildlife Journal* 13(1): 7–10.

Hall RR. 1951. American Weasels. Lawrence: University of Kansas Press.

Kruuk H. 2006. Otters Ecology, Behaviour and Conservation. New York: Oxford University Press Inc.

Park E. 1971. The World of the Otter. New York: J.B. Lippincott.

Verts BJ. 1967. Biology of the Striped Skunk. Urbana, IL: University of Illinois Press.

PROCYONS

Evans AT, Evans RH. 1995. Rearing Raccoons for Release: Part II: Rehabilitation and Diet. *Veterinary Technician* 6(6):296–306.

Goldman EA. 1950. Raccoons of North and Middle America. U.S. Department of Interior, U.S. Fish and Wildlife Services, North American Fauna 60. Washington, DC.

Rue LL, III. 1994. The World of the Raccoon. Springville, CA: Wild Ones Animal Books.

Stuewer FW. 1943. Raccoons: Their Habits and Management in Michigan. *Michigan Ecol Monograph*, 13: 203–57.

WILDLIFE REHABILITATION ORGANIZATIONS

Basically Bats Wildlife Conservation Society, Inc.
106 Spooner Rd., Hawthorne, FL 32640
Nonprofit organization devoted to bat rehabilitation, research, education, and conservation; includes resources and contacts and promotes public awareness
www.basicallybats.org

BCI: Bat Conservation International
P.O. Box 162603, Austin, TX 78716
Phone: (512) 327-9721
www.batcon.org
Bat information, their conservation, and how to get involved.

IWRC: International Wildlife Rehabilitation Council
P.O. Box 8187, San Jose, CA 95155
Phone: (408) 271-2685
www.office@iwrc-online.org
Membership, training, education, and support for wildlife rehabilitators, literature catalogues, non-releasable animal placement, job line, symposium information, online training, standards, rehabilitation links.

NOS: National Opossum Society, Inc.
P.O. Box 21197, Catonsville, MD 21228
www.opossum.org
Annual subscription

NWRA: National Wildlife Rehabilitation Association
2625 Clearwater Rd. Suite 110, St. Cloud, MN 56301
Phone: (320) 230-9920
nwra@nwrawildlife.org
Membership, training, education, and support for wildlife rehabilitators, NWRA/IWRC Minimum Standards, state and federal permit agency listings, career page, baby animal care, publications, literature order reprints, upcoming events, and symposium.

REHABILITATION BOOKS, MANUALS, AND CDs

These books can be purchased from the IWRC or NWRA web sites or the other book companies listed on the product source pages.

General Rehabilitation Topics

Adams P, Johnson V, Goodrich P, Haas R. 1991. Wild Animal Care and Rehabilitation Manual. Kalamazoo Nature Center. Kalamazoo: Beech Leaf Press.

Fowler ME. 1983. Restraint and Handling of Wild and Domestic Animals. Ames: Iowa State University Press.

IWRC—Basic Wildlife Rehabilitation 1AB Skills Seminar, 5th ed. rev. By Jan White, DVM. An interpretation of existing biological and veterinary literature for the wildlife rehabilitator. Includes anatomy, physiology, calculating drug dosages, nutrition, housing, release, euthanasia, and more.

Moore AT, Joosten S. 1995b. NWRA—Principles of Wildlife Rehabilitation, The Essential Guide for Novice and Experienced Rehabilitators. St. Cloud: National Wildlife Rehabilitators Association.

NWRA Quick Reference, 3rd ed. 2006. By E.A. Miller, DVM. Includes a glossary, abbreviations, tables, calculations, drug dosing, fluid charts, infant developing, and anatomy pertaining to wildlife.

NWRA—Principles of Wildlife Rehabilitation, The Essential Guide for Novice and Experienced Rehabilitators. By Adele T. Moore and Sally Joosten. Printed by Burgess International Group Inc., Edina, MN.

NWRA/IWRC Minimum Standards for Wildlife Rehabilitation. Includes basic housing requirements for mammals and birds, euthanasia standards, and disease transmission (available free on IWRC/NWRA web site).

Raley P. 1991. Primer of Wildlife Care and Rehabilitation. Troy: Brukner Nature Center.

White J. 2000. IWRC—Basic Wildlife Rehabilitation 1AB Skills Manual. Suisun, CA: International Wildlife Rehabilitation Council.

Wild Animal Care and Rehabilitation Manual, 4th ed. 1991. Kalamazoo Nature Center, 7000 North Westedge Ave., Kalamazoo, MI 49007; phone (616) 381-1574; fax (616) 381-2557.

Wild Mammal Babies, The First 48 hours and Beyond. 2007. pp 448. By Irene Ruth and Deborah Gody; to order call 603-239-7338.

Wildlife Care Basics for Veterinary Hospitals—Before the Rehabilitator Arrives. By Irene Ruth: The Fund for Animals National Headquarters; Urban Wildlife Program; phone 203-393-1050.

Wildlife Neighbors: The Humane Approach to Living with Wildlife. 1997. Edited by John Hadidian, Guy R. Hodge, and John W. Grandy. The Humane Society of the United States.

Mammal Rehabilitation

Bats in Captivity. 1995. By Susan M. Barnard. Now available free of charge online at www.basically-bats.org/onlinebook.htm.

Complete Rehabilitation Guide for North American Bats. By Amanda Lollar, Barbara French, and Patricia Winters.

Merritt JF. 1987. Guide to the Mammals of Pennsylvania. Pittsburgh: University of Pittsburgh Press.

North American River Otter, Lontra canadensis, Husbandry Notebook, 2nd ed. 2001. By Janice Reed-Smith. John Ball Zoological Gardens, Grand Rapids, MI.

Opossum Orphan Care Training Manual. 1995. By Paula Taylor of the Opossum Society of the U.S., 14 pp; guides new opossum rehabilitators through the rearing process: Wildlife Publications.

Stinky Business: How to Rehabilitate Skunks, 3rd ed. By Share Bond, 117 p, Contact: skunks10@aol.com.

Squirrel Rehabilitation Handbook. 2003. By Shirley J and Allan M. Casey, 265pp. Sold only to permitted wildlife rehabilitators and subpermittees; order form available at www.ewildagain.org.

Avian Rehabilitation

Care and Rehabilitation of Injured Owls, 4th ed., 1987. By Katherine Mckeever. The Owl Rehabilitation Research Foundation, Vineland, Ontario, Canada.

Raptors in Captivity: Guidelines for Care and Management. 2007. By Lori R. Arent. The Raptor Center at the University of Minnesota; NWRA website.

Raptor Rehabilitation: A Manual of Guidelines. 1993. By Mathias Engelmann and Pat Marcum. The Carolina Raptor Center.

Hand-rearing Birds. 2007. By Laurie Gage, DVM, and Rebecca Duerr, DVM. 488pp. Wildlife Publications.

Rehabilitation and Conservation of Chimney Swifts. 4th ed. 2004. By Paul and Georgean Kyle; available (at no charge) online at www.chimneyswifts.org.

Reptile Rehabilitation

Turtle Husbandry for Wildlife Rehabilitators CD. 2006. By Harriet Forrester. NWRA website.

Wildlife Veterinary Topics

Wildlife Under the Microscope CD ROM. 2006. By S. Porter, VMD. 15 power point programs: microscopy, parasitology, mycology, necropsy, effusions, etc. Available on NWRA website.

Willowbrook Wildlife Center's Pharmaceutical Index, 3rd ed. 2000. By Catherine M. Brown. DVM, MSC. 187pp. Medical wildlife formulary published by the Willowbrook Wildlife Foundation, NWRA website.

Topics in Wildlife Medicine, Vol 1, Clinical Pathology, 2005, and Vol 2, Emergency and Critical Care, 2007. By Florina S. Tseng, DVM, and Mark A. Mitchell, DVM, MS, PhD. NWRA website.

Medical Management of Birds of Prey: A Collection of Notes on Selected Topics. 1993. By Patrick Redig, DVM, PhD. University of Minnesota.

Field Manual of Wildlife Diseases: National Wildlife Health Center. www.nwhc.usgs.gov; available for free download (43MB).

WEBSITES USEFUL TO REHABILITATORS

- CDC: Diseases and zoonotics, www.cdc.gov/nczved
- National Wildlife Health Center: Invaluable site for wildlife disease information, emerging diseases, wildlife health news updates, www.nwhc.usgs.gov
- NetVet: Links to hundreds of veterinary medical and animal resources related sites, www.netvet.wustl.edu
- Southeastern Cooperative Wildlife Disease Study (SCWDS): Current news on wildlife diseases, diagnostic services, education, zoonotics, www.vet.uga.edu/scwds
- Merck Veterinary Manual: Free electronic manual online version, www.merck.com
- Internet Center for Wildlife Damage Management: Tips on dealing with urban wildlife, www.icwdm.org/default.asp

- Tri-State Bird Rescue and Research Center: Wild bird care, tips on living with wildlife, oil spill response, www.tristatebird.org
- USFandW home page: www.fws.gov
- Wildlife Rehabilitation Information Directory: Books, resources, supplies, rehabilitation law, information on nuisance wildlife, locating a rehabilitator, helping wildlife, links, and information for the rehabilitation professional, www.tc.umn.edu/~devo0028/index.htm
- Songbird Diet Website: Excellent site with detailed information on songbird natural and captive diets, www.snowcrest.net/kellyj/wildbirdcare/group2.htm
- The Smithsonian National Museum of Natural History-North American mammal species database: www.mnh.si.edu/mna
- Animal Diversity Web: University of Michigan Museum of Zoology, http://animaldiversity.ummz.umich.edu/site/index.html
- Squirrel Tales: Squirrel rehabilitation, care, and information site: www.squirreltales.org
- The International Otter Survival Fund (IOSF): River otter rehabilitation, care, conservation, and information, www.otter.org
- WildAgain Wildlife Rehab, Inc.: Resources and tools for wildlife rehabilitators, teleclass training, seminars on wildlife homeopathy and squirrel rehabilitation, publications, squirrel care, articles for free, download on wildlife rehabilitation and homeopathy, www.ewildagain.org
- The National Opossum Society: Opossum care and information, www.opossum.org

INTERNET LISTSERVE FOR PROFESSIONAL WILDLIFE REHABILITATORS

- Wildlife Rehabilitation (WLREHAB): To Subscribe, send an e-mail to: listserve@listserv.nodak.edu with a blank subject line and text that reads: subscribe WLREHAB.

Supplies Necessary for an Exotic Practice

3.5 to 5 red French rubber catheters
Drinking water bottles
Electrocautery unit
Avian feeding formulas
2 to 3.5 mm endotracheal tubes
Feeding tubes
Gavage needles of various sizes
Gram scale
Gram stain kit
Heat lamps
Heated cages
Heating pads
Incubators
Induction chamber/oxygen cage
Instrument pack with small hemostats, scissors, forceps, and needle holders

Isoflurane or sevoflurane precision vaporizer
Microdrip IV sets and pumps
Microtainer blood collection tubes
Mouth speculum (stainless steel and rubber)
Nasolacrimal cannulas
Nolvasan solution and scrub
Perches of different sizes
Rigid endoscope
Small anesthesia masks (cones)
Small hand towels
Small nonrebreathing circuit
Small rebreathing bag for an anesthesia machine
Sterile cotton tip applicators
Uncuffed endotracheal tubes
Wing trimming scissors

Index

Page references in *italics* refer to figures.
Page references in **bold** refer to tables.